Coding for Pediatrics 2022

A MANUAL FOR PEDIATRIC DOCUMENTATION AND PAYMENT

For Use With AMA *CPT* 2022

27th EDITION

Author
Committee on Coding and Nomenclature (COCN)
American Academy of Pediatrics
Linda D. Parsi, MD, MBA, CPEDC, FAAP, Editor
Cindy Hughes, CPC, CFPC, Consulting Editor
Becky Dolan, MPH, CPC, CPEDC, Staff Editor

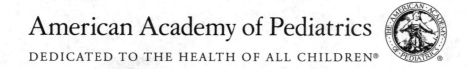

American Academy of Pediatrics
DEDICATED TO THE HEALTH OF ALL CHILDREN®

American Academy of Pediatrics Publishing Staff

Mary Lou White, *Chief Product and Services Officer/SVP, Membership, Marketing, and Publishing*

Mark Grimes, *Vice President, Publishing*

Mary Kelly, *Senior Editor, Professional/Clinical Publishing*

Laura Underhile, *Editor, Professional/Clinical Publishing*

Jason Crase, *Senior Manager, Production and Editorial Services*

Leesa Levin-Doroba, *Production Manager, Practice Management*

Peg Mulcahy, *Manager, Art Direction and Production*

Maryjo Reynolds, *Marketing Manager, Practice Publications*

Published by the American Academy of Pediatrics
345 Park Blvd
Itasca, IL 60143
Telephone: 630/626-6000
Facsimile: 847/434-8000
www.aap.org

The American Academy of Pediatrics is an organization of 67,000 primary care pediatricians, pediatric medical subspecialists, and pediatric surgical specialists dedicated to the health, safety, and well-being of all infants, children, adolescents, and young adults.

While every effort has been made to ensure the accuracy of this publication, the American Academy of Pediatrics does not guarantee that it is accurate, complete, or without error.

The recommendations in this publication do not indicate an exclusive course of treatment or serve as a standard of medical care. Variations, taking into account individual circumstances, may be appropriate. Vignettes are provided to illustrate correct coding applications and are not intended to offer advice on the practice of medicine.

Any websites, brand names, products, or manufacturers are mentioned for informational and identification purposes only and do not imply an endorsement by the American Academy of Pediatrics (AAP). The AAP is not responsible for the content of external resources. Information was current at the time of publication.

This publication has been developed by the American Academy of Pediatrics. The contributors are expert authorities in the field of pediatrics. No commercial involvement of any kind has been solicited or accepted in development of the content of this publication. Disclosures: Ms Arnold disclosed a consulting relationship with Thermo Fisher Scientific. Dr Lago disclosed an employee relationship with Cotiviti, Inc. Dr Parsi disclosed an ownership and consulting relationship with The PEDS MD Company and is part of the Mead Johnson Speaker Bureau.

Please visit www.aap.org/cfp or www.aap.org/errata for an up-to-date list of any applicable errata for this publication.

Special discounts are available for bulk purchases of this publication. Email Special Sales at nationalaccounts@aap.org for more information.

Printed in the United States of America

CPT copyright 2021 American Medical Association (AMA). All rights reserved.

Fee schedules, relative value units, conversion factors, and/or related components are not assigned by the AMA, are not part of *CPT*, and the AMA is not recommending their use. The AMA does not directly or indirectly practice medicine or dispense medical services. The AMA assumes no liability for data contained or not contained herein.

CPT is a registered trademark of the AMA.

This publication has prior approval of the American Academy of Professional Coders (AAPC) for 4.0 continuing education units. Granting of this approval in no way constitutes endorsement by AAPC of the publication content or publication sponsor.

11-35R   1 2 3 4 5 6 7 8 9 10

MA1029
ISBN: 978-1-61002-550-8
eBook: 978-1-61002-551-5
ISSN: 1537-324X

2021–2022 Committee on Coding and Nomenclature (COCN)

Eileen D. Brewer, MD, FAAP, Chairperson

Margie C. Andreae, MD, FAAP

Joel F. Bradley, MD, FAAP

Mark Joseph, MD, FAAP

David M. Kanter, MD, MBA, CPC, FAAP, Immediate Past Chairperson

S. Kalyan Katakam, MD, MPH, FAAP

Steven E. Krug, MD, FAAP

Edward A. Liechty, MD, FAAP

Jeffrey F. Linzer Sr, MD, FAAP

Linda D. Parsi, MD, MBA, CPEDC, FAAP

Renee F. Slade, MD, FAAP

Liaisons

Kathleen K. Cain, MD, FAAP
AAP Section on Administration and Practice Management

Kathryn B. Lalor, MD, FAAP
AAP Section on Early Career Physicians

Benjamin Shain, MD, PhD
American Academy of Child and Adolescent Psychiatry

Samuel D. Smith, MD, FAAP
American Pediatric Surgical Association

2021–2022 AAP Coding Publications Editorial Advisory Board

Linda D. Parsi, MD, MBA, CPEDC, FAAP, Editor in Chief

Cheryl Arnold, MHSA, FACMPE

Greg Barabell, MD, CPC, FAAP

Vita Boyar, MD, FAAP

Joel F. Bradley, MD, FAAP

Ryan Hensley, MD, CPC, CPEDC, FAAP

David M. Kanter, MD, MBA, CPC, FAAP

S. Kalyan Katakam, MD, MPH, FAAP

Steven E. Krug, MD, FAAP

Jamie C. Lago, MD, CPC, FAAP

Edward A. Liechty, MD, FAAP

Jeffrey F. Linzer Sr, MD, FAAP

Richard A. Molteni, MD, FAAP

Karen Nauman, MD, FAAP

Piedade Oliveira-Silva, MD, FAAP

Julia M. Pillsbury, DO, FAAP

Renee F. Slade, MD, FAAP

Karla Nickolas Swatski, MD, FAAP

Sanjeev Y. Tuli, MD, FAAP

AAP Staff

Becky Dolan, MPH, CPC, CPEDC

Teri Salus, MPA, CPC, CPEDC

Linda Walsh, MAB

Disclaimer

Every effort has been made to include the new and revised 2022 *Current Procedural Terminology* (CPT®); *International Classification of Diseases, 10th Revision, Clinical Modification* (ICD-10-CM); and Healthcare Common Procedure Coding System (HCPCS) codes, their respective guidelines, and other revisions that might have been made. Due to our publishing deadlines and the publication date of the American Medical Association *CPT*, additional revisions and/or additional codes may have been published subsequent to the date of this printing. It is the responsibility of the reader to use this manual as a companion to the *CPT, ICD-10-CM*, and HCPCS publications. Vignettes are provided throughout this publication to illustrate correct coding applications. They are not intended to offer medical advice on the practice of medicine. Further, it is the reader's responsibility to access the American Academy of Pediatrics website (www.aap.org/cfp or www.aap.org/errata) routinely to find any corrections due to errata in the published version. At the time of publication, codes for services related to COVID-19 diagnosis, testing, and immunization were frequently changing. Please see www.aap.org/coding for updates.

Copyright Acknowledgment

Current Procedural Terminology (CPT®) is a listing of descriptive terms and 5-digit numeric identifying codes and modifiers for reporting medical services and procedures performed by physicians. This presentation includes only the *CPT* descriptive terms, numeric identifying codes, and modifiers for reporting medical services and procedures that were selected by the American Academy of Pediatrics (AAP) for inclusion in this publication. The inclusion of a *CPT* service or procedure description and its code number in this publication does not restrict its use to a particular specialty group. Any procedure or service in this publication may be used to report the services provided by any qualified physician or, when appropriate, other qualified health care professional.

The American Medical Association (AMA) and the AAP assume no responsibility for the consequences attributable to or related to any use or interpretation of any information or views contained in or not contained in this publication.

Any 5-digit numeric *CPT* code, service descriptions, instructions, and/or guidelines are copyright 2021 (or such other date of publication of *CPT* as defined in the federal copyright laws) AMA. All rights reserved.

The most current *CPT* is available from the AMA.

No fee schedules, basic unit values, relative value guides, conversion factors or scales, or components thereof are included in *CPT*.

Equity, Diversity, and Inclusion Statement

The American Academy of Pediatrics is committed to principles of equity, diversity, and inclusion in its publishing program. Editorial boards, author selections, and author transitions (publication succession plans) are designed to include diverse voices that reflect society as a whole. Editor and author teams are encouraged to actively seek out diverse authors and reviewers at all stages of the editorial process. Publishing staff are committed to promoting equity, diversity, and inclusion in all aspects of publication writing, review, and production.

Contents

Foreword VII

Acknowledgments IX

How to Use This Manual XI

PART 1: CODING BASICS AND BUSINESS ESSENTIALS

Chapter 1
The Basics of Coding 3

Chapter 2
Coding Edits and Modifiers 23

Chapter 3
Coding to Demonstrate Quality and Value 53

Chapter 4
The Business of Medicine: Working With Current and Emerging Payment Systems 67

Chapter 5
Preventing Fraud and Abuse: Compliance, Audits, and Paybacks 89

Chapter 6
Evaluation and Management Documentation Guidelines Other Than Office and Other Outpatient Services 107

PART 2: PRIMARILY FOR THE OFFICE AND OTHER OUTPATIENT SETTINGS

Chapter 7
Office and Other Outpatient Evaluation and Management Services 141

Chapter 8
Preventive Services 171

Chapter 9
Consultation, Residential, and Non–face-to-face Evaluation and Management Services 203

Chapter 10
Surgery, Infusion, and Sedation in the Outpatient Setting 227

Chapter 11
Common Non-facility Testing and Therapeutic Services 257

Chapter 12
Management of Chronic and Complex Conditions 285

Chapter 13
Qualified Nonphysician Health Care Professional Services 309

Chapter 14
Mental and Behavioral Health Services 327

PART 3: PRIMARILY FOR HOSPITAL SETTINGS

Chapter 15
Hospital Care of the Newborn 359

Chapter 16
Noncritical Hospital Evaluation and Management Services 377

Chapter 17
Emergency Department Services 401

Chapter 18
Critical and Intensive Care 423

Chapter 19
Common Surgical Procedures and Sedation in Facility Settings 447

PART 4: DIGITAL MEDICINE SERVICES

Chapter 20
Telemedicine Services 485

Chapter 21
Remote Data Collection and Monitoring Services 497

APPENDIXES

I. Quick Reference to 2022 *ICD-10-CM* Pediatric Code Changes 511

II. Quick Reference to 2022 *CPT®* Pediatric Code Changes 514

III. Vaccine Products: Commonly Administered Pediatric Vaccines 518

IV. Test Your Knowledge! Answer Key 522

INDEXES

Subject Index 527

Code Index 537

AAP/Bright Futures "Recommendations for Preventive Pediatric Health Care" (Periodicity Schedule) .... Insert

This publication has prior approval of the American Academy of Professional Coders (AAPC) for 4.0 continuing education units (CEUs). Granting of this approval in no way constitutes endorsement by the AAPC of the publication, content, or publication sponsor. To earn your CEUs, complete the 40-question quiz online (www.aap.org/cfp). Click on "2022 AAP CEU Quiz."

The following online-exclusive content can be accessed at www.aap.org/cfp:
- 2021 Telemedicine Services
- AAP Position on Medicare Consultation Policy
- Care Management Tracking Worksheet Template
- Care Plan Oversight Billing Worksheet Template
- Codes for Skin Grafts of Infants & Children
- Coding Education Quiz/Continuing Education Units/Answer Key
- Commonly Administered Pediatric Vaccine Updates
- Emergency Department Services: Continuum Models for Asthma, Head Injury, and Laceration
- Evaluation and Management Key Components
- FAQ: Immunization Administration
- General Documentation Checklist
- Global Per Diem Critical Care Codes: Direct Supervision and Reporting Guidelines
- Medicare Requirements for Incident-to Services by Nonphysician Health Professionals and Clinical Staff
- Oops We've Overpaid You: How to Respond to Payer Audits
- RUC Survey Times for Subsequent Hospital Care and Critical Care Services
- Sample Audit Log
- Screening Laboratory Tests and Codes

Foreword

The American Academy of Pediatrics (AAP) is pleased to publish the 27th edition of *Coding for Pediatrics*—an instructional manual and reference tool for use by primary care pediatricians, pediatric subspecialists, and others involved in the provision of care to children. This manual supports the delivery of quality care to children by providing the pediatric practitioner with the knowledge to best support appropriate business practices. This edition includes the 2022 *Current Procedural Terminology* (*CPT®*) and *International Classification of Diseases, 10th Revision, Clinical Modification* (*ICD-10-CM*) code changes with guidelines for their application.

This edition introduces a wide range of new codes and guidelines, including principal care management services provided for management of a single complex chronic condition and cardiac catherization performed for the evaluation of congenital heart defects. In addition, this manual provides pediatric-specific guidance to coding for all evaluation and management (E/M) services by providing guidance and examples of documentation and code selection using the 1995 and 1997 E/M documentation guidelines and the distinctly different guidelines for office and other outpatient E/M services.

Please note that coding and guideline changes related to the 2019 COVD-19 public health emergency continued to occur during development of this manual. The AAP has maintained an up-to-date document detailing the changes at https://downloads.aap.org/AAP/PDF/COVID%202020.pdf.

For ease of reference, *Coding for Pediatrics 2022* is divided into the following parts:

- **Part 1: Coding Basics and Business Essentials** includes information on code sets, compliance, and business topics such as billing and payment methodologies.
- **Part 2: Primarily for the Office and Other Outpatient Settings** includes information on coding and billing of services such as office visits, outpatient consultations, and preventive services.
- **Part 3: Primarily for Hospital Settings** includes information on coding for inpatient and observation services, including newborn care and surgical procedures.
- **Part 4: Digital Medicine Services** includes discussion of the evolving codes for reporting telemedicine services and remote monitoring and interpretation of patient data.
- Quick references to *CPT* and *ICD-10-CM* code changes applicable to pediatrics are provided in **appendixes I and II**. A table of pediatric vaccine product codes can be found in **Appendix III**.
- A **continuing education quiz** to earn 4.0 continuing education units from the American Academy of Professional Coders is available online at www.aap.org/cfp.
- Supplemental material providing a wealth of information can be found on the *Coding for Pediatrics* website (www.aap.org/cfp), including a documentation checklist and tracking worksheets for care management and care plan oversight services.

Each chapter includes "Test Your Knowledge!" questions (answers can be located in **Appendix IV**). Additionally, resources for more information on each chapter's contents can be located at the end of chapter.

As in previous years, the AAP is also pleased to also offer *Coding for Pediatrics 2022* as an eBook.

Coding for Pediatrics 2022 does not replace *CPT, ICD-10-CM*, or the Healthcare Common Procedure Coding System; rather, it supplements those manuals. Every effort has been made to include the 2022 codes and their respective guidelines; however, revised codes and/or guidelines may have been published subsequent to the date of this printing. Errata to this manual will be posted as appropriate on the *Coding for Pediatrics* website (www.aap.org/cfp or www.aap.org/errata).

The AAP actively works with the American Medical Association (AMA) *CPT* Editorial Panel and the AMA/Specialty Society Relative Value Scale Update Committee (RUC) to develop pediatric specialty codes and assign them appropriate relative value units. Since 1995, the AAP has contributed to the process that evaluates and reviews changes to the Medicare Resource-Based Relative Value Scale (RBRVS). Pediatricians have been actively involved in the AMA RUC Practice Expense Review Committee to review direct practice expenses for all existing codes. As importantly, the AAP is represented on the AMA *CPT* Editorial Advisory Panel and on the *ICD-10-CM* Editorial Advisory Board. The AAP continues to be involved in all areas of payment. The AAP Committee on Coding and Nomenclature oversees all areas of coding as they relate to pediatrics, including *CPT* procedure coding, *ICD-10-CM* diagnosis coding, and the valuation of *CPT* services through the Medicare RBRVS.

The AAP will continue to request new code changes and attempt to expeditiously notify membership of changes through various means. *AAP Pediatric Coding Newsletter*™—a monthly newsletter available in print and online—provides up-to-date coding and payment information. The newsletter and other online resources can be accessed through the AAP newsletter website (https://coding.aap.org). Other resources include coding seminars presented at the AAP National Conference & Exhibition; webinars (located at https://coding.solutions.aap.org); instructional materials in *AAP News,* including the Coding Corner; *Pediatric ICD-10-CM: A Manual for Provider-Based Coding; Pediatric Office-Based Evaluation and Management Coding: 2021 Revisions; Pediatric Coding Basics: An Introduction to Medical Coding;* and various quick reference cards. The use of these resources should provide pediatricians with the skills needed to report their services appropriately. The AAP Health Care Financing Strategy staff stands ready to assist with coding problems and questions not covered in this manual. The AAP Coding Hotline can be contacted at https://form.jotform.com/Subspecialty/aapcodinghotline.

Acknowledgments

Coding for Pediatrics 2022, 27th Edition, is the product of the efforts of many dedicated individuals.

Our mission is to make coding easier to understand so that pediatric providers can continue to serve children well. We have sought to make this book easier to understand by categorizing care areas and by using many examples (vignettes) of different coding situations. This knowledge is key to helping all pediatric providers stay in compliance and correctly code with confidence. We hope you enjoy reading this book, and we will continue to strive to always serve you with excellence.

This work has been made immeasurably easier and the final edition dramatically improved by the dedicated work of many collaborators. First and foremost, I must thank Cindy Hughes, CPC, CFPC, consulting editor, for her professional input. Additionally, I must thank the Committee on Coding and Nomenclature (COCN) support staff at the American Academy of Pediatrics (AAP), particularly Becky Dolan, MPH, CPC, CPEDC, staff editor, for her many excellent suggestions as well as for reviewing major portions of the project. Thank you also to Teri Salus, MPA, CPC, CPEDC, for her review of new *Current Procedural Terminology* (*CPT*®) codes and suggestions for changes to content. I would also like to thank the members of COCN and the AAP Coding Publications Editorial Advisory Board. The members of these committees have each contributed extensive time in reviewing and updating content of the manual. We want to especially thank the following reviewers:

Cheryl Arnold, MHSA, FACMPE
Greg Barabell, MD, CPC, FAAP
Vita Boyar, MD, FAAP
T. Ryan Hensley, MD, CPC, CPEDC, FAAP
David M. Kanter, MD, MBA, CPC, FAAP
S. Kalyan Katakam, MD, MPH, FAAP
Jamie C. Lago, MD, CPC, FAAP
Edward A. Liechty, MD, FAAP
Richard A. Molteni, MD, FAAP
Julia M. Pillsbury, DO, FAAP
Renee F. Slade, MD, FAAP
Karla Nickolas Swatski, MD, FAAP
Sanjeev Y. Tuli, MD, FAAP

None of this work is possible without the support of the COCN members who work tirelessly to develop and value codes and fight for pediatrics "at the table." The committee strives to keep pediatrics at the forefront of coding and valuation. The excellent teams listed as follows are truly experts in these areas and are devoted to representing the AAP and its members:

CPT Team
Joel F. Bradley, MD, FAAP (*CPT* Advisor)
Renee F. Slade, MD, FAAP (*CPT* Alternate Advisor)
Teri Salus, MPA, CPC, CPEDC (AAP Staff to *CPT*)

American Medical Association/Specialty Society Relative Value Scale Update Committee (RUC) Team
Steven E. Krug, MD, FAAP (RUC Advisor)
Margie C. Andreae, MD, FAAP (RUC Representative)
Eileen D. Brewer, MD, FAAP (RUC Alternate Representative)
Linda Walsh, MAB (AAP Staff to RUC)

International Classification of Diseases (ICD) Team
Jeffrey F. Linzer Sr, MD, FAAP (AAP Representative to *ICD*)
Edward A. Liechty, MD, FAAP (AAP Alternate Representative to *ICD*)
Becky Dolan, MPH, CPC, CPEDC (AAP Staff to *ICD*)

I am most grateful to the invaluable input of the following AAP committees and individuals: the Committee on Medical Liability and Risk Management, specifically Richard L. Oken, MD, FAAP, and AAP staff Julie Ake, senior health policy analyst; the Private Payer Advocacy Advisory Committee, specifically Sue Kressly, MD, FAAP; and the Section on Neonatal-Perinatal Medicine coding trainers. In addition, we reached out to other AAP members for their expertise on specific content areas; thank you to Sergio Bartakian, MD, FAAP, for his review and contributions to the discussion of cardiovascular procedure codes.

This project would not have been completed were it not for the outstanding work of AAP staff. In Membership, Marketing, and Publishing, Mary Kelly, senior editor, professional/clinical publishing; Laura Underhile, editor, professional/clinical publishing; Jason Crase, senior manager, production and editorial services; Peg Mulcahy, manager, art direction and production; Leesa Levin-Doroba, production manager, practice management; and Maryjo Reynolds, marketing manager, practice publications, deserve special recognition for their outstanding skill and dedication to this project. At the AAP, I am especially appreciative of the support and professional expertise of Linda Walsh, MAB, senior manager, healthy policy and coding, and AAP staff support to the AAP COCN, dedicated advocates for all of us who provide medical care to children. A special thank-you to our AAP Board of Directors reviewers, Sara (Sally) Goza, MD, FAAP, immediate past president, and Jeannette Gaggino, MD, FAAP. We are so grateful to have their leadership and review for this manual!

Finally, we all would like to give a big thank-you to all our readers, billers, coders, medical team, and dedicated pediatric providers who work tirelessly around the clock to provide the best care to all children. Your work inspires us to work very hard behind the scenes to provide you the latest and most accurate coding information. We are always open to ideas to better serve you and welcome your suggestions. By all of us working together, we can accomplish the highest standards of care and be a voice for our children and their future.

Respectfully,
Linda D. Parsi, MD, MBA, CPEDC, FAAP
Editor

How to Use This Manual

Step 1. Use either the Table of Contents or Index to locate information on specific services, codes, or broader subjects.	**Contents** An Introduction to the Official Code Sets 5 Telling the Encounter Story 5
Step 2. Use chapter content to review code descriptors and instructions for reporting. Before reporting, verify current codes and complete selection and reporting instructions in the appropriate code set manual or application.	**99464** Attendance at delivery (when requested by the delivering physician or other qualified health care professional) and initial stabilization of newborn Attendance at delivery (**99464**) is not reported when hospital-mandated attendance is the only underlying basis for providing the service.
Step 3. Examples are used as guidance on meeting the criteria specified by codes and reporting instructions. However, note that codes must be assigned based on the service provided and supporting documentation.	➤ **The pediatrician administers 3 injections of allergen extract for a patient with allergic rhinitis due to pollen.** The extract was prepared and supplied by an allergist. The pediatrician will report code **95117** with *ICD-10-CM* code **J30.1**.
Step 4. Note key points of information highlighted in each chapter.	If the physician performs the venipuncture as a convenience or because staff is not trained in the procedure, code **36415** is reported because the physician's skill was not required.
Step 5. Resources for additional information are listed at the end of each chapter as well as online at www.aap.org/cfp.	CHAPTER 7. OFFICE AND OTHER OUTPATIENT EVALUATION AND MANAGEMENT SERVICES 169 **Resources** **Documentation** American Academy of Pediatrics Initial History Questionnaire Documentation Form for office or outpatient visits (available for purchase at http://shop.aap.org) **Examples of Office E/M Code Levels** "Office E/M 2021: Level 2 Visits," August 2020 *AAP Pediatric Coding Newsletter* (https://coding.solutions.aap.org/article.aspx?articleid=2765198; subscription required) "Office E/M 2021: Level 3 Visits," September 2020 *AAP Pediatric Coding Newsletter* (https://coding.solutions.aap.org/article.aspx?articleid=2765216; subscription required) "Office E/M 2021: Level 4 Visits," October 2020 *AAP Pediatric Coding Newsletter* (https://coding.solutions.aap.org/article.aspx?articleid=2765225; subscription required) "Office E/M 2021: Level 5 Visits," November 2020 *AAP Pediatric Coding Newsletter* (https://coding.solutions.aap.org/article.aspx?articleid=2765232; subscription required) **Guidelines for Office E/M Code Selection** "Retroactive Evaluation and Management Guideline Corrections Published," April 2021 *AAP Pediatric Coding Newsletter* (https://coding.solutions.aap.org/article.aspx?articleid=2765338; subscription required)
Step 6. While every effort is made to provide accurate and up-to-date coding guidance, changes do happen. Any corrections and code or instruction changes published subsequent to the date of this printing are posted online at www.aap.org/cfp or www.aap.org/errata.	American Academy of Pediatrics DEDICATED TO THE HEALTH OF ALL CHILDREN® Q Search All AAP **Coding for Pediatrics 2021** Practice Management / Coding for Pediatrics 2021 Coding for Pediatrics 2021 Welcome to the **Online Access** page for Coding for Pediatrics, 2021. To purchase the manual, click here. *Coding for Pediatrics* is an instructional manual and reference tool for use by primary

Part 1
Coding Basics and Business Essentials

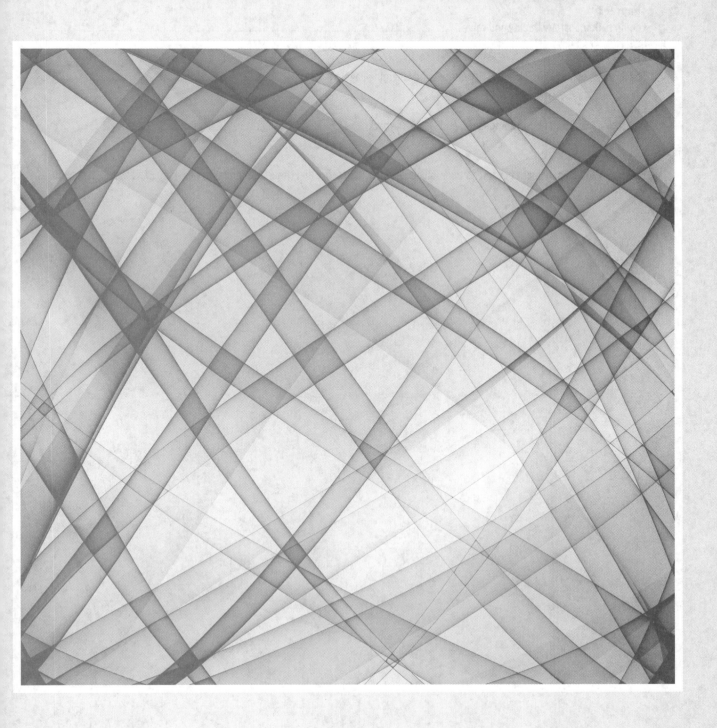

Part 1: Coding Basics and Business Essentials

Chapter 1
The Basics of Coding.. 3

Chapter 2
Coding Edits and Modifiers... 23

Chapter 3
Coding to Demonstrate Quality and Value.. 53

Chapter 4
The Business of Medicine: Working With Current and Emerging Payment Systems 67

Chapter 5
Preventing Fraud and Abuse: Compliance, Audits, and Paybacks 89

Chapter 6
Evaluation and Management Documentation Guidelines Other Than Office and Other Outpatient Services 107

CHAPTER 1

The Basics of Coding

Contents

An Introduction to the Official Code Sets 5

    Telling the Encounter Story 5

International Classification of Diseases, 10th Revision, Clinical Modification (ICD-10-CM) 6

    ICD-10-CM Guidelines 6

        Section I—Conventions, General Coding Guidelines, and Chapter-Specific Guidelines 7

        Section IV—Diagnostic Coding and Reporting Guidelines for Outpatient Services 8

    The Pathway to *ICD-10-CM* Code Selection 9

        Indexes 9

        Tabular List 9

        Diagnosis Coding Tips 10

        Appropriate Use of Unspecified Codes 11

    More About *ICD-10-CM* 12

Healthcare Common Procedure Coding System (HCPCS) 12

Current Procedural Terminology (CPT) 13

    CPT Conventions and Guidelines 13

        Provider Terminology 15

    Use of Time in Procedure Coding 15

        The Value of Documenting Time 16

National Drug Code (NDC) 18

Beyond Code Sets 19

    Who Assigns the Codes? 19

    Reporting Codes for Payment 19

        Linking the Diagnosis to the Service 21

    Other Coding and Billing Information 21

Resources 21

Test Your Knowledge! 22

An Introduction to the Official Code Sets

In the United States, the Health Insurance Portability and Accountability Act (HIPAA) of 1996 requires the use of 5 specific code sets for purposes of health care transactions. The 4 code sets primarily used by physicians are listed in **Table 1-1**. The fifth designated code set, *Code on Dental Procedures and Nomenclature* (*CDT*), is primarily used to report dental procedures to dental insurance plans.

Table 1-1. Health Insurance Portability and Accountability Act of 1996 Code Sets		
Code Set	**Used to Report**	**Examples**
International Classification of Diseases, 10th Revision, Clinical Modification (ICD-10-CM)	Diagnoses and other reasons for encounters	**Z00.110** Health examination for newborn under 8 days old **Z00.111** Health examination for newborn 8 to 28 days old
Current Procedural Terminology (*CPT*®)[a]	Most professional services, vaccine and immune globulin products, and tracking performance measurement	**99291** Critical care, evaluation and management of the critically ill or critically injured patient; first 30-74 minutes **90686** Influenza virus vaccine, quadrivalent (IIV4), split virus, preservative free, 0.5 mL dosage, for intramuscular use
Healthcare Common Procedure Coding System (HCPCS)[b]	Supplies, medications, and services (when a *CPT* code does not describe the service as covered by health plan benefits)	**S0630** Removal of sutures; by a physician other than the physician who originally closed the wound **J0171** Injection, Adrenalin, epinephrine, 0.1 mg
National Drug Code (NDC)	Specific prescription drug, vaccine, and insulin products and dosages	**00006-4047-41** RotaTeq 2-mL single-dose tube, package of 10 **60574-4114-01** Synagis 0.5-mL in 1 vial, single dose

[a] Also known as Level I of the HCPCS code set.
[b] Refers to Level II HCPCS codes assigned by the Centers for Medicare & Medicaid Services.

Each code set, other than *CDT,* is used to facilitate communication of standardized health information for purposes such as prior authorization of medical care and submission of health care claims in pediatric practice. Understanding the purpose and constructs of the 4 code sets used by physicians is important to successful interactions with health plans and supports accurate health care statistics.

New and revised codes are listed in quick references in **appendixes I** and **II**.

- Quick Reference to 2022 *ICD-10-CM* Pediatric Code Changes (effective with services provided on or after October 1, 2021)
- Quick Reference to 2022 *CPT*® Pediatric Code Changes (effective with services provided on or after January 1, 2022)

This chapter discusses pertinent guidelines and key points for accurately reporting codes. Refer to the American Academy of Pediatrics (AAP) manual, *Pediatric Coding Basics,* for more information on each code set.

Telling the Encounter Story

Because physicians do not submit full documentation, various code sets and other supportive information (eg, procedure code modifiers) tell payers what happened and what should be paid (**Table 1-2**).

Table 1-2. The Encounter Story Told Through Codes	
ICD-10-CM	Why were services rendered?
CPT/HCPCS	What services or supplies were provided?
Modifier	Was something altered or unusual?
NDC	More specific information
Associated Fees	Payment for services

Abbreviations: *CPT, Current Procedural Terminology;* HCPCS, Healthcare Common Procedure Coding System; *ICD-10-CM, International Classification of Diseases, 10th Revision, Clinical Modification;* NDC, National Drug Code.

Learning to appropriately select codes for diagnoses, services, supplies, and medications is important to support appropriate payment by health plans. In the end, the codes submitted on a claim tell the story of what happened during a patient encounter.

However, documentation of an encounter must support the codes assigned for each diagnosis and service and may be requested by a payer to support the accuracy of code assignment. The following 7 general principles of documentation apply to all services:

1. The medical record should be complete and legible.
2. The documentation of each patient encounter should include
   - Reason for the encounter and relevant history, physical examination findings, and prior diagnostic test results
   - Assessment, clinical impression, or diagnosis
   - Plan for care
   - Date and legible identity of the observer
3. If not documented, the rationale for ordering diagnostic and other ancillary services should be easily inferred.
4. Past and present diagnoses should be accessible to the treating and/or consulting physician.
5. Appropriate health risk factors should be identified.
6. The patient's progress, response to and changes in treatment, and revision of diagnosis should be documented.
7. The *Current Procedural Terminology* (CPT®) and *International Classification of Diseases, 10th Revision, Clinical Modification* (ICD-10-CM) codes reported on the health insurance claim form or billing statement should be supported by the documentation in the medical record.

International Classification of Diseases, 10th Revision, Clinical Modification (ICD-10-CM)

Physicians assign diagnoses and other reasons for encounters to which *ICD-10-CM* codes are assigned for use in payment and public health data.

Although the values assigned to procedure codes are the basis for amounts paid for services, payers are increasingly using *ICD-10-CM* codes when determining the appropriateness of services submitted on a claim (eg, level of evaluation and management [E/M] service).

Updates to *ICD-10-CM* are implemented each October 1 following publication in early to midsummer. Interim code updates may occur in April when there is a significant indication for a code to identify a new health condition. However, during the public health emergency in 2020, new codes were created and implemented on January 1 for the first time.

Oversight and resolution of coding questions related to *ICD-10-CM* is performed by the American Hospital Association (AHA) Editorial Advisory Board for *Coding Clinic for ICD-10-CM and ICD-10-PCS* and the public-private "cooperating parties": the Centers for Medicare & Medicaid Services (CMS), National Center for Health Statistics, AHA, and American Health Information Management Association. The increased granularity and specificity in *ICD-10-CM* are also at the specific request of certain medical societies. No clinical diagnosis codes are added for payment purposes.

The AAP holds a seat on the editorial advisory board. Findings are published quarterly by the AHA in *Coding Clinic*. *ICD-10-CM* codes and accompanying guidelines and findings by the editorial advisory board are part of the standard transaction code sets under HIPAA and must be recognized by all payers. For *ICD-10-CM*, the hierarchy of official coding guidelines and instructions is as follows:

1. *ICD-10-CM* alphabetic index and tabular list
2. *Official Guidelines for Coding and Reporting*
3. AHA *Coding Clinic* advice

Pediatricians with suggestions for changes to existing or new *ICD-10-CM* codes related to pediatric care are encouraged to forward their suggestions to coding staff at the AAP headquarters. The AAP staff and advisor who are involved in the process can be of great assistance. To contact the AAP Coding Staff, complete the form at https://form.jotform.com/Subspecialty/aapcodinghotline.

ICD-10-CM Guidelines

The official conventions found in the *ICD-10-CM Official Guidelines for Coding and Reporting* are outlined in sections that include descriptions of symbols, abbreviations, and other instructional notes. The guidelines are organized into 4 sections. Only sections I and IV pertain to reporting physician services. Sections II and III relate to hospital or facility technical services and are not discussed here. *ICD-10-CM* guidelines can be found in *ICD-10-CM* manuals or at www.cdc.gov/nchs/icd/icd10cm.htm.

The following excerpts from the *ICD-10-CM* guidelines provide an overview of the information pertinent to pediatric care as provided in each section of the guidelines:

Section I—Conventions, General Coding Guidelines, and Chapter-Specific Guidelines

A. Conventions

The conventions of *ICD-10-CM* include punctuation, notes, and terminology used throughout the code set.

[ ] Brackets
- Identify manifestation codes in the Alphabetic Index. For instance, otitis externa due to impetigo **L01.00** [**H62.40**] indicates that both impetigo (**L01.00**) and otitis externa in other diseases classified elsewhere (**H62.40**, unspecified ear) are used to report this condition. The index includes the default code (**H62.40**), although documentation should support the specific site of the impetigo as **H62.41**, right ear; **H62.42**, left ear; or **H62.43**, bilateral ears.
- Enclose synonyms, alternative wording, or explanatory phrases in the tabular list (eg, **S04.811** Injury of olfactory [1st] nerve, right side).

( ) Parentheses—Enclose supplementary words (ie, nonessential modifiers) that may be included in the medical record but do not affect code selection; for example, bronchiolitis (acute) (infective) (subacute) **J21.9**. If a nonessential modifier is mutually exclusive to a sub-term of the main term, the sub-term is given priority. For instance, the sub-term *influenzal* directs to see codes for influenza with respiratory manifestations overriding the nonessential modifier, *infective*.

- Dash—Indicates that additional characters are required for code completion (eg, **R10.-**). A dash is also used throughout this publication to indicate incomplete codes.

Notes
- Includes: Further defines or gives examples of the content of a category.
- Excludes1: Not coded here—used to indicate codes for conditions that would not occur in conjunction with the code category where the note is found. An exception to the *Excludes1* definition is the circumstance when the 2 conditions are unrelated to each other. If it is not clear whether the 2 conditions involving an *Excludes1* note are related, coders are instructed to query the provider.

Example

➤ *Excludes1* **notes follow J06.9 (acute upper respiratory infection, unspecified) to prohibit reporting the code in conjunction with less specific acute respiratory infection not otherwise specified (J22) or more specific codes for influenza virus with other respiratory manifestations (J09.X2, J10.1, J11.1) or streptococcal pharyngitis (J02.0).**

- Excludes2: Not included here—used to indicate codes for conditions not included in the code category where the note is found but that may be additionally reported when both conditions are present.

Example

➤ *Excludes2* **notes apply to code J02.0 (streptococcal pharyngitis).** An *Excludes2* note that applies to all codes in subcategory **J02** (**J02.0–J02.9**) indicates **J31.2** (chronic pharyngitis) is not included here, and another *Excludes2* note that applies to code **J02.0** indicates **A38.-** (scarlet fever) is not included here.

- Code first: A sequencing rule in the tabular list to report first a code for an underlying cause or origin of a disease (etiology), if known.
- Code also: An instruction that another code may be necessary to fully describe a condition. The sequence of the codes depends on the circumstances of the encounter.
- See: In the alphabetic index, this instructs that another term should be referenced to find the appropriate code.
- See also: In the alphabetic index, this instructs that another term may provide additional entries that may be useful.
- Use an additional code: A sequencing rule often found at the listing of an etiology code, this instruction directs to also report a code for the manifestation.

Terminology

- And: Means and/or when appearing in a title in *ICD-10-CM*; for example, **Q16.1**, congenital absence, atresia and stricture of auditory canal (external) includes absence, atresia, or stricture.
- Combination code: A single code that represents multiple conditions or a single condition with an associated secondary process or complication.
- First-listed diagnosis: For reporting of professional services, the diagnosis, condition, problem, or other reason for the encounter or visit shown in the medical record to be chiefly responsible for the services provided is listed first and followed by other conditions that affected management or treatment.
- NEC: Not elsewhere classifiable. Indicates a code for other specified conditions that is reported when the medical record provides detail that is not captured in a specific code.
- NOS: Not otherwise specified. Indicates a code for an unspecified condition that is reported when the medical record does not provide sufficient detail for assignment of a more specific code.
- Sequela: A late effect of an illness or injury that is no longer in the acute phase. There is no time limit on when a sequela code can be used. The residual may be apparent early, such as in cerebral infarction, or it may occur months or years later, such as that due to a previous injury.
- With and In: The classification presumes a causal relationship between the 2 conditions linked by the terms *with* or *in*. These conditions should be coded as related even in the absence of provider documentation explicitly linking them, unless the documentation clearly states that the conditions are unrelated or when another guideline exists that specifically requires a documented linkage between 2 conditions (eg, sepsis guideline for "acute organ dysfunction that is not clearly associated with the sepsis").

For conditions not specifically linked by these relational terms in the classification or when a guideline requires that a linkage between 2 conditions be explicitly documented, provider documentation must link the conditions to code them as related.

B. General Coding Guidelines

- Assign a code for signs and symptoms when no definitive diagnosis has been reached at an encounter.
- Do not report additional codes for conditions that are integral or routinely associated with a disease process (eg, wheezing in asthma).
- When the same condition is documented as acute and chronic, codes for both conditions are reported if the alphabetic index lists the conditions at the same indentation level. The acute condition is sequenced first.
- When a combination code describes 2 diagnoses, or a diagnosis and its associated manifestation or complication, report only the combination code. If a manifestation or complication is not identified in a combination code, it should be separately reported.
- When reporting a sequela (late effect) of an injury or illness, report first the current condition and then the sequela code.
- If both sides are affected by a condition and the code category does not include a code for the bilateral condition, assign codes for right and left. When a patient has a bilateral condition and each side is treated during separate encounters, assign the bilateral code for each encounter where the condition exists on both sides. Do not assign a bilateral code if the condition no longer exists bilaterally.
- Coders generally may not assume a complication of care without documentation of the cause-and-effect relationship (eg, infection in a patient with a central venous line).
- Unspecified codes are appropriately selected when information to support a more specific code was not available at the time of the encounter (eg, type of pneumonia is not known).

C. Chapter-Specific Guidelines

See guidelines for specific diagnoses and/or conditions found in each chapter of *ICD-10-CM*. Chapter guidelines are important to coding for pediatric care and need to be followed for appropriate code selection.

When selecting electronic coding applications, look for inclusion of chapter-specific guidelines when using the code search functionality. *Pediatric ICD-10-CM: A Manual for Provider-Based Coding,* a manual published by the AAP, adds chapter-specific guidance to each chapter for easy reference.

Section IV—Diagnostic Coding and Reporting Guidelines for Outpatient Services

Selecting a Code

- The coding conventions and guidelines of Section I take precedence over these outpatient guidelines.
- Never assign a code for a condition that is unconfirmed (eg, probable or rule out obstruction). Instead, assign codes for signs and symptoms (eg, vomiting, abdominal distension).

- Use codes in categories **Z00–Z99** when circumstances other than a disease or an injury are recorded as the reason for encounter.

Sequencing of Diagnosis Codes

- Physicians and other providers of professional services should list first the condition, symptom, or other reason for encounter that is chiefly responsible for the services provided. List also any coexisting conditions. However, always defer to the manual to determine if sequencing is outlined in the guidelines.

> Diagnosis codes must be appropriately linked to services on a claim to support the medical necessity of that service. See the Reporting Codes for Payment section later in this chapter for more information.

Reporting Previously Treated Conditions

- Do not code conditions that have been previously treated but no longer exist. Personal history codes **Z85–Z87** may be used to identify a patient's historical conditions. Codes for family history that affects current care are also reported (**Z80–Z84**).
- Report codes for chronic or recurring conditions as many times as the patient receives care for each condition.

Reporting Diagnoses for Diagnostic Examinations

- The condition, symptoms, or other reason for a diagnostic examination or test should be linked to the service. For laboratory or radiology testing in the absence of related conditions, signs, or symptoms, report code **Z01.89**, encounter for other specified special examinations.
- When diagnostic tests have been interpreted by a physician and the final report is available at the time of coding, code any confirmed or definitive diagnosis(es) documented in the interpretation. Do not code related signs and symptoms as additional diagnoses.

Reporting Preoperative Evaluations

- When the reason for an encounter is a preoperative evaluation, a code from subcategory **Z01.81-**, encounter for pre-procedural examinations, is reported first, followed by codes for the condition that is the reason for surgery and codes for any findings of the preoperative evaluation.
- Please see **Chapter 9** for discussion of reporting health examinations (preventive care).

The Pathway to *ICD-10-CM* Code Selection

To correctly select codes in *ICD-10-CM*, it is important to recognize and follow instructions found in the alphabetic index and tabular list to locate the most specific code for documented diagnoses. These are the prevailing instructions for reporting that are supplemented by the guidelines and guidance published in AHA *Coding Clinic for ICD-10-CM*.

Indexes

Code selection begins in the alphabetic index, table of drugs and chemicals (eg, to report an adverse effect or poisoning), and/or table of neoplasms. The instructions (eg, instructions to see other terms) in the index will direct to the most specific code in the tabular list. An external cause of injuries index is also useful for locating codes to describe causes such as animal bites, falls, or motor vehicle accidents.

Tabular List

The tabular list is the end point for code selection. It is an alphanumeric list of *ICD-10-CM* codes structured as an indented list of 22 chapters with further divisions, including blocks, categories, subcategories, and codes.

> Look for instructional notes at each division within the tabular list (ie, chapter, block, category, or code), as these give important guidance to correct code selection.

The *ICD-10-CM* tabular list displays codes in an indented format to help users identify complete codes in each category or subcategory of codes. Only complete codes are reported.

Examples of category, subcategory, and complete codes follow:

Category	**P08**	Disorders of newborn related to long gestation and high birth weight
Code	**P08.0**	Exceptionally large newborn baby
Code	**P08.1**	Other heavy for gestational age newborn
Subcategory	**P08.2**	Late newborn, not heavy for gestational age
Code	**P08.21**	Post-term newborn
Code	**P08.22**	Prolonged gestation of newborn

Some code categories include instruction to add a seventh character. When required, assignment of the seventh character is based on whether the patient is undergoing active treatment (ie, services to establish a pattern of healing) and not on whether the provider is seeing the patient for the first time over the course of treatment for an injury.

Examples of the seventh characters that apply to most injuries (**A**, **D**, and **S**) are included in **Table 1-3**. Categories for traumatic fractures have additional seventh character values (eg, **C**, initial encounter for open fracture type IIIA, IIIB, or IIIC).

Table 1-3. Examples of Seventh Characters A, D, and S
When selecting a seventh character to indicate the type of encounter, a helpful mnemonic for the seventh character is A as active treatment/management, D as during healing, and S as scars and other sequela.

A Initial Encounter (Active Care)	D Subsequent Encounter (During Routine Healing Phase)	S Sequela (Late Effect)
A physician repairs a laceration to the face (active treatment).	A pediatrician removes facial sutures placed by an emergency department physician.	A pediatrician evaluates a complaint of scar contracture that resulted from repair of a facial laceration.
S01.81XA Laceration without foreign body of other part of head, initial encounter	**S01.81XD** Laceration without foreign body of other part of head, subsequent encounter	**L90.5** Scar conditions and fibrosis of skin **S01.81XS** Laceration without foreign body of other part of head, subsequent encounter. NOTE: Sequela (eg, scar) must always be reported first.

Refer to the AAP manuals *Pediatric Coding Basics* and *Pediatric ICD-10-CM* for more information on codes and code selection.

Diagnosis Coding Tips

- Specificity in coding is important to demonstrating the reason for a service or encounter, including the nature or severity of conditions managed. See further discussion of this important topic in the Appropriate Use of Unspecified Codes section later in this chapter.
- Physicians and other practitioners should become familiar with the documentation elements that are captured in *ICD-10-CM* code categories for conditions commonly seen in their practice. For example, when documenting care for otitis media, key documentation elements include whether the condition
  — Affects the right, the left, or both ears
  — Is acute, acute recurrent, or chronic
  — Is suppurative or nonsuppurative
  — Is with or without spontaneous rupture of the tympanic membrane

  Exposure to or use of tobacco is also reported in conjunction with otitis media.
- Pay close attention to the terminology for nonspecific diagnoses. For example, the diagnosis "reactive airways disease" is to be coded as asthma per the guidelines.

  In children treated for an asthma-like condition who have not been diagnosed with asthma, it may be more appropriate to report the signs or symptoms as the primary diagnosis.
- When testing is performed to rule out or confirm a suspected diagnosis or condition on a patient with a sign(s) or symptom(s), it is considered a diagnostic examination and is not screening. Therefore, the code that explains the reason for the test (ie, sign or symptom) should be reported.

Examples

➤ **A chest radiograph is ordered due to positive purified protein derivative testing.** Code **R76.11** (nonspecific reaction to tuberculin skin test without active tuberculosis) is assigned on the order to indicate the reason for testing.

➤ **A tuberculin purified protein derivative test is performed to screen for tuberculosis in a patient with no symptoms and no known exposure.** Code **Z11.1** (encounter for screening for respiratory tuberculosis) is assigned as the reason for the test.

- If, after evaluation and study of a suspected condition, there is no diagnosis or there are no signs or symptoms that are appropriate, report the codes for observation and evaluation for suspected conditions not found.

   Codes for observation and evaluation for suspected conditions not found in a neonate (*ICD-10-CM* codes **Z05.0–Z05.9**) are distinct from those for reporting suspected conditions not found in older children and adults (*ICD-10-CM* code **Z03.89**).
- Use aftercare codes (**Z42–Z49**, **Z51**) for patients who are receiving care to consolidate treatment or managing residual conditions.
- Conditions that were previously treated and no longer exist cannot be reported. Therefore, it is correct coding to report care following completed treatment with *ICD-10-CM* code **Z09**, encounter for follow-up examination after completed treatment for conditions other than malignant neoplasm.
   — Personal history codes (**Z86.-**, **Z87.-**) may be used to provide additional information on follow-up care.
   — If a payer does not accept follow-up care codes as primary and requires that the service be reported with the diagnosis code that reflects the condition that had been treated, report the follow-up care codes as secondary. However, get the payer's policy in writing and inquire why it is not following coding guidelines.

Example

➤ **A patient is seen to follow up on otitis media with effusion, which has now resolved.** The physician reports codes **Z09** and **Z86.69** (personal history of other diseases of the nervous system and sense organs) in lieu of the code for otitis media with effusion (no longer applicable).

- Do not select a diagnosis code that is "close to" the diagnosis or condition documented in the medical record. For example, do not report unspecified joint pain (**M25.50**) if the diagnosis is right knee pain (**M25.561**). Modify code selection methods to support correct code assignment.
- Pay attention to age factors within certain code descriptors. For example, report *ICD-10-CM* code **R10.83** for infantile colic and *ICD-10-CM* code **R10.84** for colic in a child older than 12 months.
- There is no limit to the number of diagnosis codes that can be documented.
   — Space is only allotted for up to 12 codes on the CMS-1500 paper claim form and each service line may be connected to 1 to 4 of the included codes. You may submit as many claim forms as necessary to report the diagnoses.
   — Electronic claims in HIPAA version 5010 may also include up to 12 diagnosis codes.
- "Recurrent" is not defined by *ICD-10*. Therefore, to use a recurrent code, the documentation should reflect that a practitioner believes it to be a recurrence.
- "Confirmed" influenza or other conditions do not require a positive laboratory test result or other test. What is required is that the practitioner, through training and experience, believes the patient has the condition based on clinical assessment and documents the condition in the chart.
- Do not report "suspected" or "rule out" diagnoses for physician services. Code to the nearest clinical certainty, which may be signs or symptoms. Exposure to communicable disease (category **Z20**) may be reported when a patient has known or suspected exposure or when a disease is endemic but ruled out after evaluation.

Appropriate Use of Unspecified Codes

Unspecified codes are valid *ICD-10-CM* codes used to report conditions for which a more specific diagnosis has not yet been determined and/or testing to determine a more specific diagnosis would not be medically necessary. However, misuse of unspecified codes may result in claim denials and unnecessary delays in receiving prior authorizations for testing or procedures.

   Do not report the default code (first code listed in the alphabetic index) when more detail about the patient's condition(s) should be documented to support another, more specific code. For example, do not report **J45.909** for unspecified asthma, uncomplicated, for reevaluation of asthma, which includes clinical classification of intermittent, mild-persistent, moderate-persistent, or severe-persistent asthma. The diagnosis code reported should reflect what is known at the end of the current encounter. Unspecified codes are not appropriate when information to support a more specific code would generally be known (eg, laterality, type of attention-deficit/hyperactivity disorder).

CPT copyright 2021 American Medical Association. All rights reserved.   ●=New code   ▲=Revised code   #=Re-sequenced code   +=Add-on code   ★=Telemedicine

Examples of unspecified codes that may be acceptable are as follows:
- Viral intestinal infection, unspecified (**A08.4**)
- Infectious gastroenteritis and colitis, unspecified (**A09**)
- Acute pharyngitis, unspecified (**J02.9**)
- Pneumonia, unspecified organism (**J18.9**)
- Sprain of unspecified site of right knee (**S83.91X-**)

The following examples of unspecified codes indicate inappropriate coding due to failure to document information (eg, location) that would typically be known at the time of the encounter and/or inappropriate code selection:
- Acute suppurative otitis media without spontaneous rupture of eardrum, unspecified ear (**H66.009**)
- Otitis media, unspecified, unspecified ear (**H66.90**)
- Cutaneous abscess of limb, unspecified (**L02.419**)
- Extremely low birth weight newborn, unspecified weight (**P07.00**)

In short, unspecified codes are necessary and should be reported when appropriate. Physicians must document in enough detail to capture what is known at the time of the encounter, and codes selected must reflect the documented diagnosis(es). If, at the time of code selection, documentation does not appear to include information that would be known at the time of the encounter, it is appropriate for coders to query the physician for more information and/or request an addendum to the documentation to more fully describe the conditions addressed at the encounter.

More About *ICD-10-CM*

The AAP *Pediatric ICD-10-CM: A Manual for Provider-Based Coding* (available through https://shop.aap.org) is a condensed version of the entire *ICD-10-CM* manual and provides only the guidelines and codes that are applicable and of importance to pediatric practitioners. The manual was designed for use in conjunction with the complete *ICD-10-CM* code set. The *ICD-10-CM* codes are found at www.cdc.gov/nchs/icd/icd10cm.htm.

AAP Pediatric Coding Newsletter™ provides timely articles on diagnosis coding for pediatric conditions. Subscriptions are available through https://shop.aap.org.

Healthcare Common Procedure Coding System (HCPCS)

The Healthcare Common Procedure Coding System (HCPCS) includes Level I codes (*CPT*) and Level II codes (CMS national codes). HCPCS Level II codes are the standardized coding system for describing and identifying health care services, equipment, and supplies (eg, **Q4011**, cast supplies, short arm cast, pediatric [0–10 years], plaster) that are not identified by HCPCS Level I (*CPT*) codes. To differentiate discussion of *CPT* and HCPCS Level II codes, the term HCPCS typically is used in reference to Level II codes unless otherwise stated.

HCPCS codes may be reported when the narrative differs from the *CPT* code for the service. Payer policies, particularly Medicaid plan policies, often drive the decision between reporting with *CPT* versus HCPCS. For instance, *CPT* does not include a code for removal of sutures by a physician other than the physician who repaired the wound and instructs to report an E/M service for encounters for suture removal. HCPCS includes code **S0630** (removal of sutures by a physician other than the physician who originally closed the wound). When allowed or required by a payer, code **S0630** may be reported in lieu of an E/M service for suture removal.

HCPCS **J** codes (eg, **J0696**, injection, ceftriaxone sodium, per 250 mg) represent medications only and not the administration of the medication.
- The term *injection* is included in the descriptor to specify that the medication code is reported for the medication when provided via injection or infusion and not oral or topical applications.
- Separate procedure codes, typically *CPT* codes, are used to report each medication administration by injection (**96372**) or infusion.
- HCPCS codes for drugs specify the unit of measure for each unit reported on the claim (eg, 250 mg of ceftriaxone sodium is reported with 1 unit on the claim line reporting provision of the medication). (See the National Drug Code [NDC] section later in this chapter for information on reporting units of service in conjunction with NDC reporting.)

> Do not report the number of milligrams (mg) as the unit of service on a claim. Reporting 900 mg of ceftriaxone sodium with 900 units would be incorrect; 900 mg of ceftriaxone sodium is reported with 4 units (rounding up is allowed by Medicare; other payers may require 3.6 units).

New permanent HCPCS codes are released by the CMS each November for implementation on January 1 of each year. However, temporary HCPCS codes may be implemented on a quarterly basis. Temporary codes are added to address the need for a reporting mechanism prior to the annual update (eg, to meet the requirements of a legislative mandate or to add a new product).

Current Procedural Terminology (CPT)

CPT is published annually by the American Medical Association (AMA). *CPT* codes are Level I codes of HCPCS but are commonly treated as a separate code set. This is the primary procedural coding system for professional services by physicians and other qualified health care professionals (QHPs). *CPT* codes are commonly included in electronic health record (EHR) systems, but instructions for reporting may not be included. *CPT* manuals and code applications or software provide important instructions for appropriate code selection.

CPT codes are generally updated annually with release of new codes each fall to allow physicians and payers to prepare for implementation on January 1 of each year.

- Exceptions include the vaccine, toxoid, immune globulin, serum, and recombinant product codes, which are updated twice annually (January and July) and may be released earlier when specific criteria for rapid release are met. Newly released vaccine codes are posted to www.ama-assn.org/practice-management/cpt/category-i-vaccine-codes.
- New vaccine codes released July 1 are implemented on January 1, and vice versa.
- New molecular pathology tier 2 codes and codes for multianalyte assays with algorithmic analyses are updated 3 times per year (April 1, October 1, January 1). Proprietary laboratory analyses codes are released quarterly (July 1, October 1, January 1, and April 1).
- Category II *CPT* codes (supplemental tracking used for performance measurement) are released online up to 3 times a year, with an effective date of 3 months after release, at www.ama-assn.org/practice-management/cpt/category-ii-codes.

See Chapter 3 for more discussion and illustration of Category II codes.

- Category III *CPT* codes (emerging technology, services, procedures, and service paradigms) are released biannually with an implementation date 6 months after the release date. For instance, a code released on January 1, 2022, is implemented on July 1, 2022, and published in *CPT 2023.* The most recent Category III code listing is found at www.ama-assn.org/practice-management/cpt/category-iii-codes.

Category III *CPT* codes are not assigned relative value units (RVUs), and payment for these services is based strictly on payer policies. If you are performing any procedure or service identified with a Category III *CPT* code, work with your payers to determine their coverage and payment policies.

The AMA hosts a website devoted to *CPT,* www.ama-assn.org/practice-management/cpt, with information on code development and maintenance, summaries of recent *CPT* Editorial Panel actions, and newly released codes.

CPT Conventions and Guidelines

CPT includes an index of procedures used to find codes and code ranges to help guide the user to the correct section(s) of codes.

- Terms in the index include procedures and services, organs and anatomic sites, conditions, synonyms, eponyms, and abbreviations (eg, EEG).
- Codes should not be selected from the index without verification in the main text of the manual.

CPT also includes specific guidelines that are located at the beginning of each section and additional prefatory instructions for categories of codes throughout the CPT manual.

- Code-specific instructions often follow a code in parentheses (referred to as *parenthetical instructions*).
- While code selection is often incorporated in EHRs, knowledge of and access to *CPT* guidelines is important to correct coding. Correct coding is important to obtaining correct claims payment. Always read the applicable guidelines and instructions before selecting a code.

Additional guidance can be found in *CPT Assistant,* a monthly newsletter published by the AMA that provides additional information about the intended use of codes, the related guidelines, and parenthetical instructions. Although widely considered authoritative, *CPT* instructions, guidelines, and *CPT Assistant* are not part of the HIPAA standard transaction code sets. All payers must accept *CPT* codes but are not required to adhere to the published *CPT* guidelines and instructions. Where payer policy differs from *CPT,* payer contracts typically require adherence to payer policy.

Example

➤ **A health plan policy does not allow separate payment for vision screening in conjunction with a routine child health examination even though *CPT* instructs that the screening is separately reported.** Although the health plan may deny charges associated with a vision screening, the plan must not reject the claim due to inclusion of a vision screening code (eg, **99173**, screening test of visual acuity, quantitative, bilateral).

Appendixes in *CPT* provide clinical examples of E/M services; quick references to modifiers; a summary of new, revised, and deleted codes; add-on and modifier-exempt codes; and other procedure code references. Based on changes to the coding manual, the appendixes may vary from year to year.

As shown in **Table 1-4**, symbols are used throughout *CPT* to code characteristics such as new or revised codes, new instructions, and other important characteristics of a code (eg, a code placed out of numeric sequence).

Symbol	Description
●	A bullet at the beginning of a code indicates a new code for the current year.
▲	A triangle means the code descriptor has been revised.
+	A plus sign means the code is an add-on code.
Ø	A null sign means the code is a "modifier **51** exempt" code and, therefore, does not require modifier **51** (multiple procedures) even when reported with other procedures.
⚡	The lightning bolt identifies codes for vaccines that are pending US Food and Drug Administration approval.
#	The pound symbol is used to identify re-sequenced codes that are out of numerical sequence. Related codes are placed in an appropriate location, making it easier to locate a procedure or service.
★	A star means the service represented by the code is included in Appendix P of the *CPT* manual as a code to which modifier **95** (synchronous telemedicine service) may be appended to indicate the service was rendered via real-time telemedicine services.

Table 1-4. *Current Procedural Terminology* Symbols

Some key *CPT* instructions are
- In the *CPT* code set, the term *procedure* is used to describe services, including diagnostic tests. The section of the book in which a code is placed is not indicative of whether the service is a surgery or not a surgery for insurance or other purposes.
- Select the code for the procedure or service that accurately identifies the service performed.
  - Do not select a code that merely approximates the service provided.
  - If no specific code exists, report the service using the appropriate unlisted procedure code. Unlisted procedure codes are provided in each section of *CPT* (eg, **99429**, unlisted preventive medicine service). When reporting an unlisted procedure code, medical records will need to be submitted to the health plan to identify the service rendered (attach to the claim to avoid delay caused by a health plan request for the records).
  - In some cases, a modifier may be used to indicate a reduced, discontinued, or increased procedural service.
- Many diagnostic services require a technical and professional component.
  - It is important to understand that the technical component (eg, obtaining an electrocardiogram) leads to results or findings.
  - The interpretation and creation of a report of the results or findings is a professional service. Some services specifically require a professional's interpretation and report.
  - Other services include only a technical component and require only documentation of the results or findings (eg, scoring of a developmental screening instrument).
  - Codes and modifiers exist to report the technical or professional component when the complete service is not provided by the same individual or provider (eg, facility provides technical component and physician provides professional component).

Never report a code for a global service without a modifier when only the technical or professional component is provided. See Chapter 2 for discussion of appropriate modifiers (eg, 26, TC).

- Add-on codes (marked with a + before the code) are always performed in addition to a primary procedure and are never reported as stand-alone services. Add-on codes describe additional intraservice work and are not valued to include preservice and post-service work like most other codes.

Example

99291   Critical care, evaluation and management of the critically ill or critically injured patient; first 30–74 minutes
+99292   each additional 30 minutes (List separately in addition to code for primary service)

Code **99292** is never reported in the absence of code **99291** on the same date of service.

Provider Terminology

Throughout the *CPT* code set, the use of terms such as *physician, QHP,* or *individual* is not intended to indicate that other entities may not report the service. In selected instances, specific instructions may define a service as limited to certain professionals or to other entities (eg, hospital, home health agency).

Of particular importance to correct reporting of services that include clinical staff and other nonphysician providers (NPPs) is identifying the providers included when terms such as *physician or other QHP* and *qualified, nonphysician health care professional* are used in *CPT* and/or payer instruction.

CPT provides definitions of providers as follows:

- Physician or other QHP: an individual who is qualified by education, training, licensure/regulation (when applicable), and facility privileging (when applicable) who performs a professional service within his or her scope of practice and independently reports that professional service

    Codes in the E/M section are reported only by a physician or QHP whose scope of practice includes E/M (eg, nurse practitioner, physician assistant). In contrast, assessment and management codes are provided in the Medicine section for reporting services by nonphysician health care professionals such as physical or occupational therapists and speech-language pathologists who may independently provide and report these services.
- Clinical staff member: a person who works under the supervision of a physician or other QHP and who is allowed by law, regulation, and facility policy to perform or assist in the performance of a specific professional service but does not individually report that professional service

    Services by clinical staff are performed under the supervision of a physician or QHP and are reported by the supervising physician or QHP.

    Note: CPT does not include any requirements for licensure but, rather, advises physicians to follow state regulations and the related scopes of practice defined by regulations (eg, regulations defining services that require a nursing license).

Coding for services by clinical staff and qualified nonphysician health care professionals is discussed in Chapter 13.

Use of Time in Procedure Coding

Most procedures and services in *CPT* are described by specific components of physician work (eg, **94011**, measurement of spirometric forced expiratory flows in an infant or child through 2 years of age). However, time (especially intraservice time) is also used as a proxy for physician/QHP work. Many services are reported based solely on time of service or, as in the case of many E/M services, may be reported based on key components of work (ie, history, examination, and medical decision-making [MDM]) *or* time (see discussion of each type of E/M service for specifications).

CPT provides general and category-/code-specific instructions for reporting services based on time. An understanding of these instructions is key to selecting codes that most accurately capture the services provided. This chapter will review the general guidelines for reporting time. Service-specific instructions and examples are also provided throughout this manual to help illustrate time-based coding.

Different categories of services use time differently. It is important to review the instructions for each category.

CPT copyright 2021 American Medical Association. All rights reserved.   ●=New code   ▲=Revised code   #=Re-sequenced code   +=Add-on code   ★=Telemedicine

Time-Based Coding Examples

➤ Moderate (conscious) sedation services are reported based on 15-minute time increments of intraservice time, beginning with administration of a sedating agent(s) and ending after the procedure is completed and the physician or QHP providing the sedation is no longer in personal continuous face-to-face contact with the patient.

➤ Intra-arterial and intravenous infusions are reported based on time and whether the infusion is the initial infusion service or a subsequent infusion service.

➤ Chronic and principal care management services are reported based on time spent in a calendar month by clinical staff or personally spent by the reporting physician or QHP. Each code has minimum time requirements, and some codes have limitations on the number of units reported per calendar month.

The Value of Documenting Time

Failure to document time of service may be costly even when it is possible to report a service without documenting time.

Example

➤ A pediatrician documents an established patient office or other outpatient visit with low-complexity MDM. The pediatrician also documents that a total of 35 minutes was spent in activities related to the care of the individual patient on the date of the visit, including extended time spent in counseling the patient's parents on the child's diagnosis and plan of care.

   Teaching Point: For office or other outpatient E/M services, a level of service is selected based on the level of MDM or the total time spent on the date of a visit by the physician or QHP in provision of that service to the individual patient. If time were not documented, the low-complexity MDM would support code 99213 (level 3 established patient office visit). However, documentation of 35 minutes' total physician time on the date of the visit would support code 99214.

   Code 99213 has 2.65 non-facility total RVUs, while code 99214 is assigned 3.76 non-facility total RVUs (2021 Medicare non-geographically adjusted). Persistent failure to document the time of E/M services may result in significant loss of otherwise earned revenue. For example, a payer contract allows $40 per RVU, so a practice is paid $106 ($40 × 2.65) for code 99213 and $150.40 ($40 × 3.76) for code 99214. Therefore, $44.40 of potential revenue is lost due to lack of documentation; if 99213 is reported 10 times when 99214 is supported, $444 of potential revenue is lost.

Failure to document time also eliminates the possibility of reporting prolonged services and may negatively affect the level of service reported when multiple episodes of care occur on the same date (eg, multiple hospital care services). Routinely noting the time spent face-to-face (outpatient) or on a patient's unit or floor (observation and inpatient) and, for services other than office or other outpatient services (99202–99205, 99212–99215), those instances when more than 50% of that time is spent in counseling and/or coordination of care allows for recognition of occasions where reporting based on time is most advantageous.

General Guidelines

CPT provides overall instructions for time-based reporting in the "Instructions for Use of the CPT Codebook" found in the Introduction of the coding manual. These instructions are followed for reporting time-based services when there are no section guidelines, prefatory instructions, parenthetical instructions, or specified time requirements in code descriptors (see examples in **Table 1-5**).

Table 1-5. *Current Procedural Terminology* Time Rules	
Time Rules	**Examples**
Midpoint rule: A unit of time is attained when the midpoint is passed (eg, a code described as 60 minutes may be reported when 31 minutes have elapsed). The midpoint rule is not applied when *CPT* includes category- or code-specific instructions to the contrary. When codes are ranked in sequential typical times and the actual time is between 2 typical times, the code with the typical time closest to the actual time is used. If the actual time of service falls exactly between the typical times of 2 codes, report the code with the lower typical time (ie, the midpoint must be passed to report the greater service).	99401 Preventive medicine counseling and/or risk factor reduction intervention(s) provided to an individual (separate procedure); approximately 15 minutes 99402 approximately 30 minutes 99403 approximately 45 minutes 99404 approximately 60 minutes At least 8 minutes of preventive medicine counseling are required to support code 99401 (midpoint of 7½ minutes is passed). The midpoints between sequential codes 99401–99404 are also 8 minutes. Services of at least 23 minutes may be reported with 99402 in lieu of 99401. See code 99403 for 38–52 minutes or 99404 for >53 minutes of service.
Code descriptor describes required time.	99238 Hospital discharge day management; 30 minutes or less 99239 more than 30 minutes
Prefatory instruction overrides midpoint rule.	Code 99291 is reported once for the first 30–74 minutes of critical care on a given date even if the time spent is not continuous on that date. *Critical care of <30 minutes' total duration on a given date is reported with an E/M code other than 99291.*

Abbreviations: *CPT, Current Procedural Terminology*; E/M, evaluation and management.

Section and prefatory instructions, code descriptors, and parenthetical instructions override the general instruction for time-based reporting.

- If your EHR or other coding reference does not include the prefatory and parenthetical instructions provided in *CPT,* code verification by a second party prior to billing may be necessary. Alternatively, it may be possible to insert instructions in the form of notes or alerts in an EHR.
- Some payers may require that the typical time assigned to a service be met or exceeded rather than approximated as allowed for some services by *CPT.*
- It is important to note that a code that is reported "per day" or for services "on the same date" is not reported for all services in a 24-hour period but, rather, all services on a single calendar date.

Examples

99463   Initial hospital or birthing center care, per day, for E/M of normal newborn infant admitted and discharged on the same date

99468   Initial inpatient neonatal critical care, per day, for the E/M of a critically ill neonate, 28 days of age or younger

- Time is the physician's or other reporting provider's time, unless otherwise stated. Time spent by clinical staff is reported only when specified in *CPT* or allowed under incident-to policy established by a payer.

See Chapter 13 for information on reporting services incident to a physician's service.

Documentation of Time

- Documentation of time spent providing services should be evident in the medical record for each service reported based on time (ie, total minutes of service or start and stop times).
- Documentation of time may be automated in an EHR, but physicians should be able to demonstrate that the EHR functionality captures the correct time for code selection as specified by *CPT.* For instance, only time for which the physician or QHP devotes full attention to providing hourly critical care services to a patient is counted toward the time of hourly critical care services (99291, 99292). Time spent in any separately reportable procedure (eg, 31500, endotracheal

intubation) is not included in the time of hourly critical care services. Documentation should clearly reflect the total times and activities of each service.

- When multiple services are provided on the same date, the time spent in time-based services must be clearly distinguished from time spent providing other services.
- In addition to documentation of total time or start and stop times of service, documentation should clearly support the service reported. For example, documentation of counseling should include discussion of diagnosis and treatment options, patient and/or caregiver questions and concerns addressed, shared decision-making for a plan of care, and any social determinants of health that affect care and were addressed (eg, advice to enroll in a prescription discount program).
- All documentation must be signed or electronically authenticated with the name and credentials of the physician or other provider of care and date of service.

Key Takeaways for Reporting Time

Examples of time-based reporting are included throughout this manual to further the understanding of time-based reporting. The examples emphasize some key tips for reporting based on time.

National Drug Code (NDC)

NDCs are universal product identifiers for prescription drugs including vaccines and insulin products. Codes are 10-digit, 3-segment numbers that identify the product, labeler, and trade package size. Medicare, Medicaid, and other government payers (eg, Tricare), as well as some private payers, require the use of NDCs when reporting medication and vaccine product codes.

- The HIPAA standards for reporting NDCs do not align with the 10-digit format; they require an 11-digit code.
  — Conversion to an 11-digit code in 5-4-2 format is required.
  — Leading zeros are added to the appropriate segment to accomplish the 5-4-2 format, as illustrated in **Table 1-6**.

  It is important to verify each payer's requirements for NDC reporting. A payer may require either of the following:
- The NDC that is provided on the outer packaging when a vaccine or other drug is supplied in bulk packages
- The NDC from the vial that was administered

  When reporting NDCs
- A qualifier (N4) precedes the NDC number on the claim form (eg, N400006404720).
- The correct number of NDC units must also be included on claims.
  — The NDC units are often different from HCPCS or *CPT* units.
  — For most payers, NDC units are reported as grams (GR), milligrams (ME), milliliters (ML), or units (UN).
  — The qualifiers GR, ME, ML, and UN are reported before the number of NDC units on a claim to indicate the measure.

Example

➤ **A claim for supply of a 0.2-mL, single-dose, prefilled applicator of influenza vaccine would include 1 unit of service on the claim line with *CPT* code 90672 and ML02 units on the NDC line for this service (example NDC claim line: N466019030701 ML02).**

Table 1-6. National Drug Code Format Examples		
Product	10-digit NDC Format	11-digit NDC Format (Added 0 [zero] is <u>underscored.</u>)
RotaTeq 2-mL single-dose tube, package of 20	0006-4047-20 (4-4-2)	<u>0</u>0006-4047-20 (5-4-2)
FluMist Quadrivalent 0.2-mL applicator, package of 10	66019-307-10 (5-3-2)	66019-<u>0</u>307-10 (5-4-2)
Synagis 0.5-mL in 1 vial, single dose	60574-4114-1 (5-4-1)	60574-4114-<u>0</u>1 (5-4-2)
Abbreviation: NDC, National Drug Code.		

If you are not currently reporting vaccines with NDCs, be sure to coordinate the requirements with your billing software company. For more information on NDCs, visit www.fda.gov/drugs/informationondrugs/ucm142438.htm for updates.

Beyond Code Sets

Who Assigns the Codes?

- Diagnoses should be assigned by the clinician (ie, pediatrician, pediatric nurse practitioner, or physician assistant) indicating a principal (primary) diagnosis that best explains the reason with the highest risk of morbidity or mortality for the patient encounter.
- All contributing (secondary) diagnoses that help explain the medical necessity for the episode of care should also be listed. However, only those conditions that specifically affect the patient's encounter should be listed.
- Code assignment may take place in conjunction with documentation or later, depending on the workflow processes of the practice.

> Documentation of diagnoses, signs and symptoms, or other reasons for a service is not accomplished through code assignment. Per official guidance from *Coding Clinic*, selection of a code cannot replace a written diagnostic statement. Multiple clinical conditions may be represented by a single diagnosis code, and more than 1 code may be required to fully describe a condition. Codes should be assigned to the documented diagnostic statement.

- When codes are selected by physicians at the time of EHR documentation, it is advisable to have trained administrative staff verify that the codes are selected in compliance with *ICD-10-CM* guidelines and conventions. Electronic health records often fail to show complete code descriptors and/or *ICD-10-CM* instructions (eg, exclusion notes).
- Assignment of the specific diagnosis code by clinical or administrative staff should be done under the physician's or reporting provider's supervision.
- The first-listed code on the claim should be the principal reason for the service unless the tabular instructions direct to "code first" another reason (eg, code first routine child health examination [**Z23**] when immunizations are provided at the time of a preventive E/M service [**Z00.121**, **Z00.129**]).
- Verification of the levels of service, need for modifiers, and compliance with *CPT* and payer policies is advised prior to billing.
- For those practices using a printed encounter form, including 50 to 100 of the most commonly used diagnoses *and* their respective codes on the outpatient encounter form allows the physician or other QHP to mark the appropriate code(s), indicating which is primary.
  - If a specific diagnosis code is not included on the form, write it in.
  - Do not select a diagnosis code that is "closest to" the diagnosis.
  - The AAP has developed a *Pediatric Office Superbill* (an encounter form including *ICD-10-CM* codes).

Reporting Codes for Payment

In addition to establishing standard code sets, HIPAA also established electronic transaction standards for patient benefit inquiries and submission of health claims and related reports.

- Claims for professional services are typically submitted electronically in a format referred to as 837P (professional claim) as currently configured in version 5010A1.
- Paper claim form submissions using the National Uniform Claim Committee 1500 claim form, version 02/12 (1500 form), are allowed for providers who meet an exception to the HIPAA requirements for electronic claim submission (eg, provider with <10 full-time employees).
  - Paper claims submission increases the length of time between submission and payment and increases the chance of error in either completion of the form or claims processing. Because of this, few physicians routinely submit paper claims, and it is advisable to submit electronic claims whenever possible.
  - The 1500 form contains the same information as an electronic claim and is valuable for demonstrating how codes and other information necessary for claims processing must be relayed to payers. An example of a completed 1500 form is found in **Figure 1-1**.

Figure 1-1. Example of a Completed 1500 Form

Example 1500 Claim Form

HEALTH INSURANCE CLAIM FORM
APPROVED BY NATIONAL UNIFORM CLAIM COMMITTEE (NUCC) 02/12

ABC Health Plan
123 Money St.
Anywhere, AK 00000

PICA	
1. Type	MEDICAID [X]
1a. INSURED'S I.D. NUMBER	123456789
2. PATIENT'S NAME	Smith, Boy
3. PATIENT'S BIRTH DATE	11 22 2021 SEX M [X]
4. INSURED'S NAME	Smith, Momma
5. PATIENT'S ADDRESS	123 Main St.
6. PATIENT RELATIONSHIP TO INSURED	Self [X]
7. INSURED'S ADDRESS	
CITY	Anywhere STATE KS
8. RESERVED FOR NUCC USE	
ZIP CODE	12345 TELEPHONE (555) 5555555
9. OTHER INSURED'S NAME	Smith, Poppa
10. IS PATIENT'S CONDITION RELATED TO:	
11. INSURED'S POLICY GROUP OR FECA NUMBER	98765432102
a. OTHER INSURED'S POLICY OR GROUP NUMBER	45612378900
a. EMPLOYMENT?	YES [ ] NO [X]
a. INSURED'S DATE OF BIRTH	01 01 1992 SEX F [X]
b. RESERVED FOR NUCC USE	
b. AUTO ACCIDENT?	YES [ ] NO [X] PLACE (State)
b. OTHER CLAIM ID	
c. RESERVED FOR NUCC USE	
c. OTHER ACCIDENT?	YES [ ] NO [X]
c. INSURANCE PLAN NAME OR PROGRAM NAME	Good Health Plan
d. INSURANCE PLAN NAME OR PROGRAM NAME	Another Good Plan
10d. CLAIM CODES	
d. IS THERE ANOTHER HEALTH BENEFIT PLAN?	YES [X] NO [ ] If yes, complete items 9, 9a, and 9d.

READ BACK OF FORM BEFORE COMPLETING & SIGNING THIS FORM.
12. PATIENT'S OR AUTHORIZED PERSON'S SIGNATURE: SIGNED Signature on file DATE 02/22/2022
13. INSURED'S OR AUTHORIZED PERSON'S SIGNATURE: SIGNED Signature on file

14. DATE OF CURRENT ILLNESS, INJURY, or PREGNANCY (LMP)
15. OTHER DATE
16. DATES PATIENT UNABLE TO WORK IN CURRENT OCCUPATION
17. NAME OF REFERRING PROVIDER OR OTHER SOURCE
18. HOSPITALIZATION DATES RELATED TO CURRENT SERVICES
19. ADDITIONAL CLAIM INFORMATION
20. OUTSIDE LAB? $ CHARGES

21. DIAGNOSIS OR NATURE OF ILLNESS OR INJURY ICD Ind. 0
A. Z00.129 B. Z23

22. RESUBMISSION CODE ORIGINAL REF. NO.
23. PRIOR AUTHORIZATION NUMBER

24.	A. DATE(S) OF SERVICE From / To	B. PLACE OF SERVICE	C. EMG	D. CPT/HCPCS	MODIFIER	E. DIAGNOSIS POINTER	F. $ CHARGES	G. DAYS OR UNITS	H. EPSDT	I. ID QUAL	J. RENDERING PROVIDER ID. #
1	02 22 22 02 22 22	11		99391	25	A	111.00	1		NPI	1234567890
	N44928105105 ML05										
2	02 22 22 02 22 22	11		90698		AB	200.00	1		NPI	1234567890
	N400006404741 ML2										
3	02 22 22 02 22 22	11		90680		AB	200.00	1		NPI	1234567890
	N400005197105 ML05										
4	02 22 22 02 22 22	11		90670		AB	200.00	1		NPI	1234567890
5	02 22 22 02 22 22	11		90460		AB	150.00	3		NPI	1234567890
6	02 22 22 02 22 22	11		90461		AB	100.00	4		NPI	1234567890

25. FEDERAL TAX I.D. NUMBER 12-4567897 EIN [X]
26. PATIENT'S ACCOUNT NO. 11111
27. ACCEPT ASSIGNMENT? YES [X] NO [ ]
28. TOTAL CHARGE $ 961.00
29. AMOUNT PAID $
30. Rsvd for NUCC Use

31. SIGNATURE OF PHYSICIAN OR SUPPLIER INCLUDING DEGREES OR CREDENTIALS
Signature on file 02232022
32. SERVICE FACILITY LOCATION INFORMATION
Pediatric Practice
111 Some Street
Anywhere, US 99999
33. BILLING PROVIDER INFO & PH # (555) 5555555
Pediatric Practice
111 Some Street
Anywhere, US 99999
a. 01233456789

NUCC Instruction Manual available at: www.nucc.org PLEASE PRINT OR TYPE APPROVED OMB-0938-1197 FORM 1500 (02-12)

Sidebar: CARRIER — PATIENT AND INSURED INFORMATION — PHYSICIAN OR SUPPLIER INFORMATION

Vertical left margin: Chapter 1. The Basics of Coding

Linking the Diagnosis to the Service

- Every claim line for a physician service must be linked to the appropriate *ICD-10-CM* code that represents the reason for the service.
  - Each *ICD-10-CM* code is placed in a diagnosis field labeled 21A–L.
  - A diagnosis pointer in field 24E indicates which diagnosis code relates to each service line by indicating the letter of the related diagnosis field. More than 1 diagnosis field may be linked to a service.
- When using an EHR, physicians should list the primary diagnosis in the EHR first and make certain the software knows that it should be reported as the first listed. In addition, the EHR should be able to link diagnosis codes to the appropriate services.
- The diagnosis code may be the same for each service performed.

Example

➤ **If a child is diagnosed with a urinary tract infection, the code for urinary tract infection (*ICD-10-CM* code N39.0) should be linked to the E/M service (eg, 99213) and to a performed dipstick urinalysis without microscopy (81002).**

Other Coding and Billing Information

Correct code assignment and claim completion are important steps in compliant and effective practice management. However, many other processes and policies are required. Please see **Chapter 4** for additional guidance on coding and billing procedures.

Resources

AAP Coding Assistance and Education

AAP Coding Hotline (https://form.jotform.com/Subspecialty/aapcodinghotline)

AAP *Coding for Pediatrics* Online

www.aap.org/cfp

AAP Initial History Questionnaire

Available for purchase at https://shop.aap.org

AAP *Pediatric Coding Newsletter*

ICD-10-CM collection (https://coding.solutions.aap.org/icd10.aspx; subscription required)

Current Procedural Terminology (CPT)

American Medical Association *CPT* general information (www.ama-assn.org/practice-management/cpt-current-procedural-terminology)
Category II code changes (*CPT* Category II codes alphabetical clinical topics listing: www.ama-assn.org/practice-management/cpt/category-ii-codes)
Category III code list (www.ama-assn.org/practice-management/cpt/category-iii-codes)
Newly released vaccine codes (www.ama-assn.org/practice-management/cpt/category-i-vaccine-codes)

ICD-10-CM Code Files and Guidelines

National Center for Health Statistics *ICD-10-CM* (www.cdc.gov/nchs/icd/icd10cm.htm)

American Academy of Pediatrics *Pediatric ICD-10-CM: A Manual for Provider-Based Coding* (available for purchase at https://shop.aap.org)

National Drug Codes

US Food and Drug Administration National Drug Code Directory (www.fda.gov/drugs/informationondrugs/ucm142438.htm)

Test Your Knowledge!

1. **Which of the following means "not included here" in *International Classification of Diseases, 10th Revision, Clinical Modification (ICD-10-CM)*?**
   a. Excludes1
   b. See also
   c. Excludes2
   d. Use an additional code

2. **Which of the following best describes the meaning of seventh character D?**
   a. Delayed treatment
   b. Subsequent care during the healing phase
   c. Care due to an unanticipated complication
   d. Care due to a sequela or late effect

3. **Which of the following is a guideline for time in *Current Procedural Terminology*?**
   a. Documentation of time must always include the exact start and stop times of the service.
   b. All evaluation and management services include clinical staff time.
   c. The midpoint rule applies to all time-based services.
   d. Category- or code-specific instructions are followed in lieu of the midpoint rule.

4. **Which of the following is true of Health Insurance Portability and Accountability Act of 1996 standards for reporting National Drug Codes (NDCs)?**
   a. NDCs are reported only for injectable medications.
   b. NDCs must be submitted on a claim with 11 digits in 5-4-2 format.
   c. All payers require the NDC from the outer packaging of products purchased in bulk packaging.
   d. The NDC is reported in lieu of a Healthcare Common Procedure Coding System code for a product.

5. **Which of the following is true of the *ICD-10-CM* code set?**
   a. The diagnosis code may be the same for each service performed.
   b. All codes are updated on January 1 of each year.
   c. Listing *ICD-10-CM* codes in the patient record is the equivalent of documenting diagnoses or reasons for an encounter.
   d. *ICD-10-CM* codes do not affect whether a claim for a service is paid or denied.

CHAPTER 2

Coding Edits and Modifiers

Contents

Coding Edits 27

National Correct Coding Initiative (NCCI) Edits 27

Procedure-to-Procedure Edits 27

Appropriate NCCI Modifiers 27

Medically Unlikely Edits 28

Keeping Up to Date With the NCCI 29

Reviewing and Using These Edits 30

Current Procedural Terminology Modifiers 30

22—Increased Procedural Services 31

24—Unrelated E/M Service by the Same Physician or Other Qualified Health Care Professional During a
Postoperative Period 32

25—Significant, Separately Identifiable E/M Service by the Same Physician or Other Qualified Health Care
Professional on the Same Day of the Procedure or Other Service 32

26—Professional Component 34

Professional, Technical, or Global Services 34

Reporting Modifier 26 34

32—Mandated Services 35

33—Preventive Services 35

47—Anesthesia by Surgeon 36

50—Bilateral Procedure 36

51—Multiple Procedures 37

52—Reduced Services 38

53—Discontinued Procedure 38

54—Surgical Care Only 39

55—Postoperative Management Only 39

56—Preoperative Management Only 39

57—Decision for Surgery 40

58—Staged or Related Procedure or Service by the Same Physician or Other Qualified Health Care
Professional During the Postoperative Period 40

59—Distinct Procedural Service 41

62—Two Surgeons 42

63—Procedure Performed on Infants Less Than 4 kg 42

66—Surgical Team 43

76—Repeat Procedure or Service by Same Physician or Other Qualified Health Care Professional 43

77—Repeat Procedure or Service by Another Physician or Other Qualified Health Care Professional 44

78—Unplanned Return to the Operating/Procedure Room by the Same Physician or Other Qualified
Health Care Professional Following Initial Procedure for a Related Procedure During the Postoperative Period 44

79—Unrelated Procedure or Service by the Same Physician or Other Qualified Health Care Professional
During the Postoperative Period 44

80—Assistant Surgeon 45

81—Minimum Assistant Surgeon 45

82—Assistant Surgeon (When Qualified Resident Surgeon Not Available) 45

90—Reference (Outside) Laboratory 45

91—Repeat Clinical Diagnostic Laboratory Test 45

92—Alternative Laboratory Platform Testing 45

95—Synchronous Telemedicine Service Rendered via a Real-time Interactive Audio and Video
Telecommunications System 46

99—Multiple Modifiers 46

Healthcare Common Procedure Coding System Modifiers 46

    Anatomical Modifiers 46

    X {E, P, S, U} Modifiers.. 47

    CR—Catastrophe/Disaster Related 47

    EP—Service Provided as Part of Medicaid Early and Periodic Screening, Diagnostic, and Treatment
    (EPSDT) Program 47

    GA—Waiver of Liability Statement Issued as Required by Payer Policy, Individual Case......................... 48

    GU—Waiver of Liability Statement Issued as Required by Payer Policy, Routine Notice.......................... 48

    GX—Notice of Liability Issued, Voluntary Under Payer Policy 48

    GC—This Service Has Been Performed in Part by a Resident Under the Direction of a Teaching Physician.................... 48

    GE—This Service Has Been Performed by a Resident Without the Presence of a Teaching Physician Under
    the Primary Care Exception 48

    GT—Via Interactive Audio and Video Telecommunication Systems... 48

    JW—Drug Amount Discarded/Not Administered to Any Patient... 48

    KP—First Drug of a Multiple Drug Unit Dose Formulation 49

    KQ—Second or Subsequent Drug of a Multiple Drug Unit Dose Formulation.. 49

    QW—Clinical Laboratory Improvement Amendments–Waived Tests 49

    RT, LT—Right and Left Side 49

    X1–X5 Patient Relationship Modifiers 50

Resources... 50

Test Your Knowledge! 51

Coding edits and modifiers are important tools for getting paid correctly for physician services. Coding edits are used by all payers in electronic claims adjudication to determine which reported services are payable on the same date or what number of units are allowed based on payment policies. Physicians use modifiers to communicate information to payer systems about the service described by a procedure code. Modifiers are used to indicate either a change in the way a service was provided or additional information, such as laterality of a body site or services provided that may be separately reported in addition to other services due to certain circumstances (eg, a significant problem was addressed at an encounter for a routine child health examination).

Coding Edits

National Correct Coding Initiative (NCCI) Edits

The National Correct Coding Initiative (NCCI) edits were developed for use by the Centers for Medicare & Medicaid Services (CMS) in adjudicating Medicare claims, and all Medicaid programs use a Medicaid-specific version of the NCCI edits. The NCCI edits frequently form the basis for proprietary claim editors used by private payers.

The NCCI edits

- Have been developed based on *Current Procedural Terminology* (*CPT*®) code descriptors and instructions, coding guidelines developed by national medical societies (eg, American Academy of Pediatrics [AAP]), Medicare billing history, local and national Medicare carrier policies and edits, and analysis of standard medical and surgical practice.
- Are used by payers in the claim processing system for physician services as well as to promote correct coding.
- Include 2 types of edits: procedure-to-procedure edits and Medically Unlikely Edits (MUEs).
- Physicians should not inconvenience patients or increase risks to patients by performing services on different dates of service to avoid MUE or NCCI procedure-to-procedure edits.
  - This instruction comes from the Medicaid NCCI manual and prohibits practice policies that focus on achieving maximum payment.
  - Delaying patient care to avoid code edits could be seen as an abusive billing practice; policies or practices that might be perceived in this way should be avoided.

Procedure-to-Procedure Edits

- Identify code pairs that normally should not be billed by the same physician or physicians of the same group practice and same specialty (*provider* is used in NCCI manuals) for the same patient on the same date of service.
- Include edits based on services that are mutually exclusive based on code descriptor or anatomical considerations (**Table 2-1**), services that are considered to be inherent to each other, and edits based on coding instructions.
  - If 2 codes of an edit are billed by the same provider for the same patient for the same date of service without an appropriate modifier, only the column 1 code is paid.
  - If clinical circumstances justify appending the appropriate modifier to the column 2 code, payment of both codes may be allowed. (The Medicaid NCCI will allow payment when an NCCI modifier is appended to either code in a code pair.)

> The Centers for Medicare & Medicaid Services allows physicians to append modifiers 59, XE, XP, XS, and XU to either the column 1 or column 2 code when reporting 2 codes paired by the Medicare National Correct Coding Initiative (NCCI) edits. Other payers may adopt this policy or require the modifier be appended to the code in column 2 of the NCCI edit file.

Appropriate NCCI Modifiers

Modifier indicators are assigned to every code pair identified in the NCCI. They dictate whether modifiers are needed or will be accepted to override the edit. These indicators are

0   Under no circumstance may a modifier be used to override the edit.
1   An appropriate modifier may be used to override the edit.
9   This edit was deleted prior to its effective date or there is, essentially, no edit.

Refer to **Table 2-1** for examples.

Chapter 2. Coding Edits and Modifiers

Table 2-1. Examples of Medicaid National Correct Coding Initiative Edits			
Column 1 Comprehensive Code	**Column 2 Component Code**	**Modifier Indicator**	**Effective Date**
99221 Initial hospital or birthing center care, per day, for evaluation and management of normal newborn infant	**99462** Subsequent hospital care, per day, for evaluation and management of normal newborn	0	10/1/2010
The NCCI edits preclude any payment for the column 2 code because the services are mutually exclusive. Each code represents all normal newborn care on a single date of service by 1 physician or physicians of the same specialty and group practice.			
10121 Incision and removal of foreign body, subcutaneous tissues; complex	**10120** Incision and removal of foreign body, subcutaneous tissues; simple	1	10/1/2010
The component code (10120) would be denied unless a modifier indicating a distinct procedural service (eg, 59) is appended (eg, 10120 59). Medicaid payment policy allows both services only if the incisions and removals are from separate noncontiguous sites or the occurred at separate encounters.			
99221–99223 Initial hospital care, per day	**99217** Observation care discharge day management	0	10/1/2010
The NCCI edits preclude any payment for the component code (ie, column 2 code 99217). When a patient is transferred to inpatient status following observation care on the same date, only the initial hospital care is reported.			
10120 Incision and removal of foreign body, subcutaneous tissues; simple	**99212** Office or other outpatient visit for the E/M of an established patient with straightforward MDM or 10-19 minutes of total time is spent on the date of the encounter.	1	10/1/2020
The component code (99212) would be denied if modifier 25 (significant, separately identifiable E/M service) were not appended to it. E/M codes must require significant and separate MDM or time beyond that included in the preservice and post-service work of a procedure performed at the same encounter.			
Be aware that the higher valued service may be the component code and would be denied without the application of the correct modifier.			
Abbreviations: E/M, evaluation and management; MDM, medical decision-making; NCCI, National Correct Coding Initiative.			

- Only certain modifiers can be used to override edits when the service or procedure is clinically justified, and they may be used only on the code pairs that are assigned the 1 indicator. See **Table 2-2** for a list of modifiers that override NCCI edits.
- The CMS now allows modifiers **59**, **XE**, **XS**, **XP**, or **XU** (individually discussed later in this chapter) on column 1 and 2 codes.
- For overrides of other mutually exclusive edits or correct coding edits, the appropriate modifier is always appended to the code that appears in column 2 because that is considered the bundled or exclusive procedure.
- To append the appropriate modifier and override an edit, it is imperative that the conditions of that modifier are met.

Medically Unlikely Edits

The *National Correct Coding Initiative Policy Manual for Medicaid Services* describes MUEs as unit of service edits that were established by the CMS to prevent payment for an inappropriate number or quantity of the same service (eg, accidental reporting of 100 rather than 10 units). An MUE for a Healthcare Common Procedure Coding System (HCPCS) or *CPT* code is the maximum number of units of service, under most circumstances, allowable by the same provider for the same beneficiary on the same date of service.

Medicaid MUEs

- Are applied separately to each line of a claim. If the unit of service on a line exceeds the MUE value, the entire line is denied.
- Are coding edits rather than medical necessity edits.
- May be established based on claims data.
- May limit units of service based on anatomical structures.
- May limit the number of units of service based on *CPT* code descriptors or *CPT* coding instructions.
- Are published on the CMS Medicaid NCCI website at www.medicaid.gov/medicaid/program-integrity/ncci/index.html.

Table 2-2. Modifiers That Can Be Used to Override National Correct Coding Initiative Edits

24	Unrelated E/M service by the same physician or other QHP during a postoperative period	F6	Right hand, second digit
25	Significant, separately identifiable E/M service by the same physician or other QHP on the same day of the procedure or other service	F7	Right hand, third digit
57	Decision for surgery	F8	Right hand, fourth digit
58	Staged or related procedure or service by the same physician or other QHP during the postoperative period	F9	Right hand, fifth digit
59	Distinct procedural service	LC	Left circumflex, coronary artery
78	Unplanned return to the OR by the same physician or other QHP following initial procedure for a related procedure during the postoperative period	LD	Left anterior descending coronary artery
79	Unrelated procedure/service by the same physician or other QHP during the postoperative period	LM	Left main coronary artery
91	Repeat clinical diagnostic laboratory test	LT	Left side
E1	Upper left, eyelid	RC	Right coronary artery
E2	Lower left, eyelid	RI	Ramus intermedius coronary artery
E3	Upper right, eyelid	RT	Right side
E4	Lower right, eyelid	TA	Left foot, great toe
FA	Left hand, thumb	T1	Left foot, second digit
F1	Left hand, second digit	T2	Left foot, third digit
F2	Left hand, third digit	T3	Left foot, fourth digit
F3	Left hand, fourth digit	T4	Left foot, fifth digit
F4	Left hand, fifth digit	T5	Right foot, great toe
F5	Right hand, thumb	T6	Right foot, second digit
		T7	Right foot, third digit
		T8	Right foot, fourth digit
		T9	Right foot, fifth digit
		XE	Separate encounter (different session)
		XP	Separate practitioner
		XS	Separate structure (site/organ)
		XU	Unusual nonoverlapping service

Abbreviations: E/M, evaluation and management; OR, operating/procedure room; QHP, qualified health care professional.

- Are published with an *edit rationale* for each HCPCS and *CPT* code.
  - The MUE value assigned for code 96110 (developmental screening, per instrument) is 3 based on CMS NCCI policy. (No further explanation of this rationale is provided in the current Medicaid or Medicare NCCI manuals but may be based on historical claims data.)
  - The MUE value assigned to code 96127 (brief emotional/behavior assessment, per instrument) is 2 based on the nature of the service or procedure (typically determined by the amount of time required to perform a procedure/service or clinical application of a procedure/service).
- Are applied separately to each claim line for a service when modifiers (eg, 59, 76, 77, anatomical) cause the same HCPCS or *CPT* code to appear on separate lines of a claim.

It is important to recognize that the use of modifiers to override the MUE must be justified based on correct selection of the procedure code, correct application of the number of units reported, medical necessity and reasonableness of the number of services, and, if applicable, reason the physician's practice pattern differs from national patterns.

Keeping Up to Date With the NCCI

Medicaid and Medicare NCCI edits are updated quarterly. Each Medicare NCCI version ends with .0 (point zero), .1, .2, or .3 indicating its effective dates.

- Versions ending in .0 (point zero) are effective from January 1 through March 31 of that year.
- Versions ending in .1 are effective from April 1 through June 30 of that year.
- Versions ending in .2 are effective from July 1 through September 30 of that year.
- Versions ending in .3 are effective from October 1 through December 31 of that year.

The CMS releases the Medicare NCCI edits free of charge on its website (www.cms.gov/NationalCorrectCodInitEd/NCCIEP/list.asp). Medicaid NCCI files are published separately free of charge at www.medicaid.gov/medicaid/program-integrity/ncci/edit-files/index.html.

- Although many of the Medicaid edits mirror Medicare edits, this is not always the case. The CMS has instructed that use of the appropriate NCCI file is important to correct coding.

- Online NCCI edits are posted in spreadsheet form, which allows users to sort by procedure code and effective date.
- There is a "Find" tool that allows users to look for a specific code. The edit files are indexed by procedure code ranges for simplified navigation.
- Policy manuals that explain the rationale for edits and correct use of NCCI-associated modifiers are published to the web pages listed previously (see "Reference Documents" link on the Medicaid NCCI page).
  — Updated manuals for the year ahead are published annually in late fall.
  — Changes in the manual are shown in red font for easy identification.
  — Be sure to update your NCCI edit files quarterly and review changes to the NCCI manual each year.

Practice management and electronic health record software may also contain tools for identifying codes affected by NCCI edits.

Reviewing and Using These Edits

1. Be aware of all coding edits that are applicable to your specialty; as each update replaces the former edits, it is important to review them quarterly. Always look for new or deleted edits. Updated files can be found at www.aap.org/coding under the "Coding Resources, National Correct Coding Initiative (NCCI) Edits" tab.
2. Pay close attention to the modifier indicator because it may have changed from the last quarterly update. For example, a code set that initially would not allow override with a modifier may now subsequently allow one, or vice versa.
3. Pay attention to the effective date and deletion date of each code set. The edits are applicable only if they are effective. The effective date is based on the date of service, not the date the claim was submitted. Sometimes a pair is retroactively terminated. If so, you may resubmit claims for payment if the date of service is within the filing time frame of the payer.
4. Use modifiers as appropriate.
   a) Modifiers should be used only when applicable based on coding standards, when medically justified or necessary, and when supported by medical record documentation (progress notes, procedure notes, diagrams, or pictures) or, as previously mentioned, when dictated by payers.
   a) Refer to the CMS written guidelines (because they are very explicit about billing surgical procedures) or to your payer's provider manual.
5. When billing surgical procedures, you may need to look at several different codes for possible edits. Be sure to always use the code that is reflective of the total service performed.
6. Appeal denied payment for services for which there is no edit and the policy manual and/or payment policies do not preclude reporting, for which a reported modifier should have allowed payment, and/or for which the edit is inconsistent with *CPT* guidelines. Having knowledge of how this system works is to your benefit when appealing the denial.
7. Some payers have developed or adopted coding edit programs that are different from and often more comprehensive than the NCCI.
   a) If a payer policy differs from the CMS NCCI policy and is not clearly defined in its provider manual, refer to the payer's website.
   a) Make sure you get policies in writing for the services you commonly perform. Your contracts with health plans should be explicit regarding how you will receive initial and updated policies.
8. Report the services provided correctly based on *CPT* code guidelines (unless a payer has clearly stated otherwise).

Current Procedural Terminology Modifiers

CPT defines a *modifier* as an indicator that a service or procedure has been altered by some specific circumstance but not changed in its basic code definition. Modifiers are also used to show compliance with payment policy. Medical record documentation must always support the use of the modifier.

In addition to *CPT* modifiers, the CMS maintains a list of modifiers for use with HCPCS and *CPT* codes. Most state Medicaid programs and many commercial payers recognize HCPCS modifiers as well.

When are modifiers needed? In brief, a modifier or combination of modifiers is appended to a procedure code when it is necessary to add context of how or when the service was provided. Context often affects payment, such as when a bilateral procedure is reported with a code that does not indicate unilateral or bilateral. By appending modifier **50** (bilateral procedure), the claim for services provides context allowing claims adjudication systems to process for payment at a higher rate (typically 150% of the allowable amount for the unilateral service). Examples of information provided by modifiers include

- A service provided on the same date or within the global period of a previous service is unrelated, more extensive, performed on a different body area, or performed at separate encounters.
- A face-to-face service was provided via telemedicine using real-time, interactive communication technology.

- The same service was repeated on the same date.
- An evaluation and management (E/M) service that might otherwise be considered part of another service is significantly beyond the typical preservice and/or post-service components of the other service.
- The units of services provided were medically necessary but exceed the payer's unit of service edits.
- A service that may be provided for diagnostic or preventive purposes was provided for preventive purposes.

Payers use coding edits (ie, paired codes and/or unit of service limitations) to aid in automated claims adjudication. Modifiers play an important role in this process.

- When a modifier is appropriately applied to 1 code in a pair of codes reported by a physician on 1 date of service or to a code for services that exceed the units of service typically allowed by payer edits, the payer may allow charges that would otherwise be denied as bundled or non-covered.

The Health Insurance Portability and Accountability Act of 1996 requires recognition of all *CPT* modifiers, but payers may have their own payment and billing policies for the use of modifiers that can vary from *CPT* guidelines.

- Know and understand their policies. This is important to capturing all payments allowed under your contract.
- If payment is denied inappropriately because of nonrecognition or the incorrect application of a modifier, you should appeal the denied services.
- For additional assistance, contact the AAP Coding Hotline (https://form.jotform.com/Subspecialty/aapcodinghotline).

Some modifiers are used exclusively with E/M services, and others are reported only with surgical or other procedures. Refer to **Table 2-3** to review modifiers used with E/M service codes and those used only for other services. Multiple modifiers can be appended to a single *CPT* or HCPCS code.

Table 2-3. Modifiers and Evaluation and Management Services

24,25,57	E/M-only modifiers
22,26,47,50,51,52,53,54,55,56,58,59,62,63,66,76,77,78,79,80,81, 82,91	Procedure-only modifiers (Do not append to E/M services.)
32,33,92,95,96,97,99	Either E/M or procedures

Abbreviation: E/M, evaluation and management.

22—Increased Procedural Services

- Modifier **22** is used to report procedures when the work required to provide a service is substantially greater than typically required.
- Modifier **22** is only appended to anesthesia, surgery, radiology, laboratory, pathology, and medicine codes.
- Documentation must clearly reflect the substantial additional work and the reason for the additional work (eg, increased intensity, time, technical difficulty of procedure, severity of patient's condition, physical and mental effort required).
  - It is important that the documentation is specific. For instance, documentation that a procedure took longer than 1 hour is less supportive than documentation that the procedure took a total of 85 minutes or lasted from 9:15 to 10:40 am.
  - Reporting of additional diagnosis codes to support the increased work is also important.
- Most payers will require that a copy of the medical record documentation be sent with the claim when modifier **22** is reported.
- For an electronic claim, indicate "additional documentation available on request" in the claim level loop (2300 NTE) or in the line level loop (2400 NTE) segment. If the payer allows electronic claim attachments, follow the payer's instructions to submit the procedure note and, if necessary, a physician statement about the increased difficulty of the procedure.

Examples—Modifier 22

➤ **The physician required 45 minutes to perform a simple repair of a 1-cm laceration on a 2-year-old because the child was combative and several stops and starts were necessary.**

12011 22 (simple repair superficial wound of face; ≤2.5 cm)

➤ **An appendectomy is performed on a morbidly obese 12-year-old.** The surgery is complicated and requires additional time because of the obesity.

    44950 22 (appendectomy)

24—Unrelated E/M Service by the Same Physician or Other Qualified Health Care Professional During a Postoperative Period

> **For more information on global surgery guidelines, see chapters 10 and 19.**

- Modifier **24** is appended to an E/M code when the physician or other qualified health care professional (QHP) who performed a procedure provides an unrelated E/M service during the postoperative period.
- The CMS has its own system for definition of global periods, and many payers will follow those guidelines or assign a specific number of follow-up days for surgical procedures.

    Link the appropriate *International Classification of Diseases, 10th Revision, Clinical Modification* (ICD-10-CM) code to the E/M visit to support that the service was unrelated to the surgical procedure. Do not report the surgical diagnosis code if it was not the reason for the encounter.

Example—Modifier 24

➤ **A physician sees a 10-year-old established patient for follow-up of stable mild persistent asthma and performs a level 3 established patient office or other outpatient E/M service.** Eight days prior to this visit, the physician had performed a simple removal of a subcutaneous foreign body (by incision), which was reported with **10120**. The CMS has assigned a 10-day global postoperative period to code **10120** indicating that payment for all follow-up visits within that period related to that surgical service are included under the code.

ICD-10-CM	CPT
J45.30 (mild persistent asthma, uncomplicated)	**99213 24** (established office/outpatient E/M)

25—Significant, Separately Identifiable E/M Service by the Same Physician or Other Qualified Health Care Professional on the Same Day of the Procedure or Other Service

- Modifier **25** is appended only to an E/M service, and only when *all of the following are true:*
  - A separate service identified by a separate procedure code is performed by the same physician or other QHP, or by a physician or other QHP of the same specialty and group.
  - The patient's condition requires a significant E/M service (**99202–99499**) above and beyond the other service provided or beyond the usual preoperative and postoperative care associated with the procedure that was performed.
  - The service is separately identifiable in the documentation of the encounter(s).
- Different diagnoses are not required for reporting of the E/M service on the same date.
- The performed and documented E/M components must support the level of service reported and be separately identifiable from the procedure or other service documentation whether documented in 1 combined note or separate notes.
- *CPT* procedure codes include evaluative elements routinely performed prior to the procedure and the routine postoperative care. An assessment of the problem with an explanation of the procedure to be performed is considered inherent to the procedure and should not be reported separately with an E/M service code.
- When appropriate, modifier **25** may be reported on more than 1 E/M service for a single encounter. An example would be reporting a preventive medicine service (eg, **99393 25**) along with a problem-oriented service (eg, **99212 25**) in addition to giving the patient vaccines with counseling (eg, **90460**). See example on next page.
- **DO *NOT* USE MODIFIER 25 WHEN**
  - **The medical record does not support both services.**
  - **A problem encountered during a preventive medicine visit is insignificant or incidental (eg, minor diaper rash, renewal of prescription medications without reevaluation) or did not require additional work to perform the key components (ie, history, physical examination, and, importantly, medical decision-making [MDM], or time) of the E/M service.**

— The E/M service is a routine part of the usual preoperative and postoperative care.
— Modifier **57** (decision for surgery) is more appropriate. The ultimate decision on whether to use modifier **25** or **57** requires knowledge of payer policies. (See modifier **57** later in this chapter.)

Examples—Modifier 25

➤ **An E/M service is performed on a 6-year-old established patient.** The patient also is immunized against influenza, with counseling performed by the pediatrician.

ICD-10-CM	CPT
Appropriate diagnosis code for problem addressed **Z23** (encounter for immunization)	**99212–99215 25** (established patient E/M visit, office) **90694** (influenza virus vaccine, quadrivalent [aIIV4], inactivated, adjuvanted, preservative free, 0.5 mL dosage, for intramuscular use) **90460** (administration of first or only vaccine component, patient age ≤18 years, with physician counseling)

Teaching Point: *CPT* requires that modifier **25** be appended to a significant and separately identifiable E/M service when also reporting the administration of a vaccine or for a therapeutic injection (**96372**).

➤ **A 12-year-old established patient is seen for his preventive medicine visit.** The patient complains of increased asthma symptoms. Medical decision-making is moderate for management of moderate persistent asthma with worsening symptoms requiring adjustment to the dose of the control medication, supporting code **99214**. He has not yet received his tetanus, diphtheria, and acellular pertussis (Tdap) or meningococcal (MenACWY-D) intramuscular vaccines. The physician counsels the parents on the risks and protection from each of the diseases. The Centers for Disease Control and Prevention (CDC) Vaccine Information Statements are given to the parents and the nurse administers the vaccines.

ICD-10-CM	CPT
Z00.121 (well-child check with abnormal findings) **Z23** (encounter for immunization)	**99394 25** (preventive medicine visit, established patient, age 12 through 17 years) **90715** (Tdap, 7 years or older, intramuscular) **90734** (MenACWY-D) **90460** × 2 units **90461** × 2 units
J45.40 (moderate persistent asthma, uncomplicated	**99214 25** (office/outpatient E/M, established patient)

Teaching Point: Medical record documentation supports that a significant, separately identifiable E/M service was provided and is reported in addition to the preventive medicine service. Modifier **25** is appended to code **99214** to signify that it is significant and separately identifiable from the preventive medicine service. Modifier **25** is also appended to code **99394** to signify it is significant and separately identifiable from immunization administration (required by payers that have adopted Medicare and Medicaid bundling edits).

> See Chapter 9 for additional examples and guidelines for reporting a preventive medicine visit and a problem-oriented visit on the same day of service.

➤ **A patient is scheduled for removal of impacted cerumen following use of softening drops as directed at a prior visit.** The physician takes a problem-focused history from the patient, who has no other complaints; examines the affected ear; and determines that manual extraction is necessary, explaining the procedure, risks, and benefits. A combination of irrigation and removal using instrumentation is successful in clearing the ear canal.

Chapter 2. Coding Edits and Modifiers

ICD-10-CM	CPT
H61.2- (impacted cerumen, addition character is needed to report laterality)	**69210** (removal impacted cerumen requiring instrumentation, unilateral)

Teaching Point: An E/M service with modifier **25** is *not* reported. A separate charge for an E/M service is reported only when the E/M service is significant and separately identifiable from the preservice work of a procedure reported on the same date.

See chapters 10 and 19 for more information on reporting an evaluation and management service on the date of a procedure.

26—Professional Component

Professional, Technical, or Global Services

Certain procedures (eg, cardiac tests, radiographs, surgical diagnostic tests) are broken down into professional and technical components. *CPT* has a modifier for the professional component (**26**) but does not have a modifier for reporting only the technical component. That falls under the HCPCS modifier set (modifier **TC**).

- Professional component only: The physician who does not supply the equipment but performs the written interpretation and report of a service with professional and technical components should report the service with modifier **26** appended to the appropriate *CPT* code.

    The professional component includes the physician work (eg, interpretation of the test, written report).

- Technical component only: Most payers recognize modifier **TC** (technical component only). The facility or provider who owns the equipment and is responsible for the overhead and associated costs would report the same procedure code with modifier **TC** appended.

- Technical and professional components (global): If a service includes a professional and technical component and the physician owns the equipment, employs the staff to perform the service, and interprets the test, the procedure is reported *without a modifier*.

Reporting Modifier 26

- When reporting the professional component of diagnostic tests, interpretation should be documented in a report similar to that which is typical for the physicians who predominantly provide the service. This report should include *all of the following:*
    — Indication(s) for testing
    — Description of test
    — Findings
    — Limitations (when applicable)
    — Impression or conclusion
- If the report of a physician's interpretation is included in the documentation of another service (eg, office visit), it is important that the report is distinct and complete.
- The professional component is not reported when a physician reviews a test and notes agreement with the interpreting physician or when only a quick read without formal interpretation is provided.
- Some codes were developed to distinguish between technical and professional components (eg, routine electrocardiogram [ECG] codes **93000–93010**). Modifier **26** is not appropriate when reporting codes that distinguish professional and technical components and may result in a denial of the charge.

Examples—Modifier 26

➤ **A pediatrician interprets and creates a report of the findings from a radiograph of the foot that was produced by an outpatient radiology practice and transmitted electronically to the pediatrician. The pediatrician's order was for imaging without interpretation and report, so there is no other interpretation and report (ie, a radiologist will not also interpret and report).**

    73620 26 (x-ray foot, 2 views)

    The physician reports modifier **26**, indicating professional component only, because the hospital provided the technical component.

➤ **A pediatrician electronically accesses the image of a foot radiograph that was taken at the outpatient department of the hospital and will be interpreted by a radiologist at that facility. The pediatrician notes findings in the patient's records.**

   The pediatrician's review of the radiograph is not separately reported when a radiologist will provide a final interpretation and report. The physician did not perform the interpretation and report that constitutes the professional component of the foot radiograph. However, the physician's review of the image increases the level of MDM in a related E/M service.

➤ **A cardiologist performs transthoracic echocardiography with spectral and color-flow Doppler on a patient in the hospital.**

   The cardiologist would report code 93306 26 (echocardiography, transthoracic, real-time with image documentation [2D], includes M-mode recording, when performed, complete, with spectral Doppler echocardiography, and with color-flow Doppler echocardiography), and the hospital would report code 93306 TC.

32—Mandated Services

- Modifier 32 is appended to services (eg, second opinion) that are mandated by a third-party payer or governmental, legislative, or regulatory requirements.
- The modifier may be reported with codes for E/M services (eg, for second opinion required by a payer).
- Modifier 32 would be used when, for example, radiological services are requested from a worker's compensation carrier, laboratory testing (eg, drug tests) is requested by a court system, or a physical therapy assessment is requested by an insurer.

Example—Modifier 32

➤ **A Medicaid managed care organization requires modifier 32 to indicate off-schedule provision of a routine child health examination for purposes of clearance to attend child care or preschool.** A pediatrician provides an age- and gender-appropriate preventive E/M service to an established 3½-year-old patient who will be entering the Head Start program.

ICD-10-CM	CPT
Z02.0 (encounter for examination for admission to educational institution)	99392 32 (established patient preventive service, age 1–4 years)

33—Preventive Services

CPT modifier 33 is used to communicate to payers that a preventive medicine service (defined by the Patient Protection and Affordable Care Act [PPACA] provisions; the 4 categories are listed as follows) was performed on a patient enrolled in a health care plan subject to the preventive service coverage requirements of the PPACA and, therefore, should not be subject to cost sharing.

- The appropriate use of modifier 33 will reduce claim adjustments related to preventive services and facilitate correct payments to members.
- Modifier 33 should only be appended to codes represented in 1 or more of the following 4 categories:
  - Services rated A or B by the US Preventive Services Task Force
  - Immunizations for routine use in children, adolescents, and adults as recommended by the Advisory Committee on Immunization Practices of the CDC
  - Preventive care and screenings for children as recommended by Bright Futures (AAP) and newborn testing (American College of Medical Genetics and Genomics)
  - Preventive care and screenings provided for women supported by the Health Resources and Services Administration
- **DO *NOT* USE MODIFIER 33**
  - **When the *CPT* code(s) is identified as inherently preventive (eg, preventive medicine counseling)**
  - **When the service(s) is not indicated in the categories noted previously**
  - **With an insurance plan that continues to implement the cost-sharing policy on preventive medicine services**
- Check with your payers before reporting modifier 33 to verify any variations in reporting requirements.

Example—Modifier 33

➤ **A 17-year-old established patient is seen for an office visit and requests contraception.** The physician determines the patient is not pregnant but has been sexually active with multiple partners and would like contraception. The physician then spends approximately 15 minutes discussing contraception and risks of sexually transmitted infection (STI) with the patient. Point-of-care HIV-1 and HIV-2 testing is conducted with negative results. Specimen is collected for chlamydia and gonorrhea screening by an outside laboratory. The patient chooses oral contraception, which is prescribed.

ICD-10-CM	CPT
Z30.09 (encounter for other general counseling and advice on contraception) **Z11.4** (encounter for screening for HIV) **Z11.3** (encounter for screening for STI)	**99401** (preventive counseling, approximately 15 minutes) **86703 33 92** (antibody; HIV-1 and HIV-2; single assay)

Teaching Point: Append modifier **33** to code **86703** to indicate the test was performed as a preventive service because, although recommended as a preventive service, the test is also used for diagnostic purposes. Modifier **92** is reported to indicate use of the HIV test kit (not all payers recognize modifier **92**). Code **99401** is reported for 8 to 23 minutes of service based on the midpoint rule for billing based on time (ie, time is met when the midpoint is passed). Typically, health plans cover services related to contraception (eg, **99401**) without cost to the patient.

47—Anesthesia by Surgeon

● Modifier **47** is used only when a physician performing a procedure *also personally performs* the regional and/or general anesthesia. The physician performing the procedure may not report codes **00100–01999** for anesthesia services. Instead, modifier **47** is appended to the code for the procedure performed.
● When performed, a code for regional anesthesia (nerve block) may be reported to indicate the site of the block.
● Modifier **47** is considered informational by many payers and does not affect payment.
  — Medicaid considers all anesthesia (other than moderate conscious sedation) provided by the same physician performing a procedure to be included in the procedure.
  — Other payers may restrict use of modifier **47** to specific procedure codes and provide specific reporting instructions. Be sure to verify payer policy prior to reporting.
● **DO *NOT* USE MODIFIER 47 WHEN**
  — **Administering local anesthesia because it is considered inherent to the procedure**
  — **Performing moderate (conscious) sedation**

> For more information on reporting moderate sedation, see chapters 10 and 19.

Example—Modifier 47

➤ **The surgeon performs a nerve block on the brachial plexus (64415) and removal of a ganglion cyst on the wrist (25111).**
  25111 47 and **64415**
  The regional anesthesia is separate from the procedure.

50—Bilateral Procedure

● Modifier **50** is used to identify bilateral procedures that are performed at the same session.
● It is used only when the services and/or procedures are performed on identical anatomical sites, aspects, or organs.
● Modifier **50** is not appended to any code with a descriptor that indicates the procedure includes bilateral, "one or both," or "unilateral or bilateral."
● The Medicare Physician Fee Schedule Relative Value Files (www.cms.gov/Medicare/Medicare-Fee-for-Service-Payment/PhysicianFeeSched/PFS-Relative-Value-Files.html) include a column (Column Z, BILAT SURG) that identifies codes that may be reported with modifier **50**. Procedures with a 1 indicator can be reported with modifier **50**.

Many private payers also publish lists of codes that may be reported as bilateral procedures.

- When the *CPT* code descriptor indicates a bilateral procedure and only a unilateral procedure is performed, modifier **52** (reduced services) should be appended to the procedure code.
- For Medicaid claims that require use of modifier **50**, only report 1 unit of service on the line item for the bilateral procedure.

Examples—Modifier 50

➤ **A physician performs bilateral tympanostomy with insertion of ventilating tubes under general anesthesia.**
   64936 50 (tympanostomy [requiring insertion of ventilating tube], general anesthesia)

➤ **A physician performs bilateral nasal endoscopy.**
   Modifier **50** would not be appended to code **31231** (nasal endoscopy, diagnostic, unilateral or bilateral [separate procedure]) because the code descriptor indicates a unilateral or bilateral procedure. (Modifier **52** is also not required for reporting a unilateral service when the code descriptor includes unilateral or bilateral.)

Coding Conundrum: Modifier 50

Nearly all payers now follow *Current Procedural Terminology* guidelines and Medicaid National Correct Coding Initiative (NCCI) instruction for bilateral surgical procedures. The NCCI edits require that bilateral surgical procedures (for which there is no code specifying a bilateral procedure) be reported with modifier **50** and 1 unit of service.

Example: Report removal of foreign bodies from both ears with code **69200 50** with 1 unit.

Bilateral diagnostic procedures may be reported with 2 units of service on 1 claim line, 1 unit of service and modifier **50** on 1 claim line, or 1 unit of service and modifier **RT** on 1 claim line plus 1 unit of service and modifier **LT** on a second claim line.

Example: Report bilateral x-rays of clavicles with one of the following methods:
73000 (radiologic examination; clavicle, complete) × 2 units
73000 50 × 1 unit
73000 RT × 1 unit and **73000 LT** × 1 unit

51—Multiple Procedures

- When multiple procedures or services are reported, payers usually reduce the payment for the second and each additional code by 50% because there is some resource cost duplication when multiple procedures are done at the same visit or session. Medicare and some state Medicaid programs follow this policy.
- Some payers, including Medicare administrative contractors, have advised against reporting this modifier, as their systems automatically assign multiple service reductions to the appropriate services. In these cases, the system ignores modifier **51**. Follow payer guidance for reporting modifier **51**.
- When required, modifier **51** is appended to additional procedures(s) or service(s) when multiple procedures are performed at the same session by the same individual or individuals in the same group practice. The primary procedure or service is reported first without a modifier.
- Although many claims adjudication systems now automatically identify the primary procedure, it is advisable that the first-reported service is that with the highest relative value, followed by additional services appended with modifier **51**, when applicable.

For information on multiple surgery indicators and adjustments, see Chapter 12, Section 40.6, of the *Medicare Claims Processing Manual* at www.cms.gov/Regulations-and-Guidance/Guidance/Manuals/Downloads/clm104c12.pdf.

- **DO *NOT* USE MODIFIER 51 WHEN**
  - **Reporting add-on procedures codes (identified with the + symbol) that are exempt from modifier 51 because the services are always performed in addition to a primary service.**
  - **Reporting *CPT* codes identified with the symbol Ø (exempt from modifier 51) because they have no associated preservice or post-service valuation and are already reduced (see Appendix E in *CPT* for a list of these codes).**
  - **Different providers perform the procedures.**

— **Two or more physicians perform different and unrelated procedures (eg, multiple trauma) on the same patient on the same day (unless one of the physicians performs multiple procedures).**
— **Reporting E/M services, physical medicine and rehabilitation services, or provision of supplies (eg, vaccines).**

Example—Modifier 51

➤ **A child undergoes adenoidectomy and bilateral myringotomy with tube placement at the same surgical session. The surgeon reports**

69436 50   Tympanostomy (requiring insertion of ventilating tube), general anesthesia
42830 51   Adenoidectomy, primary; younger than age 12

Teaching Point: Code **69436** is reported first because it carries the highest relative value when reported with modifier **50** (7.17 non-facility total relative value units [4.78 times 150%] vs 6.33 for code **42830**). Modifier **51** is appended to code **42830**. If the myringotomy was a unilateral procedure, code **42830** would be listed first and modifier **51** appended to code **69436** (with no modifier **50**).

52—Reduced Services

- Modifier **52** is used when a service or procedure is partially reduced or eliminated (ie, procedure started but discontinued) at the discretion of the physician or other QHP.
- Modifier **52** is not used when a procedure is canceled prior to the induction of anesthesia and/or surgical preparation in the operating room.
- The diagnosis code linked to the procedure reported with modifier **52** should reflect why the procedure was reduced.
- When reporting a reduced service or a procedure code with modifier **52**, do not reduce your normal fee. Let the payer reduce the payment based on its policy.

Examples—Modifier 52

➤ **A physician begins a circumcision (54150) on a 3-day-old boy.** The physician elects to perform the circumcision without a dorsal penile or ring block. In this circumstance, modifier **52** would be reported with code **54150** to indicate the service was reduced from its full descriptor based on the physician's discretion.

➤ **A peripherally inserted central venous catheter (PICC) without a subcutaneous port is inserted with imaging guidance, but tip location is not confirmed by imaging.**

ICD-10-CM	CPT
J13 (pneumonia due to *Streptococcus pneumoniae*)	36572 52 (PICC insertion without subcutaneous port, with imaging guidance; younger than 5 years of age)

Teaching Point: Code **36572** includes confirmation of the tip location. Therefore, modifier **52** would be appended when performed without confirmation of catheter tip location.

53—Discontinued Procedure

- Modifier **53** signifies that a procedure was terminated (ie, started but discontinued) due to extenuating circumstances or circumstances in which the well-being of the patient was threatened (eg, patient is at risk or has unexpected, serious complications, such as excessive bleeding or hypotension) during a procedure.
- It is not used to report the elective cancellation of a procedure prior to the patient's anesthesia induction and/or surgical preparation in the operating suite.
- The diagnosis code should reflect the reason for the termination of the procedure.
- Most payers will require that operative or procedure reports be submitted with the claim.

Chapter 2. Coding Edits and Modifiers

Examples—Modifier 53

➤ **An unsuccessful attempt is made to place a central line in the right subclavian vein.** The line is successfully placed in the left subclavian vein.

> 36555 53 RT (insertion non-tunneled centrally inserted central venous catheter; younger than 5 years)
> 36555 LT
>
> *Note:* Some payers do not recognize modifiers RT and LT. See the descriptions and use of these modifiers in the Healthcare Common Procedure Coding System Modifiers section later in this chapter.

➤ **A physician begins a circumcision (54150) on a 3-day-old boy.** During the procedure, the physician notices the neonate is showing signs of respiratory distress. Due to the severity of the situation, the physician decides not to continue with the procedure.

> 54150 53 (circumcision, using clamp or other device with regional dorsal penile or ring block)
>
> In this circumstance, the physician would link diagnosis codes Z41.2 (encounter for routine and ritual male circumcision) and P22.9 (respiratory distress, newborn) to indicate why the procedure was discontinued. When reporting a procedure with modifier 53, it is important to indicate why the procedure was discontinued.

54—Surgical Care Only

Modifier 54 is appended to the surgery procedure code when the physician does the procedure but another physician or other QHP (not of the same group practice) accepts a transfer of care and provides preoperative and/or postoperative management.

55—Postoperative Management Only

Modifier 55 is appended to the surgical code to report that only postoperative care is performed because another physician or other QHP of another group practice has performed the surgical procedure and transferred the patient for postoperative care.

56—Preoperative Management Only

Modifier 56 is appended to the surgical code when only the preoperative care and evaluation are performed because another physician or other QHP of another group practice has performed the surgical procedure. This modifier is seldom applicable.

Coding Conundrum: Modifiers 54, 55, and 56

Modifiers 54, 55, and 56 typically are used to report surgical procedures that have a global period of 10 to 90 days. They are not reported with procedures that have 0-day global periods. It is important to learn which guidelines are followed by your major payers. When reporting these modifiers, coordination and communication between the physicians and their billing staff is imperative.

For more information on global surgery guidelines, see **chapters 10** and **19.**

Examples—Modifiers 54 and 55

➤ **An emergency department (ED) physician provides initial care for a Colles fracture of the right radius and instructs the patient to follow up with a primary care or orthopedic physician for care during the global period.** The ED physician reports an ED E/M service (99281–99285) with modifier 57 (decision for surgery) and code 25600 with modifier 54.

> 25600 54   Closed treatment of distal radial fracture (eg, Colles or Smith type) or epiphyseal separation, includes closed treatment of fracture of ulnar styloid, when performed; without manipulation
>
> The primary care or orthopedic physician who assumes management of the patient's fracture care will report code 25600 55.
>
> **Teaching Point:** If a physician's initial fracture care is limited to stabilization pending referral for definitive treatment, only the E/M and any splinting or casting and supplies are reported. The physician who will provide definitive fracture care will report a fracture care code without a modifier.

CPT copyright 2021 American Medical Association. All rights reserved.   ●=New code   ▲=Revised code   #=Re-sequenced code   +=Add-on code   ★=Telemedicine

➤ **A child is admitted to the hospital by the pediatrician for intravenous antibiotics for a deep abscess on the right leg.** On the second day of the hospital stay, a surgeon is called in and performs an incision and drainage of the abscess (includes follow-up care within 90 days following the procedure). The child is discharged on day 3 and seen in follow-up by the pediatrician.

Surgeon reports

ICD-10-CM	CPT
L02.415 (cutaneous abscess of right lower limb)	**27603 54** (incision and drainage with surgical care only)

Pediatrician reports

ICD-10-CM	CPT
L02.415	**27603 55** (incision and drainage with postoperative management only)

57—Decision for Surgery

- Modifier **57** is appended to an E/M service that resulted in the initial decision to perform the surgery or procedure.
- Appending modifier **57** to the E/M service indicates to the payer that the E/M service is not part of the global period. The global period for surgical procedures is assigned by the CMS, private payers, or state Medicaid and not by the American Medical Association.
- Many payers will follow the CMS Medicare payment policy that allows reporting of modifier **57** only when the visit on the day before or day of surgery results in a decision to perform a surgical procedure that has a 90-day global period (major procedure).
- Know commercial and state Medicaid policies, maintain a written copy of the policy, and adhere to the policy.

Examples—Modifier 57

➤ **A 10-year-old is seen by the pediatrician for the evaluation of pain in her foot and arm after a fall.** Radiograph reveals a metatarsal fracture, and the decision is made to treat the closed fracture. Arm injuries are limited to bruising and abrasions.

Code **28470** (closed treatment, metatarsal fracture; without manipulation) has an assigned global surgery period of 90 days. The appropriate E/M code (**99202–99215 57**), based on the medical necessity and performance and documentation of the required MDM, would be reported in addition to code **28470**. An E/M code with modifier **57** is reported only by the physician or a physician of the same specialty and group practice of the physician who performs the procedure. Other physicians providing E/M services on the day before or day of a procedure would not append modifier **57**.

➤ **A circumcision is performed on the day of discharge on a 2-day-old born in the hospital, delivered vaginally.**

ICD-10-CM	CPT
Z38.00 (single liveborn infant, delivered vaginally) **Z41.2** (encounter for routine male circumcision)	**99238 25** (hospital discharge management) **54150** (circumcision using clamp/device with dorsal penile or ring block)

Teaching Point: The procedure has a 0-day global period. Per CMS guidelines, modifier **25** would be appended to the E/M service instead of modifier **57**.

58—Staged or Related Procedure or Service by the Same Physician or Other Qualified Health Care Professional During the Postoperative Period

- Modifier **58** is used to indicate that a procedure or service performed during the postoperative period was planned or anticipated (ie, staged), was more extensive than the original procedure, or was for therapy following a surgical procedure.

- Modifier **58** is a recognized modifier under the NCCI.
- Typically, payers recognize modifier **58** only when there is a global surgical period associated with the procedure code.
- **DO *NOT* REPORT MODIFIER 58 WHEN**
  - **Treatment of a problem requires a return to the operating/procedure room (eg, unanticipated clinical condition) (see modifier 78).**
  - **Reporting procedures that include as part of their *CPT* descriptor "one or more visits" or "one or more sessions."**

Examples—Modifier 58

➤ **An excision of a malignant lesion (1 cm) on the leg is performed.** The pathology report indicates that the margins were not adequate, and a re-excision is performed 1 week later. The excised diameter is less than 2 cm.

    11602 58 (excision, malignant lesion including margins, leg; excised diameter 1.1–2.0 cm) for the second excision
    Note: The first excision would be reported using code **11601** (margin diameter 0.6–1.0 cm).

➤ **A physician replaces a cast during the global period of fracture care.** (Only the first cast is included in the code for fracture care. See more on fracture care in **Chapter 10**.)

    29000–29799 58 (appropriate casting code)

59—Distinct Procedural Service

> **Never use modifier 59 in place of modifier 25 or on an evaluation and management service.**

- Modifier **59** is used to identify procedures or services, other than E/M services, that are not normally reported together but are appropriate under the circumstances.
- Report modifier **59** only when no other modifier better describes the reason for separately reporting a service that might otherwise be bundled with another procedural service on the same date.
- Never append modifier **59** to bypass payer edits without clinical justification.
- See HCPCS modifiers **XE**, **XP**, **XS**, and **XU** for potential alternatives to modifier **59**.
- Per *CPT*, modifier **59** represents one of the following conditions of a procedure:
  - The procedure was provided at a different session from another procedure.
  - The procedure was a different procedure or surgery.
  - The procedure involved a different site or organ system.
  - The procedure required a separate incision or excision.
  - The procedure was performed on a separate lesion or injury (or area of injury in extensive injuries).

Example—Modifier 59

➤ **Three behavioral health assessment instruments are completed and scored during one encounter to assess symptoms of depression, mood and feelings, and anxiety.**

    96127 × 2 (brief emotional/behavioral assessment [eg, depression inventory, attention-deficit/hyperactivity disorder (ADHD) scale], with scoring and documentation, per standardized instrument)
    96127 59 × 1 (third assessment instrument)
    Modifier **59** would be appended to the code for the third assessment instrument to reflect that 3 distinct assessment instruments were scored and documented. Medicaid NCCI MUEs limit units of **96127** to 2 units per claim, but modifier **59** may be appended to units on an additional line to indicate additional instruments were necessary.

CPT copyright 2021 American Medical Association. All rights reserved.   ●=New code   ▲=Revised code   #=Re-sequenced code   +=Add-on code   ★=Telemedicine

Coding Conundrum: Modifier 51 (Multiple Procedures) or 59 (Distinct Procedural Service)?

Modifier 51 is most often used on surgical procedures that are performed during the same session and through the same incision. This modifier identifies potentially overlapping or duplicative relative value units related to the global surgical package or the technical component of certain services (eg, radiology services). Not all payers recognize or require modifier 51.

Modifier 59 is used to identify distinct and independent procedures that are not normally reported together but are appropriate to the clinical circumstances. They are typically unrelated procedures or services performed on the same patient by the same provider on the same day on different anatomical sites or at different encounters. This is a modifier of last resort. When another modifier, such as 51, is more appropriate, it should be reported in lieu of modifier 59.

62—Two Surgeons

- Modifier 62 is used when 2 surgeons work together as primary surgeons performing a distinct part(s) of a procedure. Do not use modifier 62 when 1 surgeon assists another.
- Each surgeon should report his or her distinct operative work by adding modifier 62 to the procedure code and any associated add-on code(s) for that procedure as long as both surgeons continue to work together as primary surgeons.
- Each surgeon should report the co-surgery once using the same procedure code.
- If an additional procedure(s) (including an add-on procedure[s]) is performed during the same surgical session, a separate code(s) may also be reported without modifier 62 added.
- Column AB (CO SURG) of the Medicare Physician Fee Schedule (Resource-Based Relative Value Scale [RBRVS]) identifies procedures that may or may not be performed by co-surgeons. Indicator 1 is assigned to those procedures for which co-surgery is allowed under the Medicare program. See www.cms.gov/Medicare/Medicare-Fee-for-Service-Payment/PhysicianFeeSched/PFS-Relative-Value-Files.html.

Example—Modifier 62

➤ **A neurosurgeon and general surgeon work together to place a ventriculoperitoneal shunt.**

Both physicians would report code 62223 62 with the same diagnosis code. The operative note must include the name of each surgeon, specific role of each surgeon, and necessity for 2 surgeons. Each surgeon should dictate his or her own operative report.

Most payers will require authorization prior to the procedure.

63—Procedure Performed on Infants Less Than 4 kg

- Modifier 63 is used to report procedures performed on neonates and infants up to a *present body weight of 4 kg* that involve significantly increased complexity and physician work commonly associated with these patients.
- Unless otherwise designated, this modifier may only be appended to procedures or services listed in the 20100–69990 code series and codes 92920, 92928, 92953, 92960, 92986, 92987, 92990, 92997, 92998, 93312–93318, 93452, 93505, 93593–93598, 93563–93564, 93568, 93580, 93582, 93590–93592, 93615, and 93616.
- Use of modifier 63 may require submission of an operative note with the claim. The operative note should include the patient's weight. It is also beneficial to report the patient's weight on the claim.
- **DO *NOT* REPORT MODIFIER 63**
  — **When the code is included in Appendix F, as codes in this appendix were valued to include the increased complexity and physician work associated with modifier 63**
  — **With any *CPT* codes listed in the E/M Services, Anesthesia, Radiology, Pathology/Laboratory, or Medicine sections (other than those previously identified from the Medicine/Cardiovascular section).**
  — **When the *CPT* code includes a parenthetical instruction prohibiting reporting modifier 63**

Examples—Modifier 63

➤ **A surgeon performed a right and left heart catheterization through normal native connections on a 4-week-old who weighed 3.1 kg with positive findings of congenital anomalies.**

93596 26 63 (right and left heart catheterization for congenital heart defect[s] including imaging guidance by the proceduralist to advance the catheter to the target zone[s]; normal native connections)

Because the procedure may be performed on patients weighing more than 4 kg, the complexity and work associated with performing the procedure on an infant weighing up to 4 kg *was not* included in the valuation assigned to code 93596.

➤ **A repair of patent ductus arteriosus by ligation is performed on an infant weighing less than 4 kg.**

33820 63 (repair of patent ductus arteriosus; by ligation)

66—Surgical Team

- Modifier **66** is appended to the basic procedure code when highly complex procedures (requiring the concomitant services of several physicians or other QHPs, often of different specialties, plus other highly skilled, specially trained personnel and various types of complex equipment) are carried out under the surgical team concept.
- Each surgeon reports modifier **66**.
- Each surgeon should dictate his or her own operative report and it should reflect the medical necessity for team surgery.
- Column AC (TEAM SURG) of the Medicare Physician Fee Schedule (RBRVS) identifies procedures that may or may not be performed by a team of surgeons. Indicator 1 is assigned to those procedures for which team surgery is allowed under the Medicare program.
- The operative notes are usually required by the payer.
- If a surgeon is assisting another surgeon, modifier **80**, **81**, or **82** would be more applicable.

Example—Modifier **66**

➤ **Multiple surgeons perform different portions of an organ transplant.**

Each physician would report his or her services with modifier **66** appended to the procedure code.

76—Repeat Procedure or Service by Same Physician or Other Qualified Health Care Professional

- Modifier **76** is used when a procedure or service is repeated by the same physician or other QHP subsequent to the original procedure or service. Use of this modifier may prevent denial as a duplicate service line.
- The repeat procedure may be performed on different days. (Payer guidance may vary.)
- This modifier is appended to non-E/M procedure codes only and is not reported when the code definition indicates a repeat procedure.
- The use of this modifier advises the payer that this is not a duplicate service. (See modifier **91** for repeat clinical diagnostic laboratory test.)
- The CMS only recognizes this modifier on ECGs and radiographs or when a procedure is performed in an operating room or other location equipped to perform procedures. State Medicaid programs or other commercial payers may follow this guideline. Check with payers to determine their policy on use of the modifier.

Examples—Modifier **76**

➤ **You see a patient in your office with severe asthma and give 3 nebulized albuterol treatments and steroids over the course of the visit.**

Report **94640** 3 times with modifier **76** appended to the second and third codes (ie, **94640** × 1, **94640 76** × 1, **94640 76** × 1). Only report **94640 76** with 3 units if directed to do so by payer policy because most payers will deny based on the lack of an initial service (ie, code reported without modifier **76**).

The Medicare and Medicaid NCCI manuals contradict *CPT* instruction for code **94640**, stating that *CPT* code **94640** should only be reported once during a single patient encounter regardless of the number of separate inhalation treatments that are administered. Follow individual payer guidance.

➤ **The same physician performs re-reduction (closed treatment with manipulation) of radial and ulnar shaft fractures within the global period of the initial closed treatment of the fractures.**

Re-reduction: **25565 76** (closed treatment of radial and ulnar shaft fractures; with manipulation)

77—Repeat Procedure or Service by Another Physician or Other Qualified Health Care Professional

- Modifier **77** is used when a procedure or service is repeated by another physician or health care professional subsequent to the original procedure or service. Be sure that the same code(s) is reported by each physician to avoid denials when reporting modifier **77**.
- Payers may require documentation to support the medical necessity of performing the same service or procedure on the same day or during the global surgical period (if applicable).

Example—Modifier 77

➤ **An orthopedic physician performs re-reduction (closed treatment with manipulation) of radial and ulnar shaft fractures. The initial closed treatment of the fractures was reported by a physician of another specialty or other group practice.**

Re-reduction: **25565 77** (closed treatment of radial and ulnar shaft fractures; with manipulation)

78—Unplanned Return to the Operating/Procedure Room by the Same Physician or Other Qualified Health Care Professional Following Initial Procedure for a Related Procedure During the Postoperative Period

- Modifier **78** is used when another procedure is unplanned and related to the initial procedure, requires a return to the operating or procedure room, and is performed during the postoperative period of the initial procedure by the same physician.
- The related procedure might be performed on the same day or any time during the postoperative period. (For repeat procedures, see modifier **76**.)
- Link the appropriate diagnosis code(s) that best explains the reason for the unplanned procedure.

Examples—Modifier 78

➤ **A pediatric surgeon returns to the operating room to stop bleeding from an abdominal procedure performed earlier in the day.**

35840 78 (exploration for postoperative hemorrhage, thrombosis, or infection; abdomen)
The second procedure will usually be paid only for the intraoperative service, not the preoperative or postoperative care already paid in the original procedure.

➤ **An incision and drainage of a deep abscess in the pelvis area 6 days following excision of a lipoma is performed.**

26990 78 (incision and drainage, pelvis area; deep abscess)

79—Unrelated Procedure or Service by the Same Physician or Other Qualified Health Care Professional During the Postoperative Period

- The physician may need to indicate that the performance of a procedure or service during the postoperative period was unrelated to the original procedure. This circumstance may be reported by using modifier **79**.
- The diagnosis must identify the reason for the new procedure within the global period. (For repeat procedures by the same physician on the same day, see modifier **76**.)

Example—Modifier 79

➤ **An adolescent patient requires an emergency appendectomy within 90 days of undergoing left inguinal hernia repair.**

44970 79 (laparoscopy, surgical, appendectomy)

Chapter 2. Coding Edits and Modifiers

80—Assistant Surgeon

- Modifier 80 is used when the assistant surgeon assists the surgeon during the entire operation. Note: Modifier 62, not 80, is used when 2 surgeons work together as primary surgeons performing a distinct part(s) of a procedure.
- The primary surgeon reports the appropriate *CPT* code for the procedure and the assistant surgeon reports the same code with modifier 80 appended. Some payers require modifier AS (assistant at surgery) in lieu of 80 when other QHPs (ie, physician assistant, nurse practitioner, or clinical nurse specialist) act as assistant surgeon.
- Payers vary on payment rules. The CMS establishes guidelines for payment of assistant surgery for each procedure code. Most payers, including the CMS, will not pay for nonphysician surgery technicians in this role.
- Many payers require documentation to support the necessity of an assistant surgeon.

81—Minimum Assistant Surgeon

- Modifier 81 is used when an assistant surgeon is required for a short time and minimal assistance is provided.
- The assistant surgeon reports the same procedure code as the surgeon with modifier 81 appended.
- Many payers require documentation to support the use of an assistant surgeon for only a portion of a procedure.

82—Assistant Surgeon (When Qualified Resident Surgeon Not Available)

- Modifier 82 is used in teaching hospitals when a resident surgeon is not available to assist the primary surgeon.
- The unavailability of a qualified resident surgeon is a prerequisite for the use of modifier 82 appended to the usual procedure code number(s).

Modifiers 80, 81, and 82

The Medicare Physician Fee Schedule includes in column AA (ASST SURG) indicators identifying procedures that may or may not be billed by an assistant surgeon. Indicator 1 is assigned to those procedures for which an assistant surgeon is allowed to bill under the Medicare program.

90—Reference (Outside) Laboratory

- Modifier 90 is used to indicate that a laboratory service is being billed by the physician but performed at an outside laboratory.
- Modifier 90 indicates pass-through billing in that the payer will pay the physician for the laboratory service and the laboratory will charge the physician.
- Many payers do not accept modifier 90 and require that the laboratory performing the service bill directly to the health plan for the services. Check with your payers prior to utilizing modifier 90.

91—Repeat Clinical Diagnostic Laboratory Test

- Modifier 91 is used to indicate it is necessary to repeat the same laboratory test on the same day to obtain subsequent test results.
- Modifier 91 is only reported when the laboratory test is performed more than once on the same patient on the same day.
- Modifier 91 cannot be reported when repeat tests are performed to confirm initial results, because of testing problems with the specimen or equipment, or for any reason when a normal one-time, reportable result is all that is required.

Example—Modifier 91

➤ **In the course of treatment for hypoglycemia by administration of oral carbohydrate, a patient had 3 blood glucose determinations (82947) done on the same day in the same office.**

   82947 91 × 3 units of service

92—Alternative Laboratory Platform Testing

- Modifier 92 is used to indicate that laboratory testing was performed using a kit or transportable instrument that wholly or in part consists of a single-use, disposable analytic chamber.
- This modifier is not required or acknowledged by all payers.
- *CPT* instructs to report this modifier with HIV test codes 86701–86703 and 87389.

●=New code ▲=Revised code #=Re-sequenced code +=Add-on code ★=Telemedicine

95—Synchronous Telemedicine Service Rendered via a Real-time Interactive Audio and Video Telecommunications System

Modifier **95** is used to indicate a service was rendered via real-time (synchronous) interactive audio and video telecommunications system. This modifier is not applied if the communication is not real-time interactive audio and video.

Codes to which modifier **95** may be applied are found in Appendix P of *CPT* and are preceded by a star symbol in the *CPT* manual.

Appendix P codes that may be of particular interest to pediatricians include

- New and established patient office or other outpatient E/M services (**99202–99205, 99212–99215, 99417**)
- Subsequent hospital care (**99231–99233**)
- Inpatient and outpatient consultations (**99241–99245, 99251–99255**)
- Subsequent nursing facility care (**99307–99310**)
- Individual behavior change interventions (**99406–99409**)
- Transitional care management services (**99495, 99496**)

> **For more information on reporting synchronous telemedicine services, see Chapter 20.**

For a full listing of codes that may be reported for telemedicine services, see Appendix P in your *CPT* reference.

99—Multiple Modifiers

CPT instructs that modifier **99** is reported under certain circumstances when 2 or more modifiers are required to completely describe a service. However, current paper and electronic claims allow listing of up to 4 modifiers per claim line, and payers often instruct to report modifier **99** only when more than 4 modifiers are required on a single code.

Follow individual payer instructions regarding use of modifier **99** and placement of additional modifiers on the claim (eg, in narrative field 19 of the paper claim form).

> **For more information on reporting modifiers, see "When Are Modifiers Necessary?" in the November 2016 *AAP Pediatric Coding Newsletter*™ (https://coding.solutions.aap.org/article.aspx?articleid=2571212; subscription required).**

Healthcare Common Procedure Coding System Modifiers

The HCPCS modifiers are used to report specific information not conveyed in code descriptors or by *CPT* modifiers, such as

CR	Catastrophe/disaster related
E1	Upper left eyelid
QW	Performance of tests waived by Clinical Laboratory Improvement Amendments (CLIA)
RT	Right side
SL	State-supplied vaccine
TC	Technical component only
XE	Procedural services performed at separate encounters on the same date

Medicaid programs often use a variety of HCPCS modifiers for state-defined purposes. See your state Medicaid provider manual for information on HCPCS modifiers and definitions assigned in your state (eg, modifier **SY** [persons who are in close contact with member of high-risk population] may be used with codes for certain immunizations). Be sure to review the list of HCPCS modifiers in your HCPCS reference.

Anatomical Modifiers

An anatomical modifier may be reported to identify specific sites, such as right foot, fifth digit (**T9**).
- The anatomical-specific modifiers are designated as appropriate modifiers under NCCI edits and are listed in the Appropriate NCCI Modifiers section earlier in this chapter.
- The Medicaid NCCI manual indicates that procedures performed on fingers should be reported with modifiers **FA** and **F1–F9**, and procedures performed on toes should be reported with modifiers **TA** and **T1–T9**. See also modifiers for eyelids (**E1–E4**) and coronary arteries (**LC, LD, LM, RC, RI**).

MUE values for many finger and toe procedures are 1 (one) based on use of these modifiers for clinical scenarios in which the same procedure is performed on more than 1 finger or toe. (See the Medically Unlikely Edits section earlier in this chapter for more information.)

Example—Anatomical Modifiers

➤ **A physician performs nail avulsion (11730) on the patient's right ring finger and evacuation of blood under nail (11740) on the patient's right middle finger.**

    11730 F8 (avulsion, nail plate, partial or complete, simple; single–right hand, 4th digit)
    11740 F7 (evacuation of subungual hematoma–right hand, 3rd digit)
    Note: Some payers may require that modifier 59 (distinct procedural service) or XS (separate structure) be reported. Verify coding edits and payer policy before reporting.

X {E, P, S, U} Modifiers

Modifiers XE, XP, XS, and XU more specifically identify reasons for separate reporting of procedures or services that otherwise may be identified by *CPT* modifier 59.

XE	Separate encounter (different operative session)
XP	Separate practitioner
XS	Separate structure (site/organ)
XU	Unusual nonoverlapping service

- As payer adoption and guidance on use of these modifiers may vary, it is important to verify individual payer policy before reporting.
- As the XE, XP, XS, and XU modifiers are more specific, payers may require reporting in lieu of modifier 59.
- Modifiers XE, XP, XS, and XU should not be appended to an E/M code.
- Do not append modifier 59 and the XE, XP, XS, and XU modifiers to the same service line of a claim (ie, single code).
- While accepted by most payers, few resources are available to describe appropriate reporting of these modifiers.
- National Correct Coding Initiative edits are not yet updated to require modifiers XE, XP, XS, and XU in lieu of modifier 59 for specific code pairs.

Learn more about modifiers XE, XP, XS, and XU in the July 2020 *AAP Pediatric Coding Newsletter* article, "Modifiers: Do You Use 59 or XE, XP, XS, XU?" (https://coding.solutions.aap.org/article.aspx?articleid=2765192; subscription required).

CR—Catastrophe/Disaster Related

Modifier CR is used based on payer instruction during a federal- or state-declared disaster or public health emergency to indicate a service was provided in a manner or under circumstances for which payment may otherwise be prohibited by government statute or payer policies.

Example—Modifier CR

➤ **A well-child examination is conducted via telemedicine on a patient in her home during a public health emergency.** Per payer policy, the service requires a comprehensive, unclothed physical examination. A waiver has been issued allowing billing for the incomplete preventive E/M service with modifier CR (eg, 99391 CR). Payer policy may require an in-person visit within a specified period.

EP—Service Provided as Part of Medicaid Early and Periodic Screening, Diagnostic, and Treatment (EPSDT) Program

Some Medicaid and private payers require the use of modifier EP to denote services that are provided to covered patients as part of the Early and Periodic Screening, Diagnostic, and Treatment (EPSDT) program services required in the state.

Modifier EP can be appended to the preventive medicine service (eg, 99392) or screening services, such as developmental screening (96110).

Chapter 2. Coding Edits and Modifiers

Example—Modifier EP

➤ **A 9-month-old established patient presents for her routine preventive medicine service.** As part of her state EPSDT services, she receives an age-appropriate history and physical examination, preventive counseling, and anticipatory guidance. A standardized developmental screening, which is required of EPSDT services, is also completed and scored.

 99391 EP (preventive medicine service, established patient <1 year)
 96110 EP (developmental screening)

GA—Waiver of Liability Statement Issued as Required by Payer Policy, Individual Case

GU—Waiver of Liability Statement Issued as Required by Payer Policy, Routine Notice

GX—Notice of Liability Issued, Voluntary Under Payer Policy

Modifiers **GA**, **GU**, and **GX** may or may not be recognized by Medicaid and private payers when reporting services that are not covered under the patient's benefit plan. Follow individual payer policies regarding provision and reporting of advance notice of noncoverage to patients/responsible parties.

GC—This Service Has Been Performed in Part by a Resident Under the Direction of a Teaching Physician

- Modifier **GC** indicates a teaching physician is certifying that the service was rendered in compliance with the CMS requirements for services reported by teaching physicians.
- Requirements for reporting modifier **GC** may vary among commercial health plans. This modifier is typically informational, meaning it does not affect the amount paid for a service.
- If the service was provided solely by the teaching physician, the claim should not be billed with the **GC** modifier.

GE—This Service Has Been Performed by a Resident Without the Presence of a Teaching Physician Under the Primary Care Exception

- Modifier **GE** indicates a teaching physician is certifying that the service was rendered in compliance with the CMS primary care exception rule. Please see **Chapter 6** for discussion of this rule.
- Requirements for reporting modifier **GE** may vary among Medicaid and commercial health plans. This modifier is typically informational, which means it does not affect the amount paid for a service.

GT—Via Interactive Audio and Video Telecommunication Systems

Modifier **GT** indicates that a face-to-face service was provided via a telecommunication system that included audio and video components. This modifier preceded *CPT* development of modifier **95** (telemedicine via audiovisual technology) and is reported in lieu of **95** when specified in payer policy (eg, appended to a code not included in *CPT* Appendix P).

JW—Drug Amount Discarded/Not Administered to Any Patient

- Practice administrators may use as a tool to internally track wasted drugs and vaccines.
- This modifier is reported on claims only when allowed or required by certain payers.
- Medicare requires use of modifier **JW** on codes for the unused portion of a drug or biological from a single-dose vial or package. Medicaid plans may also require reporting of modifier **JW**.
  - Report only when the full amount of a single-dose vial is not used due to patient indications (eg, patient requires lower dose) and required by a payer.
  - Report only when the amount of drug wasted is equal to at least 1 billing unit (ie, do not report wastage when 7 mg of a 10-mg vial is administered and the billing unit is 10 mg, as the remaining 3 mg is already accounted for in the billing unit).
  - Never report for discarded amounts from a multidose vial.
  - Never report modifier **JW** for overfill wastage (ie, an excess amount placed in the single-dose vial by the manufacturer to ensure that an adequate amount can be drawn into the syringe for use).

- Modifier **JW** is not applicable for reporting the following circumstances. However, some practices use the modifier for internal tracking of drug waste.
  - A parent decides to forego an immunization after the vaccine had been drawn up. Report on a claim only when specifically allowed by payer policy. Practices should keep a log of all wasted vaccines.
  - The vial is dropped, and the medication must be discarded.
  - A vaccine is discarded due to temperature out of range during storage.

> Learn more in the July 2020 *AAP Pediatric Coding Newsletter* article, "Coding for Vaccines Not Administered" (https://coding.solutions.aap.org/article.aspx?articleid=2765196; subscription required).

KP—First Drug of a Multiple Drug Unit Dose Formulation

KQ—Second or Subsequent Drug of a Multiple Drug Unit Dose Formulation

Some payers require only the distinct National Drug Code for each vial administered and do not require use of modifiers **KP** and **KQ**. When required by a payer, append modifier **KP** to the procedure code to indicate either of the following:

- When reporting the first drug in a multiple drug formulation compounded from drugs supplied in a unit dose form
- When reporting the first dose of a single drug supplied in a unit dose form when the total dose is greater than the amount supplied in a single vial or container

Append modifier **KQ** to the procedure code to indicate either of the following:

- When reporting the second drug in a multiple drug formulation compounded from drugs supplied in a unit dose form
- When reporting the second dose of a single drug supplied in a unit dose form when the total dose is greater than the amount supplied in a single vial or container

Example—Modifier KP

- **An infant requires administration of 150-mg palivizumab to prevent serious lower respiratory tract disease caused by respiratory syncytial virus (RSV). Two single-dose vials (one 100 mg and one 50 mg) are administered.**

  90378 KP × 2 units 100-mg single-dose vial (RSV, monoclonal antibody, recombinant, for intramuscular use, 50 mg, each)

  90378 KQ × 1 unit 50-mg single-dose vial

QW—Clinical Laboratory Improvement Amendments–Waived Tests

- The CLIA-waived tests are those commonly done in a laboratory or an office that are considered simple and low risk.
- One common test in the *CPT* **80000** series that is CLIA waived is the rapid strep test (**87880**).
- Laboratories and physician offices performing waived tests may need to append modifier **QW** to the *CPT* code for CLIA-waived procedures. The use of modifier **QW** is payer specific.
- Some of the CLIA-waived tests are exempt from the use of modifier **QW** (eg, **81002**, **82272**). To review the list of CLIA-waived procedures, go to www.cms.gov/clia.

RT, LT—Right and Left Side

- Modifiers **RT** and **LT** are used for information only and do not affect payment of a procedure unless otherwise specified by a payer.
- Used to identify procedures performed on the left or right side of the body.
- Some plans allow modifiers **RT** and **LT** in place of modifier **50**, but be sure of payer policy for reporting bilateral diagnostic procedures.

Some payers may require that modifier **59** (distinct procedural service) be reported in addition to or in lieu of the laterality modifiers.

Example—Modifiers RT and LT

➤ **Radiographs of the left elbow and wrist are ordered.**

  73110 LT (radiologic examination, wrist; complete, minimum of 3 views)

  73080 LT (radiologic examination, elbow; complete, minimum of 3 views)

X1–X5 Patient Relationship Modifiers

- Modifiers X1–X5 were introduced for voluntary identification of the reporting physician or practitioner's relationship to a patient during an episode of care.

X1	Continuous/broad services
X2	Continuous/focused services
X3	Episodic/broad services
X4	Episodic/focused services
X5	Only as ordered by another clinician

- At this time, there is no requirement to report modifiers X1–X5, and there is no effect on payment whether these modifiers are used or not used.
- In the future, the patient relationship modifiers are intended for use in value-based payment methodologies where the cost of care and outcomes may be attributed to specific physicians and other providers of care.

For more information on value-based payment methodologies, see Chapter 3.

Resources

AAP Coding Hotline

American Academy of Pediatrics Coding Hotline (https://form.jotform.com/Subspecialty/aapcodinghotline)

Assistant Surgeon Procedure Identification

Medicare Physician Fee Schedule Relative Value Files (www.cms.gov/Medicare/Medicare-Fee-for-Service-Payment/PhysicianFeeSched/PFS-Relative-Value-Files.html; see Column AA [ASST SURG] in the file applicable to the date of service).

Bilateral Procedure Identification

Medicare Physician Fee Schedule Relative Value Files (www.cms.gov/Medicare/Medicare-Fee-for-Service-Payment/PhysicianFeeSched/PFS-Relative-Value-Files.html; see Column Z [BILAT SURG] in file applicable to date of service).

CLIA-Waived Tests

Medicare list of CLIA-waived tests (www.cms.gov/clia)

Co-surgery and Team Surgery Procedure Identification

Medicare Physician Fee Schedule Relative Value Files (www.cms.gov/Medicare/Medicare-Fee-for-Service-Payment/PhysicianFeeSched/PFS-Relative-Value-Files.html; see Column AB [CO SURG] or Column AC [TEAM SURG] in the file applicable to the date of service).

Global Period of Procedures

"The Surgical Package and Related Services," May 2018 *AAP Pediatric Coding Newsletter* (https://coding.solutions.aap.org/article.aspx?articleid=2679119; subscription required)

Modifier Use

"When Are Modifiers Necessary?" November 2016 *AAP Pediatric Coding Newsletter* (https://coding.solutions.aap.org/article.aspx?articleid=2571212; subscription required)

"Modifiers: Do You Use 59 or XE, XP, XS, XU?" July 2020 *AAP Pediatric Coding Newsletter* (https://coding.solutions.aap.org/article.aspx?articleid=2765192; subscription required)

"Coding for Vaccines Not Administered," July 2020 *AAP Pediatric Coding Newsletter* (https://coding.solutions.aap.org/article.aspx?articleid=2765196; subscription required)

Multiple Surgery Indicators and Adjustments

Medicare Claims Processing Manual, Chapter 12, Section 40.6 (www.cms.gov/Regulations-and-Guidance/Guidance/Manuals/Downloads/clm104c12.pdf)

National Correct Coding Initiative Edits

Medicaid NCCI website (www.medicaid.gov/medicaid/program-integrity/ncci/index.html)

Medicare NCCI website (www.cms.gov/NationalCorrectCodInitEd/NCCIEP/list.asp)

NCCI file links from AAP (www.aap.org/coding; see the "Coding Resources, National Correct Coding Initiative (NCCI) Edits" tab)

Test Your Knowledge!

1. **A National Correct Coding Initiative modifier indicator of 0 indicates which of the following?**
    a. No modifier is necessary to receive payment for each service reported.
    b. Only modifier 59 will override the edit for this code pair.
    c. The edit for this code pair cannot be overridden with a modifier.
    d. All of the above

2. **Which of the following is described by modifier 26?**
    a. The reporting physician provided the professional and technical components.
    b. The reporting physician provided only the technical component.
    c. The reporting physician provided only the professional component.
    d. An unrelated evaluation and management (E/M) service was provided in addition to this service.

3. **Which of the following modifiers is not required on claims to some payers?**
    a. 50, bilateral procedure
    b. 54, surgical care only
    c. 51, multiple procedures
    d. 77, repeat procedure or service by another physician or other qualified health care professional

4. **Which modifier indicates that a second physician provided assistance throughout a procedure?**
    a. 66
    b. 63
    c. 80
    d. 81

5. **Which of the following is indicated by modifier 95?**
    a. A service was provided by telephone.
    b. The physician provided a significant and separately identifiable E/M service.
    c. Real-time audiovisual technology was used to provide a service.
    d. The physician provided postoperative management only.

Coding to Demonstrate Quality and Value

Contents

Quality and Performance Measurement 55

CPT® Category II Codes: Performance Measure Codes 55

Hierarchical Condition Categories 56

Healthcare Effectiveness Data and Information Set (HEDIS) 57

    Effectiveness of Care 57

    Access/Availability of Care 57

    Utilization 57

    Risk-Adjusted Utilization 57

    Measures Collected Using Electronic Clinical Data Systems 57

    Why HEDIS Matters to Pediatricians 58

    What Is a Pediatrician's Role in HEDIS? 58

        Medical Record Requests 59

Consumer Assessment of Healthcare Providers and Systems 59

Medicaid and Children's Health Insurance Program Quality Measures 60

Coding and Documentation for Performance Measures 61

        Effectiveness of Care 63

Resources 65

Test Your Knowledge! 65

Chapter 3. Coding to Demonstrate Quality and Value

Quality and Performance Measurement

Quality and performance measurement are important aspects of the pediatric medical home and the movement from payment by fee for service alone to value-based payment. Performance measures are developed by national organizations, including the National Committee for Quality Assurance (NCQA), and based on quality indicators currently accepted and used in the health care industry. Physicians who have successfully participated in quality measurement may see incentive payments, such as per-member/per-month payments, annual incentives, or a percentage of savings.

> For more information on value-based payment and other emerging payment models, see Chapter 4.

Physicians, payers, and accreditation organizations may use codes or claims data as a first line of quality measurement. When diagnosis or procedure codes provide necessary information for reviewing quality performance data, more time-consuming and costly medical record review may be avoided.

In January 2017, the American Academy of Pediatrics (AAP) published a policy statement, "A New Era in Quality Measurement: The Development and Application of Quality Measures" (http://pediatrics.aappublications.org/content/139/1/e20163442). This policy statement includes the following recommendation to national policy makers:

> "Quality measures, as much as possible, should be reportable by either *International Classification of Diseases, 10th Revision, Clinical Modification,* or *Current Procedural Terminology*® category II codes to reduce burden on pediatric health care providers. However, the inclusion of measures that also capture patient-centered perspectives on care is essential."

Clinical registries and other electronic data may also be used in quality measurement. This chapter discusses 3 ways that correct coding may support performance measurement.
- *Current Procedural Terminology* (*CPT*) Category II codes
- Hierarchical condition categories (HCCs)
- Codes that may support specific performance measures

Also discussed in this chapter are other measures that affect the perceived quality and/or value of care, such as surveys of patient/caregiver perception of care received from physicians and other qualified health care professionals (QHPs), and how practices can affect those perceptions.

> Following the public health emergency for COVID-19, use of telemedicine has expanded and performance measures may now include services provided via telemedicine. See guidance from health plans for those measures that may be met during telemedicine services.

CPT® Category II Codes: Performance Measure Codes

When codes are used to collect quality and performance measurement data, one category of *Current Procedural Terminology* (*CPT*) codes that is useful for conveying this information is *CPT* Category II. Category II codes were developed and are used by physicians and hospitals to report performance measures and certain aspects of care not yet included in performance measures.

Category II codes may or may not be used by payers in pediatric performance measurement. Assignment of Category II codes also allows internal monitoring of performance, patient compliance, and outcomes.

Category II codes
- Are intended for reporting purposes only.
- Describe clinical conditions (including complete performance measurements sets) and screening measures.
- Have no relative values on the Medicare Physician Fee Schedule (Resource-Based Relative Value Scale).
- Are reported on a voluntary basis.
- Are reported in addition to, *not in place of,* Category I *CPT* codes.
- Describe the performance of a clinical service typically included in an evaluation and management (E/M) code or the result that is part of a laboratory procedure/test.

Category II codes are included after the Category I procedure codes in the *CPT* manual and online at www.ama-assn.org/practice-management/cpt/category-ii-codes. Also available at this link is the Alphabetical Clinic Topics Listing, an overview of the performance measures, a listing of *CPT* Category II codes that may be used with each measure, and any applicable reporting instructions. Abbreviations following code descriptors of Category II codes indicate the performance measure to which the code is associated.

Chapter 3. Coding to Demonstrate Quality and Value

Examples

3008F	Body mass index (BMI), documented (PV)
3016F	Patient screened for unhealthy alcohol use using a systematic screening method (PV) (DSP)

Hierarchical Condition Categories

Hierarchical condition categories are categories of conditions that are assigned weight values and used along with certain demographic and prescription drug claims data in calculating a patient's risk of increased health care use or risk adjustment. **Figure 3-1** shows other components of risk adjustment.

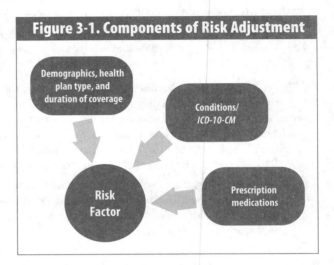

Figure 3-1. Components of Risk Adjustment

- Health plans offered to individuals under the Patient Protection and Affordable Care Act are subject to revenue adjustment based on the average risk of insured members based in part on HCCs.
- Hierarchical condition categories are also used in shared savings agreements with accountable care organizations (ACOs) and value-based payment to hospitals.
- Even if a pediatrician is not part of an ACO or alternative payment model, health plans and hospitals rely on physicians to document conditions that affect HCC assignment.

International Classification of Diseases, 10th Revision, Clinical Modification (ICD-10-CM) codes are collected from the claims submitted to health plans and used to identify HCCs. Only a small percentage of *ICD-10-CM* codes are assigned to HCCs. Examples of values assigned for certain HCCs can be found in **Table 3-1**.

Most pediatricians do not need to know the weights assigned to various conditions or how those weights are used to calculate risk adjustment factors. What pediatricians need to know is how their documentation affects risk adjustment and how risk adjustment may affect pediatricians and their patients. In addition, choosing a less-specific code than a code supported in the documentation could affect that weight.

- Payment to pediatricians may increasingly be based on quality and cost of care.

Risk adjustment is used to set the expected cost of care for a patient panel. Pediatricians will be affected (especially pediatricians whose employers may already gain or lose revenue based on risk factor adjustment). Correct

Table 3-1. Examples of US Department of Health and Human Services Hierarchical Condition Categories and Weights[a] by Plan Type (2021)

Diagnosis Category	Health Plan Type				
	Platinum	**Gold**	**Silver**	**Bronze**	**Catastrophic**
Asthma, Severe	0.868	0.640	0.484	0.249	0.246
Asthma, Except Severe	0.328	0.242	0.171	0.076	0.075
Autistic Disorder	2.812	2.539	2.353	2.147	2.144
Cleft Lip/Cleft Palate	1.322	1.114	0.987	0.824	0.822
Down Syndrome, Fragile X, Other Chromosomal Anomalies, and Congenital Malformation Syndromes	1.458	1.293	1.186	1.075	1.074
Extremely Immature Severity Level 5 (Highest)	234.247	232.335	230.986	230.901	230.901
Extremely Immature Severity Level 4	147.335	145.263	143.835	143.511	143.508
Immature Severity Level 5 (Highest)	135.262	133.350	132.009	131.845	131.843

[a] Weights attributed to hierarchical condition categories (HCCs) are one of several factors in the calculation of a risk adjustment factor. Multiple HCCs may be supported for a single patient encounter, but only the highest-valued HCC describing a condition (eg, extremely immature or immature) can be assigned to a patient.

and complete diagnosing is necessary to tell the health plan the disease burden of your patients. Showing the true nature of your patient's health status may have a short-term effect on rates paid per visit but also long-term implications in contracting with health plans.

- Patient access to care may be affected when conditions are not documented or are documented in insufficient detail.

    If risk adjustment results in lower revenue for health plans, health plan coverage and benefits will undoubtedly be affected.

     It is also important to know

- Like all health care payments, those based on HCCs are audited for accuracy. Documentation must support the *ICD-10-CM* codes used in assigning HCCs.

    Health plans may request medical records to validate *ICD-10-CM* codes supporting assigned HCCs.

- Pediatric HCC categories apply to children younger than 2 years (ie, before their second birthday) or to patients aged 2 through 20 years (ie, before their 21st birthday).

- Hierarchical condition category values are cumulative, making documentation of all diagnoses that affect management important for accurate calculation of risk.

Learn more in the July 2019 *AAP Pediatric Coding Newsletter*™ article, "Hierarchical Condition Categories: What They Are and Why They Matter to Pediatricians" (https://coding.solutions.aap.org/article.aspx?articleid=2736885; subscription required).

Healthcare Effectiveness Data and Information Set (HEDIS)

Most pediatricians should be aware of the Healthcare Effectiveness Data and Information Set (HEDIS). The NCQA describes HEDIS as a tool used by more than 90% of American health plans to measure performance on important dimensions of care and service. It is intended to allow purchasers and consumers to compare quality among health plans. The HEDIS measures are often incorporated in physician quality initiatives.

Altogether, HEDIS consists of more than 90 measures across the following 5 domains of care (not all measures apply to pediatric populations):

Effectiveness of Care

Examples of effectiveness of care measures are
- Childhood immunization status
- Immunizations for adolescents
- Appropriate testing for children with pharyngitis
- Follow-up care for children prescribed attention-deficit/hyperactivity disorder medication

Access/Availability of Care

Examples of access to and availability of care measures are
- Access to primary care practitioners for children and adolescents
- Annual dental visit

Utilization

Examples of utilization measures are
- Child and adolescent well-care visits
- Antibiotic utilization

Risk-Adjusted Utilization

An example of a risk-adjusted utilization measure is emergency department utilization.

Measures Collected Using Electronic Clinical Data Systems

- Depression screening and follow-up for adolescents and adults
- Utilization of the Patient Health Questionnaire-9 to monitor depression symptoms for adolescents and adults
- Postpartum depression screening and follow-up

To ensure HEDIS stays current, the NCQA has established an annual update to the measurement set.

Each health plan reviews a select set of measures every year. Because so many plans collect HEDIS data and the measures are so specifically defined, it is important to become familiar with the HEDIS system as it relates to quality measures and pay for performance (P4P).

Why HEDIS Matters to Pediatricians

The Centers for Medicare & Medicaid Services (CMS) has directly linked payment for health care services to patient outcomes. Consequently, health plans and providers, including physicians, are being asked to close gaps in care and improve overall quality. This focus on quality outcomes can help patients and members get the most from their benefits, which ultimately means better use of limited resources.

There are large sums of money at stake for health plans. For example, for a health plan with just 100,000 members being evaluated by HEDIS, each quality measure could mean millions in payments from federal or state agencies. When you consider that there are 20 to 25 measures directly tied to payment (depending on the health plan and population served), this is a significant amount of money! Now consider what that might look like for larger managed care organizations that have 1 million or more members enrolled. This is what keeps health care plans running. However, they cannot do it without physicians.

A fundamental concept behind P4P quality initiatives is that the plans will pay the physicians to help them attain these funds from the CMS.

What Is a Pediatrician's Role in HEDIS?

You and your office staff can help facilitate HEDIS process improvement by
- Providing appropriate care within the designated time frames.

> Attention to the time frames for providing recommended screenings and services across the patient population is important.

Example

➤ **A practice uses a reminder system to track immunizations for children younger than 24 months to avoid failure to provide the recommended immunizations on or before the second birthday.**

If patients reach 25 months of age without receiving the recommended vaccines, this negatively affects the HEDIS score for the physician until the child turns 3 years old (ie, is no longer included in the patient count for the measure).
- Documenting all care in the patient's medical record.

> When a measure is met during an inpatient or observation stay (eg, newborn immunization during the birth admission), supporting documentation may be required in the record of the primary care physician even if the care was ordered or provided by another physician or qualified health care professional.

- Watching payer guidelines for specific documentation requirements (eg, documentation of specific body mass index [BMI] percentile rather than a BMI percentile range).

> Many health plans provide specific information on documentation and codes that do or do not support HEDIS measurement.

- Not all patients will be included in a physician's patient count for HEDIS purposes, as continuous enrollment in the health plan without a gap of more than a specified number of days may be required for inclusion.

Example

➤ **The measure for appropriate prescribing for pharyngitis includes members continuously enrolled without a gap in coverage from 30 days prior to the encounter date through 3 days afterward (34 days total).**

- Accurately coding all claims. Providing information accurately on a claim may reduce the number of records requested.
  Use a full spectrum of diagnosis, procedure, and National Drug Codes to show that each measure is met. Health plans typically produce educational resources giving examples of codes that indicate a measure has been met.
- Responding to a health plan's requests for medical records in a timely fashion (typically within a week). This is required under many health plan contracts.
  Health plans typically include a specific turnaround time for providing records. The time frames are set each year.
  — January to May 15: Medical record requests will come in from the plans. All data must be gathered by the plan by May 15, with no exceptions.
  — June: The plans must report their results to the NCQA.
  — July to October: The NCQA releases the new Quality Compass (a quality comparison tool) nationwide—commercial plans in July; Medicaid and Medicare in September and October.

Medical Record Requests

Some information cannot be captured through claims data, so requests for medical records related to health plan HEDIS surveys are necessary.

- The Health Insurance Portability and Accountability Act of 1996 allows disclosure of protected health information to a health plan for the plan's HEDIS purposes as long as the period for which information is needed overlaps with the period for which the patient is or was enrolled in the health plan.
- Health plans may contract with outside vendors to conduct HEDIS record reviews.
- Providers are notified of record requests.
- The request will include a member list, the measure that is being evaluated, and the minimum necessary chart information needed.
- Data collection may vary by plan but may include fax, mail, on-site visits for large requests, remote electronic health record access, and electronic data interchange via a secure web portal.

Consumer Assessment of Healthcare Providers and Systems

The Consumer Assessment of Healthcare Providers and Systems (CAHPS) is a program developed by the Agency for Healthcare Research and Quality (AHRQ), part of the US Department of Health and Human Services, that uses surveys to capture patient experience with health care. Different surveys are used to learn about patient experiences in primary care and specialty care settings, in hospitals, and with health plans. The surveys must be conducted by approved survey vendors under a specific framework that is designed to eliminate bias in sample selection and results.

The CAHPS Clinician & Group Survey may be used to measure patient experience in primary and specialty care settings in the following categories. A version of this survey may be used by accountable care organizations to meet a requirement to measure patient experience.

- Getting timely appointments, care, and information

- How well providers communicate with patients

- Providers' use of information to coordinate patient care

The use of information to coordinate patient care can be facilitated, at least for initial referrals to other providers, by practice staff assisting patients with scheduling and transfer of relevant clinical and demographic information.

- Helpful, courteous, and respectful office staff

Physicians and other qualified health care professionals seldom make the first and last impressions on patients/caregivers. Training all office staff to be professional, respectful, and empathic to patient/caregiver concerns is necessary to support a positive image of the practice.

- Patients' rating of the provider

A rating by a patient/caregiver can be influenced by anything from a clear understanding of a plan of care to the level of customer service received from the practice's billing staff or agency. Each of the previous recommendations along with empathy for patients/caregivers who have concerns with their experience can drive a positive rating.

Health plans use a HEDIS version of CAHPS for gathering, reporting, analyzing, and acting on patient experience (CAHPS) data for Medicaid and commercial health plan members. The surveys are required by the CMS and also for health plans to receive or maintain HEDIS accreditation. The health plan surveys typically are a retrospective random sampling of patients from the prior 6 or 12 months.

These surveys measure patient experience based on the following:
- Getting needed care
- Getting care quickly
- How well doctors communicate
- Health plan customer service
- How people rated their health plan

Health plans must rely on physician practices and other sites of service to participate in quality improvement initiatives focused on patient experiences and may offer incentives to adopt policies and procedures that support an improved patient experience of care (eg, more timely access to care).

Learn more about the Consumer Assessment of Healthcare Providers and Systems at https://www.ahrq.gov/cahps/index.html.

Medicaid and Children's Health Insurance Program Quality Measures

Medicaid and the Children's Health Insurance Program (CHIP) plans select and report measures from the Core Set of Children's Health Care Quality Measures for Medicaid and CHIP (Child Core Set). The Child Core Set includes many HEDIS measures and a few measures developed by the CMS or other parties.

Examples

➤ **Percentage of newborns who did not pass hearing screening and have an audiological diagnosis no later than 3 months of age (90 days) (Centers for Disease Control and Prevention).** Specific use of the new *ICD-10-CM* code, **P09.6** (abnormal findings on neonatal screening for neonatal hearing loss) can assist in tracking these patients.

➤ **The percentage of children screened for risk of developmental, behavioral, and social delays using a standardized screening tool in the 12 months preceding or on their first, second, or third birthday (Oregon Health and Science University [formerly an NCQA measure])**

See the current set of quality measures at https://www.medicaid.gov/medicaid/quality-of-care/performance-measurement/adult-and-child-health-care-quality-measures/childrens-health-care-quality-measures/index.html.

Coding and Documentation for Performance Measures

The following are documentation and coding tips for some of the pediatric performance measures for 2021 (2022 measures were not finalized at time of publication). See guidance from health plans in your area for more specific documentation and coding guidance.

Note that each measure includes a defined patient population (eg, children who turn 2 years of age during the measurement year).

> **Healthcare Effectiveness Data and Information Set requires that measures be met within specific time frames (eg, before the second birthday). Catching up after the specified time will not be counted in the number of patients for whom the measure was met.**

Physicians and group practices may also report performance measures as part of a pediatric medical home or other quality improvement initiative using data pulled from internal administrative data (eg, number of preventive medicine service *CPT* codes reported for population of patients 3–21 years old). Pediatric medical home and quality improvement initiatives vary by state or region and may include a combination of HEDIS and other nationally recognized quality measures.

Some measures include criteria that exclude a patient from the population for the measure. For example, hospice patients and adolescents with history of anaphylactic reaction to a vaccine or its components prior to their 13th birthday may be excluded from the measure for immunizations for adolescents. *ICD-10-CM* codes such as **Z28.04** (immunization not carried out because of patient allergy to vaccine or component), **Z87.892** (personal history of anaphylaxis), and **Z88.7** (allergy status to serum and vaccine status) may be reported to indicate this patient history.

Coding Conundrum: Quality Measurement and Vaccine Refusal

Codes for patient or caregiver vaccine refusal do not exclude a patient from the population for immunization measures. This creates a dilemma for physicians whose quality scores and payment may be affected by unimmunized patients within their patient panel. Does the physician continue providing care to patients whose parents refuse immunization despite any effect on quality scores?

The American Academy of Pediatrics policy statement, "Responding to Parental Refusals of Immunization of Children" (https://pediatrics.aappublications.org/content/115/5/1428), provides the following guidance:

"In general, pediatricians should endeavor not to discharge patients from their practices solely because a parent refuses to immunize his or her child. However, when a substantial level of distrust develops, significant differences in the philosophy of care emerge, or poor quality of communication persists, the pediatrician may encourage the family to find another physician or practice. Although pediatricians have the option of terminating the physician-patient relationship, they cannot do so without giving sufficient advance notice to the patient or custodial parent or legal guardian to permit another health care professional to be secured. Such decisions should be unusual and generally made only after attempts have been made to work with the family. Families with doubts about immunization should still have access to good medical care, and maintaining the relationship in the face of disagreement conveys respect and at the same time allows the child access to medical care. Furthermore, a continuing relationship allows additional opportunity to discuss the issue of immunization over time."

Preventive Screening and Utilization Measures

Following are some examples of measures in the categories of preventive screening and utilization with tips for coding and documentation:

Well-Child Visits—First 30 Months of Life

Measurement is based on the age of the patient at 2 distinct points *during the measurement period*.

- Children who turned 15 months—6 or more well-child visits

Health plans may count normal newborn care provided during the birth admission as 1 of 6 well-child visits before 15 months. Inclusion of history from a child's birth admission (eg, date and provider of initial hospital care, hepatitis B immunization) in the patient's health record may support this and other measures.

- Children who turned 30 months—2 or more well-child visits

This measure can be met by completing each child's recommended well-child visits at 18 and 24 months or, if delayed, before the child reaches 30 months of age.

Chapter 3. Coding to Demonstrate Quality and Value

Chapter 3. Coding to Demonstrate Quality and Value

Annual Child and Adolescent Well-Care Visits

The measure applies to patients aged 3 to 21 years. To meet the measure, one comprehensive well visit must be provided during the calendar year.

Documentation of a comprehensive well visit should include specific information such as the Tanner stage, assessed skills that support the child's developmental milestones, and context of anticipatory counseling (eg, discussed diet, screen time, sleep).

A comprehensive well-care visit provided in conjunction with a physical for school or sports participation may also support this measure.

Developmental Screening in the First 3 Years of Life

This measure applies to children who reached age 1, 2, or 3 years in the measurement year and requires use of a standardized screening instrument for motor, language, cognitive, and social-emotional development (must include all skills). Developmental screening is counted in each measurement year and for the 3-year period (ie, measure counts 4 times).

ICD-10-CM code Z13.42 (encounter for screening for global developmental delays) and *CPT* code 96110 (developmental screening, with scoring and documentation, per standardized instrument) are typically reported for these services. Code 96110 alone is not sufficient because this code is also reported for screening for specific conditions (eg, autism spectrum disorder [ASD]).

Child/Adolescent Weight Assessment and Counseling for Nutrition and Physical Activity

Percentage of patients aged 3 to 17 years whose BMI was measured and documented as a BMI percentage (eg, 20%) and with documented counseling for nutrition and physical activity (a checklist of counseling topics may be acceptable).

Most health plans require physicians to report a code for the BMI percentile (Z68.51–Z68.54). The BMI value is reported as an additional code to counseling for nutrition (Z71.3) and codes for any related condition (eg, overweight, obesity).

> *International Classification of Diseases, 10th Revision, Clinical Modification (ICD-10-CM)* codes for pediatric body mass index (BMI) percentiles (Z68.51–Z68.54) are only reported in conjunction with physician documentation of a related condition (eg, overweight, obesity). If a physician is reporting codes Z68.51–Z68.54 based only on a payer's written guidance for reporting quality measures, it is advisable to keep a copy of the payer's guidance. An alternative method for reporting that the patient's BMI was documented is to report *Current Procedural Terminology* Category II code 3008F (BMI, documented) in lieu of *ICD-10-CM* codes for BMI.

Code Z71.82 (exercise counseling) is used to report counseling for physical activity.

> When obesity is diagnosed and at least 15 minutes is spent in counseling specific to the obesity, code G0447 (face-to-face behavioral counseling for obesity, 15 minutes) may be separately reportable in addition to a preventive evaluation and management (E/M) service (eg, 99383). Verify individual health plan policies to determine if benefits for counseling for obesity are separately paid on the same date as a preventive E/M service.

Immunization Status

These measures are as follows:

- Child: Patients who received all recommended immunizations on or before their second birthday. This includes administration of 2 doses of influenza vaccine in addition to other recommended immunizations.
- Adolescent: Percent of patients who are fully immunized by their 13th birthday.

> Documentation of immunizations that require a series of administrations (eg, 3 doses) should be documented as such (dose 2 of 2 or dose 2 of 3). This may be accomplished by use of a chart/template that indicates each vaccine/toxoid product administered, doses required, and the date that each dose is administered.

The following *ICD-10-CM* codes (not all-inclusive) may indicate a patient's reason for exclusion from one or more recommended immunizations.

Z87.892	Personal history of anaphylaxis
Z88.7	Allergy status to serum and vaccine
B20	Human immunodeficiency virus (HIV) disease
Z21	Asymptomatic human immunodeficiency virus (HIV) infection status
D81.9	Combined immunodeficiency, unspecified

D81.31	Severe combined immunodeficiency due to adenosine deaminase deficiency	
D84.9	Immunodeficiency, unspecified	

Lead Screening

This measure is of the percentage of children who turn 2 years old during the measurement year who had at least one capillary or venous blood test for lead poisoning (**83655 QW**).

Examples

➤ **A 23-month-old presents as a new patient for clearance to attend child care.** Records from the child's former physician indicate that a preventive E/M service was provided when the child was 18 months old and all immunizations are up to date, including 2 doses of influenza in the prior year. However, the prior preventive service was provided via telemedicine and immunizations were provided at a separate encounter. The physician identifies that screenings for lead, global development, and ASD were not performed. These are performed (with parental permission) at this encounter in addition to performing the 24-month well-child examination.

ICD-10-CM	CPT	Related HEDIS Measures
Z00.129 (encounter for routine child health examination without abnormal findings)	**99392** (periodic comprehensive preventive medicine reevaluation and management, age 1–4 years)	*Well-Child Visits in the First 30 Months of Life* Patients turning 30 months old during measurement year 2 or more comprehensive well-care visits completed between 15 and 30 months after birth
Z13.42 (encounter for screening for global developmental delays [milestones])	**96110** (developmental screening, with scoring and documentation, per standardized instrument)	*Developmental Screening in the First Three Years of Life* Once within each of the first 3 years after birth
Z13.41 (encounter for autism screening)	**96110 59** (developmental screening, with scoring and documentation, per standardized instrument)	*Not applicable—the measure for developmental screening is limited to screening for global developmental delay.*
Z13.88 (encounter for screening for disorder due to exposure to contaminants)	**36416** (collection capillary blood specimen) **99000** (handling and/or conveyance of specimen)	*Lead Screening* Patients turning 2 years old in the measurement year At least one capillary or venous lead blood test completed on or before their second birthday

The physician in this scenario has proactively provided preventive care that is recommended for this patient and, in doing so, is able to report diagnosis and procedure codes demonstrating that quality measures have been met.

Code **Z02.0** (encounter for examination for admission to educational institution) is not reported because an *Excludes1* note prohibits reporting codes in category **Z02** with codes in category **Z00**.

> **See Chapter 8 for more details on coding for preventive medicine services.**

Effectiveness of Care

Certain measures are used to determine the effectiveness of care. Some effectiveness of care measures use a combination of medical and pharmacy claims data to assess overuse or appropriate use of medications. Other measures are of the percentage of patients receiving follow-up care after new diagnoses, emergency department visits, or hospital stays. Examples of these measures include the following:

Pharyngitis and Antibiotic Prescriptions

Percentage of patients 3 years and older diagnosed with pharyngitis who were tested for streptococcus infection and, only if appropriate, prescribed an antibiotic.

Chapter 3. Coding to Demonstrate Quality and Value

Physician, pharmacy, and laboratory claims may be used for this measure. Codes for testing for streptococcal infection (eg, 87880, infectious agent antigen detection by immunoassay with direct optical [ie, visual] observation; *Streptococcus,* group A) and *ICD-10-CM* codes (eg, J02.0, streptococcal pharyngitis) are indicative of meeting this measure.

Depression Screening and Follow-up

Percentage of patients aged 12 years and older who were seen during the measurement year and were screened for depression with a structured instrument and, for positive results, for whom an appropriate follow-up was planned. Code 96127 (brief emotional/behavioral assessment using standardized instrument) may be reported for providing screening, but Healthcare Common Procedure Coding System codes are used to indicate the screening result and follow-up plan.

G8510   Screening for depression is documented as negative, a follow-up plan is not required

G8431   Screening for depression is documented as being positive AND a follow-up plan is documented

G9717   Documentation stating the patient has had a diagnosis of depression or has had a diagnosis of bipolar disorder

Example

➤ **A physician sees an established patient (aged 12 years or older) for follow-up of major depressive disorder.** The patient also complains of a runny nose and sore throat. The caregiver requests an antibiotic but is instructed that the condition is viral and to use over-the-counter medicine as necessary for the child's comfort. No antibiotic is ordered. Diagnoses are single episode of moderate major depression with improvement measured with standardized rating scale and acute nasopharyngitis. Plan is to continue antidepressant medication and reevaluate in 1 month. Home care for acute nasopharyngitis is to gargle with salt water, push fluids, and rest. The patient and caregiver are warned against use of cold and cough medications.

ICD-10-CM	CPT	Related HEDIS Measures
F32.1 (major depressive disorder, single episode, moderate) **J00** (acute nasopharyngitis)	**99214** (office or other outpatient visit for the E/M of an established patient [See full code descriptor in **Chapter 7**.])	*Appropriate Treatment for Children With Upper Respiratory Infection (URI)* Patients 3 mo–18 y with • Diagnosis of URI (includes J00, J06.0, J06.9) *and* • Not prescribed an antibiotic within 3 days of URI diagnosis
F32.1 (major depressive disorder, single episode, moderate)	**96127** (brief emotional/behavioral assessment [eg, depression inventory, attention-deficit/hyperactivity disorder (ADHD) scale], with scoring and documentation, per standardized instrument)	*Not applicable—code* 96127 *is not indicative of depression screening because* 96127 *is used to report use of a standardized instrument in diagnosis and management of other disorders in addition to depression.*
F32.1 (major depressive disorder, single episode, moderate)	**G9717** (documentation stating the patient has had a diagnosis of depression or has had a diagnosis of bipolar disorder)	*Depression screening and follow-up—code* G9717 *indicates the patient is not included in the population for whom screening is appropriate.*

Because this patient had no symptoms of a bacterial infection, the physician did not prescribe an antibiotic. This supports the measure for appropriate treatment for URI.

Reporting code G9717 removes this patient from the population measured for screening for depression and follow-up plan.

Performance measures change annually. Physician practices should maintain awareness of how health plans collect data for performance measurement and the documentation and coding practices that may reduce burdens associated with associated chart reviews. An updated Child Core Set is published on https://www.Medicaid.gov annually. Many plans publish their HEDIS measures and supporting codes, as reaching optimal HEDIS measures is important for the payers as well.

Resources

AAP Policy Statement

"A New Era in Quality Measurement: The Development and Application of Quality Measures" (http://pediatrics.aappublications.org/content/139/1/e20163442)

Consumer Assessment of Healthcare Providers and Systems (CAHPS)

AHRQ CAHPS program (https://www.ahrq.gov/cahps/index.html)

CPT Category II Codes and Alphabetical Clinical Topics Listing

www.ama-assn.org/practice-management/cpt-category-ii-codes

Hierarchical Condition Categories

"Hierarchical Condition Categories: What They Are and Why They Matter to Pediatricians," July 2019 *AAP Pediatric Coding Newsletter*™ (https://coding.solutions.aap.org/article.aspx?articleid=2736885; subscription required)

Quality Measures

National Committee for Quality Assurance (www.ncqa.org)

Medicaid and the CHIP Children's Health Care Quality Measures (https://www.medicaid.gov/medicaid/quality-of-care/performance-measurement/adult-and-child-health-care-quality-measures/childrens-health-care-quality-measures/index.html)

Vaccine Refusal

AAP clinical report, "Responding to Parental Refusals of Immunization of Children" (https://pediatrics.aappublications.org/content/115/5/1428)

Test Your Knowledge!

1. **How are hierarchical condition categories used?**
   a. To determine the value of a physician service
   b. To show performance of a Healthcare Effectiveness Data and Information Set (HEDIS) measure
   c. To calculate a patient's risk of increased health care use or risk adjustment
   d. To attribute the cost of care to a specific physician or group

2. **Which of the following is true of HEDIS measures?**
   a. HEDIS measures affect only health plans.
   b. Each health plan creates a set of unique measures.
   c. Physicians should not release medical records for HEDIS purposes due to Health Care Portability and Accountability Act of 1996 regulations.
   d. Many health plans provide specific information on documentation and codes that do or do not support HEDIS measurement.

3. **True or false? Medicaid and the Children's Health Insurance Program plans do not participate in performance measurement programs.**
   a. True
   b. False

4. **Which of the following excludes a patient from performance measurement for immunization?**
   a. Patient was a no-show for appointments.
   b. Parents refuse immunization of their child.
   c. Patient refuses immunization.
   d. Patient is allergic to the vaccine or its component.

CHAPTER 4

The Business of Medicine: Working With Current and Emerging Payment Systems

Contents

Values Assigned to Physician Services 69

    Connecting Codes to Payment and Budget 69

    Participation in Relative Value Scale Update Committee Surveys 71

Contracting and Negotiating With Payers 71

    When Negotiations Fail 72

Clean Claims to Correct Payment 73

    Capturing Charges in the Electronic Health Record 74

    Encounter Forms and Other Coding Tools 75

        Designing and Reviewing the Encounter Form 75

        Completing the Encounter Form 76

        Reviewing Assigned Codes 77

    Place of Service Codes 77

    Submitting Clean Claims 78

        Special Consideration for Medicare Claims 79

        Monitoring Claim Status 79

    Monitoring Payments 80

        Filing Appeals 81

    Documentation and Coding Audits 82

    Tools for the Pediatric Practice 82

Emerging Payment Methodologies 83

    Preparing for New Payment Models 84

        Assignment, Engagement, and Attribution of Patient Panels 84

    Accountable Care Organizations (ACOs) 86

        American Academy of Pediatrics Resources for More Information on ACOs 86

Resources 87

Test Your Knowledge! 88

Chapter 4. The Business of Medicine: Working With Current and Emerging Payment Systems

To maintain a viable practice, physicians and their staff must respond to changing payment systems and continually refine their practice management skills. This chapter's 3 sections address

- How services are currently valued and how assigned values may be used to guide practice management
- Guidelines and tools that may be used to monitor and manage charge accumulation, claims filing, review of payments, the appeals process, contract negotiations, and the use of audits to protect against lost revenue and incorrect billing practices
- Emerging payment methodologies and how these may affect traditional and newer practice models, such as accountable care organizations (ACOs)

Values Assigned to Physician Services

Connecting Codes to Payment and Budget

Before a claim is generated, a physician practice must establish fees for services that are greater than the cost of providing the service. A simple fee schedule methodology involves use of the Medicare Resource-Based Relative Value Scale (RBRVS). In 2022, most pediatric services are still valued and paid by Medicaid, Tricare, and commercial payers using a fee-for-service methodology based on the RBRVS. An understanding of how values are assigned to the codes for services, how the values relate to payment, and how this information contributes to a practice's finances is critical for the practice's financial viability and success.

The 3 components of the RBRVS are as follows:

1. *Physician work:* Physician work represents approximately 50% of the total relative value units (RVUs) assigned to most services. Work RVUs are commonly used in employment contracts as a factor in physician payment.
   - *Work* is described as time required to perform the service, mental effort and judgment, technical skill, physical effort, and psychological stress associated with concern about iatrogenic risk to the patient.
   - For most services, physician work is further broken down into *preservice, intraservice,* and *post-service* components. Correct coding requires understanding these components of work, as preservice and post-service components should not be separately reported.
     — *Preservice work:* For nonsurgical services, this preparatory non–face-to-face work includes typical review of records and communicating with other professionals. (Prolonged preservice work, such as extensive record review, may be separately reportable.) For surgical services, this includes physician work from the day before the service to the procedure but excludes the encounter that resulted in the decision for surgery or unrelated evaluation and management (E/M) services.
     — Intraservice work: For most nonsurgical services, this includes time spent by the physician or other qualified health care professional (QHP) in direct patient care activities, such as obtaining history, examining the patient, and counseling the patient and/or caregivers. Surgical intraservice work begins with incision or introduction of instruments (eg, needle, scope) and ends with closure of the incision or removal of instruments.

     A physician's intraservice time on the date of an office or other outpatient E/M service (**99202–99205, 99212–99215**) includes all time spent on the date of the encounter including pre-visit planning and post-visit work such as documenting the service provided. Certain services (eg, chronic care management) are inclusive only of intraservice time of physicians and/or clinical staff and are not valued to include preservice and post-service work.
     — *Post-service work:* Documentation of services provided is included in the post-service work of each service.
       - For nonsurgical services, post-service work includes arranging for further services, reviewing and communicating test results, preparing written reports, and/or communicating by telephone or secure electronic means. Separately reported services, such as chronic care management or care plan oversight, are not included in post-service work.
       - For surgical services, post-service work includes typical work in the procedure or operating room after the procedure has ended, stabilization of the patient in the recovery area, communications with family or other health care professionals, and visits on the day of surgery. Surgical services are also valued to include typical follow-up care for the presenting problem during a defined global period (eg, 10 or 90 days after the service).

For more on the global period for surgery, see chapters 10 and 19.

2. *Practice expense:* This component is an estimate of preservice, intraservice, and post-service clinical staff time; medical supplies; and procedure-specific and overhead equipment. Practice expense makes up about 44% of the total RVUs for most services. Practice expense varies by site of service (ie, facility vs non-facility). See the Place of Service Codes section later in this chapter for more information about how place of service affects payment.

3. *Professional liability:* This smallest component (about 4% of the total RVUs) is based on medical malpractice premium data.

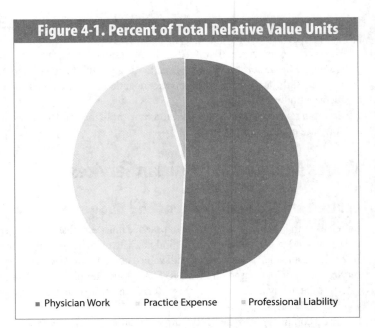

Figure 4-1. Percent of Total Relative Value Units

■ Physician Work   ■ Practice Expense   ■ Professional Liability

Figure 4-1 illustrates the percent of total RVU for each component.

Each RVU component may be independently adjusted slightly upward or downward as a function of geographic area. The Centers for Medicare & Medicaid Services (CMS) calculates Medicare payment for a procedure code by multiplying total RVUs by a dollar conversion factor (CF) that is set annually.

Example

➤ **A payer uses the 2021 Medicare Physician Fee Schedule (MPFS) as a basis for physician payment with a CF or contracted fee schedule amount of $36 per RVU.** A physician submits established patient office visit code **99214** to the payer.

The total MPFS non-facility RVUs (3.76) assigned to code **99214** are a combination of RVUs for physician work (1.92), non-facility practice expense (1.70), and professional liability (0.14). The total non-facility RVUs (3.76) are multiplied by the $36 CF to determine the allowed amount for the service.

(Total Medicare RVUs) × (Payer CF) = Allowed amount (3.76) × ($36) = $135.36

Actual payment may vary based on the patient's out-of-pocket obligation.

Medicaid fee schedules vary by state and, although often based on RVUs or the MPFS, state regulations may also designate amounts paid for specific services. Commercial payments for many procedure codes are often linked to a percentage of Medicare payment. Alternatively, payers may offer their own fee schedule (eg, a particular year's MPFS) for a practice's most used procedure codes.

- It is important to obtain the payer's fee schedule for all codes used or likely to be used by a practice (including codes for vaccines and administration) and compare these with the current year's MPFS and other published fee schedules. Although Medicare assigns a status of N (noncovered) to *Current Procedural Terminology* (*CPT*®) codes **99381–99385** and **99391–99395** in the MPFS, component RVUs are published in the MPFS allowing calculation of Medicare equivalent payments.

   Tip: If a health plan contract states that payment is based on the MPFS, it is important to verify the year of the MPFS used by the health plan because these schedules are not always current. Resetting payment according to the MPFS for the year of service may result in higher or lower payments.

- Medicaid and proposed commercial payments for pediatric preventive care can be evaluated in light of the Medicare equivalent payments.

   Tip: When reviewing a payer's fee schedule, make sure the payer also fully discloses its policies for paying for services that it considers to be *bundled* (ie, payment for 2 or more codes during the same encounter may be less than the sum of the individual payments) and those whose cost it shifts to the patient/family.

The RBRVS payment methodology may be used with practice- and physician-specific data generated from a practice's accounting and practice management systems to estimate an approximate cost of providing each service. This should result in a list of services that are each assigned a share of the practice's overhead costs as well as the margin and actual cost of providing the service.

- From the accounting system, an administrator may calculate the total practice expenses for a period, subtracting billable services that are not paid based on RVUs such as vaccines and medications.
- From the practice management system, reports may be generated to provide a total of the number of procedures billed by code, RVUs for each service, and total RVUs billed by the practice for the same period.
- By dividing total practice expenses by total RVUs, an administrator can calculate the practice cost per RVU.
- Additional calculations may be used to compare payment per RVU or per service among contracted payers. (Calculations should be viewed in context of other factors, such as history of timely and correct payment.)

> It may be important to consider several years of data to account for seasonal, year-to-year, or public health emergency impacts, which may significantly limit the accuracy of data to predict future service costs and volume.

Such calculations should be used to inform decisions on acceptance of contractual fee schedules, number of services necessary to break even or profit from provision of services, and return on investment potential for new equipment or services.

Keep in mind that some ACOs have financial agreements that require certain services be paid with a single lump payment that is then distributed among all providers of the service. To negotiate a fair portion of that lump payment, you need to know the cost of providing the service. (See the Accountable Care Organizations [ACOs] section later in this chapter.) More accurate cost estimates may be determined on an actual cost basis. However, RVU calculations are straightforward and typically provide a reasonably reliable result.

Participation in Relative Value Scale Update Committee Surveys

Pediatricians can also play a role in recommending values for services to the CMS by participation in American Academy of Pediatrics (AAP) surveys conducted through the American Medical Association/Specialty Society Relative Value Scale Update Committee (RUC). These surveys are conducted to estimate the time and complexity of performing a service in comparison with another service. American Academy of Pediatrics staff sends out requests for participation to AAP section members to allow completion by physicians who most typically perform the service being surveyed. To learn more about participation in RUC surveys, see the "Understanding the RUC Survey Instrument" video at www.youtube.com/watch?v=nu5unDX8VIs; for information on code valuation, RBRVS, and payment, see www.aap.org/en-us/professional-resources/practice-transformation/getting-paid/Coding-at-the-AAP/Pages/Code-Valuation-and-PaymentRBRVS.aspx.

Contracting and Negotiating With Payers

Participating in a payer's network typically involves entering into a contract with the payer. Physicians should not sign contracts without reading and considering the impact of entering into the contractual agreement. The payer is going to seek terms that are most favorable to its business. Negotiation is important to ensure that your practice is profitable and able to provide quality care without burdensome payer requirements (eg, policy for prepayment record review of all claims for specific services).

Negotiating payment with payers can be more successful if a practice is also prepared to provide quality of care data according to standard quality measures. Be prepared to demonstrate the cost savings that may be recognized by the plan as well as the value the practice brings to the plan in savings, quality of care data, and/or patient satisfaction.

Successful negotiation requires preparation. The following suggestions can prepare physician participation in negotiations:

- Fully read and ask questions, as necessary, about the terms of the contract: duration, fee schedule updates, types of health plans included, and how appeals are managed.
- Know a health plan's policies and procedures and their effect on pediatric services. Develop a system to monitor all updates and changes to the physician contract. Be aware of updates provided via periodic email bulletins or information posted on a payer website that practices have been instructed to review periodically. Practices must be aware that these alternative ways of disseminating payment information are often considered legal and binding.
- Know a health plan's processes to add new *CPT* codes/services and how each plan pays before determining payment policy and fee schedule amounts. (New codes are often paid at a percentage of charges, if covered at all.)
- When adding new physicians to your practice, be aware of each payer's fee schedule policies. Do not assume that the same fee schedule will be applied across all physicians in the practice (eg, a payer may assign a reduced fee schedule to new physicians or carry forward a physician's contract from a previous practice).

  Be aware of the potential that patients may incur higher out-of-pocket costs (eg, co-pays) with services by different providers within the practice. When this occurs, discussion with a health plan should include the potential effect of delayed care when the patient/family opts to wait to see a provider for whom the out-of-pocket costs are lower.

- Be aware of any accountability (eg, penalties or other effect on shared savings) that a plan attributes to the practice when patients receive care outside their plan's network without referral by physicians within the practice.
- Know *CPT* codes and modifiers and the guidelines for their use.
- Understand how the National Correct Coding Initiative (NCCI) adopted by some payers (including Medicaid) may relate to your practice.
- Understand and be able to describe the scope of services provided and the time requirements for the service.
- Be prepared to demonstrate the cost savings that may be recognized by the plan as well as the value the practice brings to the plan in savings, quality of care data, and/or patient satisfaction. *This is your leverage.*
- Monitor and know the use (distribution) of codes by each physician and, if in a group practice, for the practice as a whole.
- Identify your payer mix. Know how many patients you have in each plan and what percentage of your total patients that represents. In addition, know what percentage of RVUs each payer pays for your most frequently used codes and how these percentages compare in payment with each other. Accurate information on payer mix and potential value/loss to the practice is essential in making participation decisions.
- Know and understand the payment basis and process.
- Have specific codes or issues to discuss, not generalities (agreement with general ideas may not address specific issues).

  In negotiations

- Try to negotiate for coverage and payment of services, or, if payers refuse to cover services, get your contract amended to state that you can bill the service as non-covered. If the plan will allow for billing the patient for non-covered services, you must then advise your patients of this policy (a written notification is usually required before rendering the service).
- If the plan does agree to cover a particular service, make certain you understand how the carrier will cover and pay for the service and if there will be any restrictions or limitations.
- Keep notes during the discussion, and be certain you understand answers to any of your questions. Any specific agreements should be in writing and signed by both parties.

  Seek assistance in negotiations.

- Engage parents or employers to work in partnership to help you negotiate with a plan. Encourage parents to work through their human resources department to communicate and appeal with payers. Petitions from parents can be very effective. See the resources for health insurance education from HealthyChildren.org at www.healthychildren.org/English/family-life/health-management/health-insurance/Pages/default.aspx.

> It is important, too, to recognize that the employers in your area may offer their employees a self-funded health plan and that it is the employer who may be in control of the plan's payment rates and policies, although claims are administered by a third party (eg, health insurance company).

- Many AAP chapters have developed pediatric councils, which meet with payers to address pediatric issues. Advise your chapter pediatric council of specific issues you have experienced, and see how it can work with the plan. (The AAP chapter pediatric councils are not forums for negotiating contracts, setting fees, or discussing payments.)

  If your chapter does not have a pediatric council, this may be the right time to work with your chapter to begin developing one. To see whether your state has a pediatric council, or for more information, visit www.aap.org/en-us/professional-resources/practice-transformation/getting-paid/Pages/aap-pediatric-councils.aspx (AAP members only).

When Negotiations Fail

If the insurance company is not addressing your concerns satisfactorily, you should be willing to withdraw from its plan. Inform the payer (a formal notification process may be outlined in your contract), the patients' families, and even the state insurance commission why continued participation is impossible.

- Some reasons for withdrawal might be slow payment, excessive documentation requirements, and substandard payment compared with those of other plans.
- Many times, negotiation begins when you walk away from the table.

Clean Claims to Correct Payment

Getting paid for services provided requires a practice-wide team effort. Opportunities for lost revenue can occur anywhere between patient scheduling and posting of health plan payments (or denials). **Figure 4-2** shows steps in the revenue cycle. Even salaried physicians are affected by lost revenue and should take interest in the effectiveness of the practice's billing processes.

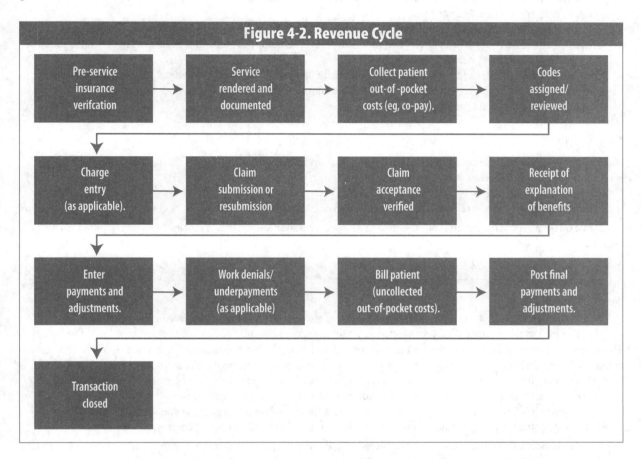

Figure 4-2. Revenue Cycle

An effective charge accumulation system, accurate billing of procedure codes, and an efficient claims filing system are necessary but not sufficient to achieve clean claim submissions. Although the physician is ultimately responsible for the accuracy of codes selected and claims submitted, it typically takes a team effort to create and maintain an effective accounts receivable system, including

- Development and use of management tools.
  - Incorporation of claims processing tools for analysis of your claims processing procedures. A self-assessment tool for improving claims processing and payment can be found at www.aap.org/en-us/Documents/ImprovingClaimsProcessing.pdf.
  - Electronic health record (EHR) and/or billing systems may include automated tools to help identify errors prior to billing, alert you to payments that do not align with contracted fees, and provide data for monitoring the time lapse from provision of service to payment.
  - Provide access to and create policy for using payer resources such as online code-checking tools that alert to coverage limitations such as bundled services or services covered only in conjunction with specific diagnoses.
- Continuing provider and staff education with constant oversight and communication with staff, payers, and patients.
  - Policies and procedures support continuous monitoring of payer communications and dissemination of information on benefit policy changes that affect coding and payment.
  - Assurance that staff assigned with responsibilities related to correct coding and billing have access to authoritative resources on coding and documentation (eg, current Medicaid NCCI edits and manual).

See chapters 2 and 5 for more information on code edits and compliant coding and billing.

- Regularly performing audits to identify potential corrective actions required to remain compliant with billing standards, coding guidelines, and federal rules and regulations (eg, Health Insurance Portability and Accountability Act [HIPAA] of 1996, Anti-Kickback Statute, False Claims Act). Audits benefit the practice by identifying
  - The number of timely and correctly submitted claims, resulting in faster and more appropriate payments and reduced practice cost of obtaining payment
  - The need for physician and staff education on coding and documentation
  - Issues for payer contract negotiations
  - Incorrect coding and related potential risk for charges of fraud or abuse
  - Areas that need written office policies and procedures (eg, pre-authorization and referral processes, claims follow-up processes, control systems)
- Procedures for efficient review of payments and potentially inappropriate denials or reductions. Timely identification of payment errors is necessary to obtain redress because contracts often specify a time limit on appeals.
- Guidance for write-offs and initiation of appeals processes.

Capturing Charges in the Electronic Health Record

Many physicians now capture encounter and billing information in the EHR. The basics of charge capture in the EHR are

- Accurate listing of diagnoses
- Selection of complete codes
- Procedure code selection based on work performed and documented

While integrating charge capture into the encounter documentation should create efficiency, there are pitfalls to be avoided.

Compliant documentation and code selection are discussed in Chapter 5.

When using an EHR, make sure that codes in the system are accurate and updated in accordance with code set updates. It is important to verify with your electronic system vendors how code updates are incorporated into the system. This might happen via scheduled upgrades that may or may not require system downtime, or it could occur via automated upgrades during night or weekend hours. It is important to make sure this information is outlined in your EHR contract.

- Code updates should be based on the effective date of changes (eg, deleted codes may be entered for charges with a date of service prior to the effective date of deletion even after the update has been made).
- Practice and billing managers must maintain contact with the system vendor's upgrade and support staff and verify what, if any, manual steps are required on the part of the practice in relation to code changes.

It is also important that code descriptors displayed in code selection are adequate for accurate code selection. Truncated descriptors may omit key information that differentiates one code from another (eg, attention-deficit hyperactivity disorder [ADHD] should provide options for predominantly hyperactive, predominantly inattentive, or combined ADHD).

Documentation of the diagnoses has been problematic in some EHR systems. As with the paper record, the physician must have the ability to fully describe patient diagnoses for each encounter (ie, not to merely select a diagnosis code).

Example

▶ 1. Recurrent otitis media with antibiotic resistance
2. Underachievement in school with grades dropping this semester
3. New symptoms of anxiety and social phobia since return to the classroom from remote learning

- Systems should not use diagnosis codes for populating the physician's diagnostic statement or assessment. Code descriptors may be generalized and do not capture the physician's differential diagnoses (eg, delayed milestone in childhood—3 years old, late talker in speech therapy; possible autism spectrum disorder—little eye contact and likes to play alone).
- The EHR should not reorder diagnoses entered by the physician. An EHR that reorders documented diagnoses (eg, alphabetically) results in noncompliance with diagnosis coding guidelines.

Physicians should list first the diagnosis and code most responsible for the encounter, followed by additional diagnoses, in compliance with coding guidelines.

- The patient problem list should not be pulled forward as the diagnoses for each encounter. Only those conditions addressed or that affected management or treatment of conditions addressed should be reported for that particular encounter.

    Follow payer guidelines for reporting diagnosis codes for chronic conditions that may be reported annually (eg, evaluating problems at preventive service visits) for purposes of risk stratification.

> **Documentation and coding to support risk adjustment are increasingly demanded by payers. Please see Chapter 3 for a discussion of appropriate coding to support risk adjustment.**

Automated code selection is also problematic. An EHR may be designed to determine the level of E/M service provided based on information documented. However, physicians must make the code determination based on the medically necessary services provided and documented and based on code selection criteria (ie, key components, medical decision-making, or time).

- Automatic population of records may result in documentation that overstates the level of work and intensity of the service provided.
- Failure to override suggested codes when appropriate may be considered an abusive practice.

When encounter data is utilized to show performance of quality metrics, it is essential that the data are configured to correctly populate reports of the patients to whom the measure applies and whether there is documentation of the outcome or process of care specified in the measure (eg, all patients aged 3–17 years and the percentage of those patients who received counseling for diet and exercise).

> **See more on compliant electronic health record documentation in Chapter 5. See also Chapter 20 for information specific to documentation and coding for telemedicine services.**

Encounter Forms and Other Coding Tools

Encounter forms are useful supplements to EHR-based code selection. They can also be used to convey codes to a billing office/system when systems are not integrated.

Designing and Reviewing the Encounter Form

The encounter form, whether electronic or printed, should be designed to help physicians and clinical staff quickly find all codes for diagnoses and services common to the practice. An encounter form or superbill should prompt recognition of separately reported services and use of diagnosis codes that most accurately describe the patient presentation.

When developing the encounter form

- Include all levels of service for each category of E/M services (eg, **99211–99215, 99221–99223**) and ensure time is listed for coding based on time. List routine health examination codes by age and new or established patient.
- List procedures (eg, laboratory) to fit your practice's workflow. For example, group codes together in the order of your workflow (eg, visit codes followed by immunization, laboratory, respiratory, etc) to maximize efficiency and your workflow.
- The printed encounter form should prompt staff for specific details of a procedure when required for code verification. For example

    Code **120**_____ Simple repair loc* _____ size _____ (*Location)

- Include the most commonly reported diagnosis codes. Consider grouping diagnosis codes by organ system, and then alphabetically, within the system.
- Leave space on the form to allow the reporting of the specific diagnosis and full *International Classification of Diseases, 10th Revision, Clinical Modification (ICD-10-CM)* codes.

Example

➤ **J45.2_**   *Asthma, mild intermittent*
 J45.3_   *Asthma, mild persistent*
 J45.4_   Asthma, moderate persistent
 J45.5_   *Asthma, severe, persistent*
   Add fifth character: 0, uncomplicated; 1, w/ (acute) exacerbation; 2, w/ status asthmaticus.

- Include the most frequently used modifiers.
- Leave space on forms to write in any services or diagnoses that are not included.
- Include add-on codes for prolonged and special services. For example

+99358	Prolonged evaluation and management service before and/or after direct patient care; first hour
99024	Postoperative follow-up visit, normally included in the surgical package, to indicate that an evaluation and management service was performed during a postoperative period for a reason(s) related to the original procedure

- Develop a separate encounter form for hospital and outpatient hospital services. Make sure it includes all the services most commonly performed in the hospital setting.

  Access to a coding application or pocket-sized reference card with required key components and/or time of services also helps promote accurate code selection in facility settings.

- When quality initiatives are dependent on codes reported (eg, codes supporting Healthcare Effectiveness Data and Information Set [HEDIS] measures), be sure that these codes are clearly indicated on the encounter form, prompted by the EHR, or provided in an easily accessible quick reference.

Encounter forms and other coding tools should be reviewed periodically and updated at the time of each code set update to ensure that most of, if not all, the services and procedures commonly performed in the practice are included and the codes are accurate.

> See Chapter 1 for the timing of updates to code sets (eg, January, April, July, October).

Completing the Encounter Form

Every practice should develop a written policy of the requirements needed to complete a form. Some points that should be part of the policy include

- The encounter form is *not* part of the medical record. Information such as the need for follow-up care, diagnostic tests, or referrals must always be documented in the medical record even if written on the encounter form.
- If you are using a printed form, services must be clearly identified (eg, circle procedure, use check mark). Procedures or diagnoses must be written on a form if they are not preprinted.

> The person providing the service (eg, physician, laboratory technologist, medical assistant) should enter procedure codes or document that service on the encounter form to ensure only the procedures performed are reported. This ensures that only work that has been performed is reported.

Example

➤ **Dr Good marks a vaccine and its administration on the encounter form when she orders the administration.** However, the parent had decided to delay the immunization until she discussed it with her spouse.

If the clinical staff (under supervision of the physician) had been responsible for reporting the service when performed, it would not have been reported.

- The physician is ultimately responsible for the services reported and billed.
- The physician should identify the diagnosis as, for example, primary or secondary.
- Diagnoses and services or procedures must be numbered and linked to each other. The EHR should not reorder the diagnoses entered by the physician because conditions must be listed in order of responsibility for the service provided.

Example

➤ **An E/M service and removal of impacted cerumen from the right ear (69210) is performed.** The physician reports the primary diagnosis (H66.001, acute suppurative otitis media without spontaneous rupture of eardrum, right ear) (field 21A) and the secondary diagnosis (H61.21, impacted cerumen, right ear) (field 21B). *ICD-10-CM* pointer A (H66.001) is linked to the office visit (99213 25) in field 24E and pointer B (H61.21) is linked to the procedure (69210) in field 24 E of the respective service lines.

See **Figure 1-1** for an example of how the linking of diagnoses to procedures appears on a claim form. An electronic claim form contains the same data in segments of loops 2300 and 2400.

- A billing manager or clerk should only add or change a service or diagnosis with the agreement of the provider of service.
- A system should be instituted to monitor and ensure capture of charges for all of the day's patient encounters (eg, cross-reference to the patient check-in records).

Reviewing Assigned Codes

A staff member who understands correct coding and reporting guidelines should always review the assigned codes before the claim is submitted to ensure that all procedures and services are captured and accurate.

For example, the reviewer should look to see that

- An administration code is reported with vaccines and/or injections. Payer instructions for reporting National Drug Codes and units are followed.
- A venipuncture or finger stick is reported with a laboratory test, when applicable. The practice's Clinical Laboratory Improvement Amendments number is included on claims for laboratory services, when required.

To learn more about requirements for in-office laboratory certification, see the article "What Is CLIA?" in the August 2019 *AAP Pediatric Coding Newsletter™* (https://coding.solutions.aap.org/article.aspx?articleid=2739279; subscription required).

- A handling fee is reported when a specimen is prepared and sent to an outside laboratory.
- A modifier is appended when appropriate (eg, modifier 25 for significant, separately identifiable E/M services).
- The office visit is reported using the correct new or established patient category of service.

See Chapter 6 for more information on new and established patients.

- The diagnoses reported as primary and secondary are appropriate and are linked to the appropriate services or procedures.
- The documentation to support each service has been completed with required dates and signatures.

Place of Service Codes

The place of service is indicated on each claim by a *place of service code* (often integrated into billing systems without need for manual entry with each charge). The place of service may appear evident when reporting codes for services such as inpatient hospital care, but this is not always the case.

- When providing services in a facility such as a hospital outpatient clinic, it is important to report the correct place of service because differences in practice expense in a facility versus a non-facility setting affect physician payment.

Example

➤ **A procedure performed in a surgical center would be paid at a lower fee schedule amount than the same procedure performed in a physician's clinic (not hospital based) because the fee schedule takes into account the overhead or practice expense of providing services (eg, procedure room, supplies, clinical staff).**

If services provided in a facility setting are reported as if provided in a physician's clinic, an overpayment may occur.

Physicians in provider-based practices (ie, those practices owned and operated as a part of a hospital) should be aware that the place of service code is especially important in this setting. Physician and practice expense portions of the patient's charges are often billed separately in provider-based practices.

- The same services provided in a provider-based practice are often costlier than those provided in an independent (physician-owned) practice. Facility fees charged by the provider are often significantly higher than the non-facility fees charged in independent practices.
- The Medicare program created place of service code 19 to define an "off-campus" hospital practice to adopt site-neutral payment for many physician services provided at provider-based practices. The rules and payment modifications have not been universally adopted, but it is important to know how your office is classified to ensure proper billing regardless. When considering purchase by a hospital system, it is important to consider the effect of billing with a different place of service code.

- The increased number of high-deductible health plans has raised awareness of the greater costs to patients when services are rendered in provider-based facilities and has prompted Medicare and some states to take action to reduce the added costs. Practices should be aware of any such restrictions that apply to billing in their locality and under payer contracts.

   Other place of service codes that may be commonly reported for pediatric services include **02**, telehealth; **03**, school; **11**, office; **12**, home; **14**, group home; **20**, urgent care facility; **21**, inpatient hospital; **22**, on campus—outpatient hospital; and **23**, emergency room—hospital.

   Place of service codes are further discussed for certain E/M services in chapters dedicated to those sites of service. See a full list of place of service codes at www.cms.gov/Medicare/Coding/place-of-service-codes/Place_of_Service_Code_Set.html.

Submitting Clean Claims

Many states have enacted laws that require prompt payment of clean claims. In general, *clean claims* are those that contain sufficient and correct information for processing without further investigation or development by the payer (definitions may vary by state).

- Submitted claims must be accurate and in accordance with the process outlined in the executed carrier or health plan agreement. Knowing a payer's claim requirements will decrease chances of denied claims.
- Make sure the practice understands payer rules, for example, for billing for nonphysician services incident to a physician's or other QHP's service.

> **See chapters 6 and 13 for more information on billing for nonphysician services.**

- Be aware of any updates issued by the carrier that affect billing and claims submission.

   Generally, a clean claim should have the following information:

- Practice information (name, address, phone, National Provider Identifier [NPI], group tax ID number)
- Patient information (patient name, birth date, policyholder, policy number, patient ID number, address)
- Codes (*CPT, ICD-10-CM,* Healthcare Common Procedure Coding System, place of service), modifiers, and service dates
- Carrier information
- Secondary and, when applicable, tertiary insurance information
- Referring physician name and NPI, if applicable
- Facility name and address, as appropriate

   If additional information is necessary to support a service or explain an unusual circumstance (eg, unlisted procedure code, unusual procedure, complicated procedure)

- Use the attachments feature of the electronic claims system, clearinghouse, or other claim attachment procedure as directed by the payer (eg, submission of attachments by online portal).

   Health plans may have specific instructions for submission of claims attachments (eg, inclusion of a unique identifier [2–50 characters] or internal control number linking the claim and attachment).

- If it is necessary, send a hard-copy claim with a cover letter and a narrative report or copy of the appropriate part of the medical record (eg, progress note, procedure note) to facilitate claim processing.
  - Any documentation (eg, coordination of benefits information, letter of medical necessity, clinical reports) should include the patient's name, service date, and policy number on each page in case the papers become separated.
  - Keep a copy of the claim and supporting information for follow-up of payment.
- When filing claims for patients with coordination of benefits, make certain all required information (ie, primary and secondary insurance information) has been obtained from the patient and claims are filed with the supporting information (eg, explanation of benefits [EOBs] or electronic remittance advice information), according to plan requirements.

   Claims should be submitted for payment as soon as possible and before the deadline for timely filing specified in the agreement.

- The optimum time for filing outpatient claims is on the day of or the day following the service but no more than 2 to 3 days from the date of service.
- Codes for services to patients with prolonged hospitalizations may be collected for 7 consecutive days before billing; in this case, claims should be filed within 2 to 3 days of the end of the service week. It is not necessary to withhold claims until the patient is discharged. It is important to know whether your EHR and billing systems limit how data is captured and reported for services that extend over consecutive dates.

Practices should monitor lag time between completion of each service and submission of a claim for the service to identify and correct any cause of delayed submission. Timely finalization of documentation is necessary to make sure that codes are supported by the documentation before claims are submitted. Many practices adopt policies for timely completion of documentation.

Policy should be adopted requiring completion of medical record documentation within a specified period to support prompt billing of services. Physicians must understand that timely completion of documentation is required for appropriate code selection, claim filing, and, ultimately, prompt payment. New entries or corrections to documentation that occur after claim submissions may affect the accuracy of codes reported.

Special Consideration for Medicare Claims

Many health plans receive Medicare claims automatically when they are the secondary payer. In this case, the explanation of Medicare benefits will indicate that the claim has been automatically crossed over for secondary consideration. Physicians and providers should look for this indication on their EOBs and should not submit a paper claim to the secondary payer.

Monitoring Claim Status

An important aspect of billing operations is prompt and routine claim monitoring. A defined process for verifying that submitted claims were received and accepted by claim clearinghouses and/or payers should be included in the practice's or billing service's written billing procedures. Steps may include (see the last item in this list if billing is outsourced or centralized outside the practice)

- Identify each type of report and/or dashboard feature of the practice's billing system for use in verifying claim submission and acceptance for processing, assigning follow-up activities for unpaid claims, and tracking average time from date of service or submission to receipt of payment.
- Assign responsibilities for verifying that electronic claim submissions were received and accepted for processing as soon after transmission as possible. Failure to verify claim acceptance by the clearinghouse and payer often leads to unrecoverable revenue because of timely filing limitations.
  - Most clearinghouses will send a report indicating acceptance or rejection of a batch of claims within minutes of transmission and a report with individual claim-level detail within 24 hours of submission.
  - It is also necessary to log in to a payer's website or system to verify receipt of claims and monitor acceptance or rejection. Errors and omissions may occur in transmission.
- Electronic claim submission reports must be promptly reviewed for rejections or denials. All rejected or denied claims must be investigated to determine what corrections or payer contact is necessary to resubmit or return the claim for readjudication (eg, when a payer system error is corrected).
- Claims should not be resubmitted without investigation, as
  - Resubmission of a claim containing errors is unlikely to result in payment.
  - Resubmission of the claim with errors may reset the aging of the claim in the billing system and result in late follow-up or denial for lack of timely filing.

Avoid potential denial of corrected claims due to duplicate charges. A claim frequency code, placed in box 22 of a CMS-1500 form or loop 2300 of an electronic 837 format, is used to indicate that a claim is a corrected (code 7) or voided (code 8) claim. Correcting or voiding a previously submitted claim typically results in either a complete replacement of a previously processed claim or voiding of the original claim from the health plan's record. See specific instructions from the health plan for full instructions when submitting a corrected claim.

- Identify staff responsible for claims follow-up and establish standards for timely follow-up on unpaid claims. System-generated reports are useful in identifying the age of claims.
- Policies and procedures should address communication with patients and responsible parties when a payer requests additional information prior to claims processing (eg, many payers will request information on other coverage and/or details of where and how an injury was sustained).

  Failure to respond to payer requests for information in a timely manner can result in delayed or denied claims payment.
- If centralized billing or an outsourced billing service is used, maintain oversight of performance by reviewing reports and taking action on any areas where potentially delayed or lost revenue are indicated. Examples of potential areas of concern include
  - Lag time between completion of documentation and submission of claims
  - Aging reports that show the average number of days since claim submission for unpaid claims is more than 45 days
  - Amounts adjusted or written off

Monitoring Payments

Develop a process to monitor the timeliness of all payments. Tips for monitoring payments include

- Identify payers who do not pay clean claims within the time frame agreed on in your contract and follow up on all late payments with the payer.
  — Check the provisions of your state prompt pay law and know the provisions for clean claims, timely filing, and penalties.
  — Report a payer's practice of late or delinquent payments to the proper agency because your practice may be entitled to payment plus interest.
- One efficiency of many electronic systems is automatic application of payments and adjustments. However, systems may apply incorrect adjustments based on payer remark codes. Staff should monitor all denials and reduced payments as appropriate and appeal incorrect adjustments when applicable.
- Review each EOB and/or remittance advice (electronic or paper) carefully to determine if the payment is correct.
  — Identify any discrepancies, such as changes to codes, payments (specifically reductions), or denials.
  — Familiarity with standard claim adjustment reason codes and remittance advice remark codes is essential to identifying denial reasons, such as a non-covered service, bundled payment, or provision of service not typical for physician specialty (not relevant for taxonomy code), and any patient responsibility for denied charges.
  — Find claim adjustment reason code and remittance advice remark code descriptions online at https://x12.org/codes.
  — Make certain that any denials or reductions in payment are not due to practice billing errors (eg, incorrect modifiers, obsolete codes) or to incorrect applications of an NCCI edit that does not pertain to pediatrics. If so, correct the errors immediately and educate staff members as appropriate to ensure correct future claim submissions.
- Review all payer explanations, particularly reasons for denials or down-coding. If the service provided is not a benefit covered by the plan, the patient should be billed directly (may need a signed waiver form).
  — Only bill patients for amounts deemed noncovered or patient responsibility by the payer and only in compliance with the health plan contract.
  — Do not bill patients for bundled services or other reduced payment due to the contract between your practice and the payer. Renegotiate your contract if payment is lower than costs of providing care.

> Billing staff must be aware of unique payment policies for health plans whose claims are processed by third-party administrators. For example, health plans A and B are employer-sponsored plans administered by insurance company A, but each plan has policies that may differ from those of health plans offered directly by insurance company A.

- If your system does not provide a variance report, compare the EOBs and/or remittance advice to a spreadsheet listing your top 40 codes and their allowable payments by carrier to monitor contract compliance. Make certain that the payment is consistent with the fee schedule, write-offs, and discounts agreed to by the practice and payer. Follow up with the payer on any discrepancies.

  Health plans may enter contracted fee schedules for each physician or provider individually, resulting in inaccurate payment for 1 or more providers in a practice.
- Maintain a log of all denials or payment reductions. This can be used as a basis for future negotiations or education of the payer. (Identify 1 individual who has billing and coding expertise to monitor as well as accept or reject denials.)
- Review your fee schedule to see if your practice is paid at 100% of the billed charges. This is an indication that your fees are below the maximum amount established by the carrier. This excludes services that are always patient responsibility (eg, form fees, cosmetic services).
- Review your fees annually and understand the Medicare RBRVS, using it to value the services you provide, as discussed in the Connecting Codes to Payment and Budget section earlier in this chapter.

> Tracking vaccine acquisition cost is very important. Costs may change during the course of the contract. Review the carrier contract for mid-contract vaccine cost changes (eg, some contracts will default to a percentage of billed charges during vaccine price transitions).

  Review your payment to ensure it exceeds your cost of providing that service, including time of clinical staff, supplies, tracking systems, and charges for electronic interfaces.
- When contracting with payers, be aware of payment options that may be specified (eg, paper checks, electronic fund transfers, virtual credit card payment). It is important to understand the pros and cons of each (eg, credit card processing fees typically apply to card-based payment). Some health plans no longer offer payment by paper check and recommend electronic fund transfer.

- *Health plans must provide payment in compliance with electronic fund transfer standards of HIPAA rather than virtual card or wire transfer when requested by a physician.* Agreements to accept electronic fund transfers should not allow health plans to debit an account without notification and consent. Banks may offer additional protections against unauthorized withdrawals.

Filing Appeals

Do not assume that the carrier's denials or audits are accurate. Be prepared to challenge the carrier and request the specific policy on which the denial is based. If you are coding correctly and in compliance with coding conventions, you should appeal all inappropriately denied claims and carrier misapplication of *CPT* coding principles. Develop a system to monitor payer updates and any changes to the provider agreement so you are aware of the current payment policies and coding edits used by the payer.

> Appealing a claim denial requires confidence that the claim was correctly coded and supported in documentation. Ongoing coding education and internal compliance reviews are necessary to support compliant claim submissions. Learn more about coding compliance in Chapter 5.

- By accepting inappropriate claim denials, a practice may be setting itself up to charges of abusive billing practices.
    If a practice recodes claims as a result of inappropriate claim denials, the resubmitted claim may not actually reflect the treatment the patient received.
    Here is a summary of basic guidelines and tips for appealing payments.
- When in contact with the payer, always document the date, name, and title of the payer representative with whom you have talked and a summary of the details of the conversation.
    - If a payer requests you submit a claim using codes or modifiers that are not consistent with clean coding standards, ask for written documentation of the direction (preferably via fax or email).
    - Address issues with the person who has the authority to make decisions to overturn denials or reductions in payment.
    - Keep an updated file with names and contact information of the appropriate personnel with each of your contracted payers.
    - Request an email or letter verifying the information provided and archive written correspondence containing payer representative advice and payer policies. If the carrier does not provide written documentation, prepare a summary and send it to your contact, stating that this will constitute the documentation of the discussion.
- Submit all appeals in writing.
    - Understand the payer's appeal process and appeal within its timeliness guidelines.
    - Format the letter to include the name of the patient, policy number, claim control number, and date of service(s) in question on each page of the letter.
    - The body of the letter should state the reason for the appeal and why you disagree with the payer's adjudication of the claim. Speak to the payer's rules/regulations regarding the decision and how your documentation supports payment.
    - Specify a date by which you expect the carrier to respond.
    - Support your case by providing medical justification and referencing *CPT* coding guidelines. If necessary, consult with the AAP Coding Hotline (https://form.jotform.com/Subspecialty/aapcodinghotline) for clarification of correct coding. It may be helpful to hire a certified coding expert with knowledge in pediatric coding to review your claims. (If hiring a full-time certified coding expert is not practical for a small practice, part-time employment or periodic consultation may be options for access to coding and compliance expertise.)
    - Consider sending correspondence to the carrier by certified mail to verify receipt. Document and retain copies of all communications with the carrier about the appeal.

> Note that some payers have multiple levels of appeal, with many initial appeals denied only because of the payer's electronic claim edits. Higher levels of appeal may be necessary for a denied claim to actually be reconsidered according to specific details about the service provided and the payer's contract or written policy.

- Maintain an appeals-pending file.
    - If there is no response from the payer within 4 weeks of the date of the letter, send a copy of the appeal letter stamped "Second Request."

Chapter 4. The Business of Medicine: Working With Current and Emerging Payment Systems

— If there is no response within 2 weeks, or if the matter continues to remain unresolved, contact the state department of insurance (or other appropriate agency in your state) to file a complaint or engage its assistance.

— Contact your AAP chapter and pediatric council, if your chapter has one, to make them aware of the situation with the payer. American Academy of Pediatrics chapter pediatric councils meet with health plans to discuss carrier policies and practices affecting pediatrics and pediatricians.

The AAP works directly with major insurance payers regarding policies that adversely effect pediatrics and pediatricians. If you receive denials, we urge you to appeal them through the individual payer's processes and include documentation and any other coding support, such as information taken directly from the *CPT* or *ICD-10-CM* manuals.

In addition, the AAP has posted a narrative that explains the appropriateness of reporting certain circumstances based on NCCI edits.

Knowing when to appeal a payer denial is just as important as knowing how to properly appeal. Writing an effective appeal letter to payers requires knowledge of *CPT* guidelines, CMS policy, and payer policy. The AAP Private Payer Advocacy Advisory Committee has developed resources to effectively respond to inappropriate claim denials, handle requests for refunds, manage private payer contracts and denials, and respond to payer audits. (See https://downloads.aap.org/AAP/PDF/PrepareYourOfficeforaPayerAuditSiteVisit.pdf.)

Documentation and Coding Audits

Medicare, state Medicaid programs, and commercial payers will audit claims as well as monitor coding profiles (especially E/M coding). Physician practices should also adopt standards for conducting internal audits or reviews. Internal audits provide important information to inform practice policy and procedures, detect missed revenue, protect against erroneous billing and poor documentation habits, and avoid issues with payers and outside auditors. Some key benefits of internal auditing are

- Identification of negative billing and revenue trends, including
  — Increased lag time between encounter and billing (eg, delays in finalization of documentation, delayed coding or billing functions, technology issues)
  — Denial or underpayment of new services or new or revised procedure codes
  — Significant unexpected increase or decrease in revenue
  — Inappropriate adjustments or write-offs of unpaid or underpaid claims that should be appealed
- Charge verification (eg, number of charges is equal to or greater than number of encounters, with exception of unbilled visits included in a global period)
- Identification of incorrect billing and coding practices
- Identification of payment that does not align with payer contract
- Identification of electronic system or workflow issues
- Identification of areas where new or additional training is necessary

See Chapter 5 for more detailed information on conducting internal audits.

Tools for the Pediatric Practice

Working with third-party payers on coding and payment issues can be a difficult task because there is little uniformity between carriers and, frequently, great inconsistencies within the same umbrella organization of carriers. The AAP Private Payer Advocacy Advisory Committee is charged with enhancing systems for members and chapters to identify and respond to issues with private carriers.

To assist the pediatric practice, the AAP has several available resources to consider.

- American Academy of Pediatrics staff is available to provide clarification on coding issues. The AAP Coding Hotline can be accessed at https://form.jotform.com/Subspecialty/aapcodinghotline.
- Claims processing tools, a collection of template letters practices can use in appealing inappropriate carrier claim denials, and other tools are available through the AAP Resources for Payment site at www.aap.org/en-us/professional-resources/practice-transformation/getting-paid/Pages/resources-for-payment.aspx (AAP members only).
- For information on pediatric councils, go to www.aap.org/en/practice-management/practice-financing/payer-contracting-advocacy-and-other-resources/aap-payer-advocacy/aap-pediatric-councils/.

- The AAP has created tools to assist practices with managed care contracting. These resources are available at www.aap.org/en/practice-management/practice-financing/payer-contracting-advocacy-and-other-resources/payer-contract-negotiations-and-payment-resources/.
- Members of the AAP are encouraged to access the AAP Coding Hotline online to report health plan issues. The information submitted is used to assist the AAP and chapters in identifying issues and facilitating public and private payer advocacy related to health plans, including discussion topics with national carriers and at chapter pediatric council meetings with regional carriers. The AAP Coding Hotline form (https://form.jotform.com/Subspecialty/aapcodinghotline) may be completed online to report insurance administrative and claim-processing concerns. The information provided will be used to assist the AAP and chapters in identifying trends and facilitating public and private sector advocacy related to health plans.
- American Academy of Pediatrics members and their staff are encouraged to attend AAP Coding Webinars, presented by pediatric coding experts.
- The *AAP Pediatric Coding Newsletter* provides articles on coding and documentation of specific services and supplies (eg, vaccines) with updates on new codes and emerging issues affecting coding and billing practices. Subscribers can access current and archived issues and coding resources at http://coding.aap.org.

Emerging Payment Methodologies

A process of transitioning from volume-based payments, such as fee for service, to value-based payments has been slowly gaining popularity in pediatrics. In the value-based model, providers are offered incentive payments based on the quality of care, outcomes, and cost containment attributable to their practice. The intent is to promote patient value and efficiency, but some risk is shifted to physician practices and there could be a lack of clarity as to how payments are actually calculated.

Important Considerations in Value-Based Payment Models

In value-based programs, it is not always transparent to families how the value is calculated (ie, how much is quality and how much is cost). When discussing such programs with payers, practices should be aware of whether immunizations and preventive care are counted in the total cost of care, or they may find that if they improve well-visit and immunization rates, the costs of those services are counted against the practice in total cost of care calculations. In addition, some payers will preferentially drive patients to high-value practices or have tiered co-payments based on practice performance.

Under these emerging payment models, practice viability will depend on how well quality, cost, and efficiency are managed. Examples of some of these newer payment models include bundled payments, shared savings, and pay for performance. Physician payments may be based on a combination of fee for service and newer payment methodologies. Emerging forms of health care financing and delivery models include ACOs and integrated delivery systems.

- *Bundled payments:* These are a type of prospective payment in which health care providers (eg, hospitals, physicians, and other health care professionals) share 1 payment for a specified range of services as opposed to each provider being paid individually. The intent of bundled payment is to foster collaboration among multiple providers to coordinate services and control costs, thereby reducing unnecessary utilization.
- *Shared savings:* Under a shared savings arrangement, providers and payers seek to deliver care at a cost that is below current budgeted amounts. The resulting savings are shared among the payer(s) and providers.
  - The contractual arrangement among the payer(s) and providers will specify how the savings are calculated and distributed.
  - Shared savings models may include upside reward exclusively or upside reward and downside risk. In an upside-reward–only arrangement, the provider only shares in any savings and is not at risk for a loss. Under reward-and-risk arrangements, the practice shares a reward if costs are less than budgeted but also would share the loss should actual total costs exceed budgeted costs.
  - Shared savings should include an up-front agreement to continue additional payments for ongoing support of infrastructure for future years when the payer may want to cut back on the shared savings margin or reduce as those savings plateau.
  - Quality metrics are typically tied to payment of shared savings, with physicians not meeting established quality benchmarks not receiving a portion of savings.

See Chapter 3 for more information on coding to support quality and performance measurement.

Chapter 4. The Business of Medicine: Working With Current and Emerging Payment Systems

- *Pay for performance:* In this arrangement, physician payments are based on a prospectively determined comparison of the provider's performance against acknowledged benchmarks. If the provider meets or exceeds those benchmarks, an enhanced payment or bonus is provided.
  — Benchmarks are often similar to the National Committee for Quality Assurance HEDIS quality metrics (some common metrics for pediatrics include rates of immunizations; rates of patient adherence to Early and Periodic Screening, Diagnostic, and Treatment visits; and rates of appropriate prescription of asthma medications).
  — Pay-for-performance arrangements often include the following 4 types of measures:
    ▪ *Structure:* Measures use of staff capabilities, policies and procedures, and systems such as EHR and computerized physician order entry
    ▪ *Process:* Determines the extent to which providers consistently give patients specific services that are consistent with recommended guidelines for care
    ▪ *Outcome:* Measures the effects that 1 or more clinical interventions have had on patients' health, health status, and function
    ▪ *Patient experience:* Measures patient-reported experience of care

Each type of measure may include additional subtypes, and payers may use composite measures (ie, 2 or more measures that result in a single score).

In considering whether to participate in one of these newer payment models, a practice needs to determine expected costs and utilization and assess whether it can deliver services under the projected budget. Using *CPT* codes and their RVUs will aid in this assessment. Projections can be made using RVUs of the services currently provided and projected to be provided. With these types of data, the practice can assess the effect of new payment methodologies to its bottom line.

In some parts of the country, practices can earn additional incentives if the total cost of care for their patients compares favorably to geographically and specialty matched peers. In addition, some payers are incentivizing around "care efficiency measures." Both of these are often risk adjusted based on claims data about the overall patient population of the practice.

Preparing for New Payment Models

The payment models discussed herein are already in place in some areas and may soon be adopted in others. Whether your practice provides primary or specialty care, there are steps that you should take to prepare for success. When payment is based on the costs of care and patient experience, practices must take responsibility for keeping costs low and quality of care and patient experience high. Steps that practices may take include

- Learning more about value-based payment options
- Generating and using reports of your costs, quality measurement, etc
- Learning who your active patients are and staying up to date through routine data analysis
  — Obtain lists of patients attributed to your practice by payers (patient panels) and reconcile to your active patient list.
  — Identify and agree on a methodology by which any disputes over attributed patient panels will be reconciled.

Assignment, Engagement, and Attribution of Patient Panels

Value-based payment may be based on the patients assigned and/or attributed to a practice (patient panel) by a payer. This may be limited to comparison of the cost of care for a physician's patient panel and other patients in a geographic area or other subset of patients. The cost of care for all attributed patients may lead to additional payment based on shared cost savings or may limit the amount of payments that the practice retains. It is important to understand the distinction between what you view as your practice panel and how the insurer views it.

It is important to differentiate assignment from engagement and attribution.

- *Assignment:* The patients the insurance company lists on your panel roster.

  For Medicaid managed care, every patient must be assigned to a provider (or provider practice) when patients are enrolled in the health plan. These patients may choose your practice or can be automatically assigned based on insurer algorithms.
- *Engagement:* Patients you have seen and with whom you have a medical home relationship.

  If you have an after-hours clinic and you see patients from other practices, it is essential you communicate to those patients that they are not part of your medical home (ie, they are part of another physician's or practice's panel).
- *Attribution:* Patients who fall into the denominator of a metric in which value (ie, payment) is assigned. Physicians should understand how health plans attribute patients to individual physicians and/or groups for purposes of performance measurement and cost of care.
  — Factors such as time of continuous enrollment with the health plan and number of visits to a provider may affect how patients are attributed.

— The CMS has initiated voluntary reporting of modifiers X1–X5, which identify the provider–patient relationship for an episode of care. Because reporting these modifiers, which were created for Medicare, is not required, adoption by other payers and physicians may be slow.

> See Healthcare Common Procedure Coding System modifiers X1–X5 in Chapter 2 for more information on these relationship modifiers.

To ensure you are engaging patients who are assigned to your practice, make sure you receive a panel roster monthly, preferably an Excel file, through the payer's portal. Identify new patients assigned to your practice and plan for what services they will need based on their age.

- Use the roster at check-in to make sure all patients seen in your medical home are assigned to you. This is just as important as identifying those you are not seeing on your roster. It will ensure you are getting credit for the quality work your office is providing.

> Know the insurer's rules for requesting a patient be removed from your roster. They may require specific documentation, such as number of outreach attempts by phone or mail, to fulfill your request.

- Track the number of patients assigned to your office each month. If there is a large increase, a group of patients from another practice may have been shifted to your practice. Consider including language in your contract that specifies that no panel transfers can be done without prior authorization of your practice.
- If the insurer is nonresponsive in working to ensure only patients who can be or are engaged are assigned, consider limiting the ages that can be assigned to your practice or closing your practice to auto-assignment altogether.

When considering overall cost of care or emergency department or hospital utilization, your full panel's costs will be assigned to your practice.

For HEDIS measures, patients must meet certain age-, utilization-, or encounter-based criteria to fall into your denominator. Knowing when they will be attributed (and show up on your "gaps in care" reports) is essential. See further discussion in **Chapter 3**. For primary care physicians, the cost of preventive services should not negatively affect the physician's calculated cost of care per patient.

Remember that your revenue comes from encounters with engaged patients regardless of assignment or attribution in a value-based payment model. Your practice will never have a 100% accurate assigned panel. The effort you put in to reaching this perfection must be balanced by what is being measured and how much payment is at risk.

Steps that may increase successful participation in value-based payment include

- Embracing automation and alternatives to paper handling and traditional office-based care.
- Seeking to remove inefficiencies by reviewing routine tasks and patient flow. Provide staff with incentives and an expectation to create consistency and efficiency.
- Learning about the communities of your patients—school and community resources, school schedules, average income and education of caregivers, urgent and emergency care utilization patterns—and using that information in providing care.
- Knowing the costs of the care you provide and order for your patients. Recognize that every provider within and outside of your practice must contribute to reducing the cost of care to reduce the practice's risk under new payment models.
  - Remember that care received in the emergency department and urgent care clinics and from subspecialists or qualified nonphysician health care professionals (eg, physical therapists) is included in the cost of care attributed to your cost to care for your patients.
  - Collaborate with subspecialists to ensure patients receive evidence-based and cost-effective care, including consideration of formulary and total cost of coordinated care.
- Considering options for adding nonphysician health care professionals, such as care coordinators, patient educators, and emotional/behavioral health specialists, to your practice. (These clinicians may also add separately reportable services under fee-for-service contracts.)
- Embedding clinical guidelines into care delivery through protocols and reminders.
- Configuring and using your EHR and other automated systems to promote efficiency (eg, display generic drugs first when brand name is entered).
- When considering an alternative payment model contract, seek expert consultation to help identify and, as necessary, negotiate points of concern within the contract.

Chapter 4. The Business of Medicine: Working With Current and Emerging Payment Systems

Other considerations for pediatricians include

- Recognizing that, depending on how the payment model is set up, managing a healthy population of patients may not result in significant cost savings.
- The ability to access and monitor patient population and performance metric data is important to successful participation in new payment methodologies. Physicians must be aware of not only the patients they are seeing but those who are not receiving preventive and/or follow-up care.
- Physicians need to understand the links between new payment methodologies and data collection to support quality metrics (eg, failure to report codes for screening services performed may result in negative performance measurement and lost opportunity for enhanced payment).
- In states where the Children's Health Insurance Program (CHIP) operates independent of a state Medicaid program, children covered by CHIP may or may not be included in new payment methodologies and/or performance measurement.

See the *AAP News* article, "PPAAC: Chapter pediatric councils work with payers on medical home programs," at www.aappublications.org/news/2016/03/18/PPAAC031816 for examples of how AAP chapters and their pediatric councils advocate for developing adequate financing for pediatric medical homes under value-based payment methodologies.

Accountable Care Organizations (ACOs)

As defined by the CMS, an ACO is an organization of health care professionals that agrees to be accountable for the quality, cost, and overall care of beneficiaries. In return, the ACO will receive incentive payments based on quality and cost containment instead of volume and intensity. Eligible providers are likely to be individual and group practices, hospitals, integrated delivery systems, and others who create a legal entity with a management structure able to deliver and report on evidence-based and informed care to a defined population, effectively engage patients, and receive and distribute shared savings.

The Patient Protection and Affordable Care Act of 2010 included a number of provisions that establish ACOs in Medicare, Medicaid, and CHIP. Federal regulations, such as anti-kickback and self-referral prohibitions, continue to be revised to allow more cooperation and technical support among ACO participants.

From a practical standpoint, an ACO is a community of physicians and other health care providers who work collaboratively to reduce health care costs and improve the quality of care for their patient population. Accountable care organization members typically focus on data sharing and care coordination to help deliver timely preventive and care management services to generate health care savings that are then shared by members of the ACO.

Most pediatric ACOs tend to be affiliated with children's hospitals and/or health plans. Commercial health insurers are actively exploring the development of ACOs and may support establishment of an ACO.

Pediatricians must be in a position to assess the ACO transition locally. More importantly, pediatricians need to be actively engaged in this transition to a new care model to ensure it best serves the needs of children and families and the pediatric health care delivery system.

American Academy of Pediatrics Resources for More Information on ACOs

When considering establishment or participation in an ACO, physicians can access the following AAP resources:

- Accountable Care Organizations (https://www.aap.org/en/practice-management/practice-financing/payment-models/accountable-care-organizations/)
- "Pediatric Accountable Care Organizations: Insight From Early Adopters" (http://pediatrics.aappublications.org/content/early/2017/01/29/peds.2016-1840)

For additional resources related to value-based payment, see the Resources section at the end of this chapter.

Resources

AAP Coding Assistance and Education

AAP Coding Hotline (https://form.jotform.com/Subspecialty/aapcodinghotline)

AAP Pediatric Coding Newsletter (https://coding.aap.org)

AAP Coding Webinars (www.aap.org/webinars/coding)

Charge Capture

AAP *Pediatric Office Superbill* (can be purchased at https://shop.aap.org/pediatric-office-superbill-2022)

Claims Processing

"Codes Assigned by Payers: CARCs and RARCs," July 2019 *AAP Pediatric Coding Newsletter* (https://coding.solutions.aap.org/article.aspx?articleid=2736881; subscription required)

Remittance advice remark codes (https://x12.org/codes/remittance-advice-remark-codes)

Coding Compliance

"Coding Compliance: Conducting Internal Audits"; "Planning Chart Audits"; and "Audit Tools: What You Need to Perform and Document Chart Audits," February 2019 *AAP Pediatric Coding Newsletter* (https://coding.solutions.aap.org/issues.aspx#issueid=937761; subscription required)

Health Insurance

Health insurance education resources from HealthyChildren.org (www.healthychildren.org/English/family-life/health-management/health-insurance/Pages/default.aspx)

Laboratory Services in the Office

"What Is CLIA?" August 2019 *AAP Pediatric Coding Newsletter* (https://coding.solutions.aap.org/article.aspx?articleid=2739279; subscription required)

Payment/Denial Advocacy

AAP Pediatric Councils (www.aap.org/en/practice-management/practice-financing/payer-contracting-advocacy-and-other-resources/aap-payer-advocacy/aap-pediatric-councils/)

AAP Coding Hotline (https://form.jotform.com/Subspecialty/aapcodinghotline)

AAP "Prepare Your Office for a Payer Audit Site Visit" (https://downloads.aap.org/AAP/PDF/PrepareYourOfficeforaPayerAuditSiteVisit.pdf)

Payment/Relative Value Units

AAP Practice Financing (www.aap.org/en/practice-management/practice-financing/)

AAP Payer Contract Negotiations and Payment Resources (www.aap.org/en/practice-management/practice-financing/payer-contracting-advocacy-and-other-resources/payer-contract-negotiations-and-payment-resources/)

"Application of the Resource-Based Relative Value Scale System to Pediatrics" (http://pediatrics.aappublications.org/content/133/6/1158.full.pdf)

"2021 RBRVS: What Is It and How Does It Affect Pediatrics?" (https://downloads.aap.org/AAP/PDF/2021%20RBRVS.pdf)

"Understanding the RUC Survey Instrument" video (www.youtube.com/watch?v=nu5unDX8VIs)

Place of Service Codes

Place of Service Code Set (www.cms.gov/Medicare/Coding/place-of-service-codes/Place_of_Service_Code_Set.html)

Value-Based Payment

AAP Value-Based and Other Alternative Payment Models (https://www.aap.org/en/practice-management/practice-financing/payment-models/value-based-and-other-alternative-payment-models/)

Accountable Care Organizations (ACOs): General Information (http://innovations.cms.gov/initiatives/ACO/index.html)

"Accountable Care Organizations (ACOs) and Pediatricians: Evaluation and Engagement," *AAP News* (www.aappublications.org/content/32/1/1.6)

"Pediatric Accountable Care Organizations: Insight From Early Adopters," *Pediatrics* (http://pediatrics.aappublications.org/content/early/2017/01/29/peds.2016-1840)

"PPAAC: Chapter pediatric councils work with payers on medical home programs," *AAP News* (www.aappublications.org/news/2016/03/18/PPAAC031816)

Test Your Knowledge!

1. **Which of the following is a step in preparing for negotiating a contract with a payer?**
   a. Know the specifics of contracts between the payer and other physicians in the area.
   b. Fully read and ask questions, as necessary, about the terms of the contract.
   c. Identify the payer's net profits from the last quarter.
   d. Sign all contracts before negotiating specific terms.

2. **Which of the following is a basic part of charge capture in the electronic health record?**
   a. Accurate listing of diagnoses
   b. Selection of complete codes
   c. Procedure code selection based on work performed and documented
   d. All of the above

3. **What is the definition of a clean claim?**
   a. It contains sufficient and correct information for processing without further investigation or development by the payer.
   b. No payer edits apply to the codes reported on the claim.
   c. A modifier is appended to all procedure codes on the claim.
   d. A claim is submitted within 10 days of the date of service.

4. **When you are appealing denial of a claim, which is not an appropriate action?**
   a. Include the name of the patient, policy number, claim control number, and date of service(s) in question on each page of the letter.
   b. State the reason for the appeal and why you disagree with the payer's adjudication of the claim.
   c. Request payer guidance on codes that are more likely to be paid.
   d. Speak to the payer's rules/regulations regarding the decision.

5. **Which of the following terms refers to the patients a payer includes on your panel roster?**
   a. Attribution
   b. Engagement
   c. Assignment
   d. Active patient list

Preventing Fraud and Abuse:
Compliance, Audits, and Paybacks

This chapter was contributed by the American Academy of Pediatrics Committee on Medical Liability and Risk Management.

Contents

Defining Medical Fraud and Abuse.. 91

    Fraud 91

    Abuse.. 92

    Kickbacks, Inducements, and Self-referrals 92

        Evolving Safe Harbors and Exceptions.. 92

    Anti-fraud and Anti-abuse Activities 93

    Areas of Specific Concern 94

Compliance Programs 94

    The 7 Elements of the Office of Inspector General Compliance Program 94

Steps to Developing a Compliance Program 95

    Written Policies and Procedures 95

    Coding and Billing 95

    Medical Record Documentation 96

    Retention of Records.. 98

    Document Advice From Payers 98

    Designate a Compliance Officer 98

    The Audit/Review Process 99

    Documentation and Coding Audits 100

    Preparing for the Audit... 100

    Performing the Audit 100

    Following the Audit.. 102

    Do Not Get Caught Without a Plan... 103

    Responding to Repayment Demands 103

    What if Your Practice Is Audited? 103

Can This Really Happen?... 104

    Explore the Need for Additional Insurance 105

Summary... 105

Resources.. 105

Test Your Knowledge! 106

Although most physicians work ethically, provide high-quality care, and submit appropriate claims for payment, unfortunately, there are some providers who exploit the health care system for personal gain. These few have necessitated an array of laws to combat fraud and abuse and protect the integrity of the health care payment system.

Just as patients put enormous trust in physicians, so do payers. Medicare, Medicaid, other federal health care programs, and private payers rely on physicians' medical judgment to treat patients with appropriate services. They depend on physicians to submit accurate and truthful claims for the services provided to their enrollees. And most physicians intend to do just that. However, the process is made more difficult by the complex and dynamic nature of payer coding and billing procedures, which, despite efforts to standardize variations, persist from carrier to carrier, policy to policy, state to state, and month to month.

This chapter outlines the importance of safeguarding the health care system from fraud and abuse, describes how compliance programs can protect medical practices from unintentional billing errors, and provides general considerations on how to respond to overpayment notices and inquiries from auditors.

Defining Medical Fraud and Abuse

The federal government has more than a dozen laws in its anti-fraud and anti-abuse arsenal. The 5 most important laws that apply to physicians are the

- False Claims Act: Prohibits and establishes penalties for submitting claims for payment to Medicare or Medicaid that you know *or should know* are false or fraudulent.
- Anti-Kickback Statute: Prohibits the knowledge and willful payment of anything of value (eg, money, trips) to induce or reward patient referrals or the generation of business involving any item or service payable by the federal health care program.
- Physician Self-Referral Law (Stark law): Prohibits physicians from referring patients to receive designated health services (DHS) payable by Medicare or Medicaid from entities with which the physician or an immediate family member has a financial relationship, unless an exception applies. The following items or services are DHS:
  — Clinical laboratory services
  — Physical therapy services
  — Occupational therapy services
  — Outpatient speech pathology services
  — Radiology and certain other imaging services
  — Radiation therapy services and supplies
  — Durable medical equipment and supplies
  — Parenteral and enteral nutrients, equipment, and supplies
  — Prosthetics, orthotics, and prosthetic devices and supplies
  — Home health services
  — Outpatient prescription drugs
  — Inpatient and outpatient hospital services
- Exclusion Authorities: Prohibits billing a federal health program (eg, Medicaid, Tricare) for any services furnished, ordered, or prescribed by an excluded individual. Physicians are also responsible for ensuring that they do not employ or contract with excluded individuals or entities who may furnish items or services that may be paid for by a federal health care program.
- Civil Monetary Penalties Law: Authorizes the US Department of Health and Human Services (HHS) to impose civil money penalties and/or exclude from the Medicare and Medicaid programs physicians who commit various forms of fraud and abuse involving Medicare and Medicaid (eg, anti-kickback violations, false claims, or submission of false information on enrollment in a federal health program).

Abiding by these laws is not just the right thing to do; violating them, even (for some) unwittingly, could result in criminal penalties, civil fines, exclusion from federal health care programs, or loss of a medical license from a state medical board. It all begins with understanding the definition of *fraud and abuse* in health care.

Fraud

Fraud is obtaining something of value through intentional misrepresentation or concealment of material facts. Examples of fraud in the physician's office may include

- Requiring that a patient return for a procedure that could have been performed on the same day
- Billing Medicare or Medicaid for services not provided, including no-shows
- Billing 1 member for services provided to another (non-covered) member
- Billing more than 1 party for the same service

●=New code   ▲=Revised code   #=Re-sequenced code   +=Add-on code   ★=Telemedicine

- Billing services under a different National Provider Identifier (NPI) (except as allowed by payer guidance) to receive payment for services that would otherwise be non-covered or paid at a lesser rate
- Taking a kickback in money, in-kind, or other valuable compensation for referrals
- Completing a certificate of medical necessity for a patient who does not need the service or who is not professionally known by the provider

Abuse

Abuse includes any practice that is not consistent with the goals of providing patients with services that

- Are medically necessary
- Meet professionally recognized standards
- Are fairly priced

  Examples of actions that will likely be considered abusive are

- Charging in excess for services or supplies
- Billing Medicare or Medicaid based on a higher fee schedule than for other patients
- Providing medically unnecessary services
- Submitting bills to Medicare or Medicaid that are the responsibility of another insurance plan
- Waiving co-payments or deductibles (except as permitted for financial hardship)
- Advertising for free services
- Coding all visits at the same level
- Unbundling claims (ie, billing separately for services that are correctly billed under 1 code)

Kickbacks, Inducements, and Self-referrals

Business arrangements in which physician practices refer business to an outside entity (eg, hospitals, hospices, nursing facilities, home health agencies, durable medical equipment suppliers, vendors) should be on a fair market value basis. Whenever a physician practice intends to enter a business arrangement that involves making referrals, legal counsel familiar with anti-kickback and physician self-referral laws should review the arrangement.

  Risk areas that may need to be addressed in policies and procedures include

- Offering inappropriate inducements to patients (eg, waiving coinsurance or deductible amounts without a good-faith determination that the patient is in financial need, failing to make reasonable efforts to collect the cost-sharing amount)
- Financial arrangements with outside entities to which the practice may refer federal health care program business
- Joint ventures with entities supplying goods or services to the physician practice or its patients
- Participation in an accountable care organization and/or compliance in the context of participation in a Medicaid Shared Savings Program
- Consulting contracts or medical directorships
- Laboratory payments based on volume of referred services
- Payments for services already covered by a federal health insurer (double-dipping)
- Office and equipment leases with entities to which the physician refers business
- Soliciting, accepting, or offering any gift or gratuity of more than nominal value to or from those who may benefit from a physician practice referral of federal health care program business

  When considering whether to engage in a particular billing practice, enter into a particular business venture, or pursue an employment, consulting, or other personal services relationship, it is prudent to evaluate the arrangement for potential compliance problems. Use experienced health care lawyers to analyze the issues and provide a legal evaluation and risk analysis of the proposed venture, relationship, or arrangement.

> **The state bar association may have a directory of local attorneys who practice in the health care field. The American Health Law Association is another resource (www.americanhealthlaw.org).**

Evolving Safe Harbors and Exceptions

In late 2020, the Office of Inspector General (OIG) and Centers for Medicare & Medicaid Services (CMS) published new safe harbors and exceptions under the physician self-referral (Stark) and anti-kickback laws to support value-based care arrangements and cybersecurity. Most of the changes were implemented on January 19, 2021. However, an important change for all group practices, related to the Physician Self-Referral Law, was delayed to January 1, 2022.

The rule before 2022 allowed a group practice to disburse profit shares of the overall profits of the group and/or productivity bonuses to a physician provided that the share was *not determined in any manner* that was directly related to the volume or value of referrals of DHS made by the physician. Designated health services are services such as routine venipuncture, laboratory, radiology, and therapy services for which a physician is prohibited from referring to an entity when the physician has a financial relationship, unless an exception applies. When an exception applies (eg, an in-office ancillary exception allows a physician to refer a patient for DHS provided within a group practice meeting certain requirements), the overall profits from DHS must *not be used* in determining physician compensation (ie, must not create a financial incentive to refer patients for DHS).

The new rule
- Clarifies that *overall profits* means the profits derived from all DHS of any component of a group that consists of at least 5 physicians, which may include all physicians in the group. If there are fewer than 5 physicians in the group, *overall profits* means the profits derived from all the DHS of the group.
- Provides 3 options each for bonuses and profit sharing, any of which will deem that bonuses or shares are not related directly to the volume or value of referrals.
  — Options for bonuses include
    1. Bonus is based on the physician's total patient encounters or relative value units.
    2. Bonus is based on the allocation of the physician's compensation that is attributable to services not DHS payable by any federal health care program or private payer.
    3. Revenues derived from DHS constitute less than 5% of the group's total revenues, and the allocated shares for each physician in the group constitute 5% or less of their total compensation from the group.
  — Options for profit sharing include
    1. Profits are divided per capita.
    2. Revenues derived from DHS are distributed according to the distribution of revenues that are attributed to services not DHS payable by any federal health care program or private payer.
    3. Revenues derived from DHS constitute less than 5% of the group's total revenues, and the allocated shares for each physician in the group constitute 5% or less of their total compensation from the group.

Please consult a health lawyer for specific advice on business arrangements that may be affected. This may be especially important when physicians are added to or leave a component of a group practice (eg, a component no longer has at least 5 physicians). State regulations may be more or less restrictive.

Anti-fraud and Anti-abuse Activities

Physician practices are subject to several levels of scrutiny for possible fraudulent activity, including the federal and state levels of government as well as private payers. Increasingly, these groups are sharing information. This means that a provider under investigation by 1 government health care program will likely be contacted by another program and possibly by private payers.
- The HHS OIG has several anti-fraud campaigns underway.
- Many states have enacted anti-fraud and anti-abuse legislation, and state Medicaid programs have established Medicaid fraud control units.
- The Medicaid program integrity provisions include activities such as
  — Increased fraud detection methods
  — Terminating providers previously terminated from other government health care programs
  — Suspending future payments based on credible allegations of fraud
  — Adopting the National Correct Coding Initiative edits

See Chapter 2 for more information on National Correct Coding Initiative edits.

In addition, Medicaid auditors have a financial incentive to find fraud. The Medicaid Recovery Audit Contractors (RAC) program allows states to hire private contractors to audit Medicaid payments and keep a percentage of what they collect. Because it is Medicaid, pediatricians may be included in RAC audits.
- Contingency fees for these contractors vary by state and range from 5.25% to 17%, with most between 9% and 13%.
- Under some circumstances, there can be bonuses paid that increase these fees to more than 20%.
- Some Medicare and Medicaid RAC programs have started to open audits of physician claims when an audit of a related hospital claim indicates a likely error (eg, lack of documentation to support an observational stay).

Chapter 5. Preventing Fraud and Abuse: Compliance, Audits, and Paybacks

It is always better to be prepared. Information on the status of state Medicaid RAC programs is available through the CMS Medicaid website, www.medicaid.gov. This site includes the name and contact information for each state's RAC and medical directors as well as information on the look-back period for audits.

Areas of Specific Concern

Many findings and initiatives put physician practices under high scrutiny for miscoded services, failure to adequately document services, and operating in a manner that conflicts with anti-kickback and self-referral laws. Examples of audit and evaluation findings include

- Specific areas of concern that affect physicians include billing for a higher level of service than was provided, billing for services by clinical staff that do not meet incident-to provisions, and physician self-referral violations.
- Several cases in recent years involved inappropriate payments or other incentives paid by laboratory companies to physicians for sending business to their laboratories.
- Analysis of claim data is increasingly combined across payers and care settings to identify physicians and other providers who are outliers in their billing and referral patterns to identify potential fraud and abuse.

The fraud and abuse control units of HHS and the US Department of Justice also continue to cross-reference enrollment information for the physicians and providers when there is history of enrollment in multiple states and/or programs. By cross-referencing enrollment data, conflicting information and/or evidence of prior revocation of eligibility to participate in federal programs may be discovered.

Compliance Programs

Does your practice have a fraud and abuse prevention compliance program? For many years, compliance programs for small practices were voluntary. This is no longer the case; they are now required, even for small practices, but they can be scalable.

A compliance program establishes strategies to prevent, detect, and resolve conduct that does not conform to

- Federal and state law
- Federal, state, and private payer health care program requirements
- The practice's own ethical and business policies

Pediatric practices benefit from having compliance initiatives because they tighten billing and coding operations and documentation. Practices with written compliance programs report having better control on internal procedures, improved medical record documentation, and streamlined practice operations.

Section 6401(a) of the Patient Protection and Affordable Care Act requires physicians and other providers and suppliers who enroll in Medicare, Medicaid, or the Children's Health Insurance Program to establish a compliance program with certain "core elements."

The 7 Elements of the Office of Inspector General Compliance Program

The 7 core elements described in the OIG guidance for compliance programs for small physician practices published in 2000 are

- Conduct internal monitoring and auditing.
- Implement written compliance and practice standards.
- Designate a compliance officer, contact, or committee.
- Conduct appropriate training and education.
- Respond appropriately to detected offenses and develop corrective action.
- Develop open lines of communication.
- Enforce disciplinary standards through well-publicized guidelines.

It is also useful to consult the *United States Sentencing Commission Guidelines Manual,* which makes it clear that an organization under investigation may be given more sympathetic treatment if a good compliance program is in place. Compliance programs not only help to prevent fraudulent or erroneous claims, but they also show that the physician practice is making a good-faith effort to submit claims appropriately. However, that would require the program to be integrated into the daily operations of the practice. It cannot be a set of policies and procedures merely kept in a binder or on a computer unrelated to actual business operations.

Here are some reasons cited by the *United States Sentencing Commission Guidelines Manual* to implement an effective compliance program.

- It may save the practice money if it prevents costly civil suits and criminal investigations.
- It sends an unambiguous message to employees that fraud and abuse will not be tolerated.

- It decreases the risk of employees suing the practice under the False Claims Act because employees will have an internal communication system for reporting questionable activities and resolving problems.
- It helps if an investigation occurs. Investigators may be more inclined to resolve the problem as a civil rather than a criminal matter, or it may lead to an administrative resolution rather than a formal false claim action.
- It may help reduce the range used for imposing fines under federal sentencing guidelines.
- It may influence an OIG decision on whether to exclude a provider from participation in federal health care programs.
- It frequently results in improved medical record documentation.
- It improves coding accuracy, reduces denials, and makes claims and payment processes more effective.
- It educates physicians and employees on their responsibilities for preventing, detecting, and reporting fraud and abuse.
- It should meet governmental requirements for practices to have a formal compliance plan.

Steps to Developing a Compliance Program

The CMS has described the steps to create an effective compliance and ethics program. A key aspect is that the organization exercises due diligence to prevent and detect criminal conduct and promotes a culture that encourages ethical conduct and a commitment to compliance with the law.

The CMS specifies that in creating the compliance program, the practice

1. Develop and distribute written policies, procedures, and standards of conduct to prevent and detect inappropriate behavior.
2. Designate a chief compliance officer and other appropriate bodies (eg, a corporate compliance committee) charged with the responsibility of operating and monitoring the compliance program and who report directly to high-level personnel and the governing body.
3. Use reasonable efforts not to include any individual in the substantial authority personnel whom the organization knew, or should have known, has engaged in illegal activities or other conduct inconsistent with an effective compliance and ethics program.
4. Develop and implement regular, effective education and training programs for the governing body; all employees, including high-level personnel; and, as appropriate, the organization's agents.
5. Maintain a process, such as a hotline, to receive complaints and adopt procedures to protect the anonymity of complainants and protect whistleblowers from retaliation. (In a small practice, a hotline could be replaced with an "anonymous fraud report box.")
6. Develop a system to respond to allegations of improper conduct and enforce appropriate disciplinary action against employees who have violated internal compliance policies, applicable statutes, regulations, or federal health care program requirements.
7. Use audits and/or other evaluation techniques to monitor compliance and assist in the reduction of identified problem areas.
8. Investigate and remediate identified systemic problems, including making any necessary modifications to the organization's compliance and ethics program.

Written Policies and Procedures

A compliance program should have written compliance standards and procedures that the practice follows. They should specifically describe the lines of responsibility for implementing the compliance program.

- Standards and procedures should reduce the likelihood of fraudulent activity while also helping to identify any incorrect billing practices.
- Policies and procedures should be updated periodically to address newly identified areas of risk, new regulations, or process changes in the practice.
- All staff should receive periodic education on policies and procedures to maintain up-to-date knowledge.

Coding and Billing

The following billing risk areas have been frequent areas of investigations and audits by the OIG and should be addressed in a good compliance program:

- Billing for items or services not provided or not provided as claimed
- Submitting claims for equipment, medical supplies, and services that are not reasonable and necessary
- Double billing or billing separately for bundled services
- Billing for non-covered services as if covered
- Known misuse of NPIs, which results in improper billing

- Misuse of modifiers
- Consistently under- or over-coding services (eg, using only 1 evaluation and management [E/M] service code within a category of service)

   Other areas that may trigger an audit include

- Profile of services reported differs from payer profiles of physicians of your specialty whose patient population has similar health care comorbidities.
- Repeated use of unspecified diagnosis codes or use of codes that are not consistent with the service or your specialty.
- Surgical services not consistent with claims submitted by a facility.
- Number of procedures or services reported exceeds the hours in a day.
- High numbers of denials.

Medical Record Documentation

One of the most important physician practice compliance issues is the appropriate documentation of diagnosis and treatment. Patients and other providers must be able to trust that information within shared records is accurate and actionable for the care of the patient.

   Compliant documentation must encompass not only what should be documented but also what must be safeguarded from inaccuracies and potential noncompliant access to or disclosure of information.

   The CMS has published guidance for physicians on detecting and responding to fraud, waste, and abuse associated with the use of electronic health records (EHRs) (www.cms.gov/Medicare-Medicaid-Coordination/Fraud-Prevention/Medicaid-Integrity-Education/documentation-matters.html). The CMS instructs that physicians should apply the compliance program components previously discussed to take preventive action to deter the inappropriate use of EHR system features or inappropriate access to patient information. This includes a written compliance plan.

   The written compliance plan should specify that medical record documentation should comply with the following documentation principles and guidelines:

- The medical record should be complete (and legible, when handwritten) and individualized for each patient encounter.
  - Do not allow cut-and-paste functionality in the EHR. Any use of copy and paste, copy forward, macros, or auto-population should be regulated by office policies that address maintenance of record integrity and supplementation via free text, where indicated.
  - Guidance from the CMS includes a decision table for ensuring proper use of EHR features and capabilities.
- Retain all signatures when there are multiple authors or contributors to a document so individual contributions are unambiguously identified.
- All staff should receive initial and periodic education on compliant medical record documentation, including, as applicable, use of EHR functionality, use of individual sign-on, and appropriate access to records. See "Coding Compliance Education: Standards and Procedures" in the March 2019 *AAP Pediatric Coding Newsletter* (https://coding.solutions.aap.org/article.aspx?articleid=2727149; subscription required) for more information on developing a compliance education program.
- Documentation should be completed at the time of service or as soon as possible afterward.
- The documentation of each patient encounter should include the reason for the encounter; any relevant history; physical examination findings; prior diagnostic test results, when pertinent; assessment, clinical impression, or diagnosis; plan of care; and date and legible identity of the observer.
- If not documented, the rationale for ordering diagnostic and other ancillary services should be easily inferred by an independent reviewer or third party.
- Past and present diagnoses and history should be accessible to the treating and/or consulting physician.
- Appropriate health risk factors should be identified. The patient's progress, their response to and any changes in treatment, and any revision in diagnosis should be documented.
- All pages in the medical record should include the patient's name and an identifying number or birth date.
- Prescription drug management should include the name of the medication, dosage, and instructions.
- Clinically important telephone calls should be documented, including date, time, instructions, patient/parent understanding of and agreement with those instructions, and follow-up.
- Anticipatory guidance, patient education, and counseling are best documented when performed.
- Any addenda should be identifiable with the author's signature and labeled with the date the addendum was made. The compliance plan should address what circumstances justify making changes to the EHR and identify who can make changes, requirements for amendments and corrections to an EHR, and what information cannot be changed (ie, author, date, and time of original note).
- Consent forms should be dated; the procedure, documented; and the form, signed by the patient or their legal representative. Documentation should include a summary of the discussion of the procedure and risks.

- All abbreviations used should be explicit.
- Patient noncompliance, including immunization refusal, should be documented, as well as discussion of the risks and adverse consequences of noncompliance.

> **The American Academy of Pediatrics offers a template for creating a form to document refusal to vaccinate at https://downloads.aap.org/ DOPCSP/SOID_RTV_form_01-2019_English.pdf and https://downloads.aap.org/DOPCSP/SOID_RTV_form_01-2019_Spanish.pdf.**

- Allergies and adverse reactions should be prominently displayed.
- Immunization and growth charts must be maintained and current.
- Problem and medication lists should be completed and current, including over-the-counter medications.
- The EHR audit log should always be enabled to ensure it creates an accurate chronological history of changes to the EHR. Practice procedures should describe any exceptions, including who can disable the log and under what circumstances this may be appropriate.

Coding Conundrum: Pitfalls of Electronic Health Record Coding

One advantage of using electronic health records (EHRs) is enhanced documentation of services. Documentation of an evaluation and management (E/M) service may be easier because of the use of templates or drop-down options, and legibility is not an issue. However, there are disadvantages to documenting in an EHR. When completing an audit, be aware of the following:

- Templates may not accurately describe pertinent patient history or abnormal findings on examination. Some EHRs do not allow free texting, thereby prohibiting more detailed, appropriate documentation. If a system does not allow free texting, work with the vendor to add this capability, or add any and all abnormal findings that might be pertinent in the template so documentation can be complete and accurate.
- Avoid templates and documentation tools that feature predefined text that may include information that is not relevant to the patient presentation and/or services rendered. Review and edit all defaulted data to ensure only patient-specific data are recorded for that visit while removing all other irrelevant data pulled in by the default template.
- Users should be familiar with the way the EHR constructs a note from the data entered into each field and how the system may be customized to enhance the final note.
- Only the history and physical examination that are pertinent to the problem or condition should be used in selection of an E/M code. Therefore, physicians should code each E/M service and override the EHR-assigned E/M code when appropriate.
- The EHR will usually capture all documentation, whether performed by ancillary staff or the provider. Make certain it is clear who documented each portion of a service. For example, if history of present illness (HPI) is documented by a nurse or medical assistant, the physician must document agreement and any additional relevant history. (Electronic health record systems include audit trails that may be used to prove who entered specific elements of documentation. It is important to understand how the practice's EHR system creates and produces an audit trail.)
- The use of a scribe to enter information relayed by a physician or provider must be clearly entered in each record, when applicable. Most payers require identification of the scribe that includes a statement such as "acting as a scribe for Dr X." The physician or provider must review the note for accuracy and cosign indicating the words and actions were accurately recorded.
- If an EHR system automatically transfers the documented review of systems (ROS) and past, family, and social history from one encounter to the next or lists every medication that has been prescribed in the past, make certain the physician reviews the information to verify it is still accurate and documents the review of the pertinent copied information to support the level of history that was necessary and performed.
- The same information may be documented in the HPI and ROS (eg, HPI, "fever of 102°F"; ROS, "fever"). The repeated comment should only be used as HPI or ROS, not both, based on the context for which it was obtained (eg, description of problem, question to better define problem). The EHR system may not differentiate and will count the redundant information twice (or more), leading to a higher level of history.
- Most EHR systems have integrated an E/M coding system using standard guidance from *Current Procedural Terminology* or the Centers for Medicare & Medicaid Services, depending on the code set you are using. However, it is always important to verify the codes automatically selected are appropriate.
- If previous diagnoses are carried over from one encounter to the next, make sure only those that are pertinent to the current visit are considered when determining the complexity of the service provided.
- List the primary diagnosis first because the EHR may report the diagnoses in the order in which they are documented.
- To support management options, it may be necessary to document the diagnoses being considered. These suspected or ruled-out diagnoses should not be reported by the EHR system in the outpatient setting.
- Make certain that any separately reportable procedure or service has documentation to support that it was performed.
- Do not depend on the software vendor to add codes to the system. Review all new, deleted, and revised codes each year. Notify the vendor if codes have not been revised and educate physicians and billing staff on their appropriate use.

Retention of Records

Policies and procedures should be written to include the creation, distribution, retention, and destruction of documents. In designing a record-retention system, privacy concerns and federal and state regulatory requirements should be taken into consideration. In addition to maintaining appropriate and thorough medical records on each patient, the OIG recommends that the system include the following types of documents:

- All records and documentation (eg, billing and claims documentation) required for participation in federal, state, and private-payer health care programs
- All records necessary to demonstrate the integrity of the physician practice's compliance process and to confirm the effectiveness of the program

  The following record-retention guidelines should be used:
- The length of time that a physician's medical record documentation is to be retained should be specified. Federal and state statutes should be consulted for specific time frames. In the event of a disparity between federal and state statutes, it is advisable to select the longer retention period.
- Consulting with an attorney or risk management department of a medical liability insurer is prudent to determine the appropriate retention period.
  - At a minimum, pediatricians may want to retain records until patients obtain the age of majority plus the statute of limitations in their jurisdiction.
  - Longer retention periods may be prudent, depending on the circumstances.
- Medical records, including electronic correspondence, should be secured against loss, destruction, unauthorized access, unauthorized reproduction, corruption, and damage.
- Policies and procedures should stipulate the disposition of medical records in the event the practice is sold or closed.

The American Academy of Pediatrics (AAP) provides free Health Insurance Portability and Accountability Act (HIPAA) of 1996 privacy and security manuals with downloadable templates, policies, and procedures at www.aap.org/en-us/professional-resources/practice-transformation/managing-practice/Pages/HIPAA-Privacy-and-Security-Compliance-Manuals.aspx.

Document Advice From Payers

A physician practice should document its efforts to comply with applicable federal, state, and private health care program requirements. For example

- When requesting advice from a government agency charged with administering a federal or state health care program or from a private payer, document and retain a record of the request and of all written or oral responses.
- Maintain a log of oral inquiries between the practice and third parties.
- Keep copies of all provider manuals, provider bulletins, and communications from payers about coding and submission of claims.

Designate a Compliance Officer

To administer the compliance program, the practice should designate an individual responsible for overseeing the program. More than one employee may be designated with the responsibility of compliance monitoring, or a practice may outsource all or part of the functions of a compliance officer to a third party. Attributes and qualifications of a compliance officer include

- Independent position to protect against any conflicts of interest from "regular" position responsibilities and compliance officer duties
- Attention to detail
- Experience in billing and coding
- Effective communication skills (oral and written) with employees, physicians, and carriers

  The primary responsibilities of a compliance officer include
- Overseeing and monitoring the implementation of the compliance program.
- Establishing methods, such as periodic audits, to improve the practice's efficiency and quality of services and reduce the practice's vulnerability to fraud and abuse.
- Revising the compliance program in response to changes in the needs of the practice or changes in the law and in the policies and procedures of government and private payer health plans.
- Developing, coordinating, and participating in a training program that focuses on the elements of the compliance program and seeks to ensure that training materials are appropriate.

- Checking the HHS OIG List of Excluded Individuals and Entities and the federal System for Award Management (https://oig.hhs.gov/exclusions/exclusions_list.asp or https://exclusions.oig.hhs.gov, and www.sam.gov/SAM) to ascertain that any potential new hires, current employees, medical staff, or independent contractors are not listed; advising management of findings; and seeing that appropriate action is taken as described in the compliance program.
- Informing employees and physicians of pertinent federal and state statutes, regulations, and standards and monitoring their compliance.
- Investigating any report or allegation concerning suspected unethical or improper business practices and monitoring subsequent corrective action, compliance, or both.
- Assessing the practice's situation and determining what best suits the practice in terms of compliance oversight.
- Maintaining records of compliance-related activities, including meetings, educational activities, and internal audits. Particular attention should be given to documenting violations found by the compliance program and documenting the remedial actions.

The Audit/Review Process

1. Obtain and review a productivity report from your billing system.
2. Calculate the percentage distribution of E/M codes within each category of service (new and established office or outpatient visits, initial observation or inpatient services, use of modifier **25**) for each physician in the practice. (Most billing software provides these calculations.)
3. Use data from a 12-month period to include seasonal trends and better reflect practice patterns.
4. Perform a comparative analysis of the distribution with each physician in the practice. Remember that data only reflect the billing patterns and not if one is more correct than another. More frequent oversight and monitoring is necessary for services provided by physicians who are new to the practice and may use documentation or coding guidance that conflicts with practice policy.
5. Review the report to ensure that all procedures performed are being captured and reported appropriately. For example, are discharge visits (**99238** and **99239**) being billed and is the number proportionate to the number of newborn and other hospital admissions performed?
6. Review the practice encounter form or code selection application to ensure that *Current Procedural Terminology* (*CPT*®) and *International Classification of Diseases, 10th Revision, Clinical Modification* (*ICD-10-CM*) codes are correct and match the corresponding description.
7. Review the actual encounter and claim form with the medical record to ensure the claim is submitted with the appropriate codes and/or modifiers. (See the Documentation and Coding Audits section later in this chapter.)
8. Review each medical record and encounter form (as applicable) with the following questions in mind:
    - Are the patient's name, identification number, and/or date of birth on every page in the medical record?
    - Does the medical record contain updated demographic information?
    - Are allergies noted and prominently displayed?
    - Is the date of service documented?
    - Was the service medically necessary?
    - Are all the services and/or procedures documented/captured on the encounter form?
    - Does the documentation support the procedure billed (eg, level and type of E/M service, administration of injection, catheterization, impacted cerumen removal)?
    - Does the documentation for the preventive medicine visit meet the requirements of the Medicaid Early and Periodic Screening, Diagnostic, and Treatment program when applicable?
    - Does the documentation support the diagnosis code(s) billed? Were diagnosis codes assigned for all conditions that required or affected management or treatment?
    - If using an EHR, does the documentation support physician review and personal documentation? For example, if the EHR always brings up the patient's history, is there a notation that the physician reviewed and, when indicated, updated the information? If not, it should not be counted as part of the service.
    - Is there a completed growth chart and immunization record?
    - Is the documentation legible?
    - Does any order for medication include the specific dosage and use?
    - Is there documentation of a follow-up plan?
    - Are diagnostic reports (eg, laboratory tests, radiograph) signed and dated to reflect review?
    - Does documentation include the name and credentials of each contributing author in a manner that reflects each author's individual contributions?

- Was an appropriate modifier reported with sufficient documentation?
- Is the documentation in compliance with Physicians at Teaching Hospitals guidelines and/or incident-to provisions as appropriate?

Documentation and Coding Audits

Medicare, state Medicaid programs, and commercial payers will audit claims as well as monitor E/M coding profiles. While the specialty-specific E/M profiles published by the CMS provide helpful information, keep in mind that these distributions only reflect code use and not code accuracy. An atypical code distribution may be the result of care for a more complex patient population than average (eg, patients with chronic diseases or with social and economic challenges). Correct coding appropriately identifies the risk stratification for your patients and may directly affect your payments.

Also, just because you got paid does not mean that payers will not retrospectively audit and demand repayment or withhold future payments, particularly if claims were processed incorrectly or in error according to your contract. Practices are advised to become familiar with state laws addressing retrospective audits and repayments and with payer procedures for repayment. Your AAP chapter or state medical society may be able to help you understand your state-specific laws.

Preparing for the Audit

Before using documentation and coding audits to reduce the practice's vulnerability to fraud and abuse, it is important to consider how your practice can best conduct and use findings of an internal audit. Individual practices must consider how to conduct audits in a manner that offers the most benefit and least disruption to the practice. **Figure 5-1** offers steps to consider when developing a chart audit process.

Performing the Audit

Make certain that the reviewer has all appropriate and necessary tools, which may include
- The CMS *Documentation Guidelines for Evaluation and Management Services* (1995 and/or 1997) that are used by the practice or physician.

> Use *Current Procedural Terminology* documentation and code selection guidelines in lieu of 1995 or 1997 when reviewing office and other outpatient evaluation and management services (99202–99215) with dates of service on and after January 1, 2021. See Chapter 7 for more information.

- Current *CPT, ICD-10-CM,* and Healthcare Common Procedure Coding System manuals.
- Access to or copies of all payer newsletters or information bulletins that outline coding and/or payment policies.
- An audit worksheet. This may be one designed by your practice, or one of many published templates may be used. Make certain the audit form used includes appropriate requirements for selection of an E/M service. Note that the CMS has never endorsed any specific audit form or coding template.

> Electronic audit programs may be purchased and offer automated report- and record-keeping functions. However, compliance managers should carefully review the program's accuracy periodically (eg, when codes or coding instructions are revised).

- A general documentation checklist of elements of documentation applicable to all records (eg, having patient identification, date, and page numbers on each page of a record), which can help with identification of missing nonclinical documentation and record authentication (an example can be found online at www.aap.org/cfp).
- A log to document findings for each provider (**Table 5-1**). This log should include a summary detail of findings for each encounter reviewed. The log and E/M audit worksheets can be used as teaching tools at the conclusion of the audit.
- Audit summary reporting forms—results by individual provider with encounter details (eg, levels of history, examination, and medical decision-making assigned versus audit finding); results by individual with codes and variances (eg, level of service and/or relative value unit variances); and report of key findings (eg, practice accuracy rates; strengths; areas of concern, including historical comparisons; recommendations for correction/improvement).

Figure 5-1. Preparing and Planning Medical Chart Audits

Focus

Focus audits on documentation and coding of the most commonly performed services, adherence to medical record standards, appropriate reporting of diagnosis codes, use of modifiers, and adherence to coding and federal guidelines (eg, Physicians at Teaching Hospitals guidelines, physician self-referral laws)

Agree

Make certain all physicians in the practice are in agreement with how any audit will be conducted and how results will be used.

Auditor

The auditor (eg, physician, physician extender, coder or other administrative employee, outside consultant, a combination thereof) must be proficient at coding, understand payer guidelines and requirements, and know medical terminology. Consider a team approach (eg, nurse and coder). If a physician is not actually performing record reviews, one should be available to assist as necessary.

Legal

- Determine if audits should be performed under the direction of a health care attorney who may offer assistance with developing an audit process and provide guidance on any internal compliance concerns discovered in the process.
- Attorney–client privilege may apply when audits are directed by an attorney.

Timing

- Determine if your audit will be retrospective (ie, performed on paid claims and services) or prospective (ie, performed on services and claims that have not yet been billed).
- Prospective reviews are recommended because any necessary corrections can be made before a claim is filed. Although a prospective review will delay claims submission and introduce additional practice expense, this practice may have a net positive financial effect.

Services

- Select the types of services to be included in the audit. For example, if the review will include only office or outpatient services, include services most frequently reported (eg, a sampling of new and established patient problem-oriented and preventive medicine visits, documentation of nebulizer treatments).
- Include newborn care, critical care, initial and subsequent observation, and inpatient services when performing an audit of inpatient services.

Number

Determine how many records or encounters will be included in the audit. Most coding consultants recommend at least 10 records per physician or provider per baseline or subsequent review (may be less for part-time providers). If a more focused review is required, the sample size may need to be increased. Medical records should be randomly selected for each E/M level of service and from different dates of service.

Schedule

Determine the frequency of audits. Large practices might consider conducting audits on a rotating schedule of one physician or provider per week or one physician or provider per month throughout the year.

Following the Audit

- Discuss audit findings with each provider.
- Educate providers and staff as necessary.
- If a problem is encountered (eg, inappropriate use of modifiers, miscoding), a more focused retrospective review should be conducted to determine how long the error has been occurring and its effect. This is especially important when reviewing claims for physicians new to the practice or when a particular coding guideline or code has changed.

Table 5-1. Sample Audit Log[a]					
Physician:		**Date:**		**Auditor:**	
Patient Name	**Patient ID**	**Date of Service**	**Reported Code**	**Audited Code**	**Comments**
Jane	4494	6/3/22	**99214**	**99213**	Total physician time not documented; MDM =**99213**; level of MDM was based on inaccurate level of problems addressed.
			J45.31	**J45.30**	Documentation did not support that asthma was exacerbated (**J45.31**); diagnosis was carried forward from prior visit.
Zach	2973	6/4/22	**90460**	**90471**	Physician counseling not documented
Gracie	43221	6/4/22	**99212**	**99202**	Patient was last seen 4 years ago by a pediatrician in the same group practice. Patient is new.

Abbreviations: ID, identification; MDM, medical decision-making.

[a] Blank sample audit log available at www.aap.org/cfp.

- If overpayments have occurred because of miscoding or billing errors, the errors should be corrected and education of appropriate staff performed. Requirements (eg, contractual, regulatory) for refunding overpayments and disclosure of errors must be understood and included in practice procedures.

> **The Patient Protection and Affordable Care Act requires any person who has received an overpayment from certain defined government health programs (including Medicaid plans) to report and return the overpayment within 60 days of the date the overpayment is identified. Always seek advice from the practice's attorney prior to disclosure or repayment.**

- If necessary, document a corrective action plan with deadlines for completion (eg, completion of education, attainment of a specified accuracy rate) and administrative sign-off verifying completion.
- Schedule follow-up audits, if indicated, to determine if problems have been resolved (eg, improved documentation, capturing procedures, correct use of modifiers).
- Determine if audits need to be performed on a quarterly or annual basis and follow through with audits on a routine basis.
- If changes need to be made to the EHR system, contact the vendor and discuss how these might be accomplished. Educate physicians and providers on the changes made or need for additional physician documentation.
- Establish or update written policies and procedures.
- Maintain records of your compliance efforts and training.
- As illustrated in **Figure 5-2**, audits are not one-time events. Depending on your practice's resources for conducting audits and education, your practice may choose to conduct small audits monthly (eg, 5 charts per provider), larger audits quarterly (eg, 10 charts per provider), or continuous prospective audit of a small number of charts weekly. There may be a period of trial and error to find what works best for your practice.

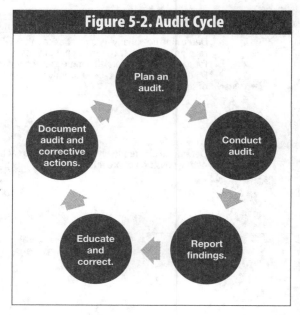

Figure 5-2. Audit Cycle

Plan an audit.

Conduct audit.

Report findings.

Educate and correct.

Document audit and corrective actions.

Do Not Get Caught Without a Plan

Most practices will never have to deal with demands for paybacks or fraud audits. Nevertheless, all practices should have a plan just in case they occur. Because time is of the essence in responding to these communications, it would be a calamity to have a letter sit on someone's desk while precious days tick away. Often, a response must be received within 30 days of the date of the request, and the paperwork demanded is not insignificant.

The first communication may be a request for repayment based on payer software analysis of claims history to detect claims paid in conflict with payment policies. It is important for all staff to be trained to recognize these requests and know to get them to the compliance officer immediately. Then, qualified staff tasked with receiving all requests for paybacks can determine the veracity of the request and, if inaccurate, act in accordance with the payer's rebuttal and appeal processes in a timely manner. Likewise, requests for records must be handled carefully and expeditiously.

Responding to Repayment Demands

In an effort to control costs and stamp out fraud, carrier claims processing and special investigative units use sophisticated software programs to identify providers with atypical coding patterns that could indicate erroneous coding and potential overpayments. For example, some carriers may flag those providers considered outliers in frequently reporting high-level E/M codes or frequent use of modifiers. They then extrapolate the alleged overpayments over several years and demand across-the-board repayments. Worse, carriers will reduce payments on future claims to correct alleged overpayments on past claims. These requests require a swift and skilled response. Usually, several thousand dollars are involved. Given the compressed timeline and dollars at stake, seeking legal advice is invaluable in these situations.

Here is some general guidance for your consideration.

- If it is truly due to a billing error by the practice, take action to correct the problem and demonstrate to the carrier how it has or will be corrected and the measures implemented to avoid the problem in the future.
- Reply in writing to inform the carrier you are willing to work with it and ask that it identify each of the claims in question as well as the specific criteria or standards it is applying to the audit.
- Make sure the practice and the carrier consistently apply current *CPT* guidelines. Reference *CPT* coding guidelines and have appropriate documentation for support. The AAP Coding Hotline can be a resource to you as well (https://form.jotform.com/Subspecialty/aapcodinghotline).
- Review your carrier contract's clauses on audits and dispute resolution as well as applicable state laws on audits and repayments with your attorney.
- Focus any overpayment recovery efforts on a case-by-case basis. Avoid unilateral take-backs by not allowing the carrier to extrapolate repayments on any or all future claims.
- Have the carrier provide documentation as proof of overpayment for each contested claim.
- Obtain and secure written documentation of all contacts with the carrier on this issue. Should a carrier payment policy require reporting that varies from *CPT* guidelines, obtain written, dated documentation from the carrier to verify that is the case. Keep this documentation permanently.
- Use legal counsel skilled in carrier contracting when negotiating contracts and confronted with repayment demands.

What if Your Practice Is Audited?

- Contact legal counsel as soon as possible. Make sure the attorney or legal practice has experience with audits. If it is a Medicaid audit, it is preferable to have an attorney with Medicaid audit experience. An audit is a complex legal process with significant consequences. It is unwise to attempt to maneuver through this process without sound legal advice.
- Designate 1 physician or staff member to serve as the primary contact with the attorney and auditors. However, keep in mind that all physicians and staff members may need to work with auditors to some extent.
- Request that the auditor provide you with an opening and closing conference. At the initial meeting, ask for the individual's credentials and job title and ask him or her to summarize the purpose of the review or audit.
- Know how far back auditors may conduct reviews, the number of records a contractor may request, the amount of time allowed to respond to each request, any rebuttal process in place, and steps necessary to appeal adverse findings.
- If the time requirements for producing copies or gathering medical records are unmanageable, contact the auditing entity and request an extension in writing. Provide a clear justification for the extension request.
- Keep copies of all written communication (eg, letters, directives, memos, emails). Keep the postmarked envelopes of all letters, including the original notice.

- Fully document all verbal communication, including time, date, persons involved, substance of the discussion, and conclusions and agreements.
- In response to requests for information, provide only the information requested and maintain copies of what you provide auditors. Before providing files, remove any information unrelated to the audit. For example, in a Medicaid audit, you could exclude information related to services provided when the patient was covered under a commercial plan or was uninsured.
- Do not alter any documents or medical records.
- Respond only to questions from the auditors; do not try to engage them in any conversations. If the auditors are conducting the review in your office, try to place them in a separate office away from patients, staff, and business operations.
- Be prepared to respond promptly to each request received. Keep a log of requests received by date, response due date, requesting party, any communication with the requestor, date of response, and outcome.
- Know HIPAA privacy regulations, documentation principles, coding guidelines, and payment policies, and verify that all supporting documentation is included in each response.
- If legibility of the record is questionable, include a transcribed copy with attestation by the author of the original document stating that the transcription is accurate and provided to ensure legibility. Any unsigned entry should also be accompanied by a separate attestation by its author.
- Copied or scanned medical records should be carefully reviewed to be sure that all pages were legibly copied (front and back, if applicable) and are straight and within the margins on the page.
- Any questions about the sufficiency of medical record documentation should be addressed with the physician or provider who ordered or documented the service prior to responding to the request for records.
  - Any corrections to an entry should be performed in a manner that maintains legibility of the original content (eg, single-line strike-through) and should be signed and dated.
  - A summary of the service provided may be included to provide more information but should be distinctly labeled as such and not as part of the original record.
- Include any policy or correspondence from the payer that was used to guide your billing and coding practices related to the service. (Archived payer manuals supportive of claims from previous years may be available on state Medicaid websites.) Clinical practice guidelines, policy statements, textbooks, and manuals may also be supportive of medical necessity.
- Send records in a manner that allows for confirmation of receipt.
- Secure a copy of auditors' contact information in case you need to follow up.
- Obtain, in writing, the expected date of a written summary of findings.

Can This Really Happen?

Conventional wisdom says that auditors will probably go after big organizations when it comes to investigating fraud and abuse, but the OIG has said repeatedly that it has zero tolerance for fraud, so, technically, everyone is at risk. Because most of the software programs used to detect unusual coding and billing patterns are based on adult services, pediatricians may be identified as outliers. As a result, valid pediatric coding may be tagged as improper and honest providers may have to respond to inappropriate recoupment requests or audits. The AAP works hard to minimize these problems and help chapters respond when state Medicaid programs target pediatric coding as inappropriate. This is an ongoing challenge.

Unfortunately, there are instances of fraud involving pediatricians. A review of past OIG reports to Congress and press releases revealed the following cases:

- A New Jersey pediatrician was found guilty of 48 counts of health care claims fraud and 1 count of Medicaid fraud for billing for more than 24 hours of services per day on 48 days despite her office being open only 3 days per week for 8 hours per day. The pediatrician was sentenced to 3 years in prison.
- A Tennessee pediatrician pleaded guilty to fraud for knowingly up-coding and billing for services that his practice had no equipment to provide. As a result, he was excluded from participating in federal health care programs for 20 years.
- A Pennsylvania pediatrician pleaded guilty to charges of health care fraud, mail fraud, and forfeiture. The pediatrician was sentenced to 8 years' incarceration and ordered to pay $7 million in restitution for submitting fraudulent claims to Medicaid, TRICARE, and private insurance companies for services not rendered.
- A Connecticut pediatrician pleaded guilty to charges of health care fraud for billing Medicaid and other insurance programs for childhood vaccines received free of charge from the joint federal/state Vaccines for Children program.
- A New York pediatrician was jailed for 37 months and fined $75,000 dollars for accepting bribes for laboratory test referrals. This was part of a $100 million fraud scheme in which 22 physician defendants have pleaded guilty.

Explore the Need for Additional Insurance

Many medical liability insurers and insurance brokers offer products to provide additional coverage for the consequences of billing errors and omissions. Pediatric practices may want to contact their insurers to see whether their current medical liability policies cover any of the following problems. If they do not, it might be worthwhile to explore insurance options for obtaining that additional protection.

- Defense coverage for a Medicaid audit
- Qui tam action (False Claims Act)
- Unintentional billing errors and omissions
- Physician Self-Referral Law (Stark) violations
- Unintentional release of medical or financial data
- Breach of computers or network security
- Data recovery
- HIPAA fines or investigation costs

Summary

These are interesting times for pediatric practices that require thoughtful preparation and ongoing concern. Learn about the fraud and abuse enforcement climate in your state. Implement an effective compliance program and follow it. Be sure your staff knows what a demand for repayment or audit notice looks like and what they need to do with it just on the off chance that something should happen. Have a response plan in place should an auditor knock on your door or a recoupment letter come in the mail. Consult with an attorney when needed. Think about the need for insurance for billing errors and omissions. Keep current with coding and billing updates.

Resources

Coding Compliance

"Coding Compliance Education: Standards and Procedures," March 2019 *AAP Pediatric Coding Newsletter* (https://coding.solutions.aap.org/article.aspx?articleid=2727149; subscription required)

Documentation

Program Integrity: Documentation Matters Toolkit (www.cms.gov/Medicare-Medicaid-Coordination/Fraud-Prevention/Medicaid-Integrity-Education/documentation-matters.html)

"What Does Your EHR Documentation Say?" March 2017 *AAP Pediatric Coding Newsletter* (https://coding.solutions.aap.org/article.aspx?articleid=2606145; subscription required)

AAP refusal to vaccinate templates (https://downloads.aap.org/DOPCSP/SOID_RTV_form_01-2019_English.pdf and https://downloads.aap.org/DOPCSP/SOID_RTV_form_01-2019_Spanish.pdf)

HHS OIG Excluded Individuals and Entities List

HHS OIG List of Excluded Individuals and Entities and the federal System for Award Management (https://oig.hhs.gov/exclusions/exclusions_list.asp or https://exclusions.oig.hhs.gov, and www.sam.gov/SAM)

Legal Advice

American Health Law Association (www.americanhealthlaw.org)

Payer Audits

AAP payer contract negotiations and payment resources (www.aap.org/en-us/professional-resources/practice-transformation/getting-paid/Pages/payer-contract-negotiations-and-payment-resources.aspx)

Medicaid RAC program (www.medicaid.gov)

Test Your Knowledge!

1. **Which law influences how a practice distributes income from designated health services?**
   a. False Claims Act
   b. Anti-kickback Statute
   c. Physician Self-Referral Law (Stark law)
   d. Civil Monetary Penalties Law

2. **Which of the following analysis of claims data may alert an auditor to possible fraud or abuse?**
   a. Analysis of claim data is combined across payers and care settings.
   b. Surgical services reported are not consistent with claims submitted by a facility.
   c. Number of services reported exceeds the hours in a day.
   d. All of the above

3. **Within which time frame must an overpayment be refunded to a Medicaid plan?**
   a. Within 60 days of the date the payment was issued
   b. Within 60 days of the date the overpayment was identified
   c. Within 6 months of the date the overpayment was identified
   d. Within 1 year of the date the payment was issued

4. **Which of the following is a recommended first step if a payer requests refunds based on extrapolation of claim data?**
   a. Request identification of each claim included in the extrapolation.
   b. Immediately refund the requested amount.
   c. Call and argue your case with the auditor.
   d. Ignore the request.

5. **True or false? Physicians in small practices do not have to be concerned about auditors because they look for fraud and abuse by only large organizations.**
   a. True
   b. False

Evaluation and Management Documentation Guidelines Other Than Office and Other Outpatient Services

Contents

Evaluation and Management (E/M) Documentation and Coding 109

   Current Procedural Terminology Guidelines 109

      New Versus Established Patients 109

   Centers for Medicare & Medicaid Services Documentation Guidelines for Evaluation and Management Services 110

Coding E/M Services From a Clinical Perspective 111

Categories of E/M Codes 111

E/M Code Components 111

   Key Components 111

   Contributory Factors 112

   Explicit Component: Time 112

1995 and 1997 Documentation Guidelines for Evaluation and Management Services 112

   I.   Introduction 112

   II.   General Principles of Medical Record Documentation 113

   III. Documentation of E/M Services 113

Split/Shared E/M Services 134

More E/M Documentation and Coding Tips 134

Teaching Physician Guidelines for Reporting E/M Services 135

   Medical Student Documentation 136

   Primary Care Exception Rule 137

Resources 138

Test Your Knowledge! 138

Evaluation and Management (E/M) Documentation and Coding

This chapter outlines the evaluation and management (E/M) guidelines for selecting codes for all E/M services *except* office and other outpatient E/M services (office E/M, **99202–99205**, **99211–99215**). Please see **Chapter 7** for guidelines for code selection and documentation of office E/M services.

For all E/M services other than office E/M services, 3 versions of E/M documentation guidelines exist, including *Current Procedural Terminology* (*CPT®*) and the 1995 and 1997 guidelines published by the Centers for Medicare & Medicaid Services (CMS). Most Medicaid and private payers allow use of either the 1995 or 1997 CMS guidelines in E/M code selection but include elements of the *CPT* guidelines for E/M services (eg, guidelines for distinguishing between new and established patients).

Separate Guidelines for Office Visits

Please see Chapter 7 for distinct documentation guidelines applicable only to office and other outpatient evaluation and management services (**99202–99205**, **99211–99215**). Codes for these services are selected based on the level of medical decision-making alone or the physician's or other qualified health care professional's total time on the date of service with no rule regarding the amount of time spent in counseling and/or coordination of care.

Current Procedural Terminology Guidelines

CPT guidelines for E/M services includes general guidelines applicable to all E/M services and separate guidelines applicable only to office and other outpatient E/M codes.

The general guidelines

- Provide expanded guidelines for topics such as distinguishing new patients from established patients, use of time in E/M code selection, and distinguishing between physicians and other qualified health care professionals (QHPs) and clinical staff.
- Are vaguer than the 1995 or 1997 guidelines for selecting a level of service based on key components. The guidelines define the components of E/M services and provide general guidance on selecting levels of history, examination, and medical decision-making (MDM) or code selection based on time.
- Includes specialty-specific clinical examples in Appendix C of the American Medical Association *CPT*.

American Medical Association clinical examples are only examples and should not be used as a basis for coding patient encounters with the same diagnosis because the selection of a code must be based on the medically necessary services performed and documented and may include clinical variations.

New Versus Established Patients

New and *established* patients are defined the same for office E/M services as other E/M services that designate new or established patient. This categorization of patients affects coding for the following services:
- Office and other outpatient E/M services (**99202–99205**, **99211–99215**)
- Domiciliary, rest home (eg, boarding home), or custodial care services (**99324–99328**, **99334–99337**)
- Home services (**99341–99345**, **99347–99350**)
- Preventive medicine services (**99381–99385**, **99391–99395**)

The criteria are as follows:
- *New patients* have not received a face-to-face professional service from the physician or QHP, or any physician or QHP of the same group practice and same exact specialty and subspecialty (eg, primary care, allergist), in the prior 3 years.
- *Established patients* have received, and a claim has been submitted for, a face-to-face professional service from a physician or QHP of the same group practice and same exact specialty within the past 3 years.

Telemedicine services (delivered via real-time audiovisual technology) are face-to-face services, even though the physician is present only by audiovisual technology. Learn more about coding for services provided via telemedicine in Chapter 20.

- Per *CPT*, a QHP working with a physician(s) and who may report E/M services is considered to be working in the exact same specialty and subspecialty as the physician(s). (Medicare assigns different specialty designations to QHPs and does not consider the specialty of the physician who provides supervision when determining whether a patient is new. Medicaid and private plans may follow either *CPT* or Medicare practices.)

- When a physician is covering for another physician of the same specialty, the patient's encounter is reported as it would have been by the physician who is not available. However, when a physician is covering for another physician of a *different* specialty, whether a patient is new or established is determined based on the rules for new and established patients.
- If a physician has moved to a different location or changed tax identification number, patients would still be considered established if they were established patients before these changes took place.

  When a new physician joins a group practice, patients who follow the physician to the new practice are considered to be established patients to any physician of the same specialty in the new practice because the patients were seen by a physician of the same specialty in the group within the past 3 years.

Examples

➤ **A physician provides an office visit to a patient who received inpatient hospital care from a physician of the same group and same exact specialty within the past 3 years. The patient is considered established at the office visit.**

➤ **A physician provided an office or other outpatient consultation to a patient within the past 3 years. Another physician in the same group but of a different specialty is asked to provide an E/M service to the patient at a group home. The patient is considered new for this encounter.**

Centers for Medicare & Medicaid Services Documentation Guidelines for Evaluation and Management Services

- Two sets of guidelines, 1995 and 1997 (see in this chapter).
- Followed by the Medicare program, most private payers, and state Medicaid programs.
- Go beyond the *CPT* definitions and guidance for selecting levels of service providing specific documentation guidance. For example
  - The chief complaint (CC), review of systems (ROS), and past, family, and social history (PFSH) may be listed as separate elements of history, or they may be included in the description of history of present illness (HPI).
  - Specific abnormal and relevant negative findings of the examination of the affected or symptomatic body area(s) or organ system(s) should be documented. A notation of "abnormal" without elaboration is insufficient.
- The CMS documentation guidelines were based on the adult population because few children are covered under the Medicare program. However, the 1995 and 1997 guidelines state that a history and/or examination performed on a pediatric patient may vary from the adult standard and yet be appropriate when considering the selection of an E/M code. As noted in the 1997 guidelines, under Section III, Documentation of E/M Services, paragraph 5:

  "These Documentation Guidelines for E/M services reflect the needs of the typical adult population. For certain groups of patients, the recorded information may vary slightly from that described here. Specifically, the medical records of infants, children, adolescents, and pregnant women may have additional or modified information recorded in each history and examination area.

  "As an example, newborn records may include under history of the present illness (HPI) the details of mother's pregnancy, and the infant's status at birth; social history will focus on family structure; family history will focus on congenital anomalies and hereditary disorders in the family. In addition, the content of a pediatric examination will vary with the age and development of the child. Although not specifically defined in these documentation guidelines, these patient group variations on history and examination are appropriate."

- The key difference between the 1995 and 1997 E/M guidelines is the physical examination component.
  - The 1997 guideline includes specific physical examination elements for a general multisystem examination and for single-system examinations (eg, cardiovascular, respiratory, skin).
  - See more in the 1995 Guidelines for Documentation of Examination and 1997 Guidelines for Documentation of Examination sections later in this chapter.

Pediatric clinical vignettes are presented throughout this manual. These, too, are only examples, and the associated *Current Procedural Terminology* codes should not be used for every patient with the same diagnosis.

Coding E/M Services From a Clinical Perspective

The definitions of the levels of service and requirements for each key component (ie, history, physical examination, and MDM) are ambiguous, and the steps defined in the requirements for selection of the code are not consistent with a physician's approach to addressing and treating an illness or problem. A physician does not enter a room and perform first a history, and then a physical examination, and finally MDM. Rather, the key components of an E/M service are performed in conjunction with one another. The MDM typically supports the level of history and/or physical examination medically necessary and is derived from the following obtained information:

- The documented CC helps to formulate the presenting problem or nature of the patient presentation.
- The level of history obtained and documented is based on the nature of the patient presentation. Concurrently, the physician is forming an impression of the problem's severity, possible diagnoses, other factors that require consideration in patient management, and a potential plan of care.
- The level of the performed physical examination is based on the presenting problem(s) and history. From the moment the physician observes the patient and while obtaining the history, the physician simultaneously is starting the physical assessment and examination (eg, general appearance). Additional history may be obtained concurrently with the examination. While performing the examination, the physician again is determining the severity or risk, need for diagnostic testing, differential diagnosis(es), and treatment plan.
- The documentation of the history, physical examination, ordered and performed diagnostic studies, assessment, and plan infer and support the complexity of MDM.

Categories of E/M Codes

There are 26 categories of E/M codes (eg, office or outpatient services, consultations, prolonged physician services, newborn care). Specific guidelines for reporting codes within these categories are described in detail in chapters of this manual devoted to E/M services provided in specific settings (eg, office, emergency department) and type of service (eg, critical care).

Many E/M codes require the performance and documentation of key components. Those E/M services that do not require the key components as the basis for code selection include those services that are

- Bundled as a daily care code (eg, pediatric and neonatal critical care)
- Bundled as a period of care (eg, transitional care management)
- Based on specific guidelines (eg, office and other outpatient, normal newborn care, preventive medicine visits)
- Based on time (eg, hourly critical care, discharge services, prolonged service)

E/M Code Components

Key Components

Most E/M services require performance and documentation of 2 or 3 of the key components (ie, history, physical examination, and MDM).

Seven Components Are Considered When Selecting the Level of Evaluation and Management Service Code

Key components: used to select a level of evaluation and management (E/M) service, using all 3 or 2 of 3
1. History
2. Examination
3. Medical decision-making

Contributory factors: may contribute to but are not required for the selection of a code. However, these usually affect the extent of the key components that are performed.
4. Counseling
5. Coordination of care
6. Nature of presenting problem

Explicit component: used to select a level of E/M service when time is the controlling factor
7. Time

Contributory Factors

CPT defines a *presenting problem* as "a disease, condition, illness, injury, symptom, sign, finding, complaint or other reason for encounter, with or without a diagnosis being established at the time of the encounter." This may be better described as patient presentation and may include psychosocial issues or ethical considerations determined by the physician or other QHP to require consideration in patient management. The nature of the patient presentation may be more extensive or different from the patient's CC (eg, adolescent girl states her reason for visit is headaches but also presents with anxiety about possible unwanted pregnancy). The nature of the presenting problem generally determines the level of history and physical examination performed and documented and supports MDM. For example, an infant with high fever and wheezing warrants a more comprehensive history and/or examination to determine the diagnosis or condition than an infant presenting with nasal congestion. This does not mean that all elements of examination, for example, require individual justification.

> **The nature of the presenting problem is defined by severity, risk, and probability of functional impairment.**

Levels of presenting problems are defined in the Risk of Significant Complications, Morbidity, and/or Mortality section later in this chapter.

Explicit Component: Time

Time shall be used as the key or controlling factor in the selection of some E/M services (those that are assigned a typical time) when more than 50% of the physician face-to-face patient and/or family encounter is spent in counseling and/or coordination of care.

See separate time instructions for services such as office or other outpatient services and critical care services.

> **See Chapter 1 for more on time-based billing.**

1995 and 1997 Documentation Guidelines for Evaluation and Management Services

It is important to note that history, MDM, and time do not vary between the 1995 and 1997 guidelines. The physical examination element is the only difference.

I.   Introduction

What is documentation and why is it important?

Medical record documentation is required to record pertinent facts, findings, and observations about an individual's health history including past and present illnesses, examinations, tests, treatments, and outcomes. The medical record chronologically documents the care of the patient and is an important element contributing to high-quality care. The medical record facilitates

- The ability of the physician and other health care professionals to evaluate and plan the patient's immediate treatment, and to monitor his/her health care over time
- Communication and continuity of care among physicians and other health care professionals involved in the patient's care
- Accurate and timely claims review and payment
- Appropriate utilization review and quality of care evaluations
- Collection of data that may be useful for research and education

An appropriately documented medical record can reduce many of the "hassles" associated with claims processing and may serve as a legal document to verify the care provided, if necessary.

What do payers want and why?

Because payers have a contractual obligation to enrollees, they may require reasonable documentation that services are consistent with the insurance coverage provided. They may request information to validate

- The site of service
- The medical necessity and appropriateness of the diagnostic and/or therapeutic services provided
- That services provided have been accurately reported

II. General Principles of Medical Record Documentation

The principles of documentation listed below *are applicable to all types of medical and surgical services in all settings.* For E/M services, the nature and amount of physician work and documentation varies by type of service, place of service, and the patient's status. The general principles listed below may be modified to account for these variable circumstances in providing E/M services.

1. The medical record should be complete and legible.
2. The documentation of each patient encounter should include
   - Reason for the encounter and relevant history, physical examination findings, and prior diagnostic test results
   - Assessment, clinical impression, or diagnosis
   - Plan for care
   - Date and legible identity of the observer
3. If not documented, the rationale for ordering diagnostic and other ancillary services should be easily inferred.
4. Past and present diagnoses should be accessible to the treating and/or consulting physician.
5. Appropriate health risk factors should be identified.
6. The patient's progress, response to and changes in treatment, and revision of diagnosis should be documented.
7. The *CPT* and *ICD-10-CM* codes reported on the health insurance claim form or billing statement should be supported by the documentation in the medical record.

III. Documentation of E/M Services

This publication provides definitions and documentation guidelines for the three key components of E/M services and for visits that consist predominantly of counseling or coordination of care. The three key components—history, examination, and medical decision making—appear in the descriptors for hospital observation services, hospital inpatient services, consultations, emergency department services, nursing facility services, domiciliary care services, and home services. While some of the text of *CPT* has been repeated in this publication, the reader should refer to *CPT* for the complete descriptors for E/M services and instructions for selecting a level of service. **Documentation guidelines are identified by the symbol •DG.**

The descriptors for the levels of E/M services recognize seven components that are used in defining the levels of E/M services. These components are

- History
- Examination
- Medical decision making
- Counseling
- Coordination of care
- Nature of presenting problem
- Time

The first three of these components (ie, history, examination, and medical decision making) are the **key** components in selecting the level of E/M services. An exception to this rule is the case of visits that consist predominantly of counseling or coordination of care; for these services, time is the key or controlling factor to qualify for a particular level of E/M service when the service is assigned a typical time.

For certain groups of patients, the recorded information may vary slightly from that described here. Specifically, the medical records of infants, children, adolescents, and pregnant women may have additional or modified information recorded in each history and examination area.

As an example, newborn records may include under history of the present illness (HPI) the details of mother's pregnancy and the infant's status at birth; social history will focus on family structure; family history will focus on congenital anomalies and hereditary disorders in the family. In addition, information on growth and development and/or nutrition will be recorded. Although not specifically defined in these documentation guidelines, these patient group variations on history and examination are appropriate.

A. Documentation of History

While the history requirements for both sets of documentation guidelines are nearly identical, the 1995 History of Present Illness (HPI) section does not state that the status of at least 3 chronic or inactive conditions supports an extended HPI. However, the CMS has published guidance stating that this is allowed.

The levels of E/M services are based on four types of history (problem focused, expanded problem focused, detailed, and comprehensive.) Each type of history includes some or all of the following elements:

- Chief complaint (CC)
- History of present illness (HPI)
- Review of systems (ROS)
- Past, family, and/or social history (PFSH)

The extent of history of present illness; review of systems; and past, family, and/or social history that is obtained and documented is dependent upon clinical judgment and the nature of the presenting problem(s). Refer to **Table 6-1** for further descriptions.

Table 6-2 *shows the progression of the elements required for each type of history. To qualify for a given type of history, all 3 elements in the table must be met. (A CC is indicated at all levels.)*

- **•DG:** *The CC, ROS, and PFSH may be listed as separate elements of history, or they may be included in the description of the history of the present illness.*
- **•DG:** *A ROS and/or a PFSH obtained during an earlier encounter does not need to be rerecorded if there is evidence that the physician reviewed and updated the previous information. This may occur when a physician updates his or her own record or in an institutional setting or group practice where many physicians use a common record. The review and update may be documented by*
  - *Describing any new ROS and/or PFSH information or noting there has been no change in the information*
  - *Noting the date and location of the earlier ROS and/or PFSH*
- **•DG:** *The ROS and/or PFSH may be recorded by ancillary staff or on a form completed by the patient. To document that the physician reviewed the information, there must be a notation supplementing or confirming the information recorded by others. The CMS now allows ancillary staff, patients, and medical students to complete documentation of any portion of the history and examination. Individual payer policies may be consistent with 1995/1997 guidelines.*
- **•DG:** *If the physician is unable to obtain a history from the patient or other source, the record should describe the patient's condition or other circumstance that precludes obtaining a history.*

Definitions and specific documentation guidelines for each of the elements of history are listed below.

Chief Complaint (CC)

The CC is a concise statement describing the symptom, problem, condition, diagnosis, physician-recommended return, or other factor that is the reason for the encounter.

•DG: *The medical record should clearly reflect the chief complaint.*

Examples: Patient is here for follow-up of attention-deficit/hyperactivity disorder following medication initiation 3 weeks ago.

Patient presents for a refill on her asthma medication.

History of Present Illness (HPI)

The HPI is a chronological description of the development of the patient's present illness from the first sign and/or symptom or from the previous encounter to the present. It includes the following elements:

- Location (*right ear, big toe, head, right lower abdomen*)
- Duration (*2 days, since last night, 1 week*)
- Timing (*persistent, occasionally, twice a week, recurrent, daily, 15 minutes after…*)
- Quality (*dull, clear, cloudy, thick, throbbing*)
- Severity (*moderate, pain scale [1–10], low grade, progressive, improving, worsening*)
- Context (*occurred when awoke from nap, while playing soccer, fell from tree*)
- Modifying factors (*took acetaminophen without relief, improved with albuterol treatment*)
- Associated signs and symptoms (*blurred vision with headache, coughing with runny nose, nausea with vomiting*)

Brief and **extended** HPIs are distinguished by the amount of detail needed to accurately characterize the clinical problem(s).

A **brief** HPI consists of one to three elements of the HPI.

•DG: *The medical record should describe one to three elements of the present illness (HPI).*

An **extended** HPI consists of four or more elements of the HPI or the status of at least three chronic or inactive conditions. *(Applies for 1995 and 1997 documentation guidelines.)*

Table 6-1. The Elements of History

History Components and Descriptions	Elements
Chief complaint (CC): The stated purpose or reason for the encounter (usually a quote of the patient's or parent's words)	Although not a defined element, a CC is required as part of the history documentation for all levels.
History of present illness (HPI): Description of the development of the present illness from the onset of the problem or symptom or from the previous encounter to the present; described with 8 specified elements or a summary of the status of 3 or more chronic or inactive conditions	● Location (specific anatomic site) ● Duration (period from onset of sign/symptom to present) ● Timing (number or frequency of occurrences of sign/symptom within the time that patient has experienced the sign/symptom) ● Quality (characterizations of sign/symptom) ● Severity (acuteness or intensity of sign/symptom) ● Context (circumstances or situation in which sign/symptom occurred) ● Modifying factors (effort taken to change the sign/symptom and its effect) ● Associated signs and symptoms (other related or additional signs/symptoms) *Alternatively,* ● Status of each of 3 or more chronic or inactive conditions (stated in 1997 guidelines; allowed under either guideline)
Review of systems (ROS): A series of questions asked to identify signs or symptoms experienced by the patient and to more clearly define the problem to help in establishing a diagnosis(es) and management options	● Constitutional (eg, fever, weight loss) ● Musculoskeletal ● Eyes ● Integumentary (skin or breast) ● Ears, nose, mouth, and throat ● Neurologic ● Cardiovascular ● Psychiatric ● Respiratory ● Endocrine ● Gastrointestinal ● Hematologic/lymphatic ● Genitourinary ● Allergic/immunologic
Past, family, and social history (PFSH): Review of medical/surgical history Review of medical events in the patient's family that may place a patient at risk Age-appropriate review of activities	Illnesses, injuries, treatments, surgeries, hospitalizations, current medications, allergies, age-appropriate immunization status, age-appropriate feeding or dietary status, pregnancy and birth history (weight, Apgar score), developmental history Health status or cause of death of family members, specific diseases of family members, hereditary disorders in the family Living arrangements; use of drugs, alcohol, and tobacco by patient or caregiver; education level; sexual history; domestic violence; other relevant social factors

Table 6-2. Progression of Elements Required for Each Type of History

History of Present Illness (HPI)	Review of Systems (ROS)	Past, Family, and/or Social History (PFSH)	Type of History
Brief (1–3 elements)	N/A	N/A	Problem focused
Brief (1–3 elements)	Problem pertinent (at least 1 system)	N/A	Expanded problem focused
Extended (4 elements or status of 3 chronic conditions)	Extended (2–9 systems)	Pertinent (1 item related to patient presentation)	Detailed
Extended (4 elements or status of 3 chronic conditions)	Complete (at least 10 of 14 systems)	Complete[a]	Comprehensive

Abbreviation: N/A, not applicable.

[a] One item from 2 areas required for established patient domiciliary and home visits, subsequent nursing home visits, or emergency department visits. One item from 3 areas required for new patient domiciliary home visits, initial nursing facility visits, observation, initial inpatient hospital visits, consultations, or comprehensive nursing facility assessments.

- **•DG 1995:** *The medical record should describe four or more elements of the present illness (HPI) or associated co-morbidities.* **The CMS has stated that the status of at least 3 chronic or inactive conditions also supports an extended HPI for 1995 documentation guidelines.**
- **•DG 1997:** *The medical record should describe at least four elements of the present illness (HPI), or the status of at least three chronic or inactive conditions.*
- *Pediatricians must review and confirm the accuracy and completeness of HPI documented by others.*
- *If the HPI summarizes the status of chronic conditions, include information such as current medications and their effects, a description of the patient's present condition (eg, stable intermittent asthma, autism spectrum disorder with improved attention and communication skills), and patient compliance with treatment plans.*

Review of Systems (ROS)

A ROS is an inventory of body systems obtained through a series of questions seeking to identify signs and/or symptoms that the patient may be experiencing or has experienced.

For purposes of ROS, the following systems are recognized:

- Constitutional symptoms (eg, fever, weight loss)
- Eyes
- Ears, nose, mouth, throat
- Cardiovascular
- Respiratory
- Gastrointestinal
- Genitourinary
- Musculoskeletal
- Integumentary (skin and/or breast)
- Neurological
- Psychiatric
- Endocrine
- Hematologic/lymphatic
- Allergic/immunologic

A **problem-pertinent** ROS inquires about the system directly related to the problem(s) identified in the HPI.

- **•DG:** *The patient's positive responses and pertinent negatives for the system related to the problem should be documented.*

An **extended** ROS inquires about the system directly related to the problem(s) identified in the HPI and a limited number of additional systems.

- **•DG:** *The patient's positive responses and pertinent negatives for two to nine systems should be documented.*

A **complete** ROS inquires about the system(s) directly related to the problem(s) identified in the HPI plus all additional body systems.

- **•DG:** *At least 10 organ systems must be reviewed. Those systems with positive or pertinent negative responses must be individually documented. For the remaining systems, a notation indicating all other systems are negative is permissible. In the absence of such a notation, at least 10 systems must be individually documented.*
- *Documentation should clarify any conflicting information between the ROS completed by the patient, family, or ancillary staff and the physician's documentation of the patient presentation (eg, ROS is negative for musculoskeletal complaints, but HPI says patient has pain in right knee).*
- *Appropriate documentation for a complete ROS (at least 10 of 14 systems) might include a checklist with documentation of "negative" or the pertinent response for each system. If a checklist is not used, documentation might indicate pertinent responses and "otherwise negative or unremarkable for all systems," pertinent responses and "all other systems reviewed and negative," or "complete ROS unchanged from previous review dated _____." Documentation of "ROS negative" is not sufficient.*
- *An ROS does not have to be recorded again on a subsequent encounter if there is documentation that the physician reviewed or updated a previous version. Documentation to reflect the subsequent review might be "ROS unchanged from most recent visit dated _____." (Tip: When history is pulled forward in the electronic health record [EHR] from a previous encounter, physicians must attest that the information has been reviewed and updated. Inconsistencies between the history pulled forward and the remainder of the encounter note may fail to represent the patient presentation and level of E/M service provided.)*

- *If a separate patient history form is used (eg, new patient history), the physician must sign and date the form to reflect his or her review. Pertinent responses to the ROS or PFSH may be documented on a separate history form, a progress note, or the signed history form.*
- *If the physician is unable to obtain a history, the record must describe the circumstance that prevents obtaining the history. In that circumstance, the history may be considered comprehensive. For example, a child is transferred to the emergency department of a children's hospital and her parents are transferred to another facility following an auto-mobile accident. In this case, if the accepting physician documents this limitation as well as any history obtained from available past medical records or the medical transport team, the history is considered comprehensive.*
- *The distinction between an HPI and ROS is often confusing. The HPI and ROS are obtained for different reasons and both contribute to the level of history performed in the selection of an E/M service code.*
- *Documentation guidelines do not directly state that a comment made under the HPI cannot be counted again in the ROS when it is repeated. However, coders and payers may refer to this as double-dipping.*

Example: HPI: "abdominal pain for 3 days"; ROS: "abdominal pain." Think about the context in which the information was obtained. If the information was gathered as a description of the development of the problem, consider it as location in the HPI. If the information was obtained to help further define the scope of the problem, consider the information as part of the ROS. Example: HPI: "location: lower abdominal pain; duration: 3 days; signs/symptoms: without nausea, vomiting, constipation; timing: not associated with eating or exercise"; ROS: "GU [genitourinary]: intermittent dysuria; constitutional: denies fever."

Past, Family, and/or Social History (PFSH)

The PFSH consists of a review of three areas

- Past history (the patient's past experiences with illnesses, operations, injuries, and treatments)
- Family history (a review of medical events in the patient's family, including diseases that may be hereditary or place the patient at risk)
- Social history (an age-appropriate review of past and current activities)
- *Like the ROS, the PFSH may be recorded by the patient or caregiver, clinical staff, or physician (or medical student if a payer follows Medicare policy). When recorded by someone other than the physician, the physician should review the documented information and correct, clarify, or supplement it as needed.*
- *The PFSH is considered a single element of the overall history.*
- *Notation of allergies without current complaint and current medications are counted as past history.*

For the categories of subsequent hospital care, follow-up inpatient consultations and subsequent nursing facility care, *CPT* requires only an "interval" history. It is not necessary to record information about the PFSH.

A **pertinent** PFSH is a review of the history area(s) directly related to the problem(s) identified in the HPI.

•**DG:**   *At least one specific item from **any** of the three history areas must be documented for a pertinent PFSH.*

A *complete* PFSH is a review of two or all three of the PFSH history areas, depending on the category of the E/M service. A review of all three history areas is required for services that by their nature include a comprehensive assessment or reassessment of the patient. A review of two of the three history areas is sufficient for other services.

•**DG:**   *At least one specific item from **two** of the three history areas must be documented for a complete PFSH for the following categories of E/M services: emergency department; subsequent nursing facility care; domiciliary care, established patient; and home care, established patient.*

•**DG:**   *At least one specific item from **each** of the three history areas must be documented for a complete PFSH for the following categories of E/M services: hospital observation services; hospital inpatient services, initial care; consultations; comprehensive nursing facility assessments; domiciliary care, new patient; and home care, new patient.*

Establishing the Level of History Performed

*The patient history may be problem focused, expanded problem focused, detailed, or comprehensive. **Table 6-2** lists required documentation elements for each level of history. To select a particular level of history, all elements of CC, HPI, ROS, and PFSH required for that level must be met.*

For example, consider a 13-year-old established patient.

- *Problem focused: "Here for stomachache. Left upper quadrant pain for 2 days."*
  - *CC: left upper quadrant*
  - *HPI: location—left upper stomachache, duration—2 days*

- *Expanded problem focused: "Here for stomachache. Generalized abdominal pain has hurt for 2 days. No diarrhea or constipation."*
  - *CC: stomachache*
  - *HPI: location—abdomen, right lower quadrant, duration—2 days*
  - *ROS: gastrointestinal (GI)*
- *Detailed: "Here for stomachache with generalized abdominal pain. Stomach has hurt on and off for a few months. Pain occurs primarily after eating, worsening over the last few days. No fever, diarrhea, or vomiting; last menstrual period 2 weeks ago and normal. Takes no medication; no known allergies."*
  - *CC: stomachache*
  - *HPI: location—abdomen, timing—on and off, duration—few months, context—after eating, severity—worsening*
  - *ROS: constitutional, GI, GU*
  - *PFSH: past medical—no medications, no allergies*
- *Comprehensive: "Here for stomachache. Complains of generalized abdominal pain on and off for a few months. Pain occurs primarily after eating, worsening over the last few days. No fever, diarrhea, or vomiting; last menstrual period 2 weeks ago and normal; no rashes; no injuries; all other systems reviewed and negative. Takes no medication, no known allergies, no exposure to illness, has excellent grades and enjoys school. Family history negative for abdominal problems or headaches."*
  - *CC: stomachache*
  - *HPI: location—abdomen, timing—on and off, duration—few months, context—after eating, severity—worsening*
  - *ROS: constitutional, GI, GU, skin, all others negative (indicates review of at least 10 of 14 systems)*
  - *PFSH: medical—no medications, no allergies, no exposure to illness; family—negative for abdominal or headache; social—excellent grades, enjoys school*

B. Documentation of Examination

The main distinction between the 1995 and 1997 documentation guidelines lies in the documentation of examination. **Table 6-3** *outlines the differences.*

Table 6-3. Comparison of 1995 and 1997 Levels of Physical Examination

Level of Examination	1995 Guidelines	1997 Guidelines
Problem focused	Limited examination of the affected area or system	Performance and documentation of 1–5 elements identified by a bullet (●) in 1 or more areas or systems
Expanded problem focused	Limited examination of the affected body area or organ system and other symptomatic or related organ system(s)	Performance and documentation of at least 6 elements identified by a bullet (●) in 1 or more areas or systems
Detailed	Extended examination of the affected body area(s) and other symptomatic or related organ system(s)	Multisystem examination—Performance and documentation of at least 2 elements identified by a bullet (●) in at least 6 areas or systems or at least 12 elements identified by a bullet (●) in at least 2 areas or systems Single organ system examination—at least 12 elements identified by a bullet (●) (Eye and psychiatric examinations require only 9.)
Comprehensive	General multisystem examination (requires 8 or more organ systems) or a complete examination of a single organ system	Multisystem examination—Examination of at least 9 organ systems or body areas with performance of all elements identified by a bullet (●) in each area/system examined. Documentation is expected for at least 2 elements identified by a bullet (●) of each area(s) or system(s). Single organ system examination—Performance of all elements identified by a bullet (●) and documentation of every element in each box with a shaded border and at least one element in a box with an unshaded border

1995 Guidelines for Documentation of Examination

The levels of E/M services are based on four types of examination that are defined as follows:

- **Problem Focused**—a limited examination of the affected body area or organ system.
- **Expanded Problem Focused**—a limited examination of the affected body area or organ system and other symptomatic or related organ system(s).
- **Detailed**—an extended examination of the affected body area(s) and other symptomatic or related organ system(s).
- **Comprehensive**—a general multisystem examination or complete examination of a single organ system.

For purposes of examination, the following **body areas** are recognized:

- Head, including face
- Neck
- Chest, including breasts and axillae
- Abdomen
- Genitalia, groin, buttocks
- Back, including spine
- Each extremity

For purposes of examination, the following **organ systems** are recognized:

- Constitutional (eg, vital signs, general appearance)
- Eyes
- Ears, nose, mouth, throat
- Cardiovascular
- Respiratory
- Gastrointestinal
- Genitourinary
- Musculoskeletal
- Skin
- Neurological
- Psychiatric
- Hematologic/lymphatic/immunologic

The extent of examinations performed and documented is dependent upon clinical judgment and the nature of the presenting problem(s). They range from limited examinations of single body areas to general multisystem or complete single organ system examinations.

- **•DG:** *Specific abnormal and relevant negative findings of the examination of the affected or symptomatic body area(s) or organ system(s) should be documented. A notation of "abnormal" without elaboration is insufficient.*
- **•DG:** *Abnormal or unexpected findings of the examination of the unaffected or asymptomatic body area(s) or organ system(s) should be described.*
- **•DG:** *A brief statement or notation indicating "negative" or "normal" is sufficient to document normal findings related to unaffected area(s) or asymptomatic organ system(s).*
- **•DG:** *The medical record for a general multisystem examination should include findings about eight or more of the 12 organ systems.*

There is no clear guidance on the distinction between a limited examination versus an extended examination. Unfortunately, this leaves room for subjectivity. The CMS does not offer guidance on this issue; however, some audit programs have attempted to quantify this.

1997 Guidelines for Documentation of Examination

The levels of E/M services are based on four types of examination

- **Problem Focused**—a limited examination of the affected body area or organ system.
- **Expanded Problem Focused**—a limited examination of the affected body area or organ system and any other symptomatic or related body area(s) or organ system(s).
- **Detailed**—an extended examination of the affected body area(s) or organ system(s) and any other symptomatic or related body area(s) or organ system(s).
- **Comprehensive**—a general multisystem examination or complete examination of a single organ system and other symptomatic or related body area(s) or organ system(s).

These types of examinations have been defined for general multisystem and the following single organ systems:

- Cardiovascular
- Ears, nose, mouth, throat
- Eyes
- Genitourinary (female)
- Genitourinary (male)
- Hematologic/lymphatic/immunologic
- Musculoskeletal
- Neurological
- Psychiatric
- Respiratory
- Skin

A general multisystem examination or a single organ system examination may be performed by any physician regardless of specialty. The type (general multisystem or single organ system) and content of examination are selected by the examining physician and are based upon clinical judgment, the patient's history, and the nature of the presenting problem(s).

The content and documentation requirements for each type and level of the 1997 examination are summarized below and described in detail in tables beginning on page 121. In the tables, organ systems and body areas recognized by *CPT* for purposes of describing examinations are shown in the left column. The content, or individual elements, of the examination pertaining to that body area or organ system are identified by bullets (●) in the right column.

Parenthetical examples, "(eg, ...)", have been used for clarification and to provide guidance regarding documentation. Documentation for each element must satisfy any numeric requirements (such as "Measurement of *any three of the following seven...*") included in the description of the element. Elements with multiple components but with no specific numeric requirement (such as "Examination of *liver* and *spleen*") require documentation of at least one component. It is possible for a given examination to be expanded beyond what is defined here. When that occurs, findings related to the additional systems and/or areas should be documented.

- **•DG:** *Specific abnormal and relevant negative findings of the examination of the affected or symptomatic body area(s) or organ system(s) should be documented. A notation of "abnormal" without elaboration is insufficient.*
- **•DG:** *Abnormal or unexpected findings of the examination of any asymptomatic body area(s) or organ system(s) should be described.*
- **•DG:** *A brief statement or notation indicating "negative" or "normal" is sufficient to document normal findings related to unaffected area(s) or asymptomatic organ system(s).*

General Multisystem Examinations

General multisystem examinations are described in detail in **Table 6-4.**

To qualify for a given level of 1997 multisystem examination, the following content and documentation requirements should be met:

- **Problem-Focused Examination**—should include performance and documentation of one to five elements identified by a bullet (●) in one or more organ system(s) or body area(s).
- **Expanded Problem-Focused Examination**—should include performance and documentation of at least six elements identified by a bullet in one or more organ system(s) or body area(s).
- **Detailed Examination**—should include at least six organ systems or body areas. For each system/area selected, performance and documentation of at least two elements identified by a bullet is expected. Alternatively, a detailed examination may include performance and documentation of at least 12 elements identified by a bullet in two or more organ systems or body areas.
- **Comprehensive Examination**—should include at least nine organ systems or body areas. For each system/area selected, all elements of the examination identified by a bullet should be performed, unless specific directions limit the content of the examination. For each of nine areas/systems, documentation of at least two elements identified by a bullet is expected.

Table 6-4. General Multisystem Examination—1997 Documentation Guidelines	
System/Body Area	**Elements of Examination**
Constitutional	• Measurement of **any three of the following seven** vital signs: 1) sitting or standing blood pressure, 2) supine blood pressure, 3) pulse rate and regularity, 4) respiration, 5) temperature, 6) height, 7) weight (may be measured and recorded by ancillary staff) • General appearance of patient (eg, development, nutrition, body habitus, deformities, attention to grooming)
Eyes	• Inspection of conjunctivae and lids • Examination of pupils and irises (eg, reaction to light and accommodation, size and symmetry) • Ophthalmoscopic examination of optic discs (eg, size, C/D ratio, appearance) and posterior segments (eg, vessel changes, exudates, hemorrhages)
Ears, Nose, Mouth, and Throat	• External inspection of ears and nose (eg, overall appearance, scars, lesions, masses) • Otoscopic examination of external auditory canals and tympanic membranes • Assessment of hearing (eg, whispered voice, finger rub, tuning fork) • Inspection of nasal mucosa, septum, and turbinates • Inspection of lips, teeth, and gums • Examination of oropharynx: oral mucosa, salivary glands, hard and soft palates, tongue, tonsils, and posterior pharynx
Neck	• Examination of neck (eg, masses, overall appearance, symmetry, tracheal position, crepitus) • Examination of thyroid (eg, enlargement, tenderness, mass)
Respiratory	• Assessment of respiratory effort (eg, intercostal retractions, use of accessory muscles, diaphragmatic movement) • Percussion of chest (eg, dullness, flatness, hyperresonance) • Palpation of chest (eg, tactile fremitus) • Auscultation of lungs (eg, breath sounds, adventitious sounds, rubs)
Cardiovascular	• Palpation of heart (eg, location, size, thrills) • Auscultation of heart with notation of abnormal sounds and murmurs Examination of: • Carotid arteries (eg, pulse amplitude, bruits) • Abdominal aorta (eg, size, bruits) • Femoral arteries (eg, pulse amplitude, bruits) • Pedal pulses (eg, pulse amplitude) • Extremities for edema and/or varicosities
Chest (Breasts)	• Inspection of breasts (eg, symmetry, nipple discharge) • Palpation of breasts and axillae (eg, masses or lumps, tenderness)
Gastrointestinal (Abdomen)	• Examination of abdomen with notation of presence of masses or tenderness • Examination of liver and spleen • Examination for presence or absence of hernia • Examination (when indicated) of anus, perineum, and rectum, including sphincter tone, presence of hemorrhoids, rectal masses • Obtain stool sample for occult blood test when indicated
Genitourinary	*Male* • Examination of the scrotal contents (eg, hydrocele, spermatocele, tenderness of cord, testicular mass) • Examination of the penis • Digital rectal examination of prostate gland (eg, size, symmetry, nodularity, tenderness) *Female* • Pelvic examination (with or without specimen collection for smears and cultures) including • Examination of external genitalia (eg, general appearance, hair distribution, lesions) and vagina (eg, general appearance, estrogen effect, discharge, lesions, pelvic support, cystocele, rectocele) • Examination of urethra (eg, masses, tenderness, scarring) • Examination of bladder (eg, fullness, masses, tenderness)

●=New code   ▲=Revised code   #=Re-sequenced code   +=Add-on code   ★=Telemedicine

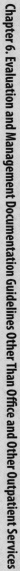

Chapter 6. Evaluation and Management Documentation Guidelines Other Than Office and Other Outpatient Services

Table 6-4 (*continued*)	
System/Body Area	**Elements of Examination**
Genitourinary (*continued*)	● Cervix (eg, general appearance, lesions, discharge) ● Uterus (eg, size, contour, position, mobility, tenderness, consistency, descent, or support) ● Adnexa/parametria (eg, masses, tenderness, organomegaly, nodularity)
Lymphatic	Palpation of lymph nodes in **two or more** areas: ● Neck ● Axillae ● Groin ● Other
Musculoskeletal	● Examination of gait and station ● Inspection and/or palpation of digits and nails (eg, clubbing, cyanosis, inflammatory conditions, petechiae, ischemia, infections, nodes) Examination of joints, bones, and muscles of **one or more of the following six areas:** 1) head and neck; 2) spine, ribs, and pelvis; 3) right upper extremity; 4) left upper extremity; 5) right lower extremity; and 6) left lower extremity. The examination of a given area includes: ● Inspection and/or palpation with notation of presence of any misalignment, asymmetry, crepitation, defects, tenderness, masses, effusions ● Assessment of range of motion with notation of any pain, crepitation, or contracture ● Assessment of stability with notation of any dislocation (luxation), subluxation, or laxity ● Assessment of muscle strength and tone (eg, flaccid, cog wheel, spastic) with notation of any atrophy or abnormal movements
Skin	● Inspection of skin and subcutaneous tissue (eg, rashes, lesions, ulcers) ● Palpation of skin and subcutaneous tissue (eg, induration, subcutaneous nodules, tightening)
Neurological	● Test cranial nerves with notation of any deficits ● Examination of deep tendon reflexes with notation of pathological reflexes (eg, Babinski) ● Examination of sensation (eg, by touch, pin, vibration, proprioception)
Psychiatric	● Description of patient's judgment and insight Brief assessment of mental status including: ● Orientation to time, place, and person ● Recent and remote memory ● Mood and affect (eg, depression, anxiety, agitation)

Single Organ System Examinations

The single organ system examinations recognized by *CPT* are described in detail (see **tables 6-5 through 6-14**). Variations among these examinations in the organ systems and body areas identified in the left columns and in the elements of the examinations described in the right columns reflect differing emphases among specialties. To qualify for a given level of single organ system examination, the following content and documentation requirements should be met:

● **Problem-Focused Examination**—should include performance and documentation of one to five elements identified by a bullet, whether in a shaded or unshaded area.

● **Expanded Problem-Focused Examination**—should include performance and documentation of at least six elements identified by a bullet, whether in a shaded or unshaded area.

● **Detailed Examination**—examinations other than the eye and psychiatric examinations should include performance and documentation of at least 12 elements identified by a bullet, whether in a shaded or unshaded area.

— Eye and psychiatric examinations should include the performance and documentation of at least 9 elements identified by a bullet, whether in a shaded or unshaded area.

● **Comprehensive Examination**—should include performance of all elements identified by a bullet, whether in a shaded or unshaded area. Documentation of every element in a shaded area and at least one element in each category in each unshaded area is expected.

Table 6-5. Cardiovascular Examination

System/Body Area	Elements of Examination
Constitutional	● Measurement of **any three of the following seven** vital signs: 1) sitting or standing blood pressure, 2) supine blood pressure, 3) pulse rate and regularity, 4) respiration, 5) temperature, 6) height, 7) weight (may be measured and recorded by ancillary staff) ● General appearance of patient (eg, development, nutrition, body habitus, deformities, attention to grooming)
Eyes	● Inspection of conjunctivae and lids (eg, xanthelasma)
Ears, Nose, Mouth, and Throat	● Inspection of teeth, gums, and palate ● Inspection of oral mucosa with notation of presence of pallor or cyanosis
Neck	● Examination of jugular veins (eg, distension; a, v, or cannon a waves) ● Examination of thyroid (eg, enlargement, tenderness, mass)
Respiratory	● Assessment of respiratory effort (eg, intercostal retractions, use of accessory muscles, diaphragmatic movement) ● Auscultation of lungs (eg, breath sounds, adventitious sounds, rubs)
Cardiovascular	● Palpation of heart (eg, location, size, and forcefulness of the point of maximal impact; thrills; lifts; palpable S3 or S4) ● Auscultation of heart including sounds, abnormal sounds, and murmurs ● Measurement of blood pressure in two or more extremities when indicated (eg, aortic dissection, coarctation) Examination of ● Carotid arteries (eg, waveform, pulse amplitude, bruits, apical-carotid delay) ● Abdominal aorta (eg, size, bruits) ● Femoral arteries (eg, pulse amplitude, bruits) ● Pedal pulses (eg, pulse amplitude) ● Extremities for peripheral edema and/or varicosities
Gastrointestinal (Abdomen)	● Examination of abdomen with notation of presence of masses or tenderness ● Examination of liver and spleen ● Obtain stool sample for occult blood from patients who are being considered for thrombolytic or anti-coagulant therapy
Musculoskeletal	● Examination of the back with notation of kyphosis or scoliosis ● Examination of gait with notation of ability to undergo exercise testing and/or participation in exercise programs ● Assessment of muscle strength and tone (eg, flaccid, cog wheel, spastic) with notation of any atrophy and abnormal movements
Extremities	● Inspection and palpation of digits and nails (eg, clubbing, cyanosis, inflammation, petechiae, ischemia, infections, Osler's nodes)
Skin	● Inspection and/or palpation of skin and subcutaneous tissue (eg, stasis dermatitis, ulcers, scars, xanthomas)
Neurological/ Psychiatric	Brief assessment of mental status including: ● Orientation to time, place, and person ● Mood and affect (eg, depression, anxiety, agitation)

System/Body Areas Not Required: Head and Face, Chest (Breasts), Genitourinary (Abdomen), and Lymphatic

CPT copyright 2021 American Medical Association. All rights reserved. ●=New code ▲=Revised code #=Re-sequenced code +=Add-on code ★=Telemedicine

Chapter 6. Evaluation and Management Documentation Guidelines Other Than Office and Other Outpatient Services

Table 6-6. Ear, Nose, and Throat Examination

System/Body Area	Elements of Examination
Constitutional	• Measurement of **any three of the following seven** vital signs: 1) sitting or standing blood pressure, 2) supine blood pressure, 3) pulse rate and regularity, 4) respiration, 5) temperature, 6) height, 7) weight (may be measured and recorded by ancillary staff) • General appearance of patient (eg, development, nutrition, body habitus, deformities, attention to grooming) • Assessment of ability to communicate (eg, use of sign language or other communication aids) and quality of voice
Head and Face	• Inspection of head and face (eg, overall appearance, scars, lesions, and masses) • Palpation and/or percussion of face with notation of presence or absence of sinus tenderness • Examination of salivary glands • Assessment of facial strength
Eyes	• Test ocular motility including primary gaze alignment
Ears, Nose, Mouth, and Throat	• Otoscopic examination of external auditory canals and tympanic membranes including pneumo-otoscopy with notation of mobility of membranes • Assessment of hearing with tuning forks and clinical speech reception thresholds (eg, whispered voice, finger rub) • External inspection of ears and nose (eg, overall appearance, scars, lesions, and masses) • Inspection of nasal mucosa, septum, and turbinates • Inspection of lips, teeth, and gums • Examination of oropharynx: oral mucosa, hard and soft palates, tongue, tonsils, and posterior pharynx (eg, asymmetry, lesions, hydration of mucosal surfaces) • Inspection of pharyngeal walls and pyriform sinuses (eg, pooling of saliva, asymmetry, lesions) • Examination by mirror of larynx including the condition of the epiglottis, false vocal cords, true vocal cords, and mobility of larynx (use of mirror not required in children) • Examination by mirror of nasopharynx including appearance of the mucosa, adenoids, posterior choanae, and eustachian tubes (use of mirror not required in children)
Neck	• Examination of neck (eg, masses, overall appearance, symmetry, tracheal position, crepitus) • Examination of thyroid (eg, enlargement, tenderness, mass)
Respiratory	• Inspection of chest including symmetry, expansion, and/or assessment of respiratory effort (eg, intercostal retractions, use of accessory muscles, diaphragmatic movement) • Auscultation of lungs (eg, breath sounds, adventitious sounds, rubs)
Cardiovascular	• Auscultation of heart with notation of abnormal sounds and murmurs • Examination of peripheral vascular system by observation (eg, swelling, varicosities) and palpation (eg, pulses, temperature, edema, tenderness)
Lymphatic	• Palpation of lymph nodes in neck, axillae, groin, and/or other location
Neurological/ Psychiatric	• Test cranial nerves with notation of any deficits Brief assessment of mental status including: • Orientation to time, place, and person • Mood and affect (eg, depression, anxiety, agitation)

System/Body Areas Not Required: Chest (Breasts), Gastrointestinal (Abdomen), Genitourinary, Musculoskeletal, Extremities, and Skin

●=New code   ▲=Revised code   #=Re-sequenced code   +=Add-on code   ★=Telemedicine

Table 6-7. Eye Examination

System/Body Area	Elements of Examination
Eyes	• Test visual acuity (does not include determination of refractive error) • Gross visual field testing by confrontation • Test ocular motility including primary gaze alignment • Inspection of bulbar and palpebral conjunctivae • Examination of ocular adnexae including lids (eg, ptosis or lagophthalmos), lacrimal glands, lacrimal drainage, orbits, and preauricular lymph nodes • Examination of pupils and irises including shape, direct and consensual reaction (afferent pupil), size (eg, anisocoria), and morphology • Slit lamp examination of the corneas including epithelium, stroma, endothelium, and tear film • Slit lamp examination of the anterior chambers including depth, cells, and flare • Slit lamp examination of the lenses including clarity, anterior and posterior capsule, cortex, and nucleus • Measurement of intraocular pressures (except in children and patients with trauma or infectious disease) Ophthalmoscopic examination through dilated pupils (unless contraindicated) of: • Optic discs including size, C/D ratio, appearance (eg, atrophy, cupping, tumor elevation), and nerve fiber layer • Posterior segments including retina and vessels (eg, exudates and hemorrhages)
Neurological/ Psychiatric	Brief assessment of mental status including: • Orientation to time, place, and person • Mood and affect (eg, depression, anxiety, agitation)

System/Body Areas Not Required: Constitutional; Head and Face; Ears, Nose, Mouth, and Throat; Neck; Respiratory; Cardiovascular; Chest (Breasts); Genitourinary; Lymphatic; Musculoskeletal; Extremities; and Skin Extremities and Skin

Table 6-8. Genitourinary Examination

System/Body Area	Elements of Examination
Constitutional	• Measurement of **any three of the following seven** vital signs: 1) sitting or standing blood pressure, 2) supine blood pressure, 3) pulse rate and regularity, 4) respiration, 5) temperature, 6) height, 7) weight (may be measured and recorded by ancillary staff) • General appearance of patient (eg, development, nutrition, body habitus, deformities, attention to grooming)
Neck	• Examination of neck (eg, masses, overall appearance, symmetry, tracheal position, crepitus) • Examination of thyroid (eg, enlargement, tenderness, mass)
Respiratory	• Assessment of respiratory effort (eg, intercostal retractions, use of accessory muscles, diaphragmatic movement) • Auscultation of lungs (eg, breath sounds, adventitious sounds, rubs)
Cardiovascular	• Auscultation of heart with notation of abnormal sounds and murmurs • Examination of peripheral vascular system by observation (eg, swelling, varicosities) and palpation (eg, pulses, temperature, edema, tenderness)
Chest (Breasts)	[See Genitourinary (female)]
Gastrointestinal (Abdomen)	• Examination of abdomen with notation of presence of masses or tenderness • Examination for presence or absence of hernia • Examination of liver and spleen • Obtain stool sample for occult blood test when indicated
Genitourinary	*Male* • Inspection of anus and perineum Examination (with or without specimen collection for smears and cultures) of genitalia including: • Scrotum (eg, lesions, cysts, rashes) • Epididymides (eg, size, symmetry, masses) • Testes (eg, size, symmetry, masses) • Urethral meatus (eg, size, location, lesions, discharge) • Penis (eg, lesions, presence or absence of foreskin, foreskin retractability, plaque, masses, scarring, deformities)

● =New code   ▲ =Revised code   # =Re-sequenced code   + =Add-on code   ★ =Telemedicine

Table 6-8 (*continued*)

System/Body Area	Elements of Examination
Genitourinary (*continued*)	Digital rectal examination including: • Prostate gland (eg, size, symmetry, nodularity, tenderness) • Seminal vesicles (eg, symmetry, tenderness, masses, enlargement) • Sphincter tone, presence of hemorrhoids, rectal masses *Female* Includes **at least seven of the following 11** elements identified by bullets: • Inspection and palpation of breasts (eg, masses or lumps, tenderness, symmetry, nipple discharge) • Digital rectal examination including sphincter tone, presence of hemorrhoids, rectal masses Pelvic examination (with or without specimen collection for smears and cultures) including: • External genitalia (eg, general appearance, hair distribution, lesions) • Urethral meatus (eg, size, location, lesions, prolapse) • Urethra (eg, masses, tenderness, scarring) • Bladder (eg, fullness, masses, tenderness) • Vagina (eg, general appearance, estrogen effect, discharge, lesions, pelvic support, cystocele, rectocele) • Cervix (eg, general appearance, lesions, discharge) • Uterus (eg, size, contour, position, mobility, tenderness, consistency, descent, or support) • Adnexa/parametria (eg, masses, tenderness, organomegaly, nodularity) • Anus and perineum
Lymphatic	• Palpation of lymph nodes in neck, axillae, groin, and/or other location
Skin	• Inspection and/or palpation of skin and subcutaneous tissue (eg, rashes, lesions, ulcers)
Neurological/ Psychiatric	Brief assessment of mental status including: • Orientation (eg, time, place, and person) • Mood and affect (eg, depression, anxiety, agitation)

System/Body Areas Not Required: Head and Face; Eyes; Ears, Nose, Mouth, and Throat; Musculoskeletal; and Extremities

Table 6-9. Hematologic/Lymphatic/Immunologic Examination

System/Body Area	Elements of Examination
Constitutional	• Measurement of **any three of the following seven** vital signs: 1) sitting or standing blood pressure, 2) supine blood pressure, 3) pulse rate and regularity, 4) respiration, 5) temperature, 6) height, 7) weight (may be measured and recorded by ancillary staff) • General appearance of patient (eg, development, nutrition, body habitus, deformities, attention to grooming)
Head and Face	• Palpation and/or percussion of face with notation of presence or absence of sinus tenderness
Eyes	• Inspection of conjunctivae and lids
Ears, Nose, Mouth, and Throat	• Otoscopic examination of external auditory canals and tympanic membranes • Inspection of nasal mucosa, septum, and turbinates • Inspection of teeth and gums • Examination of oropharynx (eg, oral mucosa, hard and soft palates, tongue, tonsils, posterior pharynx)
Neck	• Examination of neck (eg, masses, overall appearance, symmetry, tracheal position, crepitus) • Examination of thyroid (eg, enlargement, tenderness, mass)
Respiratory	• Assessment of respiratory effort (eg, intercostal retractions, use of accessory muscles, diaphragmatic movement) • Auscultation of lungs (eg, breath sounds, adventitious sounds, rubs)
Cardiovascular	• Auscultation of heart with notation of abnormal sounds and murmurs • Examination of peripheral vascular system by observation (eg, swelling, varicosities) and palpation (eg, pulses, temperature, edema, tenderness)
Gastrointestinal (Abdomen)	• Examination of abdomen with notation of presence of masses or tenderness • Examination of liver and spleen

Table 6-9 (*continued*)

System/Body Area	Elements of Examination
Lymphatic	● Palpation of lymph nodes in neck, axillae, groin, and/or other location
Extremities	● Inspection and palpation of digits and nails (eg, clubbing, cyanosis, inflammation, petechiae, ischemia, infections, nodes)
Skin	● Inspection and/or palpation of skin and subcutaneous tissue (eg, rashes, lesions, ulcers, ecchymoses, bruises)
Neurological/ Psychiatric	Brief assessment of mental status including: ● Orientation to time, place, and person ● Mood and affect (eg, depression, anxiety, agitation)

System/Body Areas Not Required: Chest (Breasts), Genitourinary, and Musculoskeletal

Table 6-10. Musculoskeletal Examination

System/Body Area	Elements of Examination
Constitutional	● Measurement of **any three of the following seven** vital signs: 1) sitting or standing blood pressure, 2) supine blood pressure, 3) pulse rate and regularity, 4) respiration, 5) temperature, 6) height, 7) weight (may be measured and recorded by ancillary staff) ● General appearance of patient (eg, development, nutrition, body habitus, deformities, attention to grooming)
Cardiovascular	● Examination of peripheral vascular system by observation (eg, swelling, varicosities) and palpation (eg, pulses, temperature, edema, tenderness)
Lymphatic	● Palpation of lymph nodes in neck, axillae, groin, and/or other location
Musculoskeletal	● Examination of gait and station Examination of joint(s), bone(s), and muscle(s)/tendon(s) of **four of the following six** areas: 1) head and neck; 2) spine, ribs, and pelvis; 3) right upper extremity; 4) left upper extremity; 5) right lower extremity; and 6) left lower extremity. The examination of a given area includes: ● Inspection, percussion, and/or palpation with notation of any misalignment, asymmetry, crepitation, defects, tenderness, masses, or effusions ● Assessment of range of motion with notation of any pain (eg, straight leg raising), crepitation, or contracture ● Assessment of stability with notation of any dislocation (luxation), subluxation, or laxity ● Assessment of muscle strength and tone (eg, flaccid, cog wheel, spastic) with notation of any atrophy or abnormal movements *Note:* For the comprehensive level of examination, all four of the elements identified by a bullet must be performed and documented for each of four anatomic areas. For the three lower levels of examination, each element is counted separately for each body area. For example, assessing range of motion in two extremities constitutes two elements.
Extremities	[See Musculoskeletal and Skin]
Skin	● Inspection and/or palpation of skin and subcutaneous tissue (eg, scars, rashes, lesions, cafe-au-lait spots, ulcers) in **four of the following six** areas: 1) head and neck, 2) trunk, 3) right upper extremity, 4) left upper extremity, 5) right lower extremity, and 6) left lower extremity. *Note:* For the comprehensive level, the examination of all four anatomic areas must be performed and documented. For the three lower levels of examination, each body area is counted separately. For example, inspection and/or palpation of the skin and subcutaneous tissue of two extremities constitutes two elements.
Neurological/ Psychiatric	● Test coordination (eg, finger/nose, heel/knee/shin, rapid alternating movements in the upper and lower extremities, evaluation of fine motor coordination in young children) ● Examination of deep tendon reflexes and/or nerve stretch test with notation of pathological reflexes (eg, Babinski) ● Examination of sensation (eg, by touch, pin, vibration, proprioception) Brief assessment of mental status including: ● Orientation to time, place, and person ● Mood and affect (eg, depression, anxiety, agitation)

System/Body Areas Not Required: Head and Face; Eyes; Ears, Nose, Mouth, and Throat; Neck; Respiratory; Chest (Breasts); Gastrointestinal (Abdomen); and Genitourinary

Table 6-11. Neurological Examination

System/Body Area	Elements of Examination
Constitutional	• Measurement of **any three of the following seven** vital signs: 1) sitting or standing blood pressure, 2) supine blood pressure, 3) pulse rate and regularity, 4) respiration, 5) temperature, 6) height, 7) weight (may be measured and recorded by ancillary staff) • General appearance of patient (eg, development, nutrition, body habitus, deformities, attention to grooming)
Eyes	• Ophthalmoscopic examination of optic discs (eg, size, C/D ratio, appearance) and posterior segments (eg, vessel changes, exudates, hemorrhages)
Cardiovascular	• Examination of carotid arteries (eg, pulse amplitude, bruits) • Auscultation of heart with notation of abnormal sounds and murmurs • Examination of peripheral vascular system by observation (eg, swelling, varicosities) and palpation (eg, pulses, temperature, edema, tenderness)
Musculoskeletal	• Examination of gait and station Assessment of motor function including: • Muscle strength in upper and lower extremities • Muscle tone in upper and lower extremities (eg, flaccid, cog wheel, spastic) with notation of any atrophy or abnormal movements (eg, fasciculation, tardive dyskinesia)
Extremities	[See Musculoskeletal]
Neurological	Evaluation of higher integrative functions including: • Orientation to time, place, and person • Recent and remote memory • Attention span and concentration • Language (eg, naming objects, repeating phrases, spontaneous speech) • Fund of knowledge (eg, awareness of current events, past history, vocabulary) Test the following cranial nerves: • 2nd cranial nerve (eg, visual acuity, visual fields, fundi) • 3rd, 4th, and 6th cranial nerves (eg, pupils, eye movements) • 5th cranial nerve (eg, facial sensation, corneal reflexes) • 7th cranial nerve (eg, facial symmetry, strength) • 8th cranial nerve (eg, hearing with tuning fork, whispered voice, and/or finger rub) • 9th cranial nerve (eg, spontaneous or reflex palate movement) • 11th cranial nerve (eg, shoulder shrug strength) • 12th cranial nerve (eg, tongue protrusion) • Examination of sensation (eg, by touch, pin, vibration, proprioception) • Examination of deep tendon reflexes in upper and lower extremities with notation of pathological reflexes (eg, Babinski) • Test coordination (eg, finger/nose, heel/knee/shin, rapid alternating movements in the upper and lower extremities, evaluation of fine motor coordination in young children)

System/Body Areas Not Required: Head and Face; Ears, Nose, Mouth, and Throat; Neck; Respiratory; Chest (Breasts); Gastrointestinal (Abdomen); Genitourinary; Lymphatic; Skin; and Psychiatric

Table 6-12. Psychiatric Examination

System/Body Area	Elements of Examination
Constitutional	• Measurement of **any three of the following seven** vital signs: 1) sitting or standing blood pressure, 2) supine blood pressure, 3) pulse rate and regularity, 4) respiration, 5) temperature, 6) height, 7) weight (may be measured and recorded by ancillary staff) • General appearance of patient (eg, development, nutrition, body habitus, deformities, attention to grooming)
Musculoskeletal	• Assessment of muscle strength and tone (eg, flaccid, cog wheel, spastic) with notation of any atrophy and abnormal movements • Examination of gait and station

Table 6-12 (*continued*)

System/Body Area	Elements of Examination
Psychiatric	• Description of speech including: rate, volume, articulation, coherence, and spontaneity with notation of abnormalities (eg, perseveration, paucity of language) • Description of thought processes including: rate of thoughts (eg, logical vs. illogical, tangential), abstract reasoning, and computation • Description of associations (eg, loose, tangential, circumstantial, intact) • Description of abnormal or psychotic thoughts including hallucinations, delusions, preoccupation with violence, homicidal or suicidal ideation, and obsessions • Description of the patient's judgment (eg, concerning everyday activities and social situations) and insight (eg, concerning psychiatric condition) Complete mental status examination including: • Orientation to time, place, and person • Recent and remote memory • Attention span and concentration • Language (eg, naming objects, repeating phrases) • Fund of knowledge (eg, awareness of current events, past history, vocabulary) • Mood and affect (eg, depression, anxiety, agitation, hypomania, lability)

System/Body Areas Not Required: Head and Face; Eyes; Ears, Nose, Mouth, and Throat; Neck; Respiratory; Cardiovascular; Chest (Breasts); Gastrointestinal (Abdomen); Genitourinary; Lymphatic; Extremities; Skin; and Neurological

Table 6-13. Respiratory Examination

System/Body Area	Elements of Examination
Constitutional	• Measurement of **any three of the following seven** vital signs: 1) sitting or standing blood pressure, 2) supine blood pressure, 3) pulse rate and regularity, 4) respiration, 5) temperature, 6) height, 7) weight (may be measured and recorded by ancillary staff) • General appearance of patient (eg, development, nutrition, body habitus, deformities, attention to grooming)
Ears, Nose, Mouth, and Throat	• Inspection of nasal mucosa, septum, and turbinates • Inspection of teeth and gums • Examination of oropharynx (eg, oral mucosa, hard and soft palates, tongue, tonsils, and posterior pharynx)
Neck	• Examination of neck (eg, masses, overall appearance, symmetry, tracheal position, crepitus) • Examination of thyroid (eg, enlargement, tenderness, mass) • Examination of jugular veins (eg, distension; a, v, or cannon a waves)
Respiratory	• Inspection of chest with notation of symmetry and expansion • Assessment of respiratory effort (eg, intercostal retractions, use of accessory muscles, diaphragmatic movement) • Percussion of chest (eg, dullness, flatness, hyper-resonance) • Palpation of chest (eg, tactile fremitus) • Auscultation of lungs (eg, breath sounds, adventitious sounds, rubs)
Cardiovascular	• Auscultation of heart including sounds, abnormal sounds, and murmurs • Examination of peripheral vascular system by observation (eg, swelling, varicosities) and palpation (eg, pulses, temperature, edema, tenderness)
Gastrointestinal (Abdomen)	• Examination of abdomen with notation of presence of masses or tenderness • Examination of liver and spleen
Lymphatic	• Palpation of lymph nodes in neck, axillae, groin, and/or other location
Musculoskeletal	• Assessment of muscle strength and tone (eg, flaccid, cog wheel, spastic) with notation of any atrophy and abnormal movements • Examination of gait and station

Table 6-13 (continued)

System/Body Area	Elements of Examination
Extremities	• Inspection and palpation of digits and nails (eg, clubbing, cyanosis, inflammation, petechiae, ischemia, infections, nodes)
Skin	• Inspection and/or palpation of skin and subcutaneous tissue (eg, rashes, lesions, ulcers)
Neurological/ Psychiatric	Brief assessment of mental status including: • Orientation to time, place, and person • Mood and affect (eg, depression, anxiety, agitation)

System/Body Areas Not Required: Head and Face, Eyes, Chest (Breasts), and Genitourinary

Table 6-14. Skin Examination

System/Body Area	Elements of Examination
Constitutional	• Measurement of **any three of the following seven** vital signs: 1) sitting or standing blood pressure, 2) supine blood pressure, 3) pulse rate and regularity, 4) respiration, 5) temperature, 6) height, 7) weight (may be measured and recorded by ancillary staff) • General appearance of patient (eg, development, nutrition, body habitus, deformities, attention to grooming)
Eyes	• Inspection of conjunctivae and lids
Ears, Nose, Mouth, and Throat	• Inspection of lips, teeth, and gums • Examination of oropharynx (eg, oral mucosa, hard and soft palates, tongue, tonsils, posterior pharynx)
Neck	• Examination of thyroid (eg, enlargement, tenderness, mass)
Cardiovascular	• Examination of peripheral vascular system by observation (eg, swelling, varicosities) and palpation (eg, pulses, temperature, edema, tenderness)
Gastrointestinal (Abdomen)	• Examination of liver and spleen • Examination of anus for condyloma and other lesions
Lymphatic	• Palpation of lymph nodes in neck, axillae, groin, and/or other location
Extremities	• Inspection and palpation of digits and nails (eg, clubbing, cyanosis, inflammation, petechiae, ischemia, infections, nodes)
Skin	• Palpation of scalp and inspection of hair of scalp, eyebrows, face, chest, pubic area (when indicated), and extremities Inspection and/or palpation of skin and subcutaneous tissue (eg, rashes, lesions, ulcers, susceptibility to and presence of photo damage) in **eight of the following 10** areas: • Head, including face • Neck • Chest, including breasts and axillae • Abdomen • Genitalia, groin, buttocks • Back • Right upper extremity • Left upper extremity • Right lower extremity • Left lower extremity *Note:* For the comprehensive level, the examination of at least eight anatomic areas must be performed and documented. For the three lower levels of examination, each body area is counted separately. For example, inspection and/or palpation of the skin and subcutaneous tissue of the right upper extremity and the left upper extremity constitutes two elements. • Inspection of eccrine and apocrine glands of skin and subcutaneous tissue with identification and location of any hyperhidrosis, chromhidroses, or bromhidrosis

System/Body Area	Elements of Examination
Table 6-14 (*continued*)	
Neurological/ Psychiatric	Brief assessment of mental status including: ● Orientation to time, place, and person ● Mood and affect (eg, depression, anxiety, agitation)

System/Body Areas Not Required: Head and Face, Respiratory, Chest (Breasts), Genitourinary, and Musculoskeletal

C. Documentation of the Complexity of Medical Decision-making

The levels of E/M services recognize four types of medical decision-making (straightforward, low complexity, moderate complexity, and high complexity). Medical decision-making refers to the complexity of establishing a diagnosis and/or selecting a management option as measured by

1. The number of possible diagnoses and/or the number of management options that must be considered
2. The amount and/or complexity of medical records, diagnostic tests, and/or other information that must be obtained, reviewed, and analyzed
3. The risk of significant complications, morbidity, and/or mortality, as well as co-morbidities, associated with the patient's presenting problem(s), the diagnostic procedure(s), and/or the possible management options.

Table 6-15 shows the progression of the elements required for each level of medical decision-making. To qualify for a given type of decision-making, **two of the three elements in the table must be either met or exceeded.**

Table 6-15. Determining Medical Decision-making

Number of Diagnoses or Management Options	Amount and/or Complexity of Data to Be Reviewed	Risk of Significant Complications, Morbidity, and/or Mortality	Type of Decision-Making
Minimal	Minimal or none	Minimal	Straightforward
Limited	*Limited*	Low	Low complexity
Multiple	Moderate	*Moderate*	*Moderate complexity*
Extensive	Extensive	High	High complexity

Each of the elements of medical decision-making is described below.

Number of Diagnoses or Management Options

The number of possible diagnoses and/or the number of management options that must be considered is based on the number and types of problems addressed during the encounter, the complexity of establishing a diagnosis, and the management decisions that are made by the physician.

Generally, decision-making with respect to a diagnosed problem is easier than that for an identified but undiagnosed problem. The number and type of diagnostic tests employed may be an indicator of the number of possible diagnoses. Problems that are improving or resolving are less complex than those that are worsening or failing to change as expected. The need to seek advice from others is another indicator of complexity of diagnostic or management problems.

●**DG:** *For each encounter, an assessment, clinical impression, or diagnosis should be documented. It may be explicitly stated or implied in documented decisions regarding management plans and/or further evaluation.*

   ● For a presenting problem with an established diagnosis the record should reflect whether the problem is: (a) improved, well controlled, resolving, or resolved; or (b) inadequately controlled, worsening, or failing to change as expected.

   ● For a presenting problem without an established diagnosis, the assessment or clinical impression may be stated in the form of a differential diagnoses or as "possible," "probable," or "rule out" (R/O) diagnoses.

● =New code   ▲ =Revised code   # =Re-sequenced code   + =Add-on code   ★ =Telemedicine

•**DG:**   *The initiation of, or changes in, treatment should be documented. Treatment includes a wide range of management options including patient instructions, nursing instructions, therapies, and medications.*

•**DG:**   *If referrals are made, consultations requested, or advice sought, the record should indicate to whom or where the referral or consultation is made or from whom the advice is requested.*

Amount and/or Complexity of Data to Be Reviewed

The amount and/or complexity of data to be reviewed is based on the types of diagnostic testing ordered or reviewed. A decision to obtain and review old medical records and/or obtain history from sources other than the patient increases the amount and complexity of data to be reviewed.

Discussion of contradictory or unexpected test results with the physician who performed or interpreted the test is an indication of the complexity of data being reviewed. On occasion the physician who ordered a test may personally review the image, tracing, or specimen to supplement information from the physician who prepared the test report or interpretation; this is another indication of the complexity of data being reviewed.

•**DG:**   *If a diagnostic service (test or procedure) is ordered, planned, scheduled, or performed at the time of the E/M encounter, the type of service (eg, lab or x-ray) should be documented.*

> **CPT** instructs that the actual performance and/or interpretation of diagnostic tests/studies during a patient encounter are not included in determining the levels of evaluation and management (E/M) services when reported separately. For example, a physician reporting interpretation and report of spirometry on the same date as an E/M service will not include the decision to perform spirometry in the medical decision-making of the E/M service.

•**DG:**   *The review of lab, radiology, and/or other diagnostic tests should be documented. An entry in a progress note, such as "WBC elevated" or "chest x-ray unremarkable," is acceptable. Alternatively, the review may be documented by initialing and dating the report containing the test results.*

•**DG:**   *A decision to obtain old records or to obtain additional history from the family, caretaker, or other source to supplement that obtained from the patient should be documented.*

•**DG:**   *Relevant findings from the review of old records and/or the receipt of additional history from the family, caretaker, or other source should be documented. If there is no relevant information beyond that already obtained, that fact should be documented. A notation of "old records reviewed" or "-additional history obtained from family" without elaboration is insufficient.*

•**DG:**   *The results of discussion of laboratory, radiology, or other diagnostic tests with the physician who performed or interpreted the study should be documented.*

•**DG:**   *The direct visualization and independent interpretation of an image, tracing, or specimen previously or subsequently interpreted by another physician should be documented.*

Risk of Significant Complications, Morbidity, and/or Mortality

The risk of significant complications, morbidity, and/or mortality is based on the risks associated with the presenting problem(s), the diagnostic procedure(s), and the possible management options.

•**DG:**   *Co-morbidities/underlying diseases or other factors that increase the complexity of medical decision making by increasing the risk of complications, morbidity, and/or mortality should be documented.*

•**DG:**   *If a surgical or invasive diagnostic procedure is ordered, planned, or scheduled at the time of the E/M encounter, the type of procedure (eg, laparoscopy) should be documented.*

•**DG:**   *If a surgical or invasive diagnostic procedure is performed at the time of the E/M encounter, the specific procedure should be documented.*

•**DG:**   *The referral for or decision to perform a surgical or invasive diagnostic procedure on an urgent basis should be documented or implied.*

Table 6-16 may be used to help determine whether the risk of significant complications, morbidity, and/or mortality is **minimal, low, moderate,** or **high.** Because the determination of risk is complex and not readily quantifiable, the table includes common clinical examples rather than absolute measures of risk. The assessment of risk of the presenting problem(s) is based on the risk related to the disease process anticipated between the present encounter and the next one. The assessment of risk of selecting diagnostic procedures and management options is based on the risk during and immediately following any procedures or treatment. *The highest level of risk in **any one category** (presenting problem(s), diagnostic procedure(s), or management options) determines the overall risk.*

An encounter resulting in multiple diagnoses/management options, limited data, and moderate risks leads to overall moderate complexity for MDM (see **Table 6-15***).*

Table 6-16. CMS Table of Risk			
Level of Risk	**Presenting Problem(s)**	**Diagnostic Procedure(s) Ordered**	**Management Options Selected**
Minimal	• One self-limited or minor problem (eg, cold, insect bite, tinea corporis)	• Laboratory tests requiring venipuncture • Chest x-rays • EKG/EEG • Urinalysis • Ultrasound, eg, echocardiography • KOH prep	• Rest • Gargles • Elastic bandages • Superficial dressings
Low	• Two or more self-limited or minor problems • One stable chronic illness (eg, well-controlled hypertension, non–insulin-dependent diabetes, cataract, benign prostatic hyperplasia) • Acute uncomplicated illness or injury (eg, cystitis, allergic rhinitis, simple sprain)	• Physiologic tests not under stress (eg, pulmonary function tests) • Non-cardiovascular imaging studies with contrast (eg, barium enema) • Superficial needle biopsies • Clinical laboratory tests requiring arterial puncture • Skin biopsies	• Over-the-counter drugs • Minor surgery with no identified risk factors • Physical therapy • Occupational therapy • Intravenous fluids without additives
Moderate	• One or more chronic illnesses with mild exacerbation, progression, or side effects of treatment • Two or more stable chronic illnesses • Undiagnosed new problem with uncertain prognosis (eg, lump in breast) • Acute illness with systemic symptoms (eg, pyelonephritis, pneumonitis, colitis) • Acute complicated injury (eg, head injury with brief loss of consciousness)	• Physiologic tests under stress (eg, cardiac stress test, fetal contraction stress test) • Diagnostic endoscopies with no identified risk factors • Deep needle or incisional biopsy • Cardiovascular imaging studies with contrast and no identified risk factors (eg, arteriogram, cardiac catheterization) • Obtain fluid from body cavity (eg, lumbar puncture, thoracentesis, culdocentesis)	• Minor surgery with identified risk factors • Elective major surgery (open, percutaneous, or endoscopic) with no identified risk factors • Prescription drug management • Therapeutic nuclear medicine • Intravenous fluids with additives • Closed treatment of fracture or dislocation without manipulation
High	• One or more chronic illnesses with severe exacerbation, progression, or side effects of treatment • Acute or chronic illnesses or injuries that pose a threat to life or body function (eg, multiple trauma, acute myocardial infarction, pulmonary embolus, severe respiratory distress, progressive severe rheumatoid arthritis, psychiatric illness with potential threat to self or others, peritonitis, acute renal failure) • An abrupt change in neurologic status (eg, seizure, transient ischemic attack, weakness, sensory loss)	• Cardiovascular imaging studies with contrast with identified risk factors • Cardiac electrophysiologic tests • Diagnostic endoscopies with identified risk factors • Discography	• Elective major surgery (open, percutaneous, or endoscopic) with identified risk factors • Emergency major surgery (open, percutaneous, or endoscopic) • Parenteral controlled substances • Drug therapy requiring intensive monitoring for toxicity • Decision not to resuscitate or to deescalate because of poor prognosis

D. **Documentation of an Encounter Dominated by Counseling or Coordination of Care**

For E/M services that are assigned a typical time of service, time (face-to-face or unit/floor) is considered the key or controlling factor in code selection when counseling and/or coordination of care dominates (more than 50%) the physician/patient and/or family encounter. Please see other chapters for discussion of the use of time for each type of E/M service.

•**DG:**   *If the physician elects to report the level of service based on counseling and/or coordination of care, the total length of time of the encounter (face-to-face or floor time, as appropriate) should be documented and the record should describe the counseling and/or activities to coordinate care.*

As of 2021, this no longer applies to **99202–99205** *or* **99212–99215.** *See* **Chapter 7.**

Split/Shared E/M Services

A split/shared E/M service is one in which a physician and a QHP from the same group practice each personally perform a medically necessary and substantive portion of 1 or more face-to-face E/M encounters on the same date. A portion of the key components of the service must be provided face-to-face by the physician to report under the physician's National Provider Identifier. Split/shared services were defined and implemented for services to Medicare beneficiaries. Private payers may adopt the same or a similar policy. The split/shared concept is applied differently for inpatient services than for services in the office or clinic setting (see **Chapter 7***).*

- When a hospital inpatient/hospital outpatient (on-campus outpatient hospital or off-campus outpatient hospital) or emergency department E/M is shared between a physician and an NPP from the same group practice and the physician provides any face-to-face portion of the E/M encounter with the patient, the service may be billed under either the physician or the NPP.
  - Payment will be made at the appropriate physician fee schedule rate based on the reporting provider entered on the claim.
  - If there was no face-to-face encounter between the patient and the physician (eg, even if the physician participated in the service by only reviewing the patient's medical record), then the service may only be billed under the NPP. Payment will be at the NPP rate (eg, 85% of physician fee schedule amount).

The following conditions apply to all split/shared services:

- *The physician and QHP must document and sign their portion of the service. A physician cannot merely sign off on the documentation of the QHP's work.*
- *If the E/M service is reported based on counseling and/or coordination of care, only the physician's time is used to select the level of service. The physician must document his or her total time spent in counseling and/or coordination of care and a summary of the issues discussed or coordination of care provided.*
- *Critical care is never a split/shared service because critical care services reflect the work of only 1 individual.*
- *Split/shared billing does not apply in the nursing or skilled nursing facility settings.*

Notice: At the time of publication, CMS has proposed, but not finalized, significant changes to the Medicare policy for split/shared visits. Please visit the American Academy of Pediatrics website (www.aap.org/cfp or www.aap.org/errata) to check for updates.

More E/M Documentation and Coding Tips

- When using an EHR system, it is important that the documentation for each encounter is unique and reflects the purpose and activity of that encounter. Use of documentation features, such as carryforward of prior history, copy and paste, and auto-completion, may lead to inaccurate documentation and wrong code assignment.

See "Coding Conundrum: Pitfalls of Electronic Health Record Coding" in Chapter 5 for more on electronic health record documentation.

- Ideally, physicians in a group practice should be consistent in their documentation policies. However, if documentation practices differ among physicians, have those differences documented in the practice's written policies.
- The code selected for a new patient will often be 1 level lower than for an established patient for the same amount of work. However, the Medicare relative value units are higher for new patient visits, compensating the physician for the extra work required.
- The American Academy of Pediatrics (AAP) has developed forms that promote good documentation of office or outpatient visits. Examples can be ordered from the AAP by calling 888/227-1770 or visiting http://shop.aap.org.

Teaching Physician Guidelines for Reporting E/M Services

> **Refer to Chapter 19 for the teaching physician guidelines for billing surgical, high-risk, or other complex procedures.**

- A teaching physician may bill for resident or fellow services if the teaching physician personally performs the key components (ie, history, physical examination, and MDM) of the service, performs the key components jointly with a resident, or personally observes the resident (in person or via real-time audiovisual communication) performing the key or critical components.

> **For teaching settings in which residency training sites are rural (outside of a metropolitan statistical area), the Centers for Medicare & Medicaid Services expanded teaching physician regulations to allow a teaching physician to use real-time audiovisual communication to interact with the resident to meet the requirement of being present for the key portion of the service, including telehealth services. This provision does not allow use of audio-only (eg, telephone) communication, and the communication must be real time, allowing the teaching physician to observe the resident who is providing the service.**

- The level of service billed will be dependent on the level of work performed and documented by the resident and the teaching physician in combination or by the teaching physician if seen independent of the resident.
- The teaching physician, resident, or nurse must document that he or she was physically present (ie, in the same room as the patient) during the key or critical portions of the service performed by the resident and participated in the management of the patient. The selected key or critical portion of the visit is at the discretion of the physician. Medicare requires that modifier **GC** (service performed in part by a resident under the direction of a teaching physician) be reported for each service unless the service is furnished under the primary care exception (reported with modifier **GE**). Other payers may or may not require a modifier.
- Time-based services (eg, face-to-face prolonged services, critical care, hospital discharge management) can only be billed when the teaching physician is present for the time required by the description of the service. This also applies to E/M visits when time is considered the key component in the selection of the E/M code (>50% of the total face-to-face visit was spent counseling and/or coordinating care). The total time spent by the teaching physician must be documented.
- The teaching physician must document the key or critical part of the service personally performed, link his or her documentation back to the resident's note, and document that the care plan was reviewed and approved. It is not necessary to repeat the resident's documentation.

> **When a resident admits a patient to the hospital without the teaching physician present and the teaching physician sees the patient later, including on the next day, the teaching physician's date of service is the day he or she saw the patient. The code reported is based on his or her personal work of obtaining a history, performing a physical examination, and participating in medical decision-making regardless of whether the combination of the teaching physician's and resident's documentation satisfies criteria for a higher level of service. For payment, the composite of the teaching physician's entry and the resident's entry must support the medical necessity of the billed service and the level of the service billed by the teaching physician.**

- The teaching physician documentation must be linked to the resident's note and all exceptions to the resident's findings must be documented. A signature alone is not acceptable documentation.
- Medicare guidelines stipulate that when documenting in an EHR, the teaching physician may use a macro (eg, predetermined text) as the required personal documentation if it is personally entered by the teaching physician. The resident or teaching physician must enter customized information to support medical necessity. If the resident and teaching physician use only macros, the documentation is not sufficient. See **Table 6-17** for minimal documentation required.

Table 6-17. Unacceptable and Minimal Acceptable Documentation by a Teaching Physician

Unacceptable	Minimal Acceptable Documentation Required Substitute the resident's name for Dr Resident.
Countersignature	"I performed a history and physical exam of the patient. Findings are consistent with Dr Resident's note. Discussed patient's management with Dr Resident and agree with the documented findings and plan of care." Signature
"Agree with above." Signature "Rounded, reviewed, agree." Signature	"I saw and evaluated the patient. I agree with the findings and the plan of care as documented in Dr Resident's note." Signature
"Patient seen with resident and evaluated." Signature "Seen and agree." Signature	"I saw the patient with Dr Resident and agree with Dr Resident's findings and plans as written." Signature
"Discussed with resident." Signature	"I was present with Dr Resident during the history and exam. I discussed the case with Dr Resident and agree with the findings and plan as documented in Dr Resident's note." Signature

Examples

➤ **A resident admits a 2-month-old at 10:30 pm.** The teaching physician's initial visit is performed the following morning at 8:00 am. The teaching physician reports an initial hospital care service based on the work personally performed that morning. The teaching physician documents, "I saw and evaluated the patient. Discussed with resident and agree with the findings and plan as documented in Dr Resident's note except as per my addendum and edits within Dr Resident's note." *Note:* Edits should be distinguishable in the note.

➤ **The teaching physician sees the same patient for follow-up inpatient care subsequent to the resident's visit.** The teaching physician documents, "I saw and evaluated the patient. Discussed with Dr Resident and agree with Dr Resident's findings and plan as documented in the resident's note."

➤ **The teaching physician and resident jointly admit on the same patient.** The teaching physician documents, "I was present with Dr Resident during the history and exam. I discussed the case with Dr Resident and agree with the findings and plan as documented in Dr Resident's note."

➤ **The teaching physician and resident jointly provide a subsequent hospital visit.** The teaching physician documents, "I saw the patient with the resident and agree with Dr Resident's findings and plan."

Medical Student Documentation

- Any contribution and participation of a student to the performance of a billable service (other than the ROS and/or PFSH, which are not separately billable but are taken as part of an E/M service) must be performed in the physical presence of a teaching physician or a resident in a service meeting the requirements set forth in this section for teaching physician billing.
- Students may document services in the medical record. However
  - The teaching physician must verify in the medical record all student documentation or findings, including history, physical examination, and/or MDM.
  - The teaching physician must personally perform (or re-perform) the physical examination and MDM activities of the E/M service being billed but may verify any student documentation in the medical record, rather than re-documenting this work.

Primary Care Exception Rule

The primary care exception rule (PCER) in the teaching physician guidelines allows teaching physicians to bill for services provided by residents under their supervision who have completed at least 6 months of approved graduate medical education (GME).

- To qualify for this exception, services must be provided in a teaching hospital ambulatory care center or clinic. If the services are provided outside a hospital, there must be a written agreement with the teaching hospital that includes a contract outlining the payment for the teaching services or written documentation that the services will be "donated." In general, this exception cannot be applied in a private physician's office.
- Preventive medicine visit codes are not included in the Medicare exception at this time. Some state Medicaid programs have granted the exemption for preventive medicine services to established patients.
- No more than 4 residents can be supervised at a time by a teaching physician. This may include residents with fewer than 6 months in a GME-approved residency program in the mix of 4 residents under the teaching physician's supervision. However, the teaching physician must be physically present for the critical or key portions of services furnished by the resident with fewer than 6 months in a GME-approved residency program. That is, the primary care exception does not apply in the case of the resident with fewer than 6 months in a GME-approved residency program.
- Patients seen should consider this practice as their primary location for health care.
- The teaching physician
  - Must be physically present in the clinic or office and immediately available to the residents and may not have other responsibilities (including supervising other personnel or seeing patients).
  - Must review the care provided (ie, history, findings on physical examination, assessment, and treatment plan) during or immediately after each visit. The documentation must reflect the teaching physician's participation in the review and direction of the services performed.

Example

➤ **The teaching physician is supervising a second-year resident in the clinic under the PCER.** An established patient is diagnosed with acute otitis media.

Unacceptable	Acceptable
Countersignature	"I reviewed Dr Resident's note and agree with Dr Resident's findings and plans as written." Signature
	"I reviewed Dr Resident's note and agree but will refer to ENT for consultation." Signature

- May only report codes **99202** and **99203** for new patient visits or **99211–99213** for established patient visits. If a higher-level E/M service is necessary and performed, the teaching physician must personally participate in the care of the patient as outlined in the guidelines. As always, code selection is based on the E/M code descriptions and documentation guidelines.
- Modifier **GE** (service performed by a resident without the presence of a teaching physician under the primary care exception) may be required by a payer that follows Medicare guidelines for teaching physician services.

*The AAP continues to advocate for the preventive medicine service codes (**99381–99385** and **99391–99395**) to be included under the PCER. In some instances, state Medicaid plans already consider preventive medicine service codes as part of their primary care exception, so be sure to check with your payers. Look for updates in the AAP Pediatric Coding Newsletter™.*

You can access the updated guidelines addressing the PCER at www.cms.gov/Outreach-and-Education/Medicare-Learning-Network-MLN/MLNProducts/MLN-Publications-Items/CMS1243499.html?DLPage=1&DLEntries=10&DLFilter=teaching%20physician&DLSort=0&DLSortDir=descending.

Resources

Evaluation and Management Coding

American Academy of Pediatrics *Pediatric Evaluation and Management: Coding Quick Reference Card* (https://shop.aap.org/pediatric-evaluation-and-management-coding-quick-reference-card-2022)

Teaching Physician and Primary Care Exception

Medicare Learning Network *Guidelines for Teaching Physicians, Interns, and Residents* booklet (www.cms.gov/Outreach-and-Education/Medicare-Learning-Network-MLN/MLNProducts/MLN-Publications-Items/CMS1243499)

Test Your Knowledge!

1. **What type of history does not require past, family, or social history?**
   a. Problem-focused history
   b. Expanded problem-focused history
   c. Interval history
   d. All of the above

2. **Using the 1995 guidelines, a general multisystem examination includes findings from how many systems?**
   a. 12
   b. At least 10
   c. 8
   d. 14

3. **Which of the following may be documented for the assessment or clinical impression of a presenting problem without an established diagnosis?**
   a. Failure to improve
   b. Stable or improving
   c. Differential diagnoses
   d. Risk of significant complications

4. **Which of the following would be insufficient to support the amount and/or complexity of data to be reviewed?**
   a. Initialing and dating the report containing the test results
   b. Documentation of "old records reviewed"
   c. Documentation of "old records reviewed, no relevant information beyond that already obtained"
   d. Documentation of "chest x-ray unremarkable"

5. **Which of the following meets the requirements for a teaching physician's observation of the key portion of an evaluation and management service provided by a resident in a rural location?**
   a. Presence via real-time audiovisual technology
   b. Presence via audio-only communication technology
   c. Presence via interactive exchange of messages
   d. Presence during chart review

Part 2
Primarily for the Office and Other Outpatient Settings

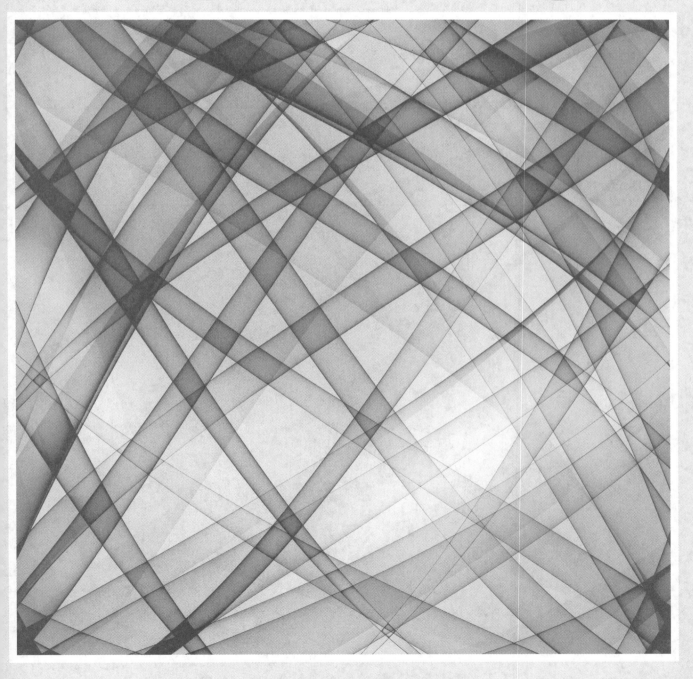

Part 2: Primarily for the Office and Other Outpatient Settings

Chapter 7
Office and Other Outpatient Evaluation and Management Services 141

Chapter 8
Preventive Services 171

Chapter 9
Consultation, Residential, and Non–face-to-face Evaluation and Management Services............................ 203

Chapter 10
Surgery, Infusion, and Sedation in the Outpatient Setting 227

Chapter 11
Common Non-facility Testing and Therapeutic Services 257

Chapter 12
Management of Chronic and Complex Conditions... 285

Chapter 13
Qualified Nonphysician Health Care Professional Services.. 309

Chapter 14
Mental and Behavioral Health Services... 327

Office and Other Outpatient Evaluation and Management Services

Contents

Overview of Office and Other Outpatient Evaluation and Management (E/M) Codes 143

    E/M Services in Urgent Care Facilities 143

Office E/M Guidelines 144

    New Versus Established Patients.. 144

    Guidelines for Selecting a Level of Office E/M Service... 145

    Visits Not Requiring a Physician's or Qualified Health Care Professional's Presence.................. 146

Time Guidelines and Application 147

Medical Decision-making (MDM): Guidelines for Selecting a Level 148

    Number and Complexity of Problems Addressed... 148

    Amount and/or Complexity of Data to Be Reviewed and Analyzed 150

    Risk of Complications and/or Morbidity or Mortality of Patient Management 153

Selection of Level 2 Through 5 Codes 155

    Office E/M Level 2 (**99202, 99212**) 157

        Time Requirements (in Lieu of MDM) 157

    Office E/M Level 3 (**99203, 99213**)... 157

        Time Requirements (in Lieu of MDM) 158

    Office E/M Level 4 (**99204, 99214**) 158

        Time Requirements (in Lieu of MDM) 159

    Office E/M Level 5 (**99205, 99215**) 160

        Time Requirements (in Lieu of MDM) 160

Prolonged Office E/M Service 160

    Prolonged Service by a Physician or Other Qualified Health Care Professional.......................... 160

    Prolonged Clinical Staff Service (**99415, 99416**)... 162

Split/Shared Office E/M Services 164

After-hours Services (**99050–99058**).. 165

    Services Provided When the Office Is Normally Closed.. 165

    Services Provided During Regularly Scheduled Evening, Weekend, or Holiday Hours 165

    Services Provided on an Emergency Basis in the Office... 166

Continuum Models: Asthma, Attention-Deficit/Hyperactivity Disorder, and Otitis Media 166

Resources... 169

Test Your Knowledge! 170

Overview of Office and Other Outpatient Evaluation and Management (E/M) Codes

This chapter provides information on reporting office and other outpatient evaluation and management (E/M) codes **99202–99205** and **99211–99215**. These codes are reported for most non-preventive E/M services in a pediatric office or outpatient clinic setting as well as in urgent care facilities. For information on other office and outpatient E/M services (eg, consultations, critical care, testing, and procedures), see **chapters 9 through 14**.

This chapter will provide important details and examples of how medical decision-making (MDM) and total time on the date of the encounter are used in selecting office E/M codes. **Table 7-1** provides an overview of the requirements for selection of each level of E/M service other than code **99211**. (Code **99211** is not included here because MDM and time are not used in support of this code.)

Table 7-1. Code Selection Overview for Office Evaluation and Management Service Levels 2 Through 5

Code		Level of Medical Decision-making	Time Spent on the Date of the Encounter[a] (minutes)
New Patient	99202	Straightforward	15–29
	99203	Low	30–44
	99204	Moderate	45–59
	99205	High	60–74
Established Patient	99212	Straightforward	10–19
	99213	Low	20–29
	99214	Moderate	30–39
	99215	High	40–54

[a] Does not include time of clinical staff. Include only time spent by the physician or other qualified health care professional directed to the individual patient's care on the date of the encounter.

E/M Services in Urgent Care Facilities

Current Procedural Terminology (*CPT*®) does not include codes specific to E/M services provided at an urgent care facility. Office E/M codes (**99202–99215**) are typically reported.

The Centers for Medicare & Medicaid Services describes an *urgent care facility* as a location, distinct from a hospital ED, an office, or a clinic, the purpose of which is to diagnose and treat illness or injury for unscheduled, ambulatory patients seeking immediate medical attention.

- Emergency department codes **99281–99285** are not reported for urgent care E/M services.
- The site of service is differentiated by the place of service code (eg, **20** for urgent care facility; **11** for office).
- Other E/M codes that may be applicable to services in an urgent care facility include
  - After-hours service codes discussed later in this chapter.
  - Healthcare Common Procedure Coding System (HCPCS) code **S9088** (services provided in an urgent care center) may be listed in addition to the codes for other services provided.
  - Some urgent care clinics also contract to bill all services under code **S9083** (global fee urgent care centers).

Some physician practices operate as a primary care pediatric practice and an urgent care center in the same location but with different tax identification numbers and insurance contracts for each. Physicians should consult a health care attorney for assistance in establishing an urgent care practice and contracting with payers to cover the additional overhead costs often applicable to urgent care (eg, extended staffing, radiology, procedural services).

It is imperative to know your contractual agreements for coding and billing as an urgent care facility or clinic versus a primary care practice, as rates of payment are typically higher for urgent care facilities and so, too, are patient co-payments. Billing and payment also vary for those urgent care facilities owned by hospitals, and guidance on billing and coding for these locations should be obtained from the compliance officer or other administrative personnel.

Office E/M Guidelines

*Please see **Chapter 6** for guidelines applicable to other categories of E/M service.*

Some *CPT* guidelines apply to all E/M services, including codes **99202–99205** and **99211–99215**. These are

- *CPT* guidelines do not establish documentation requirements or standards of care.
- Each level of E/M services may be used by all physicians and other qualified health care professionals (QHPs).
- When a category of E/M service includes codes for new and established patients, the guidelines for new versus established patients discussed in **Chapter 6** apply. See examples later in this chapter.
- When a physician or other QHP orders a test during an E/M service and an interpretation and report of the test results is reported by the same or another individual of the same specialty and same group practice, the order for the test is not counted in determining the level of MDM for a related E/M service.

> When a physician or other QHP orders and reports a separate code for a test that does not require interpretation and report (eg, laboratory tests that provide results for analysis, such as a rapid influenza test), the order for the test may be counted toward the level of MDM for the E/M service.

- The appropriate time (ie, face-to-face, unit/floor, or total time) should be documented in the medical record when it is used as the basis for code selection. Time used in selection of office E/M codes is discussed later in this chapter.
- A specifically identifiable procedure or service (ie, identified with a specific code) performed on the date of E/M services may be reported separately. Modifier **25** (significant, separately identifiable E/M service) may be required on the E/M code when codes for other physician services (eg, test interpretation and report, surgical services) are reported on the same date.

New Versus Established Patients

New and established patients are defined the same for office E/M services as other E/M services that designate new or established patient. The criteria are as follows:

- *New patients* have not received a face-to-face professional service from the physician or QHP, or any physician or QHP of the same group practice and same exact specialty and subspecialty (eg, primary care, allergist), in the prior 3 years.
- *Established patients* have received, and a claim has been submitted for, any face-to-face professional service (eg, hospital care, immunization with physician counseling) from a physician or QHP of the same group practice and same exact specialty within the past 3 years.

> Telemedicine services (delivered via real-time audiovisual technology) are face-to-face services, even though the physician is present only by audiovisual technology.

- Per *CPT,* a QHP working with a physician(s) and who may report E/M services is considered to be working in the exact same specialty and subspecialty as the physician(s). (Medicare assigns different specialty designations to QHPs and does not consider the specialty of the physician providing supervision when determining whether a patient is new. Medicaid and private plans may follow either *CPT* or Medicare practices.)

Examples

➤ **If a physician of a different specialty is covering for another physician (eg, pediatrician covering for a family physician) and has the first face-to-face contact with the other physician's established patient, the encounter is considered new.**

If a physician is covering for another physician of the same specialty, the patient's encounter is coded as it would have been by the physician who is not available. For example, an established patient for a pediatrician is seen by the on-call pediatrician. The on-call pediatrician should report that patient as established.

> Per *Current Procedural Terminology*, if a physician is covering for another physician of the same specialty, the patient's encounter is reported as it would have been by the physician who is not available.

➤ **If the physician has moved to a different location or changed his or her tax identification number, patients would still be considered established if they were established patients before these changes took place.**

When a new physician joins a group of other pediatricians, patients who follow the physician to the new practice are considered to be established patients to any of the pediatricians in the new practice because the patients were seen by a physician of the same specialty in the group within the past 3 years.

➤ **When a newborn or child is examined in the hospital (eg, nursery or emergency department [ED] care) and is subsequently examined in the office by the same physician or member of the same group and same specialty, the newborn or child is considered an established patient.**

Guidelines for Selecting a Level of Office E/M Service

The following guidelines *apply only to office E/M codes* **99202–99205** and **99212–99215**. Unlike other categories of E/M codes (eg, home visits, hospital care), office E/M codes are not chosen based on 3 key components. Use of time for code selection is also different for office E/M codes. For both new and established patient visits, the level of service is determined by either of the following:

- The level of MDM alone
- The total amount of time (face-to-face and non–face-to-face) spent by a pediatrician or other QHP on the date of service directed to care of the patient.

See **Table 7-2** for an overview of the key guidelines for code selection for office E/M services.

Table 7-2. Key Office Evaluation and Management Coding Guidelines

History and examination: Code selection is not based on the extent of history and examination. Each service includes a medically appropriate history and/or physical examination, when performed. Information supplied directly by the patient/caregiver or obtained by the care team may be reviewed and expanded on (as necessary) rather than redocumented.

Code selection: Select a code based either on MDM or the pediatrician's or QHP's total time on the date of the visit.

MDM: Four types of MDM are recognized: straightforward, low, moderate, and high.
Determine the level of MDM based on the highest 2 of 3 elements of MDM.
1. Number and complexity of problems addressed. Include problems addressed or managed by the reporting pediatrician/QHP as part of the encounter.
2. Amount and/or complexity of data reviewed and analyzed. Data include
   - Tests, documents, orders, or independent historian(s)
   - Independent interpretation of tests
   - Discussion of management/test interpretation with external physician, QHP, or appropriate source
3. Risk of complications, morbidity, and/or mortality of patient management decisions made at the visit, associated with the patient's problem(s), and the diagnostic procedure(s), treatment(s) including possible management options selected and those considered but not selected.

Time: May be used to select a code level whether or not counseling and/or coordination of care dominates the service.
- Time includes the total time on the date of the encounter (face-to-face and non–face-to-face) personally spent by the physician and/or QHP focused on the care of 1 patient.
  — Do not include time in activities performed or normally performed by clinical staff (eg, rooming the patient).
  — Time does not need to be continuous. Total all time on 1 date.
- Include the time of the following activities when performed by the reporting pediatrician/QHP:
  — Preparing to see the patient (eg, review of previous tests)
  — Obtaining and/or reviewing separately obtained history
  — Performing a medically appropriate examination and/or evaluation
  — Counseling and educating the patient/family/caregiver
  — Ordering medications, tests, or procedures
  — Referring/communicating with other QHPs (when not separately reported)
  — Documenting clinical information in the electronic or other health record
  — Independently interpreting results (when not separately reported) and communicating results to patient/family/caregiver
  — Coordinating care (when not separately reported)

Abbreviations: MDM, medical decision-making; QHP, qualified health care professional.

CPT copyright 2021 American Medical Association. All rights reserved.　　●=New code　▲=Revised code　#=Re-sequenced code　+=Add-on code　★=Telemedicine

Chapter 7. Office and Other Outpatient Evaluation and Management Services

Visits Not Requiring a Physician's or Qualified Health Care Professional's Presence

▲99211   Office or other outpatient visit for the evaluation and management of an established patient that may not require the presence of a physician or other qualified health care professional.

Services by clinical staff, such as 99211 visits, are considered incidental to a physician's or QHP's services and are reported under the supervising physician's or QHP's name and National Provider Identifier (NPI). Generally, clinical staff, such as nurses and medical assistants, are not credentialed with payers and cannot independently provide and report these services.

> Per *Current Procedural Terminology*, a *clinical staff member* is a person working under the supervision of a physician or other qualified health care professional and who is allowed by law, regulation, and facility policy to perform or assist in the performance of a specified professional service but who does not individually report that professional service.

Code 99211
- Is reported only for established patients.
- Is not reported on the same date as an office E/M service by a physician or QHP of the same group practice.
- Services are provided based on a physician's or QHP's order.
- Is reported for clinical staff assessments and other follow-up care not included in services described by other procedure codes (eg, face-to-face patient education not included in time billed as chronic care management services).
- Does not require the presence of a physician or QHP.
- Does not require MDM by a physician or QHP.
- Is not a time-based service.

Do not report 99211 for non-E/M services such as venipuncture (36415, 36416), or injections (96372) or for demonstration or teaching use of an inhalation device (94664). Do not report 99211 in conjunction with administration of immunizations (90471–90474) without separate and distinct nursing assessment and management.

Examples

➤ **An established patient presents for blood pressure and weight check.**
History: The patient is here per Dr Buena's order for follow-up on weight loss plan for obesity and hypertension. The patient is following the recommended diet and began taking yoga and martial arts lessons at the local recreation center. Mother states she feels more positive about changing the family's diet and routines now.
Physical assessment: Blood pressure is 118/70, weight is 120 pounds (down 7 pounds since last visit), and BMI is now at the 88th percentile.
Plan: Encouraged to continued diet and exercise. Patient is already scheduled to follow up with Dr Buena in 1 month. Patient and parent are instructed to call if there are any concerns prior to the follow-up visit.
Codes reported are 99211 linked to I10 (hypertension) and E66.9 (obesity, unspecified).

➤ **An established patient is provided education on use of self-injectable epinephrine by a nurse.** The supervising pediatrician reports 99211.

➤ **An established patient is seen for evaluation of reaction to a tuberculosis skin test.** A medical assistant assesses the site of the injection and finds no signs of reaction. The supervising pediatrician reports 99211.

Many payers follow Medicare policy for reporting services that are incident to a physician's service, which requires all of the following conditions:
- Clinical staff providing incident-to services must be directly or contractually employed by the practice of the reporting physician/QHP.
- The services performed are within the scope of practice of the performing clinical staff.
- The services are to an established patient in continuation of the physician's plan of care for an established problem.
- The services are provided with the supervising physician or QHP in the office suite at the time of service.

For health plans that pay for **99211** only when provided in compliance with incident-to policy, do not report **99211** when

- The patient presents with a new problem (eg, urinary tract infection) or a problem that requires new management.
- There is no supervising pediatrician or QHP in the office suite or clinic at the time of service.
- The patient is a new patient to the supervising physician or QHP.

    Check for individual health plan guidance for reporting services by clinical staff.

> **Learn more about the Medicare incident-to policy in Chapter 13.**

Time Guidelines and Application

Time may be used to select a code level in office E/M services *whether or not* counseling and/or coordination of care dominates the service. See **Table 7-1** for time ranges assigned to each office E/M code.

- Time is the physician's and/or QHP's total time on the date of service (not time in a 24-hour period).
- Both face-to-face and non–face-to-face time spent on the date of service are included in the time of the encounter. **Figure 7-1** illustrates the time included in the physician's or QHP's total time.
- The total time should be documented in the medical record when it is used as the basis for code selection. No specific verbiage is required by *CPT*.

> *Current Procedural Terminology* **does not require documentation of each segment of time spent on the date of service or any specific format of documentation. The physician must, however, document the total amount of time spent on the date of the encounter and be able to account for the time spent.**

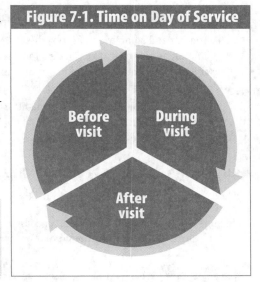

Figure 7-1. Time on Day of Service

Before visit

During visit

After visit

- No time spent by clinical staff or time spent by a physician or QHP in activities typically performed by clinical staff is included.
- When the pediatrician and a QHP meet with a patient/caregiver at the same time (split/shared visit), only the reporting individual's time is counted. *Each minute of time is counted only once.*

> A *split/shared visit* **is an evaluation and management service in which a physician and a qualified health care professional jointly provide the face-to-face and non–face-to-face work. See more information later in this chapter.**

Examples

➤ **A nurse practitioner sees an established patient for a follow-up visit due to parent concerns about the child returning to sports after sustaining a concussion.** Five minutes are spent reviewing the patient chart and accessing records from the emergency physician's initial management of the injury. History is obtained about the injury and ongoing signs and symptoms that may be related to the injury but have also occurred previously in relation to migraine headaches (10 minutes). The nurse practitioner consults the pediatrician, who joins the practitioner in answering questions and counseling the parents for another 15 minutes. The patient and parents agree to neurologic testing prior to a decision on clearance for sports. The nurse practitioner spends another 10 minutes arranging the testing and documenting the encounter. Total time on the date of the visit of 40 minutes (5 + 10 + 15 + 10).

Code **99215** (40–54 minutes) is reported. Only 15 minutes is counted by 1 individual for the time spent jointly by the pediatrician and the nurse practitioner.

A payer may allow physician reporting of split/shared visits only when following an established plan of care (ie, established problem with order for follow-up) and otherwise require reporting by the nurse practitioner.

Chapter 7. Office and Other Outpatient Evaluation and Management Services

➤ **A pediatrician spends 10 minutes reviewing laboratory results and consultation reports prior to a visit on the same date.** Later that day, a face-to-face visit with the patient and caregivers lasts 20 minutes. After the visit but on the same date, the pediatrician spends 10 minutes in discussion with a consulting subspecialist and another 10 minutes in follow-up with the caregiver and in documentation. The total time on the date of service is 50 minutes.

If the patient is a new patient, code **99204** (45–59 minutes) is reported. If the patient is established, code **99215** (40–54 minutes) is reported.

Medical Decision-making (MDM): Guidelines for Selecting a Level

Medical decision-making is the work of establishing diagnoses, assessing the status of a condition, and/or selecting a management option. As previously noted, MDM is determined by assessing the level at which 2 of 3 elements of MDM are supported in the documentation of an encounter. The 3 elements of MDM are

1. The number and complexity of problem(s) that are addressed during the encounter
2. The amount and/or complexity of data to be reviewed and analyzed
3. The risk of complications, morbidity, and/or mortality of patient management decisions made at the visit, associated with the patient's problem(s), the diagnostic procedure(s), and treatment(s)

Four types of MDM are recognized: straightforward, low, moderate, and high. Each level of MDM is based on the same criteria whether the patient is new or established. (Time and other factors considered in valuing codes differentiate new versus established patient office E/M services.)

Number and Complexity of Problems Addressed

The first step in determining the level of MDM for an encounter is identification of the number and complexity of problems addressed.

- Include all problems addressed at an encounter in the number and complexity of problems.
- Complexity is determined by the types of problems addressed.

A *problem* is a disease, condition, illness, injury, symptom, sign, finding, complaint, or other matter addressed at the encounter, with or without a diagnosis being established at the time of the encounter.

See **Table 7-3** for the levels of problems in MDM. Expanded discussion of each type of problem follows the table.

Table 7-3. Levels of Problems in Medical Decision-making	
Level	**Type of Problem**
NA	Minimal (See **99211**.)
SF	Self-limited or minor
Low	≥2 self-limited or minor problems Acute, uncomplicated illness or injury Stable chronic illness
Moderate	2 stable chronic illnesses Chronic illness with exacerbation, progression, or side effects of treatment Acute, complicated injury Acute illness with systemic symptoms Undiagnosed new problem with uncertain prognosis
High	Chronic illness with severe exacerbation, progression, or side effects of treatment Acute/chronic illness or injury posing a threat to life or bodily function
Abbreviations: NA, not applicable; SF, straightforward.	

The guidelines for office E/M services provide definitions of the types of problems that are typically addressed at these encounters. See the "Coding Conundrum: Addressed or Not Addressed" box later in this chapter for guidance on problems considered to have been addressed.

The following are definitions for the types of problems identified in each level of MDM from *CPT 2022*:

Minimal: Presence of the physician or QHP is not required, but the service is provided under the physician's or QHP's supervision (see code **99211**).

Self-limited or minor: A problem that runs a definite and prescribed course, is transient in nature, and is not likely to permanently alter health status.

Low

- Two or more self-limited or minor problems.
- Acute, uncomplicated illness or injury. A recent or new short-term problem with low risk of morbidity for which treatment is considered.
  — Little to no risk of mortality with treatment and full recovery without functional impairment is expected.
  — May be a self-limited or minor problem that is not resolving consistently with a definite and prescribed course.
  — Examples may include cystitis, allergic rhinitis, or a simple sprain.
- Stable chronic illness. A problem with an expected duration of at least 1 year or until the death of the patient where the risk of morbidity is significant without treatment.
  — *Stable* is defined by the individual patient's specific treatment goals. A patient who is not at his or her treatment goal is not stable, even if the condition has not changed and there is no short-term threat to life or function.
  — Examples of stable chronic illness may include well-controlled attention-deficit/hyperactivity disorder (ADHD), asthma, cystic fibrosis, depression, or diabetes.

> Conditions are treated as chronic whether or not stage or severity changes (eg, uncontrolled diabetes and controlled diabetes are a single chronic condition).

Moderate

- Two stable chronic illnesses.
- Chronic illness with exacerbation, progression, or side effects of treatment. Acutely worsening, poorly controlled, or progressing with an intent to control progression, *requiring additional supportive care or requiring attention to treatment for side effects* but not consideration of hospital level of care.
     Examples include non-severe exacerbation of asthma, generalized anxiety disorder now with school avoidance, and ADHD with tics secondary to treatment.
- Acute, complicated injury. Requires evaluation of body systems that are not directly part of the injured organ, extensive injury, multiple treatment options, and/or association with risk of morbidity (eg, head injury with brief loss of consciousness).
- Acute illness with systemic symptoms. An illness causing systemic symptoms and *with high risk of morbidity without treatment.*
  — For systemic general symptoms (eg, fever, body aches, fatigue) in a minor illness that may be treated to alleviate symptoms, shorten the course of illness, or prevent complications, see *self-limited or minor* or *acute, uncomplicated illness.*
  — Systemic symptoms may not be general but may be single system (eg, juvenile oligoarticular arthritis with only musculoskeletal symptoms).
  — Examples may include pyelonephritis or bacterial gastroenteritis.

> Although the risk of morbidity without treatment is a consideration in determining the nature of the problem addressed, this does not equate to the risk of mortality or morbidity of management (ie, problem risk is distinct from patient management risk).

- Undiagnosed new problem with uncertain prognosis. A problem in the differential diagnosis that represents a condition *likely to result in a high risk of morbidity without treatment.* Examples may include unexplained bruising, anterior neck mass, unexpected weight loss, and school failure.

High

- Chronic illness with severe exacerbation, progression, or side effects of treatment. Severe exacerbation or progression of chronic illness or severe side effects of treatment with significant risk of morbidity and may require hospital level of care.
- Acute or chronic illness or injury posing a threat to life or bodily function. Acute illness with systemic symptoms or an acute complicated injury, or a chronic illness or injury with exacerbation and/or progression or side effects of treatment, that poses a threat to life or bodily function in the near term without treatment.

Examples may include severe respiratory distress, psychiatric illness with potential threat to self or others, acute renal failure, or an abrupt change in neurologic status.

Coding Conundrum: Addressed or Not Addressed

A problem is addressed or managed when it is evaluated or treated at the encounter by the physician or other qualified health care professional (QHP) reporting the service.

- This includes consideration of further testing or treatment that may not be elected by virtue of risk to benefit analysis or patient, parent, guardian, or surrogate choice.
- Notation in the patient's medical record that another professional is managing the problem without additional assessment or care coordination documented does not qualify as being addressed or managed by the physician or QHP reporting the service.
- Referral without evaluation (by history, examination, or diagnostic study[ies]) or consideration of treatment does not qualify a problem as being addressed or managed by the physician or QHP reporting the service.
- Do not include problems simply listed in the medical record when determining code level if those problems were not addressed.

Determination of the type of problem addressed may require a pediatrician's clinical judgement. Coding staff should query the pediatrician when unsure of the appropriate types of problems addressed at an encounter (eg, self-limited vs acute, uncomplicated illness).

Examples

➤ **An established patient presents for evaluation of a bug bite.** The patient appears well and has a single small bump on her forearm. Patient does not indicate pain on examination. There is no sign of cellulitis or other complication. The physician explains that the bite should resolve without further treatment, but the patient may apply ice wrapped in a washcloth for itching. Patient is to return as needed or at next scheduled preventive visit.

The patient presented with a self-limiting condition with minimal risk without treatment.

Level of problems addressed ➡ Self-limited or minor

➤ **A patient with type 1 diabetes presents for follow-up.** Parents report the child has to be carefully monitored for hypoglycemia due to inattention to her glucose monitoring and request counseling to help the child achieve better control. Diagnosis is type 1 diabetes with hypoglycemic episodes.

Plan: Patient is counseled and referred to a behavioral health clinician for health behavior assessment and intervention.

Level of problems addressed ➡ Moderate

Teaching Point: The patient's diabetes is not controlled and requires additional management, so the problem is moderate. There is no severe exacerbation, progression, or side effect of treatment and no immediate threat to life or bodily function; the number and complexity of problems is not high.

Amount and/or Complexity of Data to Be Reviewed and Analyzed

Data are divided into the following 3 categories:

1. Tests, documents, orders, or independent historian(s) (Each unique test, order, or document is counted to meet a threshold number.)
2. Independent interpretation of tests that are not separately reported
3. Discussion of management or test interpretation with external physician or other QHP or appropriate source

When data are used in support of low, moderate, or high MDM, the requirements for either 1 or 2 categories of data must be met. For example, Category 1 at the limited level of data is met when a physician reviews any 2 external notes for unique sources or orders 2 tests represented by separate *CPT* codes. Instructions are provided for each level of data. Minimal or no data are required for straightforward MDM. **Table 7-4** shows the data requirements for low, moderate, and extensive data.

A decision not to order a test that was considered is counted as a test ordered when the consideration and reason for not ordering the test is documented. For example, documentation may show that a test was discussed but determined to be unnecessary or that a test that is typically performed is not indicated due to patient risk.

Table 7-4. Defining Data Required by Level of Medical Decision-making	
Limited *(Must meet the requirements of 1 of the 2 categories)*	**Category 1: Tests and documents** Any combination of 2 from the following: Review of prior external note(s) from each unique source[a] Review of the result(s) of each unique test[a] Ordering of each unique test[a]
	Category 2: Assessment requiring an independent historian(s)
Moderate *(Must meet the requirements of 1 out of 3 categories)*	**Category 1: Tests, documents, or independent historian(s)** Any combination of 3 from the following: Review of prior external note(s) from each unique source[a] Review of the result(s) of each unique test[a] Ordering of each unique test[a] Assessment requiring an independent historian(s)
	Category 2: Independent interpretation of tests performed by another physician/other qualified health care professional (not separately reported)
	Category 3: Discussion of management or test interpretation with external physician/other qualified health care professional/appropriate source (not separately reported)
Extensive *(Must meet the requirements of at least 2 out of 3 categories)*	**Category 1: Tests, documents, or independent historian(s)** Any combination of 3 from the following: Review of prior external note(s) from each unique source[a] Review of the result(s) of each unique test[a] Ordering of each unique test[a] Assessment requiring an independent historian(s)
	Category 2: Independent interpretation of tests performed by another physician/other qualified health care professional (not separately reported)
	Category 3: Discussion of management or test interpretation with external physician/other qualified health care professional/appropriate source (not separately reported)

[a] Each unique test, order, or document is counted.

Examples

➤ **A 17-year-old boy presents with need for clearance to attend a sports camp.** The patient received a preventive medicine service 3 months prior to this visit. After examination, a pediatrician clears the patient for participation.

   Level of data reviewed and analyzed ⟿ Minimal or none

   Teaching Point: Medical decision-making will likely be based on the problem addressed and risk.

➤ **A 6-year-old patient presents with a laceration of the thumb.** The patient's mother notes concern that the wound bled until pressure was held for several minutes. After evaluating the laceration, a pediatric nurse practitioner cleanses and bandages the wound.

   Level of data reviewed and analyzed ⟿ Limited

   Teaching Point: Data are low based on assessment requiring an independent historian.

An *independent historian* is an individual (eg, parent, guardian, surrogate, witness) who provides a history in addition to a history provided by a patient who is unable to provide a complete or reliable history (eg, due to developmental stage, loss of consciousness) or because a confirmatory history is judged to be necessary.

In the case where there may be conflict or poor communication between multiple historians and more than 1 historian(s) is needed, the independent historian(s) requirement is met.

➤ **A 16-year-old established patient presents for follow-up of upper respiratory symptoms.** The patient was evaluated at an urgent care practice 2 days ago, but symptoms have increased. The physician reviews records of the urgent care visit, which include a diagnosis of an upper respiratory infection. An influenza test is ordered and the result is positive.

Level of data reviewed and analyzed ⫸ Limited

Teaching Point: This is based on review of external records and order for 1 test. Note that each test is counted only once toward the level of data.

External records, communications, and/or test results are those from an external physician, qualified health care professional, facility, or health care organization. Review of all materials from any unique source counts as 1 element toward medical decision-making.

Tests include imaging, laboratory, psychometric, or physiological data. A clinical laboratory panel (eg, basic metabolic panel [80047]) is a single test because it is reported with 1 *Current Procedural Terminology* (*CPT*) code. The differentiation between single or multiple tests is defined in accordance with the *CPT* code assignment. Pulse oximetry is not counted as a test ordered or reviewed for purposes of medical decision-making.

➤ **A 10-year-old established patient presents for follow up of juvenile arthritis.** The physician reviews results of 3 tests that the physician ordered at the last encounter. Parents provide the patient's medical, family, and social history since the last visit. After evaluation, the physician advises the parents that their child should return for follow-up in 3 months. The parents advise that they will be moving out of state and request that the physician coordinate care with a physician who has agreed to assume management of the patient's juvenile arthritis. After the encounter, the physician communicates with the physician who will assume management, providing history and recommendations for ongoing management.

Level of data reviewed and analyzed ⫸ Moderate

Teaching Point: A moderate level of data is based on discussion of management with an external physician or QHP. The review of the results of the 3 tests is not counted toward the level of data because review of results of tests ordered at the previous encounter are included in that encounter, even if the review occurs on a later date or at the next visit.

An *external physician or other qualified health care professional* (QHP) is an individual who is not in the same group practice or is of a different specialty or subspecialty, including licensed professionals who are practicing independently. A facility or organizational provider, such as a hospital, nursing facility, or home health care agency, may also be an independent source.

Professionals who are not health care professionals but may be involved in the management of the patient are appropriate sources. Examples include a lawyer, case manager, or teacher. Family or informal caregivers are not appropriate sources, although they may be independent historians.

Discussion requires all of the following: an interactive and direct exchange between the reporting individual and the external physician, QHP, or other appropriate source; may be asynchronous but completed within a short period; and is used in medical decision-making for the encounter. Sending chart notes or a written exchange within chart notes is not an interactive exchange.

➤ **An established patient presents for follow-up of persistent headaches and fatigue.** Results of tests ordered at the last visit were reviewed between visits and 2 additional tests were ordered and completed prior to this visit. The physician reviews the results of the additional tests and discusses the findings and treatment recommendation with the patient and parents.

Level of data reviewed and analyzed ⫸ Low

Teaching Point: The review of 2 unique test results supports a low level of data to be reviewed and analyzed. The level of MDM for this encounter may be low, moderate, or complex depending on the nature of the problem addressed (eg, undiagnosed new problem with uncertain prognosis) and risk of morbidity from additional diagnostic testing or treatment.

In the case of tests ordered between encounters, the new test results are counted toward the level of data reviewed and analyzed.

➤ **A 15-year-old established patient presents for follow-up of type 1 diabetes with history of poor control.** The physician reviews results of 2 tests performed based on a recurring order from a prior visit (eg, repeat testing 1 week prior to each visit). Parents provide the patient's medical, family, and social history since the last visit.

    Level of data reviewed and analyzed ‖‖➡ Moderate

    Teaching Point: In the case of a recurring order, each new result may be counted toward the level of data reviewed and analyzed in the visit in which it is analyzed. Note that the original order and review of the first test results are included in the MDM of the encounter where the recurring order was initiated.

> Comparison of multiple results of the same unique test (eg, a new blood glucose result is compared to previous results) is counted as review of 1 unique test result.

➤ **A 6-year-old new patient presents with fever, cough, and vomiting for 2 days.** Parents provide history of fever as high as 102°F (38.9°C) and vomiting that may be associated with coughing. A chest radiograph and influenza test are ordered. Later that day, the pediatrician independently reviews the chest radiograph via electronic health exchange (pending receipt of the radiologist's report) and phones the parents with the results.

    Level of data reviewed and analyzed ‖‖➡ Extensive

    Teaching Point: An extensive level of data is based on orders for 2 unique tests, assessment requiring an independent historian, and independent interpretation of a test reported by another physician or QHP.

> *Independent interpretation* is the interpretation of a test for which there is a *Current Prcoedural Terminology* code and an interpretation or report is customary. This does not apply when the same physician or other qualified health care professional (QHP) (or physician or QHP of the same group practice and same specialty) is reporting or has previously reported interpretation and report for the test.
>
> An interpretation should be documented but need not conform to the usual standards of a complete report for the test (ie, notation of pertinent findings from review of an image or tracing is sufficient rather than the typical documentation completed when providing and billing for an interpretation and report).

➤ **A 6-year-old new patient presents with fever, cough, and vomiting for 2 days.** The patient is accompanied by her grandmother, who asks that the child's mother provide history by telephone. The mother speaks to the physician providing history of fever as high as 102°F (38.9°C) and vomiting that is associated with coughing. A chest radiograph and combined respiratory virus multiplex testing are ordered. Later that day, the pediatrician independently reviews the chest radiograph via electronic health exchange (pending receipt of the radiologist's report) and phones the parents with the results.

    Level of data reviewed and analyzed ‖‖➡ Extensive

    Teaching Point: The extensive level of data reviewed and analyzed is based on 2 unique tests ordered, assessment requiring an independent historian, and independent interpretation of a test by a physician not reporting a code for the interpretation and report of the findings.

> The independent history does not need to be obtained in person but does need to be obtained directly from the historian providing the independent information.

Risk of Complications and/or Morbidity or Mortality of Patient Management

Risk is the probability and/or consequences of an event. *For the purposes of MDM, a level of risk is based on consequences of the problem(s) addressed at the encounter when appropriately treated.* Risk also includes MDM related to the need to initiate or forego further testing, treatment, and/or hospitalization. For purposes of code selection, the level of risk takes into consideration the risk of morbidity from additional diagnostic testing or treatment.

    The risk of patient management criteria applies to the patient management decisions made by the reporting physician or other QHP as part of the reported encounter.

● =New code ▲ =Revised code # =Re-sequenced code + =Add-on code ★ =Telemedicine

Morbidity is a state of illness or functional impairment that is expected to be of substantial duration during which function is limited, quality of life is impaired, or there is organ damage that may not be transient despite treatment.

- Definitions of risk are based on the usual behavior and thought processes of a physician or QHP in the same specialty.
- Trained clinicians apply common meanings to terms such as *high, medium, low,* or *minimal* risk and do not require quantification for these definitions (quantification may be provided when evidence-based medicine has established probabilities).

Current Procedural Terminology does not include examples of minimal or low risk. Coders should seek guidance from a physician or other qualified health care professional if they are unsure of the risk associated with a treatment or management option. For example, a decision to use an over-the-counter medication for a patient who is younger than the age indicated on the product label may carry higher risk than use in a patient who is within the indicated age range.

- The assessment of the level of risk is affected by the nature of the event under consideration. For example, a low probability of death may be high risk, whereas a high chance of a minor, self-limited adverse effect of treatment may be low risk. Social determinants of health may also affect the risk of morbidity.

Social determinants of health are economic and social conditions that influence the health of people and communities. Examples may include food or housing insecurity.

- Risk includes the possible management options selected, and those considered but not selected, after shared MDM with the patient and/or family. For example, a decision about hospitalization includes consideration of alternative levels of care.

Shared medical decision-making is soliciting patient and/or family preferences and patient and/or family education and explaining risks and benefits of management options.

Risk levels are minimal, low, moderate, and high. **Table 7-5** provides examples of each level of risk.

Table 7-5. Examples of Levels of Risk[a]	
Minimal	Rest and drink plenty of fluids. Diaper ointment Superficial wound dressing
Low	Over-the-counter medication(s) following directions as labeled Removal of sutures Physical, language, or occupational therapy
Moderate	Prescription drug management or recommendation for off-label use of an over-the-counter medication Decision about minor surgery with identified patient or procedure risk factors Decision about elective major surgery without identified patient or procedure risk factors Diagnosis or treatment significantly limited by social determinants of health
High	Drug therapy requiring intensive monitoring for toxicity (eg, monitoring for a cytopenia in the use of an antineoplastic agent between dose cycles) Decision about hospitalization Decision about emergency major surgery (immediate or with minimal delay to allow for patient stabilization) Decision not to resuscitate or to de-escalate care because of poor prognosis

[a] Examples are subject to clinical judgment for each individual patient and encounter.

In determining risk associated with a decision about surgery, the surgical package classification does not determine if the procedure is minor or major. *Current Procedural Terminology* states that the classification of surgery into minor or major is based on the common meaning of such terms when used by trained clinicians. Risk factors are those relevant to the patient and the procedure.

Examples

➤ **A patient presents for follow-up after treatment of impetigo.** The patient appears well and parents have no complaints but need clearance to return to child care. Clearance to return to child care is provided. The patient is to follow up as needed or at next scheduled preventive visit.

    Risk ||⟹ Minimal to none

➤ **A 6-year-old boy presents with several days of increasing sneezing, itchy eyes, and fatigue.** After examination, a pediatrician recommends daily use of a nonprescription allergy medication.

    Risk ||⟹ Low

➤ **A pediatric otolaryngologist sees a 6-year-old patient who presents with recurrent otitis media and hypertrophy of adenoids.** Repeat bilateral myringotomy with tube insertion and adenoidectomy under general anesthesia is recommended, and parents agree to proceed with the procedure.

    Risk ||⟹ Moderate
    Teaching Point: Decision for major surgery supports moderate risk.

➤ **A 14-year-old presents for follow-up of asthma.** The patient's asthma is well-controlled and a refill of control medication is prescribed.

    Risk ||⟹ Moderate
    Teaching Point: The prescription medication presents a moderate risk.

➤ **A 6-month-old patient presents with fever, cough, listlessness, and poor feeding.** After examination, the pediatrician recommends hospitalization for evaluation of possible bacterial or viral infection and treatment of dehydration and respiratory distress.

    Risk ||⟹ High
    Teaching Point: The risk associated with the decision to hospitalize the ill infant is high. A decision for aggressive outpatient follow-up may also support high risk.

Selection of Level 2 Through 5 Codes

To select a code for office E/M services, you must determine which code is supported by 2 of 3 elements of MDM or the physician's or QHP's total time on the date of service. Refer to **Table 7-6** for an at-a-glance reminder of the levels of MDM or time required for each level of office E/M service.

The following pages provide an overview of a level of office E/M service with time and MDM reporting criteria and examples of each level of service. Key point to remember in code selection are as follows:

- Examples given are not clinical recommendations and levels of service supported may vary based on documentation and patient age and presentation (eg, ill appearance beyond what is typical for complaint).
- Select a code based on either total physician/QHP time on the date of service or MDM.
- The use of new versus established patient codes is based on whether the patient has received any face-to-face professional service from the same physician or a physician in the same group practice of the same exact specialty and subspecialty in the 3 years prior to the date of service.
- When selecting a code based on time, the total physician and/or QHP time spent devoted to the single patient's care must be documented in addition to the context of the care provided (eg, remarkable findings, counseling, care coordination, shared decision-making).
- When selecting a code level based on MDM as described by *CPT*, the documentation should include the medically appropriate history and examination findings and all problems, diagnoses, management, and treatment options considered.

Chapter 7. Office and Other Outpatient Evaluation and Management Services

Table 7-6. Code Selection Requirements for Office Evaluation and Management Service (Excluding 99211)

Level/Codes/ Total Time (min)[a]	Medical Decision-making (2 of 3 required: data[b], problems, risk)		
	Problems Addressed	**Data Reviewed and Analyzed[c]**	**Risk**
Straightforward *New patient* **99202** (15–29) *Established patient* **99212** (10–19)	1 self-limited or minor	Minimal or none	Minimal *Examples* • Rest and drink plenty of fluids. • Diaper ointment. • Superficial wound care.
Low *New patient* **99203** (30–44) *Established patient* **99213** (20–29)	Low—*Any 1 of* ≥2 self-limited or minor 1 stable chronic illness 1 acute, uncomplicated illness or injury	Limited (*Meet 1 of 2 categories.*) Category 1: Tests and documents (*Meet any 2.*) • Review of prior external note(s)—each unique source • Review of the result(s) of each unique test • Ordering of each unique test Category 2: Assessment requiring an independent historian(s)	Low *Examples* • Over-the-counter medication(s) • Removal of sutures • Physical, language, or occupational therapy
Moderate *New patient* **99204** (45–59) *Established patient* **99214** (30–39)	Moderate—*Any 1 of* ≥1 chronic illness with exacerbation, progression, or side effects of treatment ≥2 stable chronic illnesses 1 undiagnosed new problem with uncertain prognosis 1 acute illness with systemic symptoms 1 acute complicated injury	Moderate (*Meet 1 of 3 categories.*) Category 1: Tests and documents (*Meet any 3.*) • Review of prior external note(s)—each unique source • Review of the result(s) of each unique test • Ordering each unique test • Assessment requiring an independent historian(s) Category 2: Independent interpretation of a test performed by another physician/ other QHP[c] Category 3: Discussion of management or test interpretation with external physician/ other QHP/appropriate source	Moderate *Examples* • Prescription drug management or off-label use of over-the-counter medication • Decision about minor surgery with identified patient or procedure risk factors • Decision about elective major surgery without identified patient or procedure risk factors • Diagnosis or treatment significantly limited by social determinants of health
High *New patient* **99205** (60–74) *Established patient* **99215** (40–54)	High—*1 of* ≥1 chronic illness with severe exacerbation, progression, or side effects of treatment 1 acute or chronic illness or injury that poses a threat to life or bodily function	Extensive (*Meet 2 of 3 categories.*) Category 1: Tests and documents (*Meet any 3.*) • Review of prior external note(s) from each unique source • Review of the result(s) of each unique test • Ordering of each unique test • Assessment requiring an independent historian(s) Category 2: Independent interpretation of a test performed by another physician/ other QHP Category 3: Discussion of management or test interpretation with external physician/ other QHP/appropriate source[c]	High • Drug therapy requiring intensive monitoring for toxicity • Decision about elective major surgery with identified patient or procedure risk factors • Decision about emergency major surgery • Decision about hospitalization • Decision not to resuscitate or to de-escalate care because of poor prognosis

Abbreviation: QHP, qualified health care professional.

[a] Does not include time of clinical staff. Include only time spent by the physician or QHP directed to the individual patient's care on the date of the encounter.

[b] Each unique test, order, or document contributes to the combination of 2 or combination of 3 in Category 1.

[c] Do not count data review or communications reported with other codes (eg, test interpretation, interprofessional consultation).

Office E/M Level 2 (99202, 99212)

★99202 Office or other outpatient visit for the evaluation and management of a new patient, which requires a medically appropriate history and/or examination and straightforward medical decision making
When using time for code selection, 15–29 minutes of total time is spent on the date of the encounter.

★99212 Office or other outpatient visit for the evaluation and management of an established patient, which requires a medically appropriate history and/or examination and straightforward medical decision making
When using time for code selection, 10–19 minutes of total time is spent on the date of the encounter.

Level 2 (99202, 99212) Medical Decision-making Requirements	
Documentation must support at least 2 of 3 elements (problems, data, risk).	
Problems addressed—number and complexity	**Minimal**—1 self-limited or minor problem
Data—amount/complexity to be reviewed and analyzed	**Minimal** or none
Risk of complications and/or morbidity or mortality of patient management	**Minimal** risk of morbidity from additional diagnostic testing or treatment

Time Requirements (in Lieu of MDM)

- **99202**: 15–29 minutes total physician and/or QHP time spent on the date of the encounter
- **99212**: 10–19 minutes total physician and/or QHP time spent on the date of the encounter

Examples

➤ **A 16-year-old new patient presents with request for counseling about sexuality.** A physician spends 15 minutes answering questions and discussing sexuality in the context of the patient's relationship with a family member who is transgender. A total time of 20 minutes is spent including time spent documenting the encounter.
International Classification of Diseases, 10th Revision, Clinical Modification (ICD-10-CM): **Z70.2** (counseling related to sexual behavior and orientation of third party)
CPT: **99202** (total time 15–29 minutes) is supported by the total time of 20 minutes.

➤ **An infant presents for a follow-up visit for slow weight gain.** Parents note the patient has been nursing well. Weight gain since last check is satisfactory. Diagnosis is follow-up for infant feeding problem.
ICD-10-CM: Because the feeding problem is no longer present, a follow-up code (**Z09**) and code **Z86.898** (personal history of other specified conditions) are reported.
CPT: The resolved problem with minimal data and risk supports **99212**.

Office E/M Level 3 (99203, 99213)

★99203 Office or other outpatient visit for the evaluation and management of a new patient, which requires a medically appropriate history and/or examination and low level of medical decision making
When using time for code selection, 30–44 minutes of total time is spent on the date of the encounter.

★99213 Office or other outpatient visit for the evaluation and management of an established patient, which requires a medically appropriate history and/or examination and low level of medical decision making
When using time for code selection, 20–29 minutes of total time is spent on the date of the encounter.

Level 3 (99203, 99213) Medical Decision-making Requirements	
Documentation must support at least 2 of 3 elements (problems, data, risk).	
Problems addressed—number and complexity	**Low** (*Any 1 of the following*) ≥2 self-limited or minor problems 1 stable chronic illness 1 acute, uncomplicated illness or injury
Data—amount/complexity to be reviewed and analyzed	**Limited** (*Must meet the requirements of 1 of the 2 categories*) **Category 1:** Tests and documents (*Any combination of 2* from the following) • Review of prior external note(s) from each unique source • Review of the result(s) of each unique test • Ordering of each unique test **Category 2:** Assessment requiring an independent historian(s)
Risk of complications and/or morbidity or mortality of patient management	**Low** Examples • Over-the-counter medication(s) • Removal of sutures • Physical, language, or occupational therapy

Time Requirements (in Lieu of MDM)

- **99203**: 30–44 minutes total physician and/or QHP time spent on the date of the encounter
- **99213**: 20–29 minutes total physician and/or QHP time spent on the date of the encounter

Examples

➤ **A 6-year-old new patient presents for complaint of right ear pain.** Mother provides history of pain for 2 days. Swimmer's ear (right ear) is diagnosed. Antimicrobial ear drops are prescribed.
    ICD-10-CM: **H60.331** (swimmer's ear, right ear)
    CPT: **99203**. Low MDM is supported by the acute uncomplicated illness, data (need for independent historian), and moderate risk (prescription drug management).
    Prescription drug management alone supports moderate risk but not moderate MDM.

➤ **A 9-year-old established patient presents for follow-up of moderate intermittent asthma.** Parents are reluctant to continue daily control medication despite continued asthma symptoms when medication doses are missed. Total time of service documented is 25 minutes.
    ICD-10-CM: **J45.20** (mild intermittent asthma, uncomplicated)
    CPT: 25 minutes of physician time on the date of service supports **99213**.

➤ **An established patient presents for asthma follow-up.** Asthma control test and parent-completed symptom log indicate good control on current medication. The patient has no complaints. It is decided to continue the current plan and follow up in 3 months. Prescription is refilled. The diagnosis is intermittent asthma.
    ICD-10-CM: **J45.20** (mild intermittent asthma, uncomplicated)
    CPT: **99213** (low MDM based on 1 stable chronic condition addressed, low data [independent historian], and moderate risk [prescription drug management]) and for the separately reportable asthma control test, **96160** (administration of patient-focused health risk assessment instrument [eg, health hazard appraisal] with scoring and documentation, per standardized instrument)

Office E/M Level 4 (99204, 99214)

★**99204**   Office or other outpatient visit for the evaluation and management of a new patient, which requires a medically appropriate history and/or examination and moderate level of medical decision making
        When using time for code selection, 45–59 minutes of total time is spent on the date of the encounter.

★99214 Office or other outpatient visit for the evaluation and management of a new patient, which requires a medically appropriate history and/or examination and moderate level of medical decision making

When using time for code selection, 30–39 minutes of total time is spent on the date of the encounter.

Level 4 (99204, 99214) Medical Decision-making Requirements

Documentation must support at least 2 of 3 elements (problems, data, risk).

Problems—number and complexity of problems addressed: Moderate (*Any 1 of the following*)

≥1 chronic illness with exacerbation, progression, or side effects of treatment ≥2 stable chronic illnesses	1 undiagnosed new problem with uncertain prognosis 1 acute illness with systemic symptoms 1 acute complicated injury

Data—amount/complexity to be reviewed and analyzed: Moderate (*Must meet the requirements of at least 1 out of 3 categories*)

Category 1 (*Any combination of 3*) • Review of prior external note(s) from each unique source • Review of the result(s) of each unique test • Ordering of each unique test • Assessment requiring an independent historian(s)	**Category 2:** Independent interpretation of a test performed by another physician/other QHP (not separately reported) **Category 3:** Discussion of management or test interpretation with external physician/other QHP/appropriate source (not separately reported)

Risk of complications and/or morbidity or mortality of patient management: Moderate

• Prescription drug management
• Decision about minor surgery with identified patient or procedure risk factors
• Decision about elective major surgery without identified patient or procedure risk factors
• Diagnosis or treatment significantly limited by social determinants of health

Time Requirements (in Lieu of MDM)

- **99204**: 45–59 minutes total physician and/or QHP time spent on the date of the encounter
- **99214**: 30–39 minutes total physician and/or QHP time spent on the date of the encounter

Examples

➤ **An established patient with asthma presents with shortness of breath unrelieved by home inhalation treatment.** The patient stabilizes after an inhalation treatment in the office. New medication is prescribed. The diagnosis is exacerbation of mild persistent asthma.

ICD-10-CM: **J45.31** (mild persistent asthma with [acute] exacerbation)

CPT: Moderate MDM (exacerbation of a chronic condition with prescription drug management) supports **99214**. Spirometry and inhalation treatment are separately billed.

➤ **An established patient presents with a rash.** The pediatrician examines the patient and determines the rash is poison ivy. However, the child is under-immunized due to parents' fear of harmful effects of immunization. The pediatrician takes the opportunity to discuss how the patient is equally susceptible to serious diseases as to the poison ivy. Twenty minutes are spent in counseling the parents on risks associated with not immunizing their child and how vaccines are produced, tested, and approved. After the parents still refuse immunization at this encounter, the pediatrician requests that the parents sign and date a vaccine refusal form. The pediatrician's total time on the date of service, including documentation after the visit, is 35 minutes.

ICD-10-CM: **L23.7** (allergic contact dermatitis due to plants, except food), **Z28.3** (under-immunization), and **Z28.82** (immunization not carried out because of caregiver refusal)

CPT: **99214** is supported by the physician's total time of 35 minutes.

All of the physician's time spent in care of the 1 patient on the date of the encounter is included in the time used to select the level of service for the office visit. There is no requirement that more than 50% of that time be spent in counseling and/or coordination of care.

Office E/M Level 5 (99205, 99215)

★99205   Office or other outpatient visit for the evaluation and management of a new patient, which requires a medically appropriate history and/or examination and high level of medical decision making

> When using time for code selection, 60–74 minutes of total time is spent on the date of the encounter. (For services 75 minutes or longer, see prolonged services code **99417**.)

★99215   Office or other outpatient visit for the evaluation and management of an established patient, which requires a medically appropriate history and/or examination and high level of medical decision making

> When using time for code selection, 40–54 minutes of total time is spent on the date of the encounter. (For services 55 minutes or longer, see prolonged services code **99417**.)

Time Requirements (in Lieu of MDM)

- **99205**: 60–74 minutes total physician and/or QHP time spent on the date of the encounter
- **99215**: 40–54 minutes total physician and/or QHP time spent on the date of the encounter

Examples

➤ **A new 3-month-old patient presents for an urgent appointment with a primary care pediatrician.** The infant's presentation is consistent with possible sepsis. The decision is made to arrange for direct hospital admission by an intensivist.

> *ICD-10-CM:* Diagnosis codes are reported for the child's symptoms.
> *CPT:* **99205** is supported by the acute illness that poses a threat to life or bodily function and decision to hospitalize.

➤ **A pediatrician reviews records of a new patient with complex medical history and later that day sees the patient and assists the parents with establishing subspecialty care.** The physician's total time on the date of the visit is 60 minutes.

> *ICD-10-CM:* Appropriate codes for the diagnoses addressed at the encounter are reported.
> *CPT:* **99205** is reported based on the physician's total time on the date of the encounter.

➤ **An established patient presents with symptoms of diabetes with ketoacidosis.** Laboratory tests ordered and reviewed are a urine dipstick and basic metabolic panel. The decision is made to hospitalize for new onset type 1 diabetes with ketoacidosis.

> *ICD-10-CM:* **E10.10** is reported for type 1 diabetes with ketoacidosis without coma.
> *CPT:* **99215** is supported by the problems addressed (ie, illness with threat to life or bodily function) and risk (ie, hospitalization).

➤ **An established patient presents with fever and severe cough.** Clinical staff summon the physician to the examination room where the physician notes the patient is in respiratory failure. Less than 30 minutes are spent by the physician caring for the child before an ambulance team assumes management. The physician documents a diagnosis of respiratory failure.

> *ICD-10-CM:* **J96.00** (acute respiratory failure, unspecified whether with hypoxia or hypercapnia) or code for more specific diagnosis, when known, and **R50.9** (fever unspecified)
> *CPT:* **99205** is supported by the problems addressed (ie, illness with threat to life or bodily function) and risk (ie, hospitalization).

Prolonged Office E/M Service

Prolonged Service by a Physician or Other Qualified Health Care Professional

Prolonged service *on the date of an office E/M service* is reported with code **99417**. Codes **99354** and **99355** are not used in conjunction with codes **99202–99205** and **99211–99215**.

Chapter 7. Office and Other Outpatient Evaluation and Management Services

★+**99417**   Prolonged office or other outpatient evaluation and management service(s) beyond the minimum required time of the primary procedure which has been selected using total time, requiring total time with or without direct patient contact beyond the usual service, on the date of the primary service, each 15 minutes of total time

- Report code **99417**
  — Only when the office E/M code has been selected based on time *and only* after the minimum total time of the highest-level service (ie, **99205** or **99215**) has been exceeded by a full 15 minutes
  — When 15 minutes or more of additional time has been attained with 1 unit for each full 15 minutes beyond the minimum total time on the date of the visit
- Do not report **99417**
  — For prolonged service of less than 15 minutes on the date of the office E/M service
  — For any additional time increment of less than 15 minutes
  — For time spent performing separately reported services other than the E/M service
  — In addition to **99202–99204** or **99211–99214**
  — On the same date as **99354** and **99355**, **99358** and **99359**, or **99415** and **99416**
  — When a payer requires code **G2212** (See "Coding Conundrum: **G2212** Versus **99417**" later in this chapter.)

Table 7-7 provides the required times for reporting units of **99417** in addition to either **99205** or **99215**.

Table 7-7. Times Supporting Prolonged Service With Codes 99205 and 99215[a]

Reporting With 99205		Reporting With 99215	
Time (min)	Codes Reported	Time (min)	Codes Reported
60–74	99205	40–54	99215
75–89	99205 + 99417 × 1	55–69	99215 + 99417 × 1
90–104	99205 + 99417 × 2	70–84	99215 + 99417 × 2
≥105	99205 + 99417 × 3 plus 1 unit for each full 15-minute period beyond the first 74 minutes	≥85	99215 + 99417 × 3 plus 1 unit for each full 15-minute period beyond 119 minutes

[a] The times in this table are based on 2022 *Current Procedural Terminology* recommendations. When a payer has adopted Centers for Medicare & Medicaid Services policy, report **G2212** for each 15 minutes beyond the maximum total time in the range for **99205** (prolonged service begins at 89 minutes) and **99215** (prolonged service begins at 69 minutes) in lieu of **99417**.

For E/M services that require prolonged clinical staff time and may include face-to-face services by the physician or QHP, see codes **99415** and **99416**.

Examples

➤ **A new patient is referred following discharge from observation care for asthma.** The patient has no usual source of care and has been seen in 3 EDs for a total of 4 visits in the past year. The pediatrician spends 30 minutes prior to the face-to-face visit, on the same date, reviewing observation and ED records for the child. At the visit, the pediatrician spends 45 minutes evaluating the patient, who also has behavioral issues in school; developing a plan of care; and counseling the patient and caregiver on the plan. After the visit, the pediatrician spends 15 minutes on the same date providing instructions to the school nurse about the patient's use of a rescue inhaler and arranging for teachers to complete rating scales for ADHD. The pediatrician reports codes **99205** and **99417** × 2 for the 90 minutes devoted to the patient's care on the date of the encounter.

➤ **An established adolescent patient and her parents meet with a pediatrician to discuss newly diagnosed idiopathic scoliosis.** Because the parents do not speak fluent English, an interpreter is required. The pediatrician spends 75 minutes discussing the diagnosis and management options and coordinating care. Code **99417** × 2 units is reported in addition to **99215**.

Prolonged service by a physician or QHP on a date before or after the date of a face-to-face office E/M service (in-person or telehealth) is reported with code **99358**.

Chapter 7. Office and Other Outpatient Evaluation and Management Services

Coding Conundrum: G2212 Versus 99417

Some payers may not accept code **99417** for prolonged office evaluation and management (E/M) services. The Centers for Medicare & Medicaid Services developed an alternative code **G2212** (described below) in 2021 to require that the time of prolonged office E/M services begins when time exceeds *the higher time in the range of total time* assigned to either code **99205** or **99215** in lieu of the lower time in the range of total time as required for code **99417**.

G2212   Prolonged office or other outpatient evaluation and management service(s) beyond the maximum required time of the primary procedure which has been selected using total time on the date of the primary service; each additional 15 minutes by the physician or qualified health care professional, with or without direct patient contact

   G2212 is reported only in conjunction with **99205** (add **G2212** for total time ≥89 minutes) or **99215** (add **G2212** for total time ≥55 minutes) and only when the time requirement is met.

   In the absence of a contractual requirement to follow a payer's policy to report **G2212** in lieu of **99417**, physicians should assign code **99417** and follow *Current Procedural Terminology guidelines.*

Prolonged Clinical Staff Service (99415, 99416)

+99415   Prolonged clinical staff service (the service beyond the highest time in the range of total time of the service) during an evaluation and management service in the office or outpatient setting, direct patient contact with physician supervision; first hour

+99416   each additional 30 minutes

   Codes **99415** and **99416** are used to report 30 minutes or more of prolonged clinical staff time spent face-to-face providing care to a patient under the supervision of a physician or other QHP who has provided an office or other outpatient E/M service at the same session. See time requirements in **Table 7-8**.

Table 7-8. Level 2 Through 5 Office Evaluation and Management Times and Start of Prolonged Clinical Staff Time			
Code		**Assigned Time (min)**	**Minimum Time Required for Reporting 99415 (minutes of face-to-face clinical staff time)**
New Patient	99202	15–29	59
	99203	30–44	74
	99204	45–59	89
	99205	60–74	104
Established Patient	99212	10–19	49
	99213	20–29	59
	99214	30–39	69
	99215	40–54	84

- Report prolonged clinical staff service **99415** and **99416** in addition to office or other outpatient E/M codes **99202–99215**.
- *Never report both* prolonged office E/M service by a physician or other QHP (**99417**) and prolonged clinical staff services together.
- Codes **99415** and **99416** were assigned relative value units (RVUs) based only on clinical staff's intraservice time, as the preservice and post-service times were considered to be included in the value of the related E/M service. Relative value units (2021 non-facility practice expense only) assigned are 0.29 for **99415** and 0.15 for **99416**. When paid at a conversion rate of $36.0896 per RVU, code **99415** would be valued at $10.47 (0.29 × 36.0896) and code **99416** would be valued at $5.41 per unit (0.15 × 36.0896).

   The following guidelines apply to reporting of prolonged clinical staff services:
- A physician or other QHP must supervise the duration of prolonged clinical staff service.
- Prolonged clinical staff services are reported only when the face-to-face time spent by clinical staff is 30 minutes or more beyond the highest total time of the related E/M service on the same date.
- Do not report prolonged service of less than 30 minutes beyond the highest total time of the related E/M service.

- The total time of and medical necessity for the service must be documented.
- Time spent providing separately reported services, such as intravenous medication administration or inhalation treatment, is not counted toward the time of prolonged service.
- When not continuous, document the face-to-face time of each episode of clinical staff time.
- Report code **99416** for each additional 30 minutes of clinical staff time beyond the first hour and for the last 15 to 30 minutes of prolonged clinical staff service. Do not report **99416** for less than 15 minutes beyond the first hour or last 30-minute period.

Table 7-9 shows the calculation of units of service for codes **99415** and **99416**.

Table 7-9. How to Code Prolonged Clinical Staff Services

Minutes Beyond End Time of Office E/M Code	Code(s)
<30	Not reported separately
30–74	**99415** × 1
75–104	**99415** × 1 AND **99416** × 1
≥105 (≥1 h 45 min)	**99415** × 1 AND **99416** × 2 (and additional units for each full 30 minutes or the last 15–30 minutes)

Abbreviation: E/M, evaluation and management.

Examples

➤ **A child is seen for diarrhea and concerns of dehydration.** The physician diagnoses moderate dehydration due to viral gastroenteritis. Oral rehydration is ordered. The physician completes her documentation and selects code **99214** for service. The physician remains in the office suite while a nurse delivers and monitors a time-based oral rehydration plan using an electrolyte solution. The nurse's total direct care time is 2 hours.

ICD-10-CM: **A08.4** (viral intestinal infection, unspecified) and **E86.0** (dehydration)

CPT: E/M service by physician is reported with **99214** (includes 39 minutes); prolonged clinical staff time is reported with **99415** × 1 (first hour) and **99416** × 1 (final 30-minute period).

Teaching Point: *CPT* instructs that prolonged clinical staff time begins after the typical time of the E/M service provided by the physician and is not reported if the prolonged clinical staff time is less than 45 minutes. When a physician reports code **99214** (includes 39 minutes), prolonged clinical staff time is not reported unless clinical staff have spent at least 69 minutes in face-to-face patient care.

In this scenario, with clinical staff time of 120 minutes, the physician service includes 39 minutes, so prolonged clinical staff time is 81 minutes. The final 21 minutes is reported with code **99416** because 15 to 30 minutes beyond the previous period is separately reported.

➤ **A new patient who has been vomiting for 2 days is seen in the physician's office.** After evaluation by a physician, she is given antipyretics and fluids and then monitored and assessed by clinical staff for a total face-to-face clinical staff time of 104 minutes. After the monitoring period, the physician returns to the examination room and provides final instruction to the mother before releasing the child. The physician service includes moderate-complexity MDM (**99204**) based on key components. The physician's total time on the date of service was 45 minutes.

ICD-10-CM: **K52.9** (gastroenteritis, unspecified)

CPT: **99204** (includes 45–59 minutes) and **99415** × 1 (first hour of prolonged clinical staff time)

Teaching Point: Prolonged service by clinical staff under physician supervision is reported rather than the physician's prolonged service, as the physician's total time did not exceed the time of code **99205** (includes 60–74 minutes). Code **99415** is reported because clinical staff time of 104 minutes was more than 30 minutes beyond the 59 minutes included in code **99204**.

➤ **A physician provides treatment to an established patient with acute exacerbation of moderate persistent asthma.** Over the course of 2 hours, the patient is given fluids (oral) for mild dehydration and oxygen as needed, oral steroids, and 3 inhaled bronchodilators. Documentation supports moderate-complexity MDM and total time by the physician of 70 minutes. Clinical staff also document 60 minutes of direct patient care (eg, providing nebulizer treatments) following the physician's E/M service.

> *ICD-10-CM:* **J45.41** (acute exacerbation of moderate persistent asthma) and **E86.0** (dehydration)
> *CPT:* **99215** (includes 40–54 minutes), **99417** (additional 15 minutes), and **94640** 76 × 3 (nebulizer treatments); HCPCS codes for the medications supplied and administered (eg, **J7613** [albuterol, inhalation solution, US Food and Drug Administration–approved final product, non-compounded, administered through durable medical equipment, unit dose, 1 mg])

> **Teaching Point:** The physician's service described includes code **99215**, office or other outpatient encounter, and 1 unit of prolonged office E/M service (**99417**). Prolonged clinical staff service is not reported on the same date as prolonged service by a physician or QHP, and time spent providing separately reported services (eg, nebulizer treatment) is not included in any prolonged service time.

> Supplies related to services such as nebulizer treatment (**94640**) are included in the practice expense RVUs assigned to each code. If a payer does not base payment on RVUs, supplies may be separately reported with code **99070** (supplies and materials [except spectacles], provided by the physician or other QHP over and above those usually included with the office visit or other services rendered [list drugs, trays, supplies, or materials provided]) or specific HCPCS codes (eg, **A7003**, administration set, with small volume nonfiltered pneumatic nebulizer, disposable).

Split/Shared Office E/M Services

> **Notice: At the time of publication, CMS has proposed, but not finalized, significant changes to the Medicare policy for split/shared visits. Please visit the American Academy of Pediatrics website (www.aap.org/cfp or www.aap.org/errata) to check for updates.**

A *split/shared E/M service* is one in which a physician and a QHP from the same group practice each personally perform a medically necessary and substantive portion of 1 or more face-to-face E/M encounters on the same date. *A portion of the service must be provided face-to-face by the physician to report under the physician's NPI.*

> By reporting under the physician's NPI, a higher fee schedule amount may be paid for the service (eg, 100% vs 85% of fee schedule). Split/shared services were defined and implemented for services to Medicare beneficiaries. Private payers may adopt the same or a similar policy. The split/shared concept is applied differently for inpatient services than for services in the office setting (see **Chapter 6**).

- In the non-facility office setting (place of service 11), split/shared E/M services must meet incident-to requirements for the service to be reported under the physician's NPI.

  Incident-to services require the physician's presence in the office suite at the time of the QHP service and that the QHP provides care only in accordance with a physician's established care plan for the patient.

> **See Chapter 13 for more information on incident-to services.**

- The physician and QHP must document and sign their portion of the service. A physician cannot merely sign off on the documentation of the QHP's work.
- If the E/M service is reported based on time the physician and QHP must each document their total time spent in care of the patient on the date of the encounter. Each minute of time must be attributed to either the physician or QHP, but not both.
- Critical care is never a split/shared service because critical care services reflect the work of only one individual.

Example

➤ **The patient history and a portion of the examination are provided in the office by a nurse practitioner for an established patient in continuation of a physician's previously documented plan of care for ADHD.** The physician is consulted about concerns of increased behavioral symptoms, sees the patient face-to-face, performs a more detailed evaluation, and documents the assessment and plan of care.

●=New code   ▲=Revised code   #=Re-sequenced code   +=Add-on code   ★=Telemedicine

The total service may be reported under the physician's NPI because incident-to provisions have been met and both professionals provided face-to-face services.

After-hours Services (99050–99058)

Codes **99050–99058** are used to report services that are provided after hours or on an emergency basis and are always reported in addition to the primary service (eg, E/M service).

- Third-party payers will have specific policies for coverage and payment.
  - Some carriers pay practices for extended hours because they recognize the cost benefit realized from decreased urgent care and ED visits.
  - Communicate with individual payers to understand their definition or interpretation of the service and their coverage and payment policies.
  - As part of this negotiation and education process, it is important to demonstrate the cost savings recognized by the payer for these adjunct services.
- If appropriate, more than 1 adjunct code may be reported on the same day of service (eg, **99058** and **99051** for services provided on an emergency basis during regularly scheduled evening or weekend hours).

  Many payers will pay only for the use of a single special services code per encounter and may manually review, question, or deny payment for a claim with multiple after-hours codes.

After-hours service codes are used by physicians or other QHPs (under their state scope of practice and when billing with their own NPI) to identify the services that are adjunct to the basic services rendered. These codes

- Describe the special circumstances under which a basic service is provided.
- Are only reported in addition to an associated basic service (eg, E/M, fracture care).
- Are reported without a modifier appended to the basic service because they only further describe the services provided.

Follow individual payer policy when reporting after-hours codes in conjunction with a service provided via telemedicine.

Services Provided When the Office Is Normally Closed

99050   Service(s) provided in office at times other than regularly scheduled office hours, or days when the office is normally closed (eg, holidays, Saturday, Sunday), in addition to basic service

- Office hours must be posted. *CPT* does not define a holiday or posted office hours. While most commonly applied to evening, weekend, or holiday hours, code **99050** could be applied to services provided at the patient request on a weekday if the office is typically closed on that day.
- Code **99050** is *not* reported when a physician or other QHP is behind schedule and sees patients after posted office hours.
- The service must be requested by the patient, and the physician or other QHP must agree to see the patient.
- Documentation must indicate the time and date of the encounter and the request to be seen outside of normal posted hours.

Services Provided During Regularly Scheduled Evening, Weekend, or Holiday Hours

99051   Service(s) provided in the office during regularly scheduled evening, weekend, or holiday office hours, in addition to basic service

- Regularly scheduled office hours must be posted.
- Documentation must include the time and date of the encounter.
- Evenings and holidays are not defined by *CPT,* but holidays can generally refer to national and/or state holidays, and evenings are generally 6:00 pm and later. Check with payers for coverage and/or ability to bill patients these charges under the health plan contract.

Example

➤ **A pediatric clinic offers urgent care appointments 3 evenings a week with staffing by nonphysician QHPs (ie, nurse practitioners, physician assistants) working under general supervision.** A patient who has been seen at the clinic by Dr A within the last year is seen in the evening clinic by a nurse practitioner who documents an expanded problem-focused history and examination with low-complexity MDM with diagnosis of upper respiratory infection.

    ICD-10-CM: **J06.9** (acute upper respiratory infection, unspecified)

    CPT: **99213** (established office E/M) and **99051** (service provided in office during regularly scheduled weekend hours)

        Teaching Point: Because the office offers regularly scheduled evening hours, code **99051** is reported. The patient is established because *CPT* instructs that QHPs are considered to be of the same specialty as the physicians with whom they work in a group practice.

Services Provided on an Emergency Basis in the Office

99058   Service(s) provided on an emergency basis in the office, which disrupts other scheduled office services, in addition to basic service

- Report when an office patient's condition, in the clinical judgment of the physician, warrants the physician interrupting care of another patient to deal with the emergency.
- Code **99058** may not be reported when patients are simply fit into the schedule or for walk-ins.
- Document that the patient was seen immediately and the reason for the emergent care.

Example

➤ **A child is seen for severe exacerbation of moderate persistent asthma on a Saturday at 9:00 am.** The child arrives 30 minutes prior to the scheduled time and is immediately taken to an examination room by the triage nurse, and the physician disrupts his schedule to see the child urgently. The office is open on Saturday mornings from 8:00 am to 12:00 noon.

    ICD-10-CM: **J45.41** (moderate persistent asthma with acute exacerbation)

    CPT: **99202–99215** (new or established office E/M), **99058** (service provided on an emergency basis in office, disrupting other scheduled services), and **99051** (service provided in office during regularly scheduled weekend hours)

        Teaching Point: If the Saturday hours were for walk-in visits only (ie, no scheduled appointments), code **99058** would *not* be reported. Note that if the patient is admitted to observation or inpatient hospital care on the same date by the same physician or a physician or other QHP of the same specialty and same group practice who later sees the patient in the facility setting on the same date, all services on that date are included in the code selection for initial observation or initial hospital care.

Continuum Models: Asthma, Attention-Deficit/Hyperactivity Disorder, and Otitis Media

Continuum Model for Asthma			
Code selection at any level above **99211** *may be based on complexity of MDM or the total time spent on the date of service by the reporting physician or other qualified health care professional.* *The extent of history and examination documented does not affect code selection.*			
CPT Code and Vignette	**MDM (2 of 3 elements required)**		
99211 Nurse visit for a well 10-year-old established patient	*Time and MDM do not apply. Must indicate continuation of physician's plan of care, medical necessity, assessment, and/or education provided.* CC: Asthma care plan review Documentation of medications, peak expiratory flow, education topics reviewed, and questions answered		
CPT Code With Total Physician Time and Vignette	**Number and Complexity of Problems Addressed**	**Amount and/or Complexity of Data Reviewed and Analyzed**	**Risk of Complications and/or Morbidity or Mortality of Patient Management**
99212 (Time: 10–19 min) An 8-year-old with stable asthma presents with a single patch of poison ivy rash on her forearm.	**SF:** 1 self-limited or minor problem	**SF:** None	**SF:** Minimal risk of morbidity from treatment

Continuum Model for Asthma (*continued*)

CPT Code With Total Physician Time and Vignette	Number and Complexity of Problems Addressed	Amount and/or Complexity of Data Reviewed and Analyzed	Risk of Complications and/or Morbidity or Mortality of Patient Management
99213 (Time: 20–29 min) A 7-year-old with stable persistent asthma who is using a metered-dose steroid inhaler with β-agonist as needed returns for follow-up.	**Low:** 1 stable chronic illness	**Low:** Assessment requiring an independent historian(s)—mother provides history of asthma symptoms and medication compliance since last visit	**Moderate:** Prescription drug management
99214 (Time: 30–39 min) An 8-year-old with unstable asthma is examined because of an acute exacerbation of the disease; already receiving inhaled albuterol and inhaled steroids by metered-dose inhaler.	**Moderate:** 1 or more chronic illnesses with exacerbation, progression, or side effects of treatment	**Low:** Assessment requiring an independent historian(s)—mother provides history *Note: Spirometry and pulse oximetry provided are separately reported and not counted toward data reviewed and analyzed.*	**Moderate:** Prescription drug management
99215 (Time: 40–54 min) A 1-year-old known to have recurrent wheezing following respiratory syncytial virus bronchiolitis has had increasingly frequent attacks during the past 2 months. New infiltrates are revealed by chest radiograph (film interpreted, not separately reported). Cystic fibrosis is suspected. A sweat test is ordered.	**High:** 1 acute or chronic illness or injury that poses a threat to life or bodily function	**High:** Review of prior external note(s) from recent ED visit; order sweat test; assessment requiring independent historians (parents) and independent interpretation of radiograph performed by another physician (not separately reported)	**Moderate:** Assumes prescription drug management

Abbreviations: CC, chief complaint; CPT, *Current Procedural Terminology*; ED, emergency department; MDM, medical decision-making; SF, straightforward.

Continuum Model for Attention-Deficit/Hyperactivity Disorder

Code selection at any level above **99211** *may be based on the complexity of MDM or the total time spent by the physician or other qualified health care professional on the date of the encounter. (Code* **99211** *is not included due to lack of indication for follow-up by clinical staff.)*

CPT Code With Total Physician Time and Vignette	MDM (2 of 3 elements required)		
	Number and Complexity of Problems Addressed	Amount and/or Complexity of Data Reviewed and Analyzed	Risk of Complications and/or Morbidity or Mortality of Patient Management
99211 Nurse visit to check growth or blood pressure prior to renewing prescription for psychoactive drugs	*Time and MDM do not apply. Must indicate continuation of physician's plan of care, medical necessity, assessment, and/or education provided.* CC: Check growth or blood pressure. Documentation: Height, weight, and blood pressure. Existing medications and desired/undesired effects. Assessment: Doing well. Obtained physician approval for prescription refill. Keep appointment with physician in 1 month.		
99212 (Time: 10–19 min) 4-year-old whose parents are concerned about ADHD symptoms (ADHD is not diagnosed; parents are reassured.)	**Minimal:** 1 self-limited problem	**Limited:** Assessment requiring an independent historian	**Minimal:** Parent education
99213 (Time: 20–29 min) Initial follow-up after initiation of medication, patient responding well	**Low:** 1 stable chronic illness	**Limited:** Assessment requiring an independent historian	**Moderate:** Prescription drug management, delayed prescribing

Chapter 7. Office and Other Outpatient Evaluation and Management Services

Continuum Model for Attention-Deficit/Hyperactivity Disorder (*continued*)

CPT Code With Total Physician Time and Vignette	MDM (2 of 3 elements required)		
	Number and Complexity of Problems Addressed	Amount and/or Complexity of Data Reviewed and Analyzed	Risk of Complications and/or Morbidity or Mortality of Patient Management
99214 (Time: 30–39 min) Follow-up recent weight loss in patient with established ADHD otherwise stable on stimulant medication	**Moderate:** 1 chronic illness with side effects of treatment	**Limited:** Assessment requiring an independent historian	**Moderate:** Prescription drug management
99215 (Time: 40–54 min) Initial evaluation of patient with ADHD and new onset of suicidal ideation. Patient and mother refuse hospitalization due to cost. *Tip:* Add **99417** if time on the date of service is ≥55 minutes. Add **99058** if service(s) are provided on an emergency basis in the office, which disrupts other scheduled office services.	**High:** 1 acute or chronic illness or injury that poses a threat to life or bodily function	**Moderate:** Assessment requiring an independent historian; discussion with behavioral health specialist; psychiatric testing	**High:** Decision regarding hospitalization

Abbreviations: ADHD, attention-deficit/hyperactivity disorder; CC, chief complaint; *CPT, Current Procedural Terminology*; MDM, medical decision-making.

Continuum Model for Otitis Media

Code selection at any level above **99211** *may be based on the complexity of MDM or the total time spent by the physician or other qualified health care professional on the date of the encounter. (Code* **99211** *is not included due to lack of indication for follow-up by clinical staff.)*

CPT Code With Total Physician Time and Vignette	MDM (2 of 3 elements required)		
	Number and Complexity of Problems Addressed	Amount and/or Complexity of Data Reviewed and Analyzed	Risk of Complications and/or Morbidity or Mortality of Patient Management
99212 (Time: 10–19 min) Follow-up otitis media, uncomplicated	**Minimal:** Follow-up otitis media, evaluation of effusion and hearing	**Limited:** Tympanometry, audiometry, and/or assessment requiring an independent historian	**Minimal:** Risk associated with diagnostic testing and treatment
99213 (Time: 20–29 min) 2-year-old presents with tugging at her right ear. Afebrile. Mild otitis media.	**Low:** 1 acute, uncomplicated illness or injury	**Limited:** Assessment requiring an independent historian	**Moderate:** Prescription drug management, delayed prescribing
99214 (Time: 30–39 min) Infant presents with fever and cough and suspected third episode of otitis media within 3 months.	**Moderate:** 1 acute illness with systemic symptoms	**Limited:** Assessment requiring an independent historian	**Moderate:** Prescription drug management
99215 (Time: 40–54 min) 6-month-old presents with high fever, vomiting, and irritability. After tests, antipyretics, and fluid, infant is stable.	**High:** 1 acute illness that poses a threat to life or bodily function	**Moderate:** Orders and/or review of laboratory tests, chest radiograph, and possible lumbar puncture. Assessment requiring an independent historian.	**High:** Decision about hospitalization (Hospitalization discussed with parents and decision made for care at home with strict instructions and close follow-up.)

Abbreviations: *CPT, Current Procedural Terminology*; MDM, medical decision-making.

Resources

Documentation

American Academy of Pediatrics Initial History Questionnaire Documentation Form for office or outpatient visits (available for purchase at http://shop.aap.org)

Examples of Office E/M Code Levels

"Office E/M 2021: Level 2 Visits," August 2020 *AAP Pediatric Coding Newsletter*™ (https://coding.solutions.aap.org/article.aspx?articleid=2765198; subscription required)

"Office E/M 2021: Level 3 Visits," September 2020 *AAP Pediatric Coding Newsletter* (https://coding.solutions.aap.org/article.aspx?articleid=2765216; subscription required)

"Office E/M 2021: Level 4 Visits," October 2020 *AAP Pediatric Coding Newsletter* (https://coding.solutions.aap.org/article.aspx?articleid=2765225; subscription required)

"Office E/M 2021: Level 5 Visits," November 2020 *AAP Pediatric Coding Newsletter* (https://coding.solutions.aap.org/article.aspx?articleid=2765232; subscription required)

Guidelines for Office E/M Code Selection

"Retroactive Evaluation and Management Guideline Corrections Published," April 2021 *AAP Pediatric Coding Newsletter* (https://coding.solutions.aap.org/article.aspx?articleid=2765338; subscription required)

Medical Decision-making

"Office E/M 2021: An Overview of Medical Decision-making," February 2020 *AAP Pediatric Coding Newsletter* (https://coding.solutions.aap.org/article.aspx?articleid=2759684; subscription required)

"Office E/M 2021: Determining the Number and Complexity of Problems Addressed," April 2020 *AAP Pediatric Coding Newsletter* (https://coding.solutions.aap.org/article.aspx?articleid=2763373; subscription required)

"Office E/M 2021: Determining Levels of Amount and/or Complexity of Data," May 2020 *AAP Pediatric Coding Newsletter* (https://coding.solutions.aap.org/article.aspx?articleid=2765177; subscription required)

"Office E/M 2021: Determining the Level of Risk," June 2020 *AAP Pediatric Coding Newsletter* (https://coding.solutions.aap.org/article.aspx?articleid=2765184; subscription required)

"Office E/M 2021: Determining the Level of Medical Decision-making," July 2020 *AAP Pediatric Coding Newsletter* (https://coding.solutions.aap.org/article.aspx?articleid=2765191; subscription required)

"Office E/M 2021: Examples of Pediatric Medical Decision-making for Office Evaluation and Management Services," January 2021 *AAP Pediatric Coding Newsletter* (https://coding.solutions.aap.org/article.aspx?articleid=2765261; subscription required)

Time-Based Code Selection for Office E/M

"Documenting Total Time for Office Evaluation and Management Services," May 2021 *AAP Pediatric Coding Newsletter* (https://coding.solutions.aap.org/article.aspx?articleid=2765341; subscription required)

Prolonged Services in Conjunction With Office Visits

"2021 Prolonged Service Codes," April 2021 *AAP Pediatric Coding Newsletter* (https://coding.solutions.aap.org/article.aspx?articleid=2765337; subscription required)

Test Your Knowledge!

1. **Which of the following would be appropriately reported with code 99211?**
   a. Clinical staff provide dietary education to an established patient on a date when no physician service is provided. (Service meets incident-to requirements.)
   b. Clinical staff provide an immunization administration to an established patient.
   c. Clinical staff perform venipuncture on an established patient.
   d. Clinical staff provide an education service on the same date as a physician service.

2. **Which of the following is not an example of discussion with an external physician as defined for office evaluation and management (E/M)?**
   a. Discussion between a treating physician and a physician of a different subspecialty but in the same group practice
   b. Discussion between a treating qualified health care professional and a physician working in the same group and same specialty
   c. Discussion between a physician of a different group practice who is consulted by the treating physician
   d. Discussion between a primary care pediatrician and a licensed clinical psychologist in the same group practice

3. **Which of the following does not support a moderate number and complexity of problems addressed?**
   a. Acute illness with systemic symptoms
   b. 2 stable chronic illnesses
   c. Chronic illness with exacerbation, progression, or side effects of treatment
   d. 2 acute, uncomplicated illnesses or injuries

4. **Which of the following supports an extensive amount and/or complexity of data to be reviewed and analyzed?**
   a. Ordering 3 unique tests
   b. Ordering 3 unique tests and obtaining history from an independent historian
   c. Ordering 3 unique tests and discussing management with an external physician or external source
   d. Ordering and reviewing the results of the same 3 unique tests

5. **Which of the following supports reporting a prolonged office E/M service (99417)?**
   a. A physician's total time on the date of the encounter exceeds the minimum time of the range of total time assigned to 99205 or 99215 by 8 to 15 minutes.
   b. A physician's total time on the date of the encounter exceeds the minimum time of the range of total time assigned to 99205 or 99215 by at least 15 minutes.
   c. A physician's total time within a 24-hour period exceeds the minimum time in the range of total time assigned to 99205 or 99215 by at least 15 minutes.
   d. A physician's total time on the date of an encounter supports code 99215 and a call to the patient's caregiver on the next day lasts at least 15 minutes.

CHAPTER 8

Preventive Services

Contents

Preventive Care 173

Preventive Medicine Evaluation and Management Services 173

    ICD-10-CM Codes for Preventive Care Visits.. 175

    Quality Initiatives and Preventive Care 176

    Sports/Camp Physicals.. 177

Immunizations.. 178

    Vaccines and Toxoids 178

        New Vaccines/Toxoids.. 178

    National Drug Code 179

    Immunization Administration 179

        Coding for COVID-19 Immunization 179

        Codes **90460** and **90461** 180

        Codes **90471**–**90474** 181

        Coding for Counseling When Immunizations Are Not Carried Out 183

        Vaccines for Children Program.. 185

Screening Tests and Procedures 185

    Hearing Screening.. 185

    Vision Screening.. 186

Developmental Screening and Health Assessment 187

    Developmental Screening... 187

    Emotional/Behavioral Assessment 188

    Health Risk Assessment... 189

Prevention of Dental Caries 190

    Application of Fluoride Varnish 190

    Counseling to Prevent Dental Caries 190

    Other Codes for Prevention of Dental Caries 191

Screening Laboratory Tests... 191

Preventive Care Provided Outside the Preventive Visit 192

    Counseling and/or Risk-Factor Reduction.. 192

        Preventive Medicine, Individual Counseling Codes... 192

        Preventive Medicine, Group Counseling Codes 193

    Behavior Change Intervention 194

    Preventive Medicine Services Modifier 196

        Other Preventive Medicine Services.. 197

Reporting a Preventive Medicine Visit With a Problem-Oriented Visit 197

Resources.. 200

Test Your Knowledge! 201

Preventive Care

Preventive care is the hallmark of pediatrics. The Patient Protection and Affordable Care Act (PPACA) recognized the importance of preventive care for children and includes a critical provision that ensures that most health care plans cover, *without cost sharing*, the criterion standard of pediatric preventive care—the American Academy of Pediatrics (AAP) *Bright Futures: Guidelines for Health Supervision of Infants, Children, and Adolescents*, 4th Edition.

Coverage of and appropriate payment for these pediatric preventive services should, at a minimum, reflect the total relative value units (RVUs) outlined for the current year under the Medicare Resource-Based Relative Value Scale Physician Fee Schedule (PFS), inclusive of all separately reported codes for these services. Section 2713 of the PPACA includes the following 2 sets of services that must be provided to children without cost sharing:

1. The standard set of immunizations recommended by the Advisory Committee on Immunization Practices (ACIP) of the Centers for Disease Control and Prevention (CDC) with respect to the individual involved
2. Evidence-informed preventive care and screenings provided for in the comprehensive guidelines supported by the Health Resources and Services Administration (HRSA), which include
   - Bright Futures recommendations for preventive pediatric health care
   - Recommendations of the Advisory Committee on Heritable Disorders in Newborns and Children

The Bright Futures periodicity schedule, "Recommendations for Preventive Pediatric Health Care," is a great tool to identify recommended age-appropriate services; in addition, it can be used to identify those services that can and should be reported with their own *Current Procedural Terminology* (*CPT*®) or Healthcare Common Procedure Coding System code, and it identifies appropriate diagnosis coding. This tool can be found as an insert in this book and can be accessed online at https://downloads.aap.org/AAP/PDF/periodicity_schedule.pdf.

Although all recommended preventive services are covered, physicians and practice managers should be aware of health plan policies that may affect payment.

- Specific diagnosis codes may be required to support claims adjudication under preventive medicine benefits. Be sure to link the appropriate diagnosis to each service provided (eg, code **Z71.3**, dietary counseling, may be linked to code **99401** for a risk-factor reduction counseling visit).
- Some payers bundle certain services when the services are provided on the same date. For instance, some plans will not allow separate payment for obesity counseling on the same date as a well-child examination (health supervision visit) but will cover obesity counseling when no other evaluation and management (E/M) service is provided on the same date.
  - It is beneficial to monitor and maintain awareness of the payment policies of the plans most commonly billed by your practice.
  - Most policies are available on payers' websites with notification of changes provided in payer communications, such as electronic newsletters.

Preventive Medicine Evaluation and Management Services

Well-child or preventive medicine services are a type of E/M service and are reported with codes **99381–99395**. Most health plans provide a 100% benefit (no patient out-of-pocket cost) for the 31 recommended preventive medicine service encounters when provided by in-network providers. The selection of the pediatric-specific codes **99381–99395** is based simply on the age of the patient and whether the patient is new or established to the practice (**Table 8-1**).

In brief, an established patient has been seen (face-to-face, including via real-time audiovisual telehealth) by the physician or another physician of the same specialty and group practice within the last 3 years. Generally, other qualified health care professionals (QHPs; eg, advanced practice nurses, physician assistants) are considered to be working in the same specialty as the physicians with whom they work. Refer to **Chapter 7**, Office and Other Outpatient Evaluation and Management Services, for more information about *new* versus *established* patients.

> A neonate who received hospital newborn care by the same physician or a physician of the same specialty and same group practice will be an established patient for post-discharge care in the office or other outpatient setting.

Chapter 8. Preventive Services

Table 8-1. New and Established Preventive Medicine Codes		
Code Description **Comprehensive preventive medicine evaluation and management**	**New Patient Code**	**Established Patient Code**
infant (age <1 year)	99381	99391
early childhood (age 1–4 years)	99382	99392
late childhood (age 5–11 years)	99383	99393
adolescent (age 12–17 years)	99384	99394
age 18–39 years	99385	99395

- Most health plans will limit the benefits for preventive medicine E/M services covered in a year based on the patient's age. See **Figure 8-1** for an illustration of recommended preventive visits by age.
- Immunizations, laboratory tests, and other special procedures or screening tests (eg, vision, hearing, developmental screening) that have their own specific *CPT* codes are reported separately *in addition to* preventive medicine E/M services.
- Most payers will require reporting modifier **25** with the preventive medicine service when immunizations or other services are also performed and reported.
- A comprehensive history and physical examination must reflect an age- and a gender-appropriate history and examination and are *not* synonymous with the "comprehensive" history and examination described in the E/M documentation guidelines from the Centers for Medicare & Medicaid Services (CMS) (see **Chapter 6**, Evaluation and Management Documentation Guidelines Other Than Office and Other Outpatient Services).
- The comprehensive history performed as part of a preventive medicine visit does not require a chief complaint or history of present illness. It does require a comprehensive age-appropriate review of systems (ROS) with an updated past, family, and social history. The history should also include a comprehensive assessment or history of age-pertinent risk factors.
- Generally, the ROS of a preventive medicine service is not a list of systems with pertinent positive and negative responses but, rather, a list of inquiries and patient responses for those areas of risk identified in preventive medicine guidelines as pertinent for patients of that age and gender. However, some payers may require review of all systems regardless of age and gender (eg, required by some Medicaid plans under Early and Periodic Screening, Diagnostic, and Treatment [EPSDT] benefits).

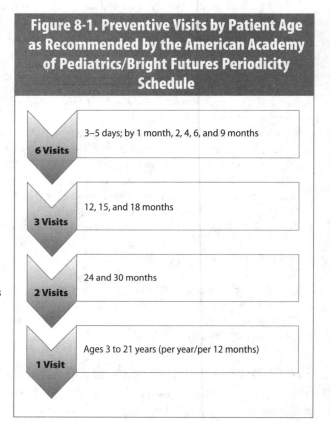

Figure 8-1. Preventive Visits by Patient Age as Recommended by the American Academy of Pediatrics/Bright Futures Periodicity Schedule

6 Visits — 3–5 days; by 1 month, 2, 4, 6, and 9 months

3 Visits — 12, 15, and 18 months

2 Visits — 24 and 30 months

1 Visit — Ages 3 to 21 years (per year/per 12 months)

The American Academy of Pediatrics (AAP) has developed an Initial History Questionnaire that promotes good documentation of preventive medicine services. Examples can be ordered from the AAP by calling 888/227-1770 or visiting https://shop.aap.org/product-list/?q=documentation%20forms. Additionally, some state Medicaid programs have developed documentation templates for preventive services delivered in their Early and Periodic Screening, Diagnostic, and Treatment program.

- Routine management of contraception is considered part of the comprehensive preventive medicine E/M service when it is provided during the well-care health supervision visit.
- A comprehensive physical examination is a multisystem examination that may include a routine pelvic and breast examination (when performed in the absence of specific symptoms of a problem) depending on the age of the patient and/or sexual history. If the pelvic examination is performed because of a gynecologic problem during a routine

preventive medicine service, it may be appropriate to report a problem-oriented E/M service in addition to the preventive medicine service when additional physician work and required key components of the E/M code are met.

- State Medicaid programs have requirements for performing, documenting, and reporting certain services in their EPSDT programs. Review your state Medicaid policies for the specific documentation and reporting requirements for services to patients in these programs.

ICD-10-CM Codes for Preventive Care Visits

International Classification of Diseases, 10th Revision, Clinical Modification (*ICD-10-CM*) well-care diagnosis codes should be linked to the appropriate preventive medicine code (**99381–99395**). *ICD-10-CM* codes for well-child examinations include developmental, hearing, and vision screening.

Z00.110	Health supervision for newborn <8 days
Z00.111	Health supervision for newborn 8–28 days old
Z00.121	Routine child health examination (≥29 days) with abnormal findings
Z00.129	Routine child health examination (≥29 days) without abnormal findings
Z00.00	Encounter for general adult medical examination without abnormal findings
Z00.01	Encounter for general adult medical examination with abnormal findings

- For the purpose of assigning codes from this category, an *abnormal finding* is a newly discovered condition on a screen or a known or chronic condition that requires attention (eg, uncontrolled, acutely exacerbated). Assign additional codes for any abnormal findings. A stable chronic condition is not considered an abnormal finding.
- An abnormal finding *ICD-10-CM* code (eg, **Z00.121**) can be linked to the procedure code for a normal screening test; the abnormality will be identified with the appropriate *ICD-10-CM* code elsewhere on the claim so the payer will be aware that the abnormality is unrelated to the screening.
- *ICD-10-CM* does not specify an age at which codes **Z00.00** and **Z00.01** are reported in lieu of codes **Z00.121–Z00.129**. The age of majority varies by state and payer, who may or may not adopt the Medicare Outpatient Code Editor assignment of age limitations (29 days–17 years) to codes **Z00.121–Z00.129**, as indicated in many *ICD-10-CM* references.
- Link routine health examination codes (eg, **Z00.129**) and code **Z23** (encounter for immunization) to the immunization administration (IA) and vaccine product codes when immunizations are administered at the preventive medicine encounter. *ICD-10-CM* instructs to report code **Z00.-** first, followed by code **Z23**.
- When an existing problem is addressed at the preventive medicine service but is not a newly discovered condition or a known or chronic condition that has increased in severity, report a routine child health examination without abnormal findings and also code the condition addressed.

> ### Preventive Services for Children With Chronic and Complex Health Care Needs
>
> Like all children, children with chronic and complex health care needs also must receive periodic preventive care visits. Preventive medicine evaluation and management (E/M) services may take longer for children who are medically complex. However, preventive E/M services are not reported based on time and prolonged service does not apply. Only report a separate E/M service on the date of a preventive E/M service when a problem is addressed that requires significant physician work (ie, medical decision-making [MDM] or time) and is separately identifiable in the documentation. A chronic medical condition that is not separately addressed with documentation of the required MDM or time spent addressing the condition does not support reporting both preventive care and a separate E/M service (eg, **99213**).
>
> See Chapter 12 for information on care management for children with complex health care needs.

Examples

➤ **A 9-year-old is seen for an established patient preventive medicine service.** The child was seen 1 month ago for mild persistent asthma and reports no increase in asthma symptoms. However, the child's mother notes that the child's rescue inhaler, which is carried to and from school, is nearing the expiration date. An age- and gender-appropriate preventive service is provided and documented. A refill prescription is ordered for the rescue inhaler. Diagnoses are well-child visit and stable mild persistent asthma.

ICD-10-CM	*CPT*
Z00.129 (routine child health exam without abnormal findings) **J45.30** (uncomplicated mild persistent asthma)	**99393** (preventive medicine visit; age 5–11)

Chapter 8. Preventive Services

Teaching Point: Because the asthma is not newly identified or failing to respond adequately to treatment, this is not an abnormal finding. However, it is appropriate to report the code for the asthma that is still present in addition to code **Z00.129**. In this example, the work of prescribing the asthma medication refill did not equate to a significant, separately identifiable E/M service.

➤ **A 9-year-old was diagnosed 8 weeks ago with mild persistent asthma.** The child presents today for a scheduled preventive service and follow-up visit. The child complains of increasing asthma symptoms and use of rescue inhaler. The patient's medications and asthma control plan are revised. The age- and gender-appropriate preventive service is also provided and documented. The diagnoses are well-child visit with abnormal findings (**Z00.121**) and mild persistent asthma with increasing symptoms and underdosing of the asthma control medication.

ICD-10-CM	CPT
Z00.121 (routine child health exam with abnormal findings) **J45.31** (mild persistent asthma with acute exacerbation)	**99393** (preventive medicine visit; age 5–11)
J45.31	**99214 25** (established patient office visit with moderate level medical decision-making [MDM])

Teaching Point: Because the asthma was inadequately controlled, the routine health examination included an abnormal finding. See more on reporting problem-oriented E/M services in conjunction with a preventive service later in this chapter. Code **J45.31** is reported once on the claim but linked to each procedure code.

Quality Initiatives and Preventive Care

Quality initiatives and measurement are becoming standard practice in health care. Many physicians have participated in quality measurement through programs such as the CMS Promoting Interoperability Programs and medical home recognition programs. In pediatrics, many quality measures are associated with preventive care (eg, provision of one meningococcal vaccine on or between the patient's 11th and 13th birthdays).

Quality measurement is also required of health plans funded by government programs or offered through health exchanges created to support health insurance adoption under the PPACA. These health plans must collect and submit Quality Rating System measure data to the CMS. This entails collecting clinical quality measures, including a subset of the National Committee for Quality Assurance Healthcare Effectiveness Data and Information Set (HEDIS) measures and a Pharmacy Quality Alliance measure. Physicians contracting with these plans may be asked to provide evidence that quality measures were met through claims data or medical records. Examples of HEDIS measures related to preventive care include

- Percentage of members who turned 15 or 30 months old during the measurement year and who had 6 or more well-child visits with a primary care provider during the first 15 months after birth *and* 2 or more well-child visits from 1 day after the child turned 15 months old to turning 30 months old
- Percentage of members 3 to 21 years of age who had at least 1 comprehensive well-care visit with a primary care provider or obstetrician-gynecologist during the measurement year
- Members 3 to 17 years of age who had an outpatient visit with a primary care provider and who had the following services in the current year:
  — Body mass index (BMI) percentile documentation
  — Counseling for nutrition
  — Counseling for physical activity

Certain preventive services, such as anticipatory guidance on healthy diet (**Z71.3**) and exercise (**Z71.82**), are components of the preventive medicine service and require no additional procedure coding for payment purposes. However, associated diagnosis and procedure codes may be reported to support quality reporting initiatives.

ICD-10-CM guidelines instruct that codes for BMI are reported when the there is an associated, reportable diagnosis (eg, overweight, obesity). However, some health plans still require this code to support quality measures in lieu of *CPT* performance measurement code **3008F** (BMI, documented). Pediatric BMI codes in category **Z68** include

Z68.51	BMI <5th percentile
Z68.52	BMI 5th–<85th percentile
Z68.53	BMI 85th–95th percentile
Z68.54	BMI ≥95th percentile

Chapter 8. Preventive Services

International Classification of Diseases, 10th Revision, Clinical Modification (ICD-10-CM) codes for pediatric body mass index (BMI) percentiles (**Z68.51–Z68.54**) are only reported in conjunction with physician documentation of a related condition (eg, overweight, obesity). If reporting codes **Z68.51–Z68.54** based on a payer's written guidance for reporting quality measures, it is advisable to keep a copy of the payer's guidance. An alternative method for reporting that the patient's BMI was documented is to report *Current Procedural Terminology* Category II code **3008F** (BMI, documented) in lieu of *ICD-10-CM* codes for BMI.

Certain other procedure codes also support quality measurement. For example, submission of claims containing codes for meningococcal (**90734, #90619**); tetanus, diphtheria, and acellular pertussis (Tdap) (**90715**); and 2 or 3 doses of human papillomavirus (HPV) vaccine (**90649–90651**) provided to an adolescent before the patient's 13th birthday is indicative of meeting the measure for the immunization of adolescents.

Example

➤ **A 12-year-old who received immunizations against Tdap (90715) and HPV (2 doses; 90651) at prior visits returns for a well-child visit.** A preventive service is provided including documentation of the child's BMI and counseling for healthy diet and exercise. The physician also counsels for immunization against meningococcal disease and recommends that a vaccine that was missed during the COVID-19 public health emergency (PHE) be administered. The meningococcal (MenACWY-D) vaccine is administered at the encounter.

ICD-10-CM	CPT
Z00.129 (routine child health examination without abnormal findings) **Z71.3** (anticipatory guidance on healthy diet) **Z71.82** (exercise counseling)	**99394** **3008F** (BMI, documented)
Z00.129 **Z23** (encounter for immunization)	**90640** (IA with physician counseling to patient ≤18 years old) **90734** (MenACWY-D vaccine product)

Teaching Point: The codes for the meningococcal vaccine product (**90734**), in addition to prior claims reported with codes for Tdap and HPV vaccines, show the recommended vaccines for patients 9 to 13 years old have been completed. To meet the measure, all vaccines must be completed by the 13th birthday.

Codes **Z13.41** (encounter for autism screening) and **Z13.42** (encounter for screening for global developmental delays [milestones]) may be used to track developmental screening measures of the Child Core Set for patients receiving benefits through their state Medicaid and Children's Health Insurance Program. Use of the Child Core Set is optional for state programs and physicians. Codes **Z13.41** and **Z13.42** may be reported at any encounter where screening is performed (eg, with or without a preventive E/M service).

It is important to note that a request for medical records is less likely when claims are submitted with procedure and diagnosis codes associated with pediatric quality measures.

See Chapter 3, Coding to Demonstrate Quality and Value, for more information on Healthcare Effectiveness Data and Information Set and quality reporting.

Sports/Camp Physicals

CPT guidelines recommend that preventive medicine service codes (**99381–99395**) be reported when possible for physicals performed to determine participation eligibility. These codes most accurately describe the services performed in that they are preventive and age appropriate in nature and physicians offer counseling on topics such as appropriate levels of exercise or injury prevention. However, the need for these services often arises after the child has had a yearly preventive medicine service, thereby rendering this service non-covered by some health plans, which allow only 1 preventive service per year. In this case, the parent may be billed if the payer contract allows because the service is non-covered.

ICD-10-CM code **Z02.5** is reported for an encounter for examination for participation in sports. If the preparticipation physical evaluation is incorporated into the annual health supervision visit, use code **Z00.121** or **Z00.129** in lieu of **Z02.5**. Any problems or conditions that are addressed during the course of the visit would also be reported.

> Codes in category **Z02** are not reported in conjunction with codes for routine child health examination (category **Z00**).

When reporting sports or camp physicals for patients who have already received a recommended preventive medicine service, check the health plan's policy on payment for these services and instructions for coding and billing. Under some Medicaid plans, school and preparticipation physical evaluations may be covered even when the child has already had an annual preventive medicine service.

Office visit codes (**99212–99215**) may be used if a problem is discovered during the service. Outpatient consultation codes (**99241–99245**) might be considered (when the health plan allows payment for these codes) if the coach or school nurse requested the physician's opinion of a suspected problem (eg, exercise cough associated with reduced performance in cold weather). The medical record must include documentation of the written or verbal request as well as a copy of the written report with the physician's opinion or advice that was sent back to the coach or school nurse.

Immunizations

Vaccine services are reported using 2 families of *CPT* codes—one for the vaccine serum (the product) and one for the services associated with the administration of the vaccine. Exceptions to this fall under those patients receiving vaccines through the Vaccines for Children (VFC) program. See the Vaccines for Children Program section later in this chapter for more details on VFC coding.

Vaccines and Toxoids

> The administration of immune globulins (including palivizumab [Synagis]) is not reported using the immunization administration codes. See codes **96365–96368**, **96372**, **96374**, and **96375**. Medications, including birth control, are reported with **96372** (therapeutic, prophylactic, or diagnostic subcutaneous or intramuscular injection).

Codes **90476–90758** are used to report the vaccine or toxoid product only. They do not include the administration of a vaccine.

- **Appendix III**, Vaccine Products: Commonly Administered Pediatric Vaccines, provides a quick reference to codes, descriptors, and the number of vaccine components for each vaccine linked to the brand and manufacturer for each.
- The exact vaccine product administered needs to be reported to meet the requirements of immunization registries, vaccine distribution programs, and reporting systems (eg, Vaccine Adverse Event Reporting System), as well as for payment.
- Codes may be specific to the product manufacturer and brand, schedule (ie, number of doses or timing), chemical formulation, dosage, and/or route of administration. When a vaccine code descriptor includes "when administered to" patients of certain ages, this is not an indication of the ages for which the product is licensed.
- Codes for combination vaccines (eg, **90707**, measles, mumps, rubella, and varicella virus vaccine) are available, as are separate codes for single-component vaccines (eg, **90716**, varicella virus vaccine).
- It is not appropriate to code each component of a combination vaccine separately using separate vaccine product codes when a combination vaccine is administered. However, if a combination vaccine is commercially available but a physician elects to administer the component vaccines due to unavailability or other clinical reason, each vaccine product administered would be separately reported.

> The word *component* refers to an antigen in a vaccine that prevents disease(s) caused by 1 organism.

New Vaccines/Toxoids

The *CPT* Editorial Panel, in recognition of the public health interest in vaccine products, has chosen to publish new vaccine product codes prior to US Food and Drug Administration (FDA) approval. The American Medical Association (AMA) uses its *CPT* site (www.ama-assn.org/practice-management/cpt/category-i-vaccine-codes) to provide updates of *CPT* Editorial Panel actions on new vaccine products. Once approved by the *CPT* Editorial Panel, vaccine/toxoid product codes are typically made available for release on a semiannual basis (July 1 and January 1). As part of the electronic distribution, there is a 6-month implementation period from the initial release date (ie, codes released on January 1 are eligible for use on July 1; codes released on July 1 are eligible for use on January 1). Codes for products pending FDA approval are indicated with a lightning bolt symbol (✐) and will be tracked by the AMA to monitor FDA approval status. The lightning bolt symbol will be removed once the FDA status changes to "approved." Refer to the AMA *CPT* site indicated earlier for the most up-to-date information on codes with this symbol. More rapid code release and implementation may occur when a government agency has identified an urgent need for a vaccine to address an emergent health issue and the FDA has granted that vaccine an expedited review process. In such cases, codes may be approved and released on an *immediate* (ie, outside the normal code consideration schedule) or *rapid* (ie, within the normal code consideration schedule but released shortly after approval with an implementation date within 3 months of release) basis.

Before administering any new vaccine product or an existing vaccine product with new recommendations, make certain the CDC, in the *Morbidity and Mortality Weekly Report,* or the AAP, in *Pediatrics,* has endorsed the use or recommendations of the vaccine. You may also want to verify with a patient's health plan that the vaccine is covered.

In the rare event that a vaccine enters the market this year and is FDA approved, recommendations for use are published by the CDC or AAP, and no code exists for the specific vaccine, use code **90749** (unlisted vaccine/toxoid) and list the specific vaccine given.

National Drug Code

Many payers, specifically Medicare, Medicaid, other government payers (eg, Tricare), and some private payers, require the use of the National Drug Code (NDC) when reporting vaccine product codes. The NDCs are universal product identifiers for medications, including vaccines. NDCs are found on outer packaging, product labels, and/or product inserts. This is discussed more fully in **Chapter 1**, The Basics of Coding.

NDCs are 10-digit, 3-segment numbers that identify the product, labeler, and trade package size. The Health Insurance Portability and Accountability Act of 1996 standards require an 11-digit code. See **Chapter 1** and **Table 1-10** for more information including how 10-digit codes are converted to the 11-digit format for reporting.

If you are not currently reporting vaccines with NDCs, be sure to coordinate the requirements with your billing software company. For more information on NDCs, visit www.fda.gov/Drugs/InformationOnDrugs/ucm142438.htm.

Immunization Administration

CPT codes **90460** and **90461** *or* **90471–90474** are reported *in addition to* vaccine/toxoid code(s) **90476–90758** for most routine childhood immunizations. Information on codes developed for administration of COVID-19 vaccines follows.

Coding for COVID-19 Immunization

Codes for the COVID-19 vaccine products and their administration were assigned specific codes by product and dose (eg, administration of first or second dose), as in the following example.

Note that, unlike other IA codes (**90460**, **90461**; **90471–90474**), codes for administration of a COVID-19 vaccine identify the specific product administered. This is in part due to federal government provision of vaccine products at no charge to the physician or other provider during the COVID-19 PHE. Some payers require reporting of the COVID-19 vaccine code with a $0.00 or $0.01 charge and the appropriate administration code, while others require only the appropriate IA code. As with any vaccine, always follow the Advisory Committee on Immunization Practices recommendations.

Example

➤ **A 16-year-old patient requests immunization against COVID-19.** The initial dose of the Pfizer-BioNTech COVID-19 vaccine is reported with

91300	Severe acute respiratory syndrome coronavirus 2 (SARS-CoV-2) (Coronavirus disease [COVID-19]) vaccine, mRNA-LNP, spike protein, preservative free, 30 mcg/0.3mL dosage, diluent reconstituted, for intramuscular use
0001A	Immunization administration by intramuscular injection of severe acute respiratory syndrome coronavirus 2 (SARS-CoV-2) (coronavirus disease [COVID-19]) vaccine, mRNA-LNP, spike protein, preservative free, 30 mcg/0.3mL dosage, diluent reconstituted; first dose

The *ICD-10-CM* code reported is **Z23** (encounter for immunization).

When the patient returns for the second dose of the same vaccine, the administration is reported with codes **91300** and **0002A** (intramuscular [IM] injection as in **0001A**, second dose). When a third dose is administered, report **91300** and **0003A** (intramuscular [IM] injection as in **0001A**, third dose).

Teaching Point: During the PHE declared in response to COVID-19, a specific set of codes were developed for COVID-19 vaccines and their administration. Vaccine codes released prior to publication in the *CPT* code set are available at www.ama-assn.org/practice-management/cpt/category-i-vaccine-codes. *CPT* Appendix Q also provides a quick reference guide to codes for COVID vaccine products and administration.

> See "AAP COVID-19 Vaccine Administration: Getting Paid" for an up-to-date discussion of coding for COVID-19 vaccines and administration (https://services.aap.org/en/pages/2019-novel-coronavirus-covid-19-infections/covid-19-vaccine-for-children/covid-19-vaccine-administration-getting-paid/).

Codes 90460 and 90461

90460   Immunization administration through 18 years of age via any route of administration, with counseling by physician or other qualified health care professional; first or only component of each vaccine or toxoid administered

+90461   each additional vaccine or toxoid component administered (report only in addition to **90460**)

When reporting codes **90460** and **90461**

- Physicians or QHPs must provide *face-to-face* counseling to the patient and/or family (patient aged 18 years or younger) at the time of the encounter for the administration of a vaccine. (See the Codes **90471–90474** section later in this chapter for IA without physician counseling or to patients older than 18 years. Also see the Coding for Counseling When Immunizations Are Not Carried Out section later in this chapter.)
- *CPT* defines a physician or other QHP as follows:

  A "physician or other qualified health care professional" is an individual who by education, training, licensure/regulation, facility credentialing (when applicable), and facility privileging (when applicable) performs a professional service within his/her scope of practice and independently reports that professional service. These professionals are distinct from "clinical staff."

- Clinical staff will not qualify to perform the counseling reported under codes **90460** and **90461**. While state scope of practice may allow certain clinical staff to perform the service, it will not qualify them to report these codes. In the absence of counseling by a physician or QHP, administration services by clinical staff are reported with codes **90471–90474**. *CPT* defines clinical staff as follows:

  A clinical staff member is a person who works under the supervision of a physician or other qualified health care professional and who is allowed by law, regulation, and facility policy to perform or assist in the performance of a specified professional service, but who does not individually report that professional service. Other policies may also affect who may report specific services.

- When a private payer contract does not allow QHPs to report services under their own name and National Provider Identifier (NPI), check with the payer to determine the eligibility of these professionals to report immunization counseling (**90460**, **90461**) and report under the name and number of the supervising physician.
- Documentation of immunization counseling should include a listing of all vaccine components with notation that counseling was provided for all listed components with authentication (electronic or written signature and date) by the physician or other QHP. Supply of the Vaccine Information Statement (VIS) without discussion of risks and benefits does not constitute counseling. Some payers require documentation of parent or caregiver questions or concerns that were addressed during counseling.
- Code **90460** is reported for the *first (or only) component of each vaccine administered* (whether single or combination) on a day of service and includes the related vaccine counseling.
- Code **90461** is only reported in conjunction with **90460** and is used to report the work of counseling for *each additional component(s) beyond the first* in a given combination vaccine. (See the Vaccines for Children Program section later in this chapter for reporting administration of vaccines containing multiple components to this program.)
- Combination vaccines are those vaccines that contain multiple vaccine components. Refer to **Appendix III**, Vaccine Products: Commonly Administered Pediatric Vaccines, for the number of components in the most commonly reported pediatric vaccines.
- The IA codes include the physician or other QHP's work of discussing risks and benefits of the vaccines, providing parents with a copy of the appropriate CDC VIS for each vaccine given, the cost of clinical staff time to record each vaccine component administered in the medical record and statewide vaccine registry, giving the vaccine, observing and addressing reactions or side effects, and cost of supplies (eg, syringe, needle, bandages).

Code **90460** is reported for each individual vaccine administered because every vaccine will have, at minimum, 1 vaccine component. For combination vaccines, code **90461** is additionally reported for counseling on each additional component. No modifier is typically required for reporting multiple units of the IA codes. Most payers advise reporting multiple units of the same service on a single line of the claim. However, individual payer guidance may vary. The AAP continues to advocate to the CMS for increased RVUs for codes **90460** and **90461**.

Append modifier **25** when a significant, separately identifiable E/M service (eg, office or other outpatient service, preventive medicine service) is performed in addition to the vaccine and toxoid administration codes. If vaccines are given during the course of a preventive medicine E/M service and another E/M service, both E/M services will need modifier **25** if required by the payer. See also the Reporting a Preventive Medicine Visit With a Problem-Oriented Visit section later in this chapter.

Examples

➤ **An adolescent presents for an influenza immunization.** After you counsel the patient, clinical staff administer an intranasal quadrivalent influenza vaccine (LAIV) at the same encounter.

Report code **90460** with 1 unit in addition to **90672** (LAIV). Code **90461** is not reported because each vaccine contains only 1 component (ie, protects against 1 disease). Link the vaccine and administration *CPT* codes to *ICD-10-CM* code **Z23** on health insurance claims.

➤ **A 6-month-old patient presents for an established patient well-baby visit.** The physician (or QHP) provides and documents the preventive medicine E/M service. The physician counsels the caregivers about recommended immunization with diphtheria and tetanus toxoids and acellular pertussis vaccine, inactivated poliovirus vaccine, and *Haemophilus influenzae* type b vaccine (DTaP-IPV/Hib); pneumococcal vaccine (PCV13); and influenza (IIV4) vaccine. The parent/guardian is given the CDC VIS and consents; the nurse prepares the vaccine. The nurse administers each vaccine, charts the required information, and accesses and enters vaccine data into the statewide immunization registry. The patient is discharged home after the nurse confirms that there are no serious immediate reactions.

ICD-10-CM	CPT
Z00.129 (encounter for routine child health examination without abnormal findings)	**99391 25** (preventive E/M service, established patient; infant [age younger than 1 year])
Z00.129 **Z23** (encounter for immunization)	**90700** (DTaP-IPV/Hib, for IM use) **90670** (PCV13, for IM use) **90685** (IIV4, split virus, preservative free, 0.25ml dose, for IM use) **90460** × 3 **90461** × 4

Teaching Point: Because the physician personally performed the counseling, code **90460** is reported for the initial component of the DTaP-IPV/Hib vaccine and each of the 2 single-component vaccines. Code **90460** is appropriate regardless of the route of administration. Code **90461** is reported for the 4 secondary components of the DTaP-IPV/Hib vaccine.

Payers who have adopted the Medicare National Correct Coding Initiative (NCCI) edits will require that modifier **25** be appended to code **99391** to signify that it was significant and separately identifiable from the IA. (For more information on NCCI edits, see **Chapter 2**, Modifiers and Coding Edits.) *ICD-10-CM* code **Z00.129** is reported first, followed by code **Z23**.

Codes 90471–90474

90471   Immunization administration (includes percutaneous, intradermal, subcutaneous, or intramuscular injections); one vaccine (single or combination vaccine/toxoid)

+90472   each additional vaccine (single or combination vaccine/toxoid)
        (List separately in addition to code for primary procedure.) (Use code **90472** in conjunction with **90460**, **90471**, or **90473**.)

Chapter 8. Preventive Services

Chapter 8. Preventive Services

90473   Immunization administration by intranasal or oral route; one vaccine (single or combination vaccine/toxoid)

+90474   each additional vaccine (single or combination vaccine/toxoid)

(List separately in addition to code for primary procedure.) (Use code **90474** in conjunction with **90460**, **90471**, or **90473**.)

Codes **90471–90474** will be reported when criteria for reporting the 2 pediatric IA codes (**90460** and **90461**) have not been met. This occurs when either of the following are true:

- The physician or QHP does not counsel the patient or family or does not document that the counseling was personally performed.
- The patient is 19 years or older.

The CMS assigned 0.49 RVUs to codes **90460**, **90471**, and **90473** and 0.37 RVUs to codes **90461**, **90472**, and **90474** in 2021 (2022 RVUs were not established at time of publication).

- Appropriate reporting of codes **90460** and **90461** in lieu of codes **90471–90474** should result in higher payment based on reporting of multiple units of code **90461** for *each additional vaccine component* versus reporting of codes **90472** and **90474** for *each additional vaccine product.*
- Individual payers may or may not assign payment values based on the RVUs published by the CMS. (Administration of vaccines provided through the VFC program is paid differently. See more about the VFC program later in this chapter.)

When reporting codes **90471–90474**

- Codes **90471–90474** are reported for each vaccine administered, whether single or combination vaccines.
- *Only one* "first" IA code (**90460**, **90471**, or **90473**) may be reported on a calendar day.

The "first" IA code can be reported from either family or either route of administration (eg, when a patient receives an immunization via injection and a second one via intranasal route, IA services can be reported with codes **90471** and **90474** or with codes **90473** and **90472**).

- If a physician personally performs counseling on one vaccine but not on another when given during the same encounter, IA will be reported using codes **90460** (and **90461** if appropriate) and either **90472** (IA, each additional vaccine via injection) or **90474** (IA, each additional vaccine via intranasal or oral route). The Medicare NCCI edits pair code **90460** with codes **90471** and **90473** and, therefore, do not allow codes from the pairs to be reported on the same day of service by the same physician or physician of the same group and specialty.

For more information on vaccine administration, please see the following examples and **Appendix III**, Vaccine Products: Commonly Administered Pediatric Vaccines:

Examples

➤ **A 4-year-old patient who was recently seen as a new patient for clearance to attend preschool returns for influenza immunization, which was not available at the time of the previous visit.** The service is scheduled with clinical staff only. The patient is noted to be in good health with no contraindications to the immunization per CDC guidelines. Next, the VIS and the antipyretic dosage for weight are reviewed with the father, who provides consent for the immunization. The influenza vaccine is administered, and the child is observed for immediate reactions prior to discharge.

ICD-10-CM	CPT
Z23 (encounter for immunization)	**90686** (influenza vaccine [IIV4], preservative free, 0.5 mL, IM) **90471** (IA, first injection)

Teaching Point: Because counseling by a physician or QHP is not provided at this encounter, code **90471** is reported in lieu of **90460**.

➤ **A 5-year-old established patient presented 2 weeks ago for her 5-year check and vaccines.** At that appointment, her physician provided counseling for each recommended vaccine component and corresponding VISs. The patient's mother asked that the vaccines be split, so only the DTaP and IPV vaccines were given at that encounter. The patient returns today and sees a nurse for an immunization-only visit to get the measles-mumps-rubella (MMR) and varicella vaccines.

ICD-10-CM	CPT
Z23 (encounter for immunization)	90707 (MMR, live) 90471 (IA, first injection) 90716 (varicella vaccine) 90472 (IA, subsequent injection)

Teaching Point: Counseling for all vaccines occurred at the last encounter and all VISs were handed out, so only administration occurred today. Immunization administration at the previous encounter would be reported with *CPT* codes 90460 × 2 and 90461 × 4 for DTaP and IPV vaccines that were administered during that encounter. However, services on this date did not include physician counseling.

> Only report codes 90460 and 90461 when physician counseling is provided on the date of vaccine administration. If vaccine administration is delayed to another date when physician counseling is not provided, report codes 90471–90474 as appropriate. There is no separate procedure code for counseling without administration during a preventive medicine service.

➤ **A 19-year-old established patient presents for college entrance examination.** In addition to providing a preventive medicine service, the physician counsels the patient on the need for meningococcal serogroup B (MenB-4C) immunization. The vaccine is administered, and a medical history and physical form provided by the college are completed.

ICD-10-CM	CPT
Z02.0 (encounter for examination for admission to educational institution)	99395 25 (preventive medicine service, established patient, 18–39 years old)
Z23 (encounter for immunization)	90620 (MenB-4C) 90471 (IA, first injection)

Teaching Point: Because the patient is older than 18 years, code 90460 cannot be reported even though the physician provided counseling for the vaccine provided. Code Z02.0 is appropriate as the reason the patient presented for the encounter. Code Z00.00 (encounter for general adult medical examination without abnormal findings) is not reported because *ICD-10-CM* excludes reporting of code Z00.00 in conjunction with codes in category Z02. Code Z00.00 is reported in lieu of Z02 when the patient receives a routine age- and gender-appropriate preventive medicine E/M service.

Coding for Counseling When Immunizations Are Not Carried Out

Pediatricians may counsel patients and caregivers on the need for immunization but decide immunization is contraindicated or not obtain consent to immunize.

> When immunization counseling takes place at the time of a preventive evaluation and management service (well-child visit) and does not result in administration, the counseling is not separately reported.

● When the purpose of the encounter is immunization counseling and immunizations are not administered, preventive medicine counseling codes (99401–99404; see further discussion later in this chapter) may be reported based on the time spent in face-to-face counseling with the patient and/or caregivers.

Codes for E/M services to address health problems (eg, 99202) may be reported in addition to 99401–99404 when preventive counseling is provided at the same encounter. Append modifier 25 (significant, separately identifiable E/M service) to the problem-oriented code (eg, 99202 25) when reporting both services at the same encounter.

Capturing the reason an immunization was not carried out begins with a code from *ICD-10-CM* category Z28, immunization not carried out, and under-immunization status.

● Under-immunization is reported with code Z28.3.

- Contraindications to immunization are captured with codes in subcategory **Z28.0-**.

Z28.01	Immunization not carried out because of acute illness of patient
Z28.02	Immunization not carried out because of chronic illness or condition of patient
Z28.03	Immunization not carried out because of immune compromised state of patient
Z28.04	Immunization not carried out because of patient allergy to vaccine or component
Z28.09	Immunization not carried out because of other contraindication

- Other codes in category **Z28** provide for reporting of immunization not carried out due to patient reasons, caregiver refusal, or other specified reason.

Z28.1	Immunization not carried out because of patient decision for reasons of belief or group pressure
Z28.20	Immunization not carried out because of patient decision for unspecified reason
Z28.21	Immunization not carried out because of patient refusal
Z28.29	Immunization not carried out because of patient decision for other reason
Z28.81	Immunization not carried out due to patient having had the disease
Z28.82	Immunization not carried out because of caregiver refusal
Z28.83	Immunization not carried out due to unavailability of vaccine

> **The American Academy of Pediatrics offers additional resources for addressing refusal to vaccinate, including a vaccine refusal form in English and Spanish (www.aap.org/en-us/advocacy-and-policy/aap-health-initiatives/immunizations/Pages/refusal-to-vaccinate. aspx).**

Examples

➤ **Parents of a 2-month-old established patient come to their physician's office to discuss immunizations.** To date, they have refused to have their infant immunized. Although the physician has discussed the need for vaccines during the infant's previous visits, the parents indicate they have further questions. The physician spends 20 minutes counseling the parents about current recommendations, safety and efficacy of vaccines, and their importance in preventing disease.

ICD-10-CM	CPT
Z71.89 (other specified counseling) **Z28.3** (personal history of under-immunization status) **Z28.82** (vaccination not carried out because of caregiver refusal)	**99401** (risk-factor reduction counseling)

Teaching Point: Because the *CPT* midpoint rule applies, code **99401** is reported for service times between 8 and 22 minutes.

➤ **An 11-year-old girl (new patient) presents to a pediatrician for a preventive medicine service.** In addition to the preventive E/M service with no abnormal findings, the physician discusses risks of the HPV vaccine and the disease for which it provides protection. The parent/guardian is given the CDC VIS. The parent/guardian consents; the nurse prepares to administer the vaccine. However, the patient refuses to be immunized. The physician returns to the examination room and provides additional counseling, but the patient continues to refuse the vaccine. The patient's mother wishes to discuss the decision with the child's father and return on a later date. A follow-up appointment is scheduled.

ICD-10-CM	CPT
Z00.129 **Z28.21** (immunization not carried out because of patient refusal)	**99383**

Teaching Point: Because no vaccine was administered, no charge for the product or the administration would be reported. Written procedures for documentation and reporting of expired and wasted vaccine doses may be required for vaccines provided under the VFC program.

When the patient returns for follow-up, the codes reported will depend on the outcome of the encounter. If the vaccine is administered after additional physician counseling at the same encounter, code **90460** would be reported in addition to the appropriate vaccine product code. If the patient returns for administration by clinical staff without additional counseling by a physician, code **90471** would be reported in lieu of **90460**. Additional counseling at the follow-up physician visit that does not result in immunization may be reported with a preventive medicine counseling code (**99401–99404**) based on the physician's face-to-face time with the patient. Do not report codes **99401–99404** on the same date as a preventive medicine E/M service (eg, **99383**).

Note that modifier **JW** (drug amount discarded/not administered to any patient) is not typically appropriate when no vaccine was administered to the patient. Modifier **JW** is used to report waste from a single-dose vial/package when the required patient dose is less than the available single-dose amount. Two claim lines report the amounts administered and wasted. Follow payer instructions for reporting wasted vaccines and use of modifier **JW**.

> For more information, see the article, "Coding for Vaccines Not Administered," in the July 2020 *AAP Pediatric Coding Newsletter* (https://coding.solutions.aap.org/article.aspx?articleid=2765196; subscription required).

Vaccines for Children Program

The VFC program makes vaccines available to children and teens up to 19 years of age who meet any of the following criteria: are enrolled in the Medicaid program (depending on the state Medicaid Managed Care), do not have health insurance, have no coverage of immunizations under their health plan, or are American Indians or Alaska Natives. Vaccines are provided at no cost to the participating physician or patient, and payment is made only for administration of the vaccine.

If reporting the VFC vaccine with administration codes and not the product code, data for the vaccine products administered must be captured for registry and quality initiatives. This can be accomplished by entering the vaccine codes with a $0 charge (if your billing system allows) and appending modifier **SL** (state-supplied vaccine) to the vaccine code. However, follow individual payer rules for reporting.

Providers are encouraged to use code **90460** for administration of a vaccine under the VFC program unless otherwise directed by a state program. If code **90461** is used for a vaccine with multiple antigens or components, it should be given a $0 value for a child covered under the VFC program. This applies to Medicaid-enrolled VFC-entitled children as well as non–Medicaid-enrolled VFC-entitled children (ie, uninsured, underinsured, and American Indian or Alaska Native children not enrolled in Medicaid).

Please be aware that some state Medicaid programs do have reporting rules that differ from VFC. *Be sure to get this policy in writing from your state Medicaid program* and follow it to avoid denied payment. The AAP continues to advocate to the CMS to allow for recognition and payment for component-based vaccine counseling and administration (ie, code **90461**). Under the current statute, administration can only be paid "per vaccine" and not component.

Participants in the VFC program should be aware of program-specific guidance, including storage of VFC vaccine separate from privately purchased vaccines. For more information on the VFC program, visit www.cdc.gov/vaccines/programs/vfc/index.html.

See "FAQ: Immunization Administration" at www.aap.org/cfp for more discussion of coding for IA.

Screening Tests and Procedures

Recommendations for age-appropriate screening services are outlined in the AAP/Bright Futures "Recommendations for Preventive Pediatric Health Care" (www.aap.org/periodicityschedule) or in your state's EPSDT plan.

When routine vision, developmental, and/or hearing screening services are performed in conjunction with a preventive medicine visit, the diagnosis code for a routine infant or child health check should be linked to the appropriate screening service. The services/codes listed as follows are examples of services that could be used to screen a patient. Some payers have specific policies that outline covered screening tools based on age; know your payer policies. For example, past a certain age, code **92567** (tympanometry) may not be covered under preventive services.

Hearing Screening

92551	Screening test, pure tone, air only
92552	Pure tone audiometry (threshold); air only (full assessment)
#92558	Evoked otoacoustic emissions, screening (qualitative measurement of distortion product or transient evoked otoacoustic emissions), automated analysis
92567	Tympanometry (impedance testing)
92568	Acoustic reflex testing, threshold portion
92583	Select picture audiometry

Chapter 8. Preventive Services

Audiometric tests require the use of calibrated electronic equipment, recording of results, and a written report with interpretation (eg, chart of hertz and decibels with pass/fail result for each ear tested and overall pass/fail result). Services include testing of both ears. If the test is applied only to 1 ear, modifier **52** (reduced services) must be appended to the code.

When hearing screening is performed in the physician office because of a failed screening in another setting (eg, school), report *ICD-10-CM* codes from category **Z01.11-**. Code **Z01.110** is reported for a normal screening result following a failed screening. Code **Z01.118** indicates a failed repeat screening. An additional code is reported to identify the abnormality found following the failed repeat screening.

> **Medicaid plans may provide specific hearing screening/testing coverage information and documentation forms/requirements.**

- Code **92551** (screening test, pure tone, air only) is used when the patient wears earphones and is asked to respond to tones of different pitches and intensities. This is a limited study.
- Code **92552** (full pure tone audiometric assessment; air only) is used when the patient wears earphones and is asked to respond to tones of different pitches and intensities. The threshold (lowest intensity of the tone heard by the patient 50% of the time) is recorded for a number of frequencies.
- Code **92558** (evoked otoacoustic emissions [OAEs] screening) is used when a probe tip is placed in the ear canal to screen for normal hearing function. Sounds that bounce back in low-intensity sound waves (ie, OAEs) are recorded and analyzed by computerized equipment and the results are automated.
- Code **92583** (select picture audiometry) is typically used for younger children. The patient is asked to identify different pictures with the instructions given at different sound intensity levels.
- Other commonly performed procedures include codes **92567** (tympanometry [impedance testing]) and **92568** (acoustic reflex testing, threshold portion). However, both codes may have limited coverage; check with payers.
- Automated audiometry testing is reported with Category III codes **0208T–0212T**. Verify individual payer payment policy before providing these services.

Examples

> **George is a 16-year-old established patient presenting for a preventive service and clearance to participate in school sports.** A complete preventive E/M service (**99394**) is provided. George has not received a hearing screening since he was 13 years old, so pure tone, air-only screening audiometry is performed (**92551**). No abnormalities are found, and George receives clearance to participate in sports. The *ICD-10-CM* code reported for each of the services is **Z00.129** (encounter for routine child health examination without abnormal findings).

> **Sally is a 6-year-old who failed a hearing screening at school and is referred to her pediatrician for additional evaluation.** Sally's parents indicate no prior concerns about her hearing, and risk-factor assessment is negative. The pediatrician chooses to perform screening audiometry (**92551**), which produces typical results. The *ICD-10-CM* code reported is **Z01.110** (encounter for hearing examination following failed hearing screening). If the MDM or total physician time (not including time of testing) supports a separate office or other outpatient E/M service, this is separately reported (eg, **99212**).

Vision Screening

99173	Screening test of visual acuity, quantitative, bilateral
99174	Instrument-based ocular screening (eg, photoscreening, automated-refraction), bilateral; with remote analysis and report
99177	with on-site analysis
0333T	Visual evoked potential, screening of visual acuity, automated, with report
0469T	Retinal polarization scan, ocular screening with on-site automated results, bilateral

- Screening test of visual acuity (**99173**) must use graduated visual stimuli that allow a quantitative estimate of visual acuity (eg, Snellen chart).
  - Code **99173** is only reported when vision screening is performed in association with a preventive medicine visit.
  - Medical record documentation must include a measurement of acuity for both eyes, not just a pass or fail score.

> Do not report code **99173** when it is performed as part of an evaluation for an eye problem or condition (eg, examination to rule out vision problems in a patient presenting with problems with schoolwork) because the assessment of visual acuity is considered an integral part of the eye examination.

- Instrument-based ocular screening (**99174**, **99177**) is used to report screening for a variety of conditions, including esotropia, exotropia, isometropia, cataracts, ptosis, hyperopia, myopia, and others, that affect or have the potential to affect vision. These tests are especially useful for screening infants, preschool patients, and those older patients whose ability to participate in traditional acuity screening is limited or very time intensive.
  - — Code **99177** specifies screening using an instrument that provides an on-site (ie, in-office) pass or fail result. The result should be documented.
  - — Code **99174** specifies the use of a screening instrument that incorporates remote analysis and report (by a physician located elsewhere).
  - — These screenings cannot be reported in conjunction with codes **92002–92700** (general ophthalmologic services), **99172** (visual function screening), or **99173** (screening test of visual acuity, quantitative) because ocular screening is inherent to these services. An AAP policy statement on instrument-based pediatric vision screening is available at http://pediatrics.aappublications.org/content/130/5/983.full.
- Vision screening performed using an automated visual evoked potential system is reported with code **0333T**. This code applies to automated screening using an instrument-based algorithm with a pass or fail result. A report of the result must be documented. Report code **95930** only for comprehensive visual evoked potential testing with physician interpretation and report.
- Retinal polarization scanning (**0469T**) is used to detect amblyopia due to strabismus and defocus. Similar to code **99177**, results of each scan are generated on-site.

Developmental Screening and Health Assessment

Standardized screening instruments (ie, validated tests that are administered and scored in a consistent or "standard" manner consistent with their validation) are used for screening and assessment purposes as reported by codes **96110** and **96127**. Health risk assessments that are patient focused (**96160**) are differentiated from those such as maternal depression screening that are caregiver focused (**96161**) for the benefit of the patient.

Developmental Screening

96110   Developmental screening with scoring and documentation, per standardized instrument

Structured screening for developmental delay is a universal recommendation of the "Recommendations for Preventive Pediatric Health Care." At 18- and 24-month visits, specifically screen for autism spectrum disorder (ASD). Global developmental screening is recommended at 9-, 18-, and 30-month visits. When reporting these screenings, code **96110** represents developmental screening with scoring and documentation per standardized instrument. (*Note:* Screening results should be documented in the patient medical record.)

ICD-10-CM codes **Z13.40–Z13.49** (eg, **Z13.42**, screening for global developmental delays [milestones]) may be reported to indicate screening for developmental disability in children when the screening is performed with or without a well-child visit at the same encounter.

Code **96110**

- Is reported only for standardized developmental screening instruments. It is not reported when the pediatrician conducts an informal survey or surveillance of development as part of a comprehensive preventive medicine service (which is considered part of the history and is not separately billed).
- Does not require interpretation and report (ie, includes scoring and documentation only).
- Is *not* reported for brief emotional or behavioral assessment; see code **96127**.
- May be reported for each standardized developmental screening instrument administered. Medicaid Medically Unlikely Edits (MUEs) allow reporting of 3 screening instruments per date of service. If use of more than 3 instruments is clinically indicated and performed, code **96110** is reported with 3 units billed on the first claim line and **96110 59** billed with 1 unit for each additional instrument reported on a separate claim line.

Example

➤ **An 18-month-old girl presents to her primary physician for an established patient well-child examination.** The mother is given standardized screening instruments for developmental status and ASD by clinical staff, who explain their purpose and how they should be completed. The nursing assistant scores the completed forms and attaches them to the child's medical chart. The physician interprets and documents the normal results of the instruments. The physician provides the recommended 18-month preventive E/M service (**99392**). The child will return for a scheduled 2-year-old preventive service.

> **Teaching Point:** Code **99392** is reported and linked on the claim form to *ICD-10-CM* code **Z00.129**. Code **96110** is reported with 2 units of service linked to *ICD-10-CM* codes **Z13.41** (autism screening) and **Z13.42** (screening for delayed milestones) to identify the reason for 2 units of service. Or, if required by a health plan, code **96110** linked to code **Z13.41** and **96110 59** (1 unit each) linked to **Z13.42** are reported on 2 separate claim lines. (For an illustration of how codes are linked on a claim form, see **Chapter 1, Figure 1-1**).

Emotional/Behavioral Assessment

96127   Brief emotional/behavioral assessment (eg, depression inventory, ADHD scale), with scoring and documentation, per standardized instrument

Code **96127**

- Is reported for standardized emotional/behavioral assessment instruments.
- Represents the practice expense of administering, scoring, and documenting each standardized instrument. No physician work value is included. Physician interpretation is included in a related E/M service.
- Is *not* reported in conjunction with preventive medicine counseling/risk-factor reduction intervention (**99401–99404**) or psychiatric or neurologic testing (**96130–96139** or **96146**).
- Can involve 2 or more separately reported completions of the same form (eg, attention-deficit/hyperactivity disorder [ADHD] rating scales by teacher and by parent). Note that MUEs limit reporting to 2 units per claim line. When reporting to payers adopting MUEs, additional units beyond the first 2 must be reported on a separate claim line with an NCCI modifier (eg, **59**, distinct procedural service). As always, documentation should support the appropriateness of the additional units of service. Note at the time of publication the AAP is working on increasing the MUE.
- Can be reported for standardized depression instruments that are required under US Preventive Services Task Force (USPSTF) and Bright Futures recommendations (see AAP/Bright Futures "Recommendations for Preventive Pediatric Health Care" [periodicity schedule] insert).

Example

➤ **A 12-year-old boy is seen for an established patient well-child health supervision.** In addition to the preventive medicine service, the physician's staff administers and scores a standardized depression screening instrument. The physician reviews the score, documents that the screening result is negative for symptoms of depression, and completes the preventive medicine service.

> The preventive medicine service code (**99394**) would be reported in addition to code **96127**. The diagnosis codes reported are **Z00.129** (encounter for routine child health examination without abnormal findings) and **Z13.31** (encounter for screening for depression). Link **Z00.129** and **Z13.31** to the claim service line for code **96127**. Inclusion of codes may support claims-based data collection for quality measurement (ie, number of adolescent patients screened for depression).

> When the physician performs further evaluation of positive screening results, leading to a diagnosis of depression, report the preventive service with abnormal findings (**Z00.121**) followed by the appropriate code for the diagnosed depression (eg, **F32.0**, major depressive disorder, single episode, mild). When appropriate, a significant and separately identifiable E/M service to evaluate and manage depression may be reported by appending modifier **25** to an office or other outpatient E/M code (eg, **99214 25**). Documentation should clearly support the MDM of the separate service or, if billing based on time, the physician's total time (not including the time spent providing the separately reported preventive medicine service and screening for depression) and a summary of the service provided (eg, education on the condition, questions answered, patient and/or caregiver concerns, management options discussed, plan of care). Link the diagnosis code for the depression to the office or other outpatient E/M code.

Health Risk Assessment

96160   Administration of patient-focused health risk assessment (eg, health hazard appraisal) with scoring and documentation, per standardized instrument

96161   Administration of caregiver-focused health risk assessment (eg, depression inventory) for the benefit of the patient, with scoring and documentation, per standardized instrument

Codes **96160** and **96161** are reported with 1 unit for each standardized instrument administered. Payer edits may limit the number of times codes **96160** and **96161** may be reported for an individual patient and/or on the same date of service. MUEs are set to 3 units for **96160** and 1 unit for **96161** per claim line. Append modifier **59** to the code for additional units on a second claim line.

> **Sparse coverage for codes 96160 and specifically 96161 has been noted by the American Academy of Pediatrics, and advocacy efforts are being made.**

Code **96160** is reported for administration of a patient-focused health risk assessment with scoring and documentation. This is differentiated from code **96161**, which is used to report a health risk assessment focused on a caregiver for the benefit of the patient (eg, maternal depression screening).

- Code **96160** cannot be used in conjunction with assessment and brief intervention for alcohol/substance abuse (**99408**, **99409**).
- Check individual payer guidance to determine if and for what purposes code **96160** is included as a covered and payable service under the payer's policies (eg, some Medicaid plans pay for adolescent health questionnaires reported with **96160**).

Code **96161** is reported for administration and scoring of a health risk assessment to a patient's caregiver. Examples are a postpartum depression inventory administered to the mother of a newborn and administration of a standardized caregiver strain instrument to parents of a child who is seriously injured or ill.

- Screening for postpartum depression is caregiver focused (sign/symptoms of depression in mother) but performed in this setting for the benefit of the infant. This service is reported as a service provided to the infant with code **96161** and the appropriate *ICD-10-CM* code for the infant's routine child health examination (eg, **Z00.129**).
- Check payer policy on adoption of code **96161** versus a requirement to report as a service to the mother (ie, to mother's health plan) with code **96127** (brief emotional/behavioral assessment [eg, depression inventory, ADHD scale], with scoring and documentation, per standardized instrument). Many Medicaid plans provide separate payment for maternal depression screening at well-child visits, but specific reporting instructions may apply. Vaccines and administration services would also be reported.

> **Avoid denials! National Correct Coding Initiative edits bundle codes 96160 and 96161 with code 96110 and with IA (90460–90474) services, but a modifier is allowed when each code represents a distinct service and is clinically appropriate. Append modifier 59 (distinct procedure) to the bundled code (second column of NCCI edits) when these services are reported on the same date to a payer that has adopted NCCI edits.**

Example

➤ **As part of a health supervision visit for a 9-month-old established patient, the physician directs clinical staff to administer a screening for postpartum depression that was not performed at the infant's 6-month visit.** Clinical staff explain the purpose of the instrument to the infant's mother. After the mother has completed the screening instrument, clinical staff score and document the result in the patient record. The mother is also asked to complete a developmental screening instrument, which is scored and documented. The physician completes the preventive medicine service with no abnormal findings and counsels the patient's mother about influenza immunization. With the mother's consent, clinical staff administer 0.25 mL of a preservative-free split-virus vaccine. Anticipatory guidance that advises the mother that her screening indicates no current signs of postpartum depression is included, along with a list of symptoms that should prompt a call to her physician. The patient is scheduled to return for a second dose of influenza vaccine in 1 month.

Chapter 8. Preventive Services

Chapter 8. Preventive Services

ICD-10-CM	CPT
Z00.129 (encounter for routine child health examination without abnormal findings)	**99393 25** (preventive medicine visit) **96110 59** (developmental screening) **96161 59** (administration of caregiver-focused health risk assessment [eg, depression inventory] for the benefit of the patient, with scoring and documentation, per standardized instrument) **90460** (IA with physician counseling) **90685** (IIV4 vaccine, split virus, preservative free, 0.25 ml dose for IM administration)

Teaching Point: NCCI edits bundle the codes shown with a modifier appended to other codes reported for this encounter (eg, **99393** is bundled to **90460**). For each of the bundled code pairs, a modifier is allowed to override the edit when both services are provided and clinically appropriate. Electronic claim scrubbers are useful for identifying and addressing NCCI edit pairs prior to claim submission. See **Chapter 2** for more on NCCI edits.

Never report *ICD-10-CM* code Z13.32 (encounter for maternal depression screen) on the baby's chart/bill.

Prevention of Dental Caries

Application of Fluoride Varnish

99188   Application of topical fluoride varnish by a physician or other qualified health care professional
- Topical fluoride application by primary care physicians is a recommended preventive service for children from birth through 5 years of age (Grade B rating by the USPSTF). This service may be covered when provided alone or in conjunction with other services. Coverage is usually limited to once every 6 months.
- *ICD-10-CM* code **Z29.3** is reported to identify an encounter for prophylactic fluoride administration. When applicable, diagnosis of dental caries may be reported as a secondary diagnosis with codes in category **K02**. Encounter for prophylactic fluoride administration is reported separately from the encounter for routine child health examination (**Z00.121** or **Z00.129**) when both services are provided at the same encounter.

Example

➤ **A 4-year-old established patient undergoes a routine preventive medicine service without abnormal findings.** In addition, a medical assistant who has been qualified by a required online training and assessment program applies fluoride varnish to the child's teeth under supervision of the pediatrician, who remains in the office suite.

The pediatrician reports code **99392** (established patient routine child health examination, age 1–4) and **99188** (application of fluoride varnish). Diagnosis code **Z00.129** (routine child health examination without abnormal findings) is linked to code **99392**. Diagnosis code **Z29.3** is linked to code **99188**. Follow payer-specific guidelines on the qualifications of the provider who performs fluoride application and other payment policy.

Although code **99188** specifies application by a physician or QHP, payers may allow billing of services by trained clinical staff under direct physician supervision (incident to). Some Medicaid plans require training of clinical staff through specific programs and documentation of training and/or certification. It is important to identify the requirements of individual payers prior to providing this service and maintain documentation demonstrating all coverage requirements were met.

Counseling to Prevent Dental Caries

Some payers will provide coverage for oral evaluation and health risk assessment or other dental preventive services when provided on the same day as a preventive medicine visit; other payers will allow services only when they are provided at an encounter separate from a preventive medicine visit. It is important to know payer requirements for reporting.

- Preventive counseling for oral health may be included as part of the preventive medicine service (**99381–99395**) or, if performed at a separate encounter, reported under the individual preventive medicine counseling service codes (**99401–99404**) or with an office or outpatient E/M service code (**99202–99215**). *ICD-10-CM* code **Z13.84** may be reported for an encounter for screening for dental disorders.

Other Codes for Prevention of Dental Caries

- *Code on Dental Procedures and Nomenclature* (*CDT*®) codes also exist for topical application of fluoride varnish and fluoride. In addition, *CDT* codes exist for nutrition counseling to prevent dental disease, oral hygiene instruction, and oral evaluations. However, acceptance of these codes by health plans may be limited to state Medicaid plans.
- For those carriers (particularly state Medicaid plans under EPSDT) that cover oral health care, some will require a modifier. These modifiers are payer specific and should only be used as directed by your state Medicaid agency or other private payer.
  - **SC** Medically necessary service or supply
  - **EP** Services provided as part of Medicaid EPSDT program
  - **U5** Medicaid Level of Care 5, as defined by each state

Screening Laboratory Tests

- A test performed in the office laboratory should be billed using the appropriate laboratory code and, if performed, the appropriate blood collection code (**36400–36416**).
- Codes **36415** (collection of venous blood by venipuncture) and **36416** (collection of capillary blood specimen [eg, finger, heel, ear stick]) are used for any age child when the physician is not needed to perform the procedure. Code **36416** is not payable by Medicare, as it is considered bundled, and many private payers follow this rule and bundle it as well.
- When a physician's skill is required to perform venipuncture (eg, access is too difficult for other staff to attain) *on a child younger than 3 years,* codes **36400–36406** are reported based on the anatomical site of the venipuncture. Report code **36400** when performed on a femoral or jugular vein, **36405** when on the scalp vein, or **36406** when another vein is accessed.
- When a physician's skill is required to perform venipuncture *on a child 3 years or older*, code **36410** (venipuncture, age 3 years and older, necessitating physician's skill, for diagnostic or therapeutic purposes [not to be used for routine venipuncture]) is reported.
- If the physician performs the venipuncture as a convenience or because staff is not trained in the procedure, code **36415** is reported because the physician's skill was not required.
- Although typically not required, some payers will require that modifier **25** be appended to the E/M code if a separate and significant E/M service is reported on the same day of service.
- Laboratories and physician offices performing waived tests may need to append modifier **QW** to the *CPT* code for Clinical Laboratory Improvement Amendments (CLIA)–waived procedures. The use of modifier **QW** is payer specific. To determine if a test is a CLIA-waived procedure, go to www.accessdata.fda.gov/scripts/cdrh/cfdocs/cfCLIA/search.cfm.
- *ICD-10-CM* allows separate reporting of special screening examinations (codes in categories **Z11–Z13**) in addition to the codes for routine child health examinations when these codes provide additional information. A screening code is not necessary if the screening is inherent to a routine examination. Payer guidelines for reporting screening examinations may vary. When specific *ICD-10-CM* codes are required to support payment for a screening service, be sure to link the appropriate *ICD-10-CM* code to the claim line for the screening service.

> A positive finding on a screening test does not change the test to a diagnostic test. When a screening test results in an abnormal finding that has been identified at the time of code assignment, list first the code for the screening or preventive service followed by a code for the abnormal finding. Failure to list the screening code first may affect the patient's out-of-pocket costs for preventive services. Please see Chapter 11 for information on coding for diagnostic tests in non-facility settings.

- To meet the HEDIS measure for percentage of children who turned 2 years of age in a measurement year and who had 1 or more capillary or venous lead blood test(s) for lead poisoning by their second birthday, a laboratory report of lead screening test result, or a note indicating the date the test was performed and the result or finding must be documented. See Chapter 3 for more information on HEDIS measures.
- A table of common pediatric screening laboratory tests and codes is included at www.aap.org/cfp.

Chapter 8. Preventive Services

Preventive Care Provided Outside the Preventive Visit

Counseling and/or Risk-Factor Reduction

Codes **99401–99404**, **99411**, and **99412** are used to report risk-factor reduction services provided for the purpose of promoting health and preventing illness or injury in persons without a specific illness.

Preventive medicine service codes (**99381–99395**) include counseling, anticipatory guidance, and/or risk-factor reduction interventions that are provided at the time of the periodic comprehensive preventive medicine examination. *CPT* states to "refer to codes **99401**–**99404**, and **99411**–**99412** for reporting those counseling/anticipatory guidance/risk-factor reduction interventions that are provided at an encounter separate from the preventive medicine examination." Therefore, according to *CPT,* do not report **99401–99404** or **99411** or **99412** in addition to **99381–99397**.

- Risk factor reduction services will vary with age and address issues such as diet, exercise, sexual activity, dental health, injury prevention, safe travel, and family problems.
- Services are reported based on time, and time should be distinctly documented (eg, 15 minutes spent in counseling about diet and exercise to reduce risk of developing diabetes).
- Counseling, anticipatory guidance, and risk-factor reduction interventions provided at the time of an initial or periodic comprehensive preventive medicine examination are components of the periodic service and not separately reported.
- Risk-factor reduction may be reported separately with other E/M services.
  - Evaluation and management services (other than preventive medicine E/M services) reported on the same day must be separate and distinct.
  - Time spent in the provision of risk-factor reduction may not be used as a basis for the selection of the other E/M code.
- When reporting a distinct E/M service, append modifier **25** to the code for the distinct E/M service.

> Payment policies for preventive medicine counseling may vary by health plan. Ideally, recommended preventive medicine counseling provided outside of a preventive evaluation and management (E/M) service (**99381–99385**, **99391–99395**) is a covered preventive service paid with no out-of-pocket cost to the patient/caregiver. It is important to know if a payer considers preventive medicine counseling bundled to a problem-oriented E/M service when provided on the same date of service. Plans may require that the preventive counseling be included in the level of problem-oriented E/M service reported in lieu of reporting the appropriate preventive counseling code. Written copies of payment policies should be documented to support billing for preventive medicine counseling as part of a problem-oriented E/M service rather than separately reporting as directed by *Current Procedural Terminology*.

Preventive Medicine, Individual Counseling Codes

Codes **99401–99404** are time-based codes. See **Table 8-2** for code descriptors, required time, and RVUs for these services.

Table 8-2. Preventive Medicine Counseling Codes and Relative Value Units			
Preventive medicine counseling and/or risk-factor reduction intervention(s) provided to an individual (separate procedure);			
Code	**Time Required**	**Total NF-RVUs**[a]	**Total F-RVUs**[a]
99401	approximately 15 minutes (8–22)	1.14	0.71
99402	approximately 30 minutes (23–37)	1.88	1.45
99403	approximately 45 minutes (38–52)	2.59	2.16
99404	approximately 60 minutes (≥53)	3.29	2.86

Abbreviations: F-RVU, facility relative value unit; NF-RVU, non-facility relative value unit; RVU, relative value unit.

[a] 2021 RVUs, not geographically adjusted.

Report codes **99401–99404**
- Based on a physician's or other QHP's face-to-face time spent providing counseling.
- For a new or an established patient.
- When the medical record includes documentation of the total counseling time and a summary of the issues discussed. Time is met when the midpoint is passed (eg, 8 minutes of service required to report a 15-minute service).

Codes **99401–99404** may be reported when expectant parents request a consultation with a pediatric physician regarding risk reduction for the fetus. However, consultation or office and other outpatient E/M services are reported when the service is requested by another physician, QHP, or an appropriate source (eg, genetic counselor). See the Expectant Parent Consultations section in **Chapter 9** for information on reporting *ICD-10-CM* and *CPT* codes for these services to the mother's health insurance.

Examples

➤ **A 7-week-old girl (established patient) is presented to a pediatrician with a scaly rash on her scalp.** The infant is examined and found to have seborrheic infantile dermatitis of the scalp and skinfolds on the extremities. The pediatrician provides information on home management and risk of yeast infection and takes the opportunity to again counsel the mother about the need for immunization against hepatitis B, which the mother has previously refused. The indications, safety, and risks are discussed for 10 minutes and the mother agrees to revisit the issue with her husband, who has been strongly opposed in the past. The pediatrician documents the separate time and context of the counseling.

ICD-10-CM	CPT
L21.0 (seborrheic infantile dermatitis)	**99212 25** (MDM: 1 self-limited problem; assessment requiring an independent historian; and minimal risk of morbidity from treatment)
Z28.3 (under-immunization status) **Z28.21** (immunization not carried out because of patient refusal)	**99401**

Teaching Point: The pediatrician's time of 10 minutes spent in preventive counseling supports reporting code **99401** because the midpoint was passed (8 minutes are required for reporting a code assigned 15 minutes). Distinct documentation of the time and work of the preventive counseling is important to support payment for both services provided.

➤ **Parents of a 6-year-old request counseling for an upcoming move to Puerto Rico.** The pediatrician spends 25 minutes reviewing CDC recommendations for immunizations and counseling for potential health hazards for the child. Any recommended vaccines are administered, and the pediatrician recommends an appointment at a travel clinic for vaccines not available in the practice (eg, dengue, typhoid).

ICD-10-CM	CPT
Z71.84 (encounter for health counseling related to travel) **Z23** (encounter for immunization), if applicable	**99402** (risk-factor reduction counseling) Codes for vaccine products and administration, as applicable

Teaching Point: The pediatrician's time of 25 minutes spent in preventive counseling supports reporting code **99402** because the midpoint between the typical times of **99401** and **99402** was passed (23 minutes). Time spent in counseling for immunizations administered at the encounter would be reported with the IA code and not included in the time of the risk-factor reduction counseling.

Preventive Medicine, Group Counseling Codes

99411   Preventive medicine counseling and/or risk factor reduction intervention(s) provided to individuals in a group setting (separate procedure); approximately 30 minutes

99412   approximately 60 minutes

- Risk factor reduction services provided to a group are reported based on time. The *CPT* midpoint rule for time applies (ie, time is met when the midpoint between the 2 codes is passed), as shown in **Table 8-3**.
- See code **99078** for reporting physician counseling to groups of patients with symptoms or an established illness. This service is reported for each participating child.

Chapter 8. Preventive Services

Table 8-3. Group Preventive Medicine Counseling Codes and Relative Value Units

Preventive medicine counseling and/or risk-factor reduction intervention(s) provided to an individual (separate procedure);

Code	Time Required	Total NF-RVUs[a]	Total F-RVUs[a]
99411	approximately 30 minutes (16–45)	0.60	0.22
99412	approximately 60 minutes (≥46)	0.75	0.37

Abbreviations: F-RVU, facility relative value unit; NF-RVU, non-facility relative value unit; RVU, relative value unit.

[a] 2021 RVUs, not geographically adjusted.

Example

➤ **A group of 10 patients aged 14 to 16 years attend a 50-minute session in the physician's office to discuss contraception and sex-related health risks.** The physician conducts the session. The session includes a 10-minute break that is not included in the time of service. Services are documented in each patient's medical record and are reported for each child.

ICD-10-CM	CPT
Z30.09 (encounter for other general counseling and advice on contraception)	**99412** (risk-factor reduction counseling, group, 60 minutes)

Teaching Point: Although 10 minutes of break time are not included in the time of the counseling service, code **99412** is supported because the midpoint between the 30 minutes assigned to **99411** and the 60 minutes assigned to **99412** is passed. Services provided to a group of patients may not be reported as individual office E/M visits (**99202–99215**) because only face-to-face time spent counseling the individual patient may be reported based on time.

Behavior Change Intervention

Behavior change interventions are for persons who have a behavior that is often considered an illness, such as tobacco use and addiction or substance use or misuse. Behavior change services may be reported when performed as part of the treatment of conditions related to or potentially exacerbated by the behavior or when performed to change the harmful behavior that has not yet resulted in illness. **Table 8-4** shows the codes and RVUs assigned to behavior change intervention codes.

Table 8-4. Behavior Change Intervention Codes

Code	Description	TNF RVUs[a]	TF RVUs[a]
99406	Smoking and tobacco use cessation counseling visit; intermediate, >3 min up to 10 min	0.45	0.36
99407	intensive, >10 min	0.83	0.74
99408	Alcohol and/or substance (other than tobacco) abuse structured screening (eg, AUDIT, DAST), and brief intervention services; 15–30 minutes	1.04	0.95
99409	>30 minutes	2.00	1.91

Abbreviations: AUDIT, Alcohol Use Disorders Identification Test; DAST, Drug Abuse Screening Test; TF, total facility; TNF, total non-facility; RVU, relative value unit.

[a] 2021 RVUs, not geographically adjusted.

Behavior change interventions involve validated interventions shown in **Figure 8-2**.
● Behavior change intervention codes **99406–99409** are reported when
  — Services are provided by a physician or QHP for patients who have a behavior that is often considered an illness (eg, tobacco use and addiction, substance use or misuse).
  — Services involve specific validated interventions, including assessing readiness for and barriers to change, advising change in behavior, providing specific suggested actions and motivational counseling, and arranging for services and follow-up care.

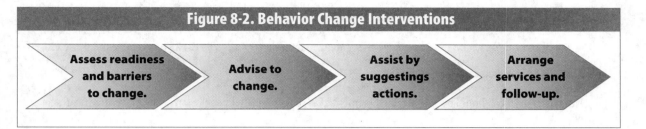

Figure 8-2. Behavior Change Interventions

Assess readiness and barriers to change. → Advise to change. → Assist by suggestings actions. → Arrange services and follow-up.

- Codes **99406–99409** include specific time requirements that must be met (eg, at least 15 minutes must be spent in counseling to support reporting of code **99408**). The *CPT* midpoint rule does not apply to codes **99406–99409**.
- Do not separately report code **96160** for screening instruments used in conjunction with codes **99408** and **99409**.
- Medical record documentation supports the total time spent in the performance of the service, and a detail of the behavior change intervention is provided.

> Behavior change intervention services cannot be performed on a parent or guardian of a patient and reported under the patient's name.

- Behavior change interventions may be reported separately with preventive medicine or other E/M services.
  - Evaluation and management services reported on the same day must be separate and distinct.
  - Time spent in the provision of behavior change intervention may not be used as a basis for the selection of the other E/M code.
- When reporting a distinct E/M service, append modifier **25** to the code for the distinct E/M service (eg, **99213 25**).

> See the Physician Group Education Services section in Chapter 11, Common Non-facility Testing and Therapeutic Services, for an example of how code **99078** is used.

Examples

➤ **During an office visit for a 17-year-old new patient for an unrelated problem, it is learned that he has been smoking for 2 years but would like to quit.** The physician spends 15 minutes discussing specific methods to overcome barriers, pharmacological options, behavioral techniques, and nicotine replacement. The patient is referred to a community support group and a follow-up visit is scheduled in 2 weeks to provide additional encouragement and counseling as needed. Diagnosis is tobacco use.

ICD-10-CM	*CPT*
Use the code appropriate for problem addressed.	**99202–99205 25** (based on service performed and documented)
Z72.0 (tobacco use) **Z71.6** (tobacco abuse counseling)	**99407**

Teaching Point: If only general advice and encouragement to stop smoking had been provided, it would be considered part of the new patient office visit. Counseling time must be documented. *ICD-10-CM* does not include a code for use of vaping products without a diagnosis of abuse or a vaping-related illness. Report **Z71.89** (other specified counseling) when counseling is focused on risks associated with vaping. See **F17.29-** for codes for nicotine dependence and vaping.

➤ **During a preventive medicine service for a 14-year-old established patient, the physician uses a structured screening tool to interview the patient about substance use.** The result is positive, and the physician spends a total of 20 minutes interviewing the patient about substance use history and counseling the patient about risks associated with alcohol and drug use, not driving or riding with someone under the influence, and seeking an agreement to avoid future use.

Chapter 8. Preventive Services

ICD-10-CM	CPT
Z00.129 (routine child health examination without abnormal findings)	**99394 25** (preventive medicine visit)
Z71.89 (other specified counseling)	**99408**

Time of counseling should be specifically documented as beginning after conclusion of the preventive medicine service.

International Classification of Diseases, 10th Revision, Clinical Modification **guidelines state that substance use codes (eg, F10.99, alcohol use, unspecified with unspecified alcohol-induced disorder) should only be assigned when the use is associated with a mental or behavioral disorder and such a relationship is documented by the provider.**

Preventive Medicine Services Modifier

33   Preventive services

Modifier **33** is used to differentiate services provided as recommended preventive care when the service might also be provided for diagnostic indications. Some payers provide a listing of services for which modifier **33** is required when provided as a preventive service.

- The appropriate use of modifier **33** will reduce claim adjustments related to preventive services and corresponding payments to members.
- Modifier **33** should only be appended to codes represented in 1 or more of the following 4 categories:
  — Services rated A or B by the USPSTF
  — Immunizations for routine use in children, adolescents, and adults as recommended by ACIP
  — Preventive care and screenings for children as recommended by Bright Futures (AAP) and newborn testing (American College of Medical Genetics and Genomics)
  — Preventive care and screenings provided for women supported by HRSA

The US Preventive Services Task Force (USPSTF) grades A and B are defined as follows:
- **Grade A: The USPSTF recommends the service. There is high certainty that the net benefit is substantial.**
- **Grade B: The USPSTF recommends the service. There is high certainty that the net benefit is moderate or there is moderate certainty that the net benefit is moderate to substantial.**

Most health plans cover preventive services with grade A or B without cost to the patient (ie, no deductible, co-pay, or coinsurance).

- **DO *NOT* USE MODIFIER 33**
  — **When the *CPT* code(s) is identified as inherently preventive (eg, preventive medicine counseling)**
  — **When the service(s) is not indicated in the categories noted previously**
  — **With an insurance plan that continues to implement the cost-sharing policy on preventive medicine services (grandfathered health plan)**
- Check with your payers before fully implementing the use of modifier **33** to verify any variations in reporting requirements. Modifier **33** *is not used for benefit determination by some payers* and may be required by others only for services that may be either diagnostic/therapeutic or preventive.

Example

➤ **A 12-year-old established patient is seen for behavioral intervention for obesity due to excess calorie intake and family history of type 2 diabetes.** The patient and her parents previously received counseling on the health risks associated with obesity and requested assistance with lifestyle changes to help the patient recover and maintain a healthy weight. The physician uses shared decision-making to develop a plan for adopting a healthier lifestyle that will lead to weight loss and improved the health status of the patient. The physician's total time on the date of service is 35 minutes.

●=New code   ▲=Revised code   #=Re-sequenced code   +=Add-on code   ★=Telemedicine

ICD-10-CM	CPT
E66.9 (obesity, unspecified) **Z68.54** (BMI ≥95th percentile) **Z83.3** (family history of diabetes mellitus)	**99214 33** (level 4 established patient office visit, total time 30–39 minutes)

Teaching Point: Modifier **33** is appended to code **99214** to indicate the preventive nature of the service, based on the USPSTF Grade B recommendation that clinicians screen for obesity in children and adolescents 6 years and older and offer to refer or refer them to comprehensive, intensive behavioral interventions to promote improvements in weight status.

Other Preventive Medicine Services

99429   Unlisted preventive medicine service

Code **99429** may be reported if these options are not suitable. If the unlisted code is used, most payers will require a copy of the progress notes filed with the claim.

Reporting a Preventive Medicine Visit With a Problem-Oriented Visit

When a problem or abnormality is addressed, *requires significant additional work* (eg, symptomatic atopic dermatitis, exercise-induced asthma, migraine headache, scoliosis), and is medically necessary, it may be reported using the office or other outpatient services codes (**99202–99205, 99212–99215**) in addition to the preventive medicine services code.

> **Know Payer Policies for Same-Day Preventive and Problem-Oriented Evaluation and Management Services**
>
> Some payers have adopted policy that problem-oriented evaluation and management (E/M) services provided on the same date as a preventive medicine E/M service will be paid at 50% of the contractual amount agreed on under the health plan contract. When reporting to these payers, be sure to include all work related to the problem-oriented encounter in determining the level of service provided. Physicians should not reduce the level of service reported.

- The presence of a chronic condition(s) in and of itself does not change a preventive medicine visit to a problem-oriented visit; nor does it unilaterally support a separate problem-oriented E/M service (**99202–99205, 99212–99215**) with the well visit, unless it is significant and has been separately addressed.
- An insignificant problem or condition (eg, minor diaper rash, stable chronic problem, renewal of prescription medications) that does not require significant MDM or time cannot be reported as a separate E/M service.
- Although a separate E/M service is not reported when a minor problem or chronic condition requires less than significant additional work, the diagnosis code for the problem or chronic condition may be reported in addition to code **Z00.121** (routine child health examination with abnormal findings).
- It is important to make parents aware of any additional charges that may occur at the preventive medicine encounter. This includes, but is not limited to, a significant, separately identifiable E/M service.
  - Some patients will be required to provide a co-payment for the non–preventive medicine visit code under the terms of their plan benefit even when there is no co-payment required for the preventive medicine visit. Legally, this co-payment cannot routinely be written off.
  - The AAP has developed a template letter that can be used to outline what may not be covered under the no-cost-sharing preventive medicine services (www.aap.org/en-us/professional-resources/practice-transformation/getting-paid/Coding-at-the-AAP/Pages/Evaluation-and-Management.aspx).

  When reporting both E/M services
- The documentation of the problem-oriented service must be distinct from that of the preventive service (even if included in the same encounter note) and clearly support the level of service reported.
- When the level of service is selected based on the physician's total time (on the date of the encounter) spent addressing the problem (not including any time spent providing the preventive service), the physician's total time spent addressing the problem must be distinctly documented in addition to documentation of the problem workup (eg, history of present illness, examination, records or test results reviewed), assessment, and plan.
- Documentation might indicate, "My total time of XX minutes was directed to activities of evaluating and managing X condition after I provided the preventive service."

Chapter 8. Preventive Services

Coding Conundrum: Reporting Evaluation and Management Services With Immunization Administration

Evaluation and management (E/M) services most often reported with the vaccine product and immunization administration (IA) include new and established patient preventive medicine visits (*Current Procedural Terminology* [*CPT*] codes 99381–99395), problem-oriented visits (99202–99215), and preventive medicine counseling services (99401–99404).

If a patient is seen for the administration of a vaccine only, it is not appropriate to report an E/M visit if it is not medically necessary, significant, and separately identifiable. The E/M service must be clinically indicated.

Payers may require modifier 25 (significant, separately identifiable E/M service by the same physician on the same day of the procedure or other service) to be appended to the E/M code to distinguish it from the administration of the vaccine.

Do not report *CPT* code 99211 (established patient E/M, minimal level, not requiring physician presence) when the patient encounter is for vaccination only because Medicare Resource-Based Relative Value Scale (RBRVS) relative values for IA codes include administrative and clinical services (ie, greeting the patient, routine vital signs, obtaining a vaccine history, presenting the Vaccine Information Statement and responding to routine vaccine questions, preparation and administration of the vaccine, and documentation and observation of the patient following administration of the vaccine). However, if the service is medically necessary, significant, and separately identifiable, it may be reported with modifier 25 appended to the E/M code (99211). The medical record must clearly state the reason for the visit, brief history, physical examination, assessment and plan, and any other counseling or discussion items. The progress note must be signed with the physician's countersignature. For more information and clinical vignettes on the appropriate use of E/M services during IA, visit www.aap.org/cfp and see "FAQ: Immunization Administration." Payers who do not follow the Medicare RBRVS may allow payment of code 99211 with IA. Know your payer guidelines, and if payment is allowed, make certain the guidelines are in writing and maintained in your office. Be aware that a co-payment may be required when the "nurse" visit is reported.

The same guidelines apply to physician visits (99202–99215).

- Modifier 25 (significant, separately identifiable E/M service by the same physician on the same day of the procedure or other service) should be appended to the problem-oriented service code (eg, 99212). If vaccines are given at the same encounter, append modifier 25 to the problem-oriented E/M service code and to the preventive medicine service code to avoid payer bundling edits that may allow payment only for IA.
- *ICD-10-CM* well-care diagnosis codes (see code list earlier in this chapter in *ICD-10-CM* Codes for Preventive Care Visits) should be linked to the appropriate preventive medicine service code (99381–99395) and the sick care diagnosis code linked to the problem-oriented service code (99202–99205, 99212–99215).

Examples

➤ **A 10-year-old boy receives a well-child (health supervision) visit.** This established patient also has previously diagnosed anxiety that is now exacerbated by health concerns of the grandmother who is his only caregiver. The grandmother notes she too is fearful about being too ill to care for her grandchild. Counseling with a licensed clinical social worker is recommended and arranged. The physician documents 20 minutes spent in counseling and coordinating care related to the patient's anxiety and the family's need for social support.

ICD-10-CM	CPT
Z00.121 (well-child check with abnormal findings) F41.96 (anxiety) Z63.79 (other stressful life events affecting family and household)	99393 (preventive medicine visit)
F41.96 (anxiety) Z63.79 (other stressful life events affecting family and household)	99213 25 (office E/M service, total physician time 20–29 minutes)

Teaching Point: Documentation should clearly support the separate time of the problem-oriented E/M service, discussion topics, and plan of care for the problems addressed.

Codes for preventive counseling and risk-factor reduction intervention (eg, 99401) are not appropriate for this example. Risk-factor reduction services are used for persons without a specific illness for which the counseling might otherwise be used as part of treatment. This patient has increased anxiety that prompts the counseling.

➤ **A 7-year-old boy with previously repaired patent ductus arteriosus is seen for a preventive medicine visit.** There are no new abnormal findings at the encounter.

ICD-10-CM	CPT
Z00.129 (well-child check without abnormal findings) **Z87.74** (personal history of [corrected] congenital malformations of heart and circulatory system)	Preventive medicine visit **New Patient** 99382 **Established Patient** 99392

Teaching Point: Because there were no current problems addressed at the encounter, only the preventive E/M code is reported. The diagnosis code for history of a congenital malformation of the heart and circulatory system may be reported as an additional diagnosis to the code for the well-child check but is not a finding of the well-child check.

See **Table 8-5** for additional illustration of coding for problem-oriented E/M services provided on the same date as preventive E/M services.

Table 8-5. Coding Continuum Model: Problem-Oriented and Preventive Evaluation and Management on the Same Date

Code selection may be based on the complexity of medical decision-making or the total time[a] spent by the physician or QHP solely devoted to the problem-oriented E/M on the date of the encounter.

CPT Code Time Vignette (Appropriate preventive E/M service codes are also reported.)	Medical Decision-making (2 of 3 elements required)		
	Number and Complexity of Problems Addressed	Amount and/or Complexity of Data Reviewed and Analyzed	Risk of Complications and/or Morbidity or Mortality of Patient Management
99212 (10–19 min) An infant is evaluated and found to have seborrheic capitis.	Minimal Self-limited problem	Limited Assessment requiring an independent historian(s)	Minimal
99213 (20–29 min) A 14-year-old presents today for a rash on bilateral forearms. Diagnosis is poison ivy.	Low 1 acute, uncomplicated illness or injury	Minimal or none	Low Home management with over-the-counter products
99214 (30–39 min)[b] A child presents with a new onset rash and history of fever and sore throat in the past week.	Moderate Acute illness with systemic symptoms and high risk of morbidity without treatment	Moderate Streptococcal test and culture Assessment requiring an independent historian(s)	Moderate Prescription of antibiotic
99215 (40–54 min)[b] A 14-year-old presents today for a previously scheduled preventive service and with complaint of stress hives. History includes recent onset of anxiety with heart palpitations and depression for which the patient is seeing a therapist. Patient admits to suicidal ideation without plan or intent. Mother provides family history, which is negative for bipolar disorder and positive for anxiety disorders.	High 1 acute or chronic illness or injury that poses a threat to life or bodily function	High Independent historian Tests ordered are CBC, thyroid function tests, comprehensive metabolic panel, electrocardiogram. Phone discussion with therapist regarding prescription of SSRI	Moderate Prescription drug management

Abbreviations: CBC, complete blood cell count; CPT, Current Procedural Terminology; E/M, evaluation and management; QHP, qualified health care professional; SSRI, selective serotonin reuptake inhibitor.

[a] Time-based E/M: Time is the total time spent in activities related to the problem-oriented E/M service by the physician or QHP on the date of the encounter. Do not include time of the preventive medicine service or time of other separately reported services.

[b] In many cases, a problem that requires higher levels of E/M service (ie, **99214** or **99215**) may warrant delay of the preventive E/M service.

Resources

Bright Futures

AAP/Bright Futures "Recommendations for Preventive Pediatric Health Care" (also see insert) (https://downloads.aap.org/AAP/PDF/periodicity_schedule.pdf)

Quality Measurement Information

US Department of Health and Human Services, Agency for Healthcare Research and Quality, National Guideline Clearinghouse (www.qualitymeasures.ahrq.gov)

CPT Category II codes (www.ama-assn.org/practice-management/cpt-category-ii-codes)

Sports/Camp Physicals

"Sports and Camp Physicals," June 2017 *AAP Pediatric Coding Newsletter* (https://coding.solutions.aap.org/article.aspx?articleid=2629481)

"Preparing for Preparticipation Physical Evaluations," July 2018 *AAP Pediatric Coding Newsletter* (https://coding.solutions.aap.org/article.aspx?articleid=2685958)

Immunization and Vaccines

Appendix III, Vaccine Products: Commonly Administered Pediatric Vaccines

AMA Category I vaccine codes (www.ama-assn.org/practice-management/cpt/category-i-vaccine-codes)

CDC VFC program (www.cdc.gov/vaccines/programs/vfc/index.html)

Vaccine Financing and Coding (www.aap.org/en/practice-management/practice-financing/coding-and-valuation/vaccine-financing-and-coding/)

AAP *Pediatric Vaccines: Coding Quick Reference Card 2022* (https://shop.aap.org/pediatric-vaccine-coding-quick-reference-chart-card-2022)

American Academy of Pediatrics Immunizations: Refusal to Vaccinate, including a vaccine refusal form in English and Spanish (www.aap.org/en-us/advocacy-and-policy/aap-health-initiatives/immunizations/Pages/refusal-to-vaccinate.aspx)

"Coding for Vaccines Not Administered," July 2020 *AAP Pediatric Coding Newsletter* (https://coding.solutions.aap.org/article.aspx?articleid=2765196; subscription required)

"AAP COVID-19 Vaccine Administration: Getting Paid" (https://services.aap.org/en/pages/2019-novel-coronavirus-covid-19-infections/covid-19-vaccine-for-children/covid-19-vaccine-administration-getting-paid/)

Laboratory Testing

Screening Laboratory Tests and Codes (www.aap.org/cfp)

US Food and Drug Administration CLIA—Clinical Laboratory Improvement Amendments Database (www.accessdata.fda.gov/scripts/cdrh/cfdocs/cfCLIA/search.cfm)

National Drug Codes

US FDA NDC directory (www.fda.gov/drugs/drug-approvals-and-databases/national-drug-code-directory)

Oral Health Preventive Services

Oral Health Coding Fact Sheet for Primary Care Physicians (https://downloads.aap.org/AAP/PDF/coding_factsheet_oral_health.pdf)

AAP Section on Oral Health state-specific information (www.aap.org/en-us/about-the-aap/Committees-Councils-Sections/Oral-Health/Map/Pages/State-Information-and-Resources-Map.aspx)

Preventive Services: Patient Education

What is Included in Preventive Medicine Encounters: Template Letter (www.aap.org/cfp)

Vision Screening

AAP Section on Ophthalmology and Committee on Practice and Ambulatory Medicine, American Academy of Ophthalmology, American Association for Pediatric Ophthalmology and Strabismus, and American Association of Certified Orthoptists "Instrument-Based Pediatric Vision Screening Policy Statement," *Pediatrics* (http://pediatrics.aappublications.org/content/130/5/983.full)

Test Your Knowledge!

1. **Which of the following is a new patient when a preventive medicine service is provided?**
   a. A newborn who was cared for by the same physician during the birth admission
   b. A child who has a new health insurance plan since the last visit
   c. A newborn who was cared for by a physician of a different group practice or different specialty during the birth admission
   d. A patient who was last seen by the physician 2 years ago

2. **Which service is reported with code 90471?**
   a. Immunization of an 18-year-old patient with physician counseling
   b. Immunization administration on a date different from the date physician counseling was provided
   c. Immunization of a patient younger than 18 years with physician counseling
   d. Immunization by injection in addition to an immunization reported with code 90473

3. **Which codes are reported when a preventive medicine service and counseling for oral health with application of fluoride varnish are provided at the same encounter?**
   a. Only a preventive medicine evaluation and management (E/M) code (eg, 99392)
   b. Code 99188 25 and a preventive medicine E/M code
   c. A preventive medicine E/M code and 99188
   d. A preventive medicine E/M code and 99401

4. **Which code is reported for use of a standardized instrument to screen for maternal depression during a newborn preventive E/M service?**
   a. 96160
   b. 96127
   c. 96110
   d. 96161

5. **To which of the following does the *Current Procedural Terminology* midpoint rule apply?**
   a. 99406, 99407
   b. 99408, 99409
   c. 99401–99404
   d. 99391–99395

Consultation, Residential, and Non–face-to-face Evaluation and Management Services

Contents

Selecting the Appropriate Evaluation and Management Codes 205

    Use of Time in Code Selection 205

Office and Outpatient Consultations (**99241–99245**) 207

    Guidelines Used by Payers That Follow Medicare Consultation Guidelines 208

    Expectant Parent Consultations 210

    Remote Interprofessional Consultations 211

        Interprofessional Consultation Reporting by an Attending/Primary Care Physician 211

        Interprofessional Consultation Reporting by a Consultant 211

Home Care Services (**99341–99350**) 213

Domiciliary, Rest Home, or Custodial Care Services (**99324–99337**) 215

Out-of-Office Service Add-on Codes (**99056–99060**) 216

Telephone Services (**99441–99443**, **98966–98968**) 217

Online Digital Evaluation and Management Services 218

    Online Digital Medical Services 218

Nursing Facility Care 219

    Initial Nursing Facility Care (**99304–99306**) 220

    Subsequent Nursing Facility Care (**99307–99310**) 221

    Nursing Facility Discharge Services (**99315**, **99316**) 222

    Annual Nursing Facility Assessment (**99318**) 222

Prolonged Services 222

    Prolonged Service With Direct Patient Contact (**99354–99357**) 222

    Prolonged Service Without Direct Patient Contact (**99358**, **99359**) 223

Critical Care (**99291**, **99292**) 223

Resources 224

Test Your Knowledge! 225

Chapter 9. Consultation, Residential, and Non–face-to-face Evaluation and Management Services

Selecting the Appropriate Evaluation and Management Codes

This chapter includes information on coding for evaluation and management (E/M) services provided in nonhospital settings (excluding office E/M services [**99202–99205**, **99211–99215**]) or non–face-to-face (ie, by telephone or online digital communication). Included here are codes for reporting

- Office and outpatient consultations (**99241–99245**)
- Home care services (**99341–99350**)
- Domiciliary, rest home, or custodial care services (**99324–99337**)
- Out-of-office service add-on codes (**99056–99060**)
- Telephone services (**99441–99443**, **98966–98968**)
- Online digital E/M services (**99421–99423**)
- Nursing facility care (**99304–99310**, **99315**, **99316**, **99318**)
- Prolonged services (**99354–99359**)
- Critical care (**99291**, **99292**)

> **See Chapter 7 for information on office and other outpatient evaluation and management (E/M) services (99202–99205, 99211–99215).**
> **See Chapter 20 for information on reporting E/M services provided via telemedicine (real-time audiovisual technology).**

Note: All E/M code descriptors and their specific instructions reflect the exclusion of references to provider/professional type, when nonessential, throughout the code set. When the word "physician" is included in a code descriptor, a qualified health care professional (QHP) working within his or her scope of practice may also provide the service.

When codes are provided for new and established patient E/M services, a new patient is one who has not received any *face-to-face* professional services within the past 3 years from the physician or another physician of the same specialty who belongs to the same group practice.

Use of Time in Code Selection

Time of service is the only basis for code selection (ie, key components do not apply) for services such as telephone or online digital E/M services and for critical care codes **99291** and **99292**. Most codes discussed in this chapter are selected based on key components or the physician's face-to-face time with the patient, but time is not always an option for code selection.

For those services for which code selection is based on either key components or time, use of time as the key controlling factor in the selection of the code, in lieu of key components, is only applicable when counseling and/or coordination of care accounts for more than 50% of the face-to-face time with the patient.

- Code selection based on time requires documentation of the total face-to-face time (may be approximate) and the percentage or number of minutes spent in counseling and/or coordination of care.
- *Current Procedural Terminology* (*CPT*®) instructs that time is met when the midpoint is passed unless code descriptors or prefatory instructions indicate otherwise. Other payers may require that the typical time specified for a service be met or exceeded.

> **See also Chapter 6 for a detailed description of evaluation and management guidelines, documentation requirements, and tips. See Chapter 12 for guidelines for reporting chronic or principal care management and other non–face-to-face services provided to manage complex and/or chronic conditions.**

Table 9-1 provides the key components and specific details on required elements within each level of history and physical examination (eg, problem focused, expanded) and medical decision-making (MDM) (eg, straightforward, moderate) for most E/M codes. Refer to this table for more information on key components when using some of the other tables in this chapter to assign codes to examples. This table can be downloaded at www.aap.org/cfp.

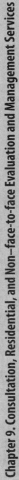

Table 9-1. Evaluation and Management Key Components

History (must meet or exceed HPI, ROS, and PFSH)	Problem Focused	Expanded	Detailed	Comprehensive
	HPI: 1–3 elements ROS: 0 PFSH: 0	HPI: 1–3 elements ROS: 1 PFSH: 0	HPI: 4+ elements or status of 3 chronic or inactive conditions ROS: 2–9 PFSH: 1	HPI: 4+ elements or status of 3 chronic or inactive conditions ROS: 10+ PFSH: 2 (established patient) or 3 (new patient)
Physical Examination	Problem Focused 1995: 1 body area/organ system 1997: Performance and documentation of 1–5 elements identified by a bullet (●) in ≥1 areas or systems	Expanded 1995: Limited examination—affected body area/organ system and 1–6 other related areas/systems 1997: Performance and documentation of at least 6 elements identified by a bullet (●) in ≥1 areas or systems	Detailed 1995: Extended examination—affected body area(s) and 1–6 other symptomatic or related organ system(s) 1997: Performance and documentation of at least 2 elements identified by a bullet (●) in at least 6 areas or systems or at least 12 elements identified by a bullet (●) in at least 2 areas or systems	Comprehensive 1995: 8+ organ systems or complete examination of a single organ system 1997: Multisystem examination—9 systems or areas with performance of all elements identified by a bullet (●) in each area/system examined Documentation of at least 2 elements identified by a bullet (●) of each area(s) or system(s) Single organ system examination—Performance of all elements identified by a bullet (●) and documentation of every element in box with shaded border and at least 1 element in box with unshaded border
Medical Decision-making (Must meet 2 of diagnoses/options, data, and risk.)	Straightforward	Low complexity	Moderate complexity	High complexity
Presenting Problem	Usually self-limited or minor severity	Usually moderate severity	Usually moderate to high severity	Usually moderate to high severity
No. of D/M Options	Minimal	Limited	Multiple	Extensive
Data	Minimal	Limited	Moderate	Extensive
Risk	Minimal	Low	Moderate	High

Abbreviations: D/M, diagnosis and management; HPI, history of present illness; PFSH, past, family, and social history; ROS, review of systems.

The examples included throughout this chapter are based on the 1995 E/M documentation guidelines. Each section includes a table illustrating key components of each type of service. Medical decision-making is listed before history and physical examination because some payers place greater emphasis on MDM than history and examination. Some payers require that the level of MDM be 1 of the 2 key components met to support the level of service for an established patient encounter.

Medical necessity for the extent of history, examination, and MDM should be evident in the documentation for each encounter. Consider only clinically indicated services when selecting the level of E/M service.

Office and Outpatient Consultations (99241–99245)

Codes **99241–99245** are used to report consultations provided in a pediatric office or outpatient clinic, a patient's home, a domiciliary, a rest home, or a custodial care home.

See codes **99251–99255** in **Chapter 16** for information on reporting consultations in nursing facility settings.

Consultations are defined by *CPT* as services provided by a physician at the request of another physician or "other appropriate source" to provide advice or opinion about the management or evaluation of a specific problem or to determine whether to accept responsibility for ongoing management of the patient's entire care or for the care of a specific condition/problem.

The "other appropriate source" is not explicitly defined in *CPT*. It may mean any interested source who seeks a medical opinion (eg, schools, juvenile court, attorney, psychologist, dentist, physician extender, occupational therapist). It does not mean the patient or family of the patient.

- Many payers require inclusion of the National Provider Identifier (NPI) of the requesting physician or other source on the claim for a consultation.
- When the source requesting a consultation does not have an NPI (eg, school counselor, teacher, attorney), verify payers' coding and billing requirements for the consultation. Claims for consultation services submitted without the NPI of the requestor may be rejected.

> **Do not report a consultation code for an encounter requested by a patient, parent, or guardian.**

Guidelines for reporting consultations include
- A physician or other appropriate source must request the consultation for opinion and/or advice (ie, with a question).
- Documentation must include
  - The request (written or verbal from the consultant; if verbal, still must be documented).
  - Name of the requesting physician or other appropriate source who requested the consultation.
  - Reason or need for the consultation (advice or opinion requested).
  - Opinion, recommendations, and services performed or ordered.
  - Written report back to the requesting physician or other appropriate source. A copy of the report must be maintained in the medical record.

> **A consultation report may be in letter form, a copy of the progress note, or a completed form (eg, preoperative form, consultation template). In a large group practice with shared medical records, it is acceptable to include the consultant's report as part of the documentation. A separate letter or report is not required.**

  - The requesting physician or other appropriate source must also document the request (even if it is a verbal request) for consultation in the patient medical record. This is not required by *CPT*, but some payers have adopted this policy to assist in review of records when it is unclear that consultation (ie, advice or opinion) was requested in lieu of a transfer of care for a particular problem.
- The consultant may initiate diagnostic or therapeutic services at the same or at a subsequent visit. Any identifiable procedures performed on or after the date of initial consultation (eg, endoscopy, cardiac catheterization, biopsy) should be reported separately.
- The management of the patient remains with the requesting or attending physician and is released in whole or in part only by the written notation of the requesting or attending physician in the medical record.
- Physicians in a group practice can provide consultations at the request of another member of the same practice if they are a different specialty or have an expertise in a specific medical area. For example, a primary care pediatrician may refer a patient to a partner, who is an allergist.
- Consultations for preoperative clearance may be reported when the surgeon requests an opinion and/or advice and a written report is sent to the requesting physician. Be aware of Medicaid program and commercial payer guidelines—some do not allow preoperative clearance consultations.
- Follow-up visits that are initiated by the physician consultant are reported using codes for established patients appropriate to the place of service (eg, office, home, domiciliary, rest home, custodial care).

- If an additional request for an opinion or advice on the same or a new problem is received from the attending physician and documented, the consultation codes may be used again.
- Consultations mandated by a third party (eg, payer, regulatory authority) are reported with modifier **32**.

Three of 3 key components must be met or exceeded when selecting the level of service for consultation services. A summary of key components for each level is in **Table 9-2**.

Chapter 9. Consultation, Residential, and Non–face-to-face Evaluation and Management Services

Table 9-2. New or Established Office/Outpatient Consultation Codes (99241–99245)			
Key Components (For a description of key components, see Table 9-1.) 3 of 3 key components must be performed to at least the degree specified under the code.			
***CPT* Code/Time**[a]	**Medical Decision-making**	**History**[b]	**1995 Examination**[c]
99241 15 min	Straightforward PP: Usually self-limited or minor	Problem-focused HPI: 1–3; ROS: 0; PFSH: 0	Problem-focused 1 body area/system
99242 30 min	Straightforward PP: Usually low to moderate severity	Expanded problem-focused HPI: 1–3; ROS: 1; PFSH: 0	Expanded problem-focused 2–7 limited
99243 40 min	Low complexity PP: Usually moderate severity	Detailed HPI: ≥4 or 3 CC; ROS: 2–9; PFSH: 1/3	Detailed 2–7 detailed
99244 60 min	Moderate complexity PP: Usually moderate to high severity	Comprehensive HPI: ≥4 or 3 CC; ROS: ≥10; PFSH: 3/3	Comprehensive ≥8 body areas/systems
99245 80 min	High complexity PP: Usually moderate to high severity	Comprehensive HPI: ≥4 or 3 CC; ROS: ≥10; PFSH: 3/3	Comprehensive ≥8 body areas/systems

Abbreviations: CC, chronic condition; *CPT, Current Procedural Terminology;* HPI, history of present illness; PFSH, past, family, and social history; PP, presenting problem; ROS; review of systems.

[a] Typical time is an average and represents a range of times that may be higher or lower depending on clinical circumstances. The presenting problem is considered to be a contributory factor and does not need to be present to the degree specified.
[b] A chief complaint is required for all levels of history.
[c] Number of body areas or organ systems examined; see **Table 9-1** for details.

Codes do not distinguish between new or established patients. Face-to-face time with the patient may be used to select the level of service when more than 50% was spent in counseling and/or coordination of care.

Guidelines Used by Payers That Follow Medicare Consultation Guidelines

It is important to check with major payers to determine if they have adopted the Medicare policy to not pay consultation codes, or if they have established their own policies and guidelines for reporting consultations. The American Academy of Pediatrics position on Medicare consultation policy is available at www.aap.org/cfp.

- If the payer does not pay for consultation codes, the consulting physician reports codes for the appropriate site of service based on the performance and documentation of the required key components or time, if appropriate (**Table 9-3**).

Table 9-3. Coding Consultations Under Medicare Rules	
New Patient	**Established Patient**
99202–99205 (office, outpatient hospital, observation)	**99212–99215** (office, outpatient hospital, observation)
99341–99345 (home visit)	**99347–99350** (home visit)
99324–99328 (domiciliary or rest home visit)	**99334–99336** (domiciliary or rest home visit)
99304–99306 (initial nursing facility care)	**99307–99310** (subsequent nursing facility care)

- Documentation of the request for consultation and a report of the results back to the referring physician are required as discussed earlier in this chapter.

Use **tables 9-2 and 9-3** to determine the appropriate consultation codes in the following examples:

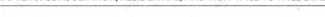

Examples

➤ **A primary care pediatrician consults an otolaryngologist for opinion on tympanostomy with tubes for treatment of chronic otitis media.** The patient is new to the otolaryngologist, who reviews and summarizes records provided by the primary pediatrician. A comprehensive history is obtained, including information from the patient's parents, who note that the patient is increasingly missing school and community events due to infections. A detailed examination is also performed, and findings of hypertrophic adenoids and resolving bilateral chronic serous otitis media are documented.

Assessment/plan: Diagnosis is chronic serous otitis media with chronic hypertrophy of adenoids; the otolaryngologist discusses treatment options with the parents, including tympanostomy with tube placement and adenoidectomy, and the parents agree. The otolaryngologist sends a report to the primary care pediatrician advising that surgery is recommended.

MDM: Moderate complexity (new problem without additional workup; old record reviewed/summarized; decision for major surgery without identified risk factors) *History:* Comprehensive *Physical examination:* Detailed	***International Classification of Diseases, 10th Revision, Clinical Modification (ICD-10-CM)*** **H65.23** (chronic serous otitis media, bilateral) **J35.2** (hypertrophy of adenoids)
	CPT **99243** or, if payer does not recognize consultations, **New Patient Office E/M** **99204** (moderate MDM—moderate number and complexity of problems and moderate amount and complexity of data reviewed and analyzed)

Teaching Point: The detailed examination limits the consultation code to **99243** because a comprehensive examination is required for **99244**. However, if a payer requires reporting an office or other outpatient E/M service in lieu of an outpatient consultation, code **99204** is supported because of the moderate level of MDM, which is based on the problems addressed (chronic otitis media with chronic adenoid hypertrophy) being of moderate complexity and a decision for major surgery without identified risk factors supporting moderate risk.

Because the code selection guidelines for office E/M services are not based on the levels of history and examination, the level of MDM alone is used in support of **99204**.

➤ **A 13-year-old boy who has obesity and Down syndrome (new patient) is referred to a cardiologist for evaluation of a murmur.** Prior to the visit but on the same date, past medical records and laboratory test results are reviewed and summarized by the cardiologist. A comprehensive history and physical examination are performed. Electrocardiogram (ECG) and echocardiogram are performed and interpreted.

Assessment/plan: Down syndrome. Patient with mitral valve prolapse with minimal regurgitation—will evaluate again in 6 months and start medication, if indicated. Obesity—dietary changes and increased exercise were recommended. A written report is sent back to the referring physician. Total face-to-face time of the consultation service was 30 minutes. Total physician time on the date of service was 60 minutes, not including time spent in interpretation and report of tests.

MDM: Moderate complexity (1 new problem with no additional workup and 1 stable chronic condition; review of laboratory test results and review and summarization of medical records) *History:* Comprehensive *Physical examination:* Comprehensive	***ICD-10-CM*** **I34.1** (nonrheumatic mitral [valve] prolapse) **E66.9** (obesity, unspecified) **Q90.9** (Down syndrome)
	CPT **99244** or, if payer does not recognize consultations, **New Patient** **99205** (60–74 minutes total time)

Chapter 9. Consultation, Residential, and Non–face-to-face Evaluation and Management Services

Teaching Point: The cardiologist evaluated the patient's murmur and addressed obesity. A cardiologist billing for interpretation and report of an ECG and/or echocardiogram will not count the test toward the data analyzed in determining the level of MDM. Where a payer requires an office E/M code in lieu of a consultation code, code **99205** is supported by the cardiologist's total time (60 minutes) on the date of the encounter. If time were used in selection of a consultation code, code **99242** would be reported for 30 minutes of face-to-face time.

➤ **A pediatrician is consulted for a 14-year-old boy who lives in a group home.** The boy has become withdrawn and disinterested in activities that he previously enjoyed. The social worker for the group home is concerned that he may need medical management of depression.

The pediatrician visits the patient at the group home and uses a standardized screening instrument to assess for depression. The score indicates moderate depression. The pediatrician obtains history and conducts an examination (10 minutes) before spending 20 minutes counseling the patient. After the visit, the pediatrician spends 10 minutes on the phone coordinating care with the social worker. The pediatrician spends another 5 minutes with the group home staff to advise of the treatment plan and address their questions about caring for the patient. Diagnosis is moderate major depressive disorder, single episode. Total time is documented as 30 minutes spent face-to-face with more than 50% spent in counseling and/or coordination of care.

ICD-10-CM	CPT
F32.1 (major depressive disorder, single episode, moderate)	The consultant reports **99242** (based on typical time of 30 minutes) or, if the payer does not recognize consultation codes, **99335** (based on typical time of 25 minutes)

Teaching Point: Levels of key components were not provided in this scenario. Time is documented with an indication that more than 50% was spent in counseling and/or coordination of care. Time on the phone with the social worker and in the office of the group home discussing care with the staff would not be attributed to the face-to-face time of the consultation service. Based on the total face-to-face time of 30 minutes, code **99242** is reported.

Coding for visits in a group home is discussed more later in this chapter.

Expectant Parent Consultations

When counseling and risk reduction interventions are provided to a mother or her fetus prior to delivery, report these services to the mother's insurance. If a family is referred by an obstetrician for an existing problem, the outpatient consultation should be reported using office-based consultation codes (**99241–99245**) or other appropriate E/M codes as directed by payer policy. (See **Chapter 16** for hospital E/M services.)

Codes 99401–99404 may be reported if a parent or family requests an appointment with a physician to discuss a risk reduction intervention (ie, seeking advice to avoid a future problem or complication). See Chapter 8 for information on coding for these services.

ICD-10-CM code **Z76.81** (expectant parent[s] pre-birth pediatrician visit) would be reported for pre-birth counseling visits in addition to other relevant *ICD-10-CM* codes as applicable. Family history codes may also be relevant for reporting the reason for pre-birth and/or preconception counseling (eg, **Z82.79**, family history of other congenital malformations, deformations, and chromosomal abnormalities).

Verification of the payer's benefit policy for these services is recommended prior to service; if non-covered, an advance beneficiary notice should be signed by the patient. An *advance beneficiary notice* or *waiver* is a written notice to the patient of noncoverage or potential out-of-pocket costs that is provided prior to delivery of a service. Verify payer requirements and applicable state regulations prior to using waivers in your practice. When used, a copy of the signed notice should be kept on file with the practice's billing records.

An encounter for a meet and greet is not considered a medically necessary service and will most likely not be covered. Check health plan contracts to determine if charging directly to the patient's caregiver is allowed and whether advance notification of noncoverage is required.

Remote Interprofessional Consultations

99446 Interprofessional telephone/Internet/electronic health record assessment and management service provided by a consultative physician including a verbal and written report to the patient's treating/requesting physician/qualified health care professional; 5–10 minutes of medical consultative discussion and review

99447 11–20 minutes of medical consultative discussion and review

99448 21–30 minutes of medical consultative discussion and review

99449 31 minutes or more of medical consultative discussion and review

#99451 Interprofessional telephone/Internet/electronic health record assessment and management service provided by a consultative physician including a written report to the patient's treating/requesting physician or other qualified health care professional, 5 or more minutes of medical consultative time

#99452 Interprofessional telephone/Internet/electronic health record referral service(s) provided by a treating/requesting physician or qualified health care professional, 30 minutes

Remote interprofessional consultations include a request by a patient's attending or primary care physician or other QHP soliciting opinion and/or treatment advice by telephone, internet, or electronic health record (EHR) from a physician with specialty expertise (ie, consultant). This consultation does not require face-to-face contact with the patient by the consultant. The patient may be in the inpatient or outpatient setting.

> See Chapter 12 for information on care management services that may include online communications.

Interprofessional Consultation Reporting by an Attending/Primary Care Physician

The treating/requesting physician or other QHP may report code **99452** or prolonged service (**99417, 99354–99357; 99358, 99359**).

- Code **99452** may be reported when 16 to 30 minutes is spent by the requesting individual in a service day preparing for the referral and/or communicating with the consultant.
- Time spent in discussion with the consultant may also be reported with prolonged service codes (in lieu of **99452**) *if the requirements for the appropriate prolonged service codes are met.*
  - Direct prolonged service code **99417** may be reported when the requesting physician has had a face-to-face encounter with the patient in the office or other outpatient setting on the same day and the physician's total time on that date extends at least 15 minutes beyond the total time of the associated E/M service (**99205, 99215**).
  - Direct prolonged service provided in conjunction with inpatient, observation, or outpatient services, except with office or other outpatient services, may be reported with codes **99354** and **99355** or **99356** and **99357**.
  - Prolonged service of more than 30 minutes in a day without the patient present is reported with codes **99358** and **99359**.

> See more on prolonged service in outpatient settings later in this chapter. For more information on prolonged office and other outpatient evaluation and management services, see Chapter 7. Coding for prolonged service in an inpatient or observation setting is reviewed in Chapter 16.

Interprofessional Consultation Reporting by a Consultant

Guidelines for the consultant reporting interprofessional telephone/internet/EHR consultations include

- Telephone/internet/EHR consultations of less than 5 minutes are not reported. For codes **99446–99449**, more than 50% of the time reported as interprofessional consultation must have been spent in medical consultative verbal or internet discussion rather than review of data (eg, medical records, test results).
- Code **99451** is reported based on the total time of review and interprofessional consultation.
- Both verbal and written reports are required for completion of the services represented by codes **99446–99449**. Only a written report is required for code **99451**.
- A single interprofessional consultation code is reported for the cumulative time spent in discussion and information review regardless of the number of contacts necessary to complete the service.
- Codes **99446–99451** are not reported more than once in a 7-day interval.
- Time spent in telephone or online consultation directly with the patient and/or family may be reported using codes **99441–99443** (telephone E/M) or **99421–99423** (online digital E/M), and the time related to these services is not included in the time attributed to interprofessional consultation services. Qualified nonphysician health care professionals (eg, therapists) report codes **98966–98968** or **98970–98972** for these services.

- When the purpose of communication is to arrange a transfer of care or face-to-face patient encounter, interprofessional consultation codes are not reported.
- Interprofessional consultation services are not reported if the consultant has provided a face-to-face service to the patient within the past 14 days or when the consultation results in scheduling of a face-to-face service within the next 14 days or at the consultant's next available appointment date.
- Time spent by the consultant reviewing pertinent medical records, studies, or other data is included in the time of the interprofessional consultation and not separately reported.
- Do not report prolonged E/M service before and/or after direct patient care (**99358**, **99359**) for any time within the service period if reporting codes **99446–99451**.
- As with all consultations, the request for advice or opinion should be documented in the patient record. For a new patient with no record, create a record to document this service.

Examples

➤ **A 10-year-old girl presents to her pediatrician to discuss new behavioral concerns that are resulting in poor academic performance and discord at home.** History and examination indicate increased anxiety and related behavioral changes since e-learning began last year. The girl and her mother complete structured screening instruments for anxiety disorders. The girl, who has predominantly inattentive attention-deficit/hyperactivity disorder (ADHD), scores just below the score indicating a generalized anxiety disorder. The diagnosis for the visit is anxiety with increased symptoms of ADHD. The physician's total time on the date of the visit is 30 minutes, including time spent arranging for a telephone consultation with a psychiatrist for advice on diagnosis and management of anxiety in the patient with preexisting ADHD.

Prior to the consultation, the psychiatrist spends 10 minutes reviewing the pediatrician's documentation of the patient's evaluation. Later that day, the pediatrician and psychiatrist spend a total of 21 minutes discussing the pediatrician's findings, diagnosis, and appropriate treatment options. The psychiatrist provides the pediatrician with a written report of the recommendations discussed. The diagnosis is adjustment disorder with anxiety complicating management of ADHD.

On a third date, the pediatrician provides a face-to-face E/M service to the patient and her parents to discuss recommendations based on the prior interprofessional consultation. A diagnosis of adjustment reaction with anxiety exacerbating ADHD and related management options are discussed. The pediatrician's total time on the date of the visit is 25 minutes.

Service	ICD-10-CM	CPT
First date of service (pediatric E/M visit)	**F41.9** (anxiety disorder, unspecified) **F90.0** (ADHD, predominantly inattentive type)	**99214** (established patient office or other outpatient visit E/M, 30–39 minutes of total time) **96127** x 2 (brief emotional/behavioral assessment using a structured instrument)
Second date (interprofessional consultation)	Both physicians report **F43.22** (adjustment disorder with anxiety) and **F90.0** (ADHD, predominantly inattentive type).	The pediatrician reports **99452** for the 21 minutes spent in interprofessional referral service.
		The psychiatrist reports **99449** (31 or more minutes of medical discussion and review).
Third date (pediatric E/M visit)	**F43.22** and **F90.0**	**99213** (established patient office or other outpatient visit E/M, 20–29 minutes of total time)

Teaching Point: In this vignette, the patient and parents are not present for the interprofessional consultation. The consultation service by the psychiatrist included 10 minutes of record review and 21 minutes of conversation with the pediatrician. If less than 50% of the psychiatrist's time was devoted to the medical consultative verbal or internet discussion, an interprofessional consultation would not be reported. The pediatrician may report code **99452** for 16 to 30 minutes of interprofessional consultation.

➤ **A hospitalized 14-year-old presents with a critical illness of undetermined cause.** An infectious process is suspected but not identified by testing. The patient's attending physician telephones an infectious disease specialist located several hours away for advice. The physicians spend 15 minutes discussing the adolescent's condition and decides on an option for further evaluation. The next day, the attending physician again consults the specialist to discuss new laboratory results and the patient's lack of improvement. The consultant spends 20 minutes on that date reviewing the patient's record and provides a written report to the attending physician via secure email.

ICD-10-CM	CPT
The infectious disease specialist reports this service with a code for either a diagnosed condition or signs and symptoms based on what is known at the conclusion of the service.	The consultant reports **99449** (interprofessional consultation, 31 minutes or more) on the date the service was completed. The pediatrician will report the appropriate E/M service on each date of service.

Teaching Point: The consulting physician reports the interprofessional consultation only once for the cumulative discussion and medical record review time. The attending physician will include this work in the per diem charge for critical care services based on the type of care rendered.

Home Care Services (99341–99350)

- For purposes of reporting home visits, *CPT* defines *home* as a private residence, temporary lodging, or short-term accommodation (eg, hotel, campground, hostel, cruise ship).
- Home visits are typically reported with place of service code **12** (home location, other than hospital or other facility, where patient receives care in a private residence).
- Place of service code **16** (temporary lodging—hotel, campground, hostel, cruise ship, or resort) may also be reported in conjunction with codes **99341–99350**.
- Medicaid plans may vary in sites of service reported as home visits.
- Do not report home visit codes for visits to patients in residential facilities or group homes. See codes for domiciliary, rest home, or custodial care services (**99324–99328** and **99334–99337**).
- Code selection is based on the performance and documentation of the required key components or on time if more than 50% of the time is spent in counseling and/or coordination of care, as seen in **tables 9-4 and 9-5**.

Table 9-4. New Patient Visits in a Home or in a Domiciliary, Rest Home, or Custodial Care

Key Components (For a description of key components, see Table 9-1.)
3 of 3 key components must be performed to at least the degree specified under the code.

CPT Code/Time[a]		Medical Decision-making	History[b]	1995 Examination[c]
Home **99341** 20 min	**DRHCC** **99324** 20 min	Straightforward PP: Usually low severity	HPI: 1–3; ROS: 0; PFSH: 0	1 body area/system
Home **99342** 30 min	**DRHCC** **99325** 30 min	Low complexity PP: Usually moderate severity	HPI: 1–3; ROS: 1; PFSH: 0	2–7 limited
Home **99343** 45 min	**DRHCC** **99326** 45 min	Moderate complexity PP: Usually moderate to high severity	HPI: ≥4 or 3 CC; ROS: 2–9; PFSH: 1/3	2–7 detailed
Home **99344** 60 min	**DRHCC** **99327** 60 min	Moderate complexity PP: Usually moderate to high severity	HPI: ≥4 or 3 CC; ROS: ≥10; PFSH: 3/3	≥8 body areas/systems

Table 9-4 (*continued*)

CPT Code/Time[a]		Medical Decision-making	History[b]	1995 Examination[c]
Home **99345** 75 min	**DRHCC** **99328** 75 min	High complexity PP: Usually patient is unstable or has developed a new problem requiring immediate physician attention.	HPI: ≥4 or 3 CC; ROS: ≥10; PFSH: 3/3	≥8 body areas/systems

Abbreviations: CC, chronic condition; *CPT, Current Procedural Terminology;* DRHCC, domiciliary, rest home, or custodial care; HPI, history of present illness; PFSH, past, family, and social history; PP, presenting problem; ROS, review of systems.

[a] Typical time is an average and represents a range of times that may be higher or lower depending on clinical circumstances. The presenting problem is considered to be a contributory factor and does not need to be present to the degree specified.

[b] A chief complaint is required for all levels of history.

[c] Number of body areas or organ systems examined; see **Table 9-1** for details.

Table 9-5. Established Patient Visits in a Home or in a Domiciliary, Rest Home, or Custodial Care

Key Components (For a description of key components, see Table 9-1.)

2 of 3 key components must be performed to at least the degree specified under the code. Some payers may require medical decision-making as 1 of the 2 components performed and documented.

CPT Code/Time[a]		Medical Decision-making	History[b]	Examination[c]
Home **99347** 15 min	**DRHCC** **99324** 20 min	Straightforward PP: Usually self-limited or minor	HPI: 1–3; ROS: 0; PFSH: 0	1 body area/system
Home **99348** 25 min	**DRHCC** **99325** 30 min	Low complexity PP: Usually low to moderate severity	HPI: 1–3; ROS: 1; PFSH: 0	2–7 limited
Home **99349** 40 min	**DRHCC** **99326** 45 min	Moderate complexity PP: Usually moderate to high severity	HPI: ≥4 or 3 CC; ROS: 2–9; PFSH: 1/3	2–7 detailed
DRHCC **99327** 60 min		Moderate complexity PP: Usually high severity	HPI: ≥4 or 3 CC; ROS: ≥10; PFSH: 3/3	≥8 body areas/systems
Home **99350** 60 min		Moderate to high complexity PP: Usually moderate to high severity	HPI: ≥4 or 3 CC; ROS: ≥10; PFSH: 2/3	≥8 body areas/systems
DRHCC **99328** 75 min		High complexity PP: Usually patient is unstable or has developed a new problem requiring immediate physician attention.	HPI: ≥4 or 3 CC; ROS: ≥10; PFSH: 3/3	≥8 body areas/systems

Abbreviations: CC, chronic condition; *CPT, Current Procedural Terminology;* DRHCC, domiciliary, rest home, or custodial care; HPI, history of present illness; PFSH, past, family, and social history; PP, presenting problem; ROS, review of systems.

[a] Typical time is an average and represents a range of times that may be higher or lower depending on clinical circumstances. The presenting problem is considered to be a contributory factor and does not need to be present to the degree specified.

[b] A chief complaint is required for all levels of history.

[c] Number of body areas or organ systems examined; see **Table 9-1** for details.

● =New code   ▲ =Revised code   # =Re-sequenced code   + =Add-on code   ★ =Telemedicine

- Travel time to and from a patient's home is assumed to be in the level of care, just as travel time to and from the hospital is included in hospital care codes and is not counted in the time spent. However, if escorting a patient to a medical facility becomes necessary, code **99082** (unusual travel) is available.
- Services provided in a patient's home by a nonphysician provider who does not have his or her own NPI may not be billed unless the physician provides direct supervision. Refer to **Chapter 13**, Qualified Nonphysician Health Care Professional Services.
- Any procedures performed by the physician may be separately reported.
- Payers may have varied policies on coverage and reporting requirements for home visits and may not use Medicare incident-to guidelines. Check with them prior to reporting this service.

Example

➤ **A pediatrician agrees to provide a home visit to a 6-year-old with symptoms of influenza or other upper respiratory illness.** The child was immunized against influenza 1 week ago during a new patient well-child (health supervision) visit. A problem-focused history and examination are documented in addition to results of a point-of-care influenza test that is positive for influenza A. The pediatrician prescribes oseltamivir. The parents are concerned that the immunization did not protect their child. The pediatrician spends 13 minutes counseling the parents about the time from immunization administration to development of immunity and potential for exposure. The total face-to-face time of the visit is 25 minutes.

ICD-10-CM	CPT
J11.1 (influenza due to unidentified influenza virus with other respiratory manifestations)	99348 (typical time 25 minutes)

Teaching Point: 13 of 25 minutes of the face-to-face visit were spent in counseling and/or coordination of care, supporting code selection based on the total face-to-face time.

Many payers require documentation of medical necessity for provision of services in the home rather than the office. Inclusion of codes that limit the patient's ability to be seen in the office or outpatient clinic may help demonstrate medical necessity.

Domiciliary, Rest Home, or Custodial Care Services (99324–99337)

- These services are provided in a facility that provides room and board and other personal assistance services (eg, assisted living facility).
- Codes **99324–99337** are not reported for patients residing in a private residence (see codes **99341–99350**).
- Codes **99324–99328** and **99334–99337** are reported for services provided in facilities assigned the following place of service codes: **13** (assisted living), **14** (group home), **33** (custodial care facility), and **55** (residential substance abuse facility).
- Prolonged services provided in a domiciliary, rest home, or custodial care are reported with codes **99354** and **99355**.

   Use **tables 9-4 and 9-5** to select codes for the following example:

Example

➤ **A pediatrician agrees to provide medically necessary services at the infirmary of a youth ranch where an established patient lives.** The patient presents with complaint of increased asthma symptoms. The pediatrician evaluates the patient and makes a change to the patient's control medication. Documentation includes a detailed interval history, detailed examination, and moderate MDM based on an established problem (moderate persistent asthma with exacerbation) and medication management.

ICD-10-CM	CPT
J45.41 (moderate persistent asthma with [acute] exacerbation)	99336 (domiciliary or rest home visit with key components as described)

Teaching Point: The history required for an established patient domiciliary or rest home visit is an interval history that does not require past, family, or social history, although these may be obtained and documented as appropriate to the patient presentation.

The place of service on this claim could be a group home (**14**) or a custodial care facility (**33**). It is important to verify the appropriate place of service for reporting, as it may affect payment and coverage.

Out-of-Office Service Add-on Codes (99056–99060)

Codes **99056–99060** are used to report services that are provided after hours or on an emergency basis and are an adjunct to the basic E/M service provided.

Third-party payers will have specific policies for coverage and payment. Communicate with individual payers to understand their definition or interpretation of the service and their coverage and payment policies. As part of this negotiation and education process, it is important to demonstrate the cost savings recognized by the payer for these adjunct services. After-hours service codes are used by physicians or other QHPs (under their state scope of practice and when billing with their own NPI) to identify the services that are adjunct to the basic services rendered. These codes

- Describe the special circumstances under which a basic procedure is performed.
- Are only reported in addition to an associated basic service (eg, home visit).
- Are reported without a modifier appended to the basic service because they only further describe the services provided.

99056 Service(s) typically provided in the office, provided out of the office at request of patient, in addition to basic service

Documentation should include the patient's request to be seen outside of the office.

99060 Service(s) provided on an emergency basis, out of the office, which disrupts other scheduled office services, in addition to basic service

Documentation should indicate that the physician was called away during scheduled office hours to attend to a patient in another location (eg, nursing facility).

Example

➤ **A physician provides care at a group home for adolescents transitioning out of foster care.** A staff member of the group home phones the physician requesting evaluation of a patient with asthma who is short of breath. The physician arrives at the group home to find an adolescent patient administering an inhalation treatment to himself due to asthma exacerbation. The patient's breathing improves and the physician obtains a detailed interval history, learning that the patient also used his emergency inhaler earlier in the day. The physician monitors the patient while reviewing the asthma control plan and then arranges for group home staff to monitor the patient for recurrent symptoms. The physician's face-to-face time with the patient is 45 minutes, with more than half spent in counseling and/or coordination of care for moderate persistent asthma with acute exacerbation.

ICD-10-CM	CPT
J45.41 (moderate persistent asthma with acute exacerbation)	**99336** (established domiciliary or rest home E/M with typical time of 40 minutes) **99056** (service[s] typically provided in the office, provided out of the office at request of patient, in addition to basic service)

Teaching Point: Payers may or may not allow payment for code **99056** when services are rendered in a domiciliary or in the patient's home. The level of E/M service was determined by time because more than 50% of the visit was spent in counseling and/or coordination of care.

Learn more about coding for special services in the May 2018 *AAP Pediatric Coding Newsletter* article, "Coding for Special Services In and Out of the Office" (https://coding.solutions.aap.org/article.aspx?articleid=2679118; subscription required).

Telephone Services (99441–99443, 98966–98968)

99441   Telephone E/M service by a physician or other qualified health care professional who may report evaluation and management services provided to an established patient, parent, or guardian not originating from a related E/M service provided within the previous 7 days nor leading to an E/M service or procedure within the next 24 hours or soonest available appointment; 5–10 minutes of medical discussion

99442   11–20 minutes of medical discussion

99443   21–30 minutes of medical discussion

98966   Telephone assessment and management services provided by a qualified nonphysician health care professional to an established patient, parent, or guardian not originating from a related assessment and management service provided within the previous 7 days nor leading to an assessment and management service or procedure within the next 24 hours or soonest available appointment; 5–10 minutes of medical discussion

98967   11–20 minutes of medical discussion

98968   21–30 minutes of medical discussion

Telephone services (99441–99443) are non–face-to-face E/M services provided to a patient using the telephone by a physician or other QHP who may report E/M services (eg, nurse practitioner, clinical nurse specialist, physician assistant).

Codes 98966–98968 are used to report telephone assessment and management services by health care professionals who may not report E/M services (eg, occupational therapists, speech-language pathologists).

Guidelines for reporting of telephone assessment and management services are the same as those for physician and QHP telephone E/M services.

Codes 99441–99443 may be reported when
- The call was initiated by an established patient or caregiver of an established patient.
- They include physician management of a new problem that does not result in an office visit within 24 hours from the telephone call or at the next available urgent visit appointment.
- They include physician management of an existing problem for which the patient was not seen in a face-to-face encounter in the previous 7 days from the telephone call (physician requested or unsolicited patient follow-up) or within the postoperative period of a performed and reported procedure.
- The physician documentation of telephone calls includes the date of the call, name and telephone number of the patient, name of person and relationship of the caller, type of service provided (eg, provide consultation or medical management, initiate or adjust therapy, report results), and the time spent in the encounter.

Codes 99441–99443 are *not* reported when
- The call results in a face-to-face encounter within 24 hours.
- There was a face-to-face encounter related to the problem in the previous 7 days from the telephone call.
- The call occurs within the postoperative period of a reported procedure.
- The call occurs within 7 days of a previously reported telephone management service.
- Care plan oversight (99339, 99340, 99374–99380), care management (99487–99490, 99439, 99491, 99437, 99424–99427), or transitional care management (99495, 99496) services are reported and the time of the calls is included as part of these services.
- Non–face-to-face communication is between the physician and other health care professionals. If applicable, the services may be reported using non–face-to-face prolonged physician service codes 99358 and 99359 or as part of care plan oversight or care management services (99339, 99340; 99374–99380; 99439, 99487–99490; 99491, 99437; 99424–99427; 99495, 99496).
- Performed by a provider who may not report E/M services. (See codes 98966–98968 for services by QHPs who may not report E/M services.)

Examples

➤ **On January 1, a pediatrician provides a telephone E/M service to a patient whose mother is concerned about the child's cough and cold symptoms.** The time of service is 10 minutes and is reportable with code 99441. The service is reported when the 7-day service period is complete and no other E/M service has been rendered.

Chapter 9. Consultation, Residential, and Non–face-to-face Evaluation and Management Services

   ● =New code   ▲ =Revised code   # =Re-sequenced code   + =Add-on code   ★ =Telemedicine

➤ **On January 3, a pediatrician provides an office visit to a child who also received a telephone E/M service due to concerns about the child's cough and cold symptoms.** The diagnosis is postnasal drip, and the mother is instructed to begin administering an over-the-counter allergy medication as per the product instructions. The office E/M service (eg, **99213**) is reported in lieu of the online digital E/M service.

Online Digital Evaluation and Management Services

Digital communication technology (eg, secure patient portals, EHR/health exchange communications) that do not meet the *CPT* definition of telemedicine are increasingly used to provide health care services. This category of services includes E/M services provided via digital communication such as secure email and interprofessional consultation via telephone, internet, and/or EHR.

Verify individual health plan policies for payment for digital medical services.

Online Digital Medical Services

#99421	Online digital evaluation and management service, for an established patient, for up to 7 days, cumulative time during the 7 days; 5–10 minutes
#99422	11–20 minutes
#99423	21 or more minutes
98970	Qualified nonphysician health care professional online digital assessment and management service, for an established patient, for up to 7 days, cumulative time during the 7 days; 5–10 minutes
98971	11–20 minutes
98972	21 or more minutes

Codes **99421–99423** are reported by physicians and other QHPs whose scope of practice includes E/M services as described by codes **99202–99499**. Codes **98970–98972** are reported by health care professionals (eg, speech or physical therapist) whose scope of practice does not include E/M services as described by codes **99202–99499**.

Online digital E/M services are different from telemedicine services. The required delivery mechanism for telemedicine (ie, synchronous audiovisual communication) is not required for online digital E/M services. Online digital E/M services may be provided using asynchronous communication such as messaging in a patient portal or via secure email.

Online digital E/M services must be patient or caregiver initiated. Online digital E/M includes

- Cumulative physician or other QHP time devoted to the patient's care over a period of 7 days whether the time is spent addressing single or multiple different problems within the 7-day period
- Cumulative service time begins at the physician's personal review of the patient's initial inquiry and includes
  - Review of patient records or data pertinent to assessment of the patient's problem
  - Physician's or QHP's personal interaction with clinical staff focused on the patient's problem
  - Development of management plans including physician or QHP generation of prescriptions or ordering of tests
  - Subsequent communication with the patient through online, telephone, email, or other digitally supported communication that does not otherwise represent a separately reported E/M service
- Permanent documentation storage (electronic or hard copy) of the encounter

Do not report online digital services
- Of less than 5 minutes' total time.
- Based on time spent by clinical staff.
- During the postoperative period of a procedure.
- If another E/M service (in person or telemedicine) for the same or related problem occurred within 7 days prior to the online digital service.

> **If a patient generates the initial online digital inquiry for a new problem within 7 days of a previous evaluation and management (E/M) visit that addressed a different problem, the online digital E/M service may be reported separately.**

- If a separately reported E/M visit occurs within 7 days following the initiation of the online service, only report one code. Combine all work of the online digital E/M service into selection of the code for the other E/M service.

Examples

➤ **On January 1, a pediatrician provides an online E/M service to a patient with a rash, which includes obtaining history, reviewing digital photographs of the rash, and advising the parent/caregiver on home treatment.** The time of service is 10 minutes and is reportable with code **99421**. The service is reported when the 7-day service period is complete and no other E/M service has been rendered.

➤ **For the same patient as in the previous example, the parent/caregiver sends a new photograph on January 3 because the parent/caregiver is concerned that the rash is not responding to treatment.** The pediatrician sees the patient in the office later that day. Code **99421** is not reported for the prior online digital E/M services, but the level of service reported for the office encounter (eg, **99213**) includes the MDM or time of the online encounters.

➤ **A patient is seen in the office by a pediatrician for complaint of a foreign body in the ear on January 9.** On January 14, the same patient receives an online digital E/M service for advice on treating a mild sunburn on the child's shoulders and face. Because the problem addressed by the online service is not related to the problem addressed at the office encounter, the online service is separately reported (eg, **99421**). Follow payer instructions for reporting an unrelated online service within 7 days of an office E/M service (eg, append modifier **XU** [unusual nonoverlapping service]).

➤ **A 10-year-old patient is seen in the office by a pediatrician for complaint of otitis media on January 9.** On January 11, a parent/caregiver contacts the pediatrician via secure email with concern that the patient's symptoms have worsened, and the pediatrician prescribes an antibiotic. Only the office encounter (eg, **99213**) is reported because the online digital E/M service is provided within 7 days for the same problem.

➤ **A patient receives an online digital E/M service on January 9.** The physician's total time spent providing the service is 10 minutes. On January 15, the same patient receives an online digital E/M service for an unrelated problem with total physician time of 15 minutes. The 2 services occurring within 7 days are combined (even though each service addressed different problems) and reported with code **99423**.

Do not include the time of separately reported online digital E/M services in the time attributed to other services (eg, care plan oversight [**99339, 99340, 99374, 99375, 99377–99380**] or chronic or principal care management services [**99487, 99489, 99490, #99439, 99491, 99424–99427, 99437**]).

Learn more about online digital and telephone services in the December 2020 *AAP Pediatric Coding Newsletter* article, "General Documentation Requirements for Digital and Telephone Evaluation and Management Services" (https://coding.solutions.aap.org/article.aspx?articleid=2765248; subscription required).

Nursing Facility Care

Nursing facility care is provided to patients who require medical, nursing, or rehabilitative services above the level of custodial care but not at the level of care available in a hospital. Place of service codes for nursing facility care were created by Medicare to differentiate between skilled nursing facility care and nursing facility care because Medicare benefits are different for patients requiring skilled nursing care. Medicaid and private payer plans may offer specific instructions on the appropriate places of service for reporting physician services provided in nursing facilities.

Examples of nursing facility services that may be provided during one admission are included in **Table 9-6**. Place of service codes for physician services provided to patients in a nursing facility are described in **Table 9-7**.

Table 9-6. Examples of Nursing Facility Evaluation and Management Services	
Service Provided	**Procedure Code(s)**
A pediatrician accepts management of a child's care following discharge from a rehabilitation hospital for brain injury due to near-drowning and provides initial care in a nursing facility. 60 minutes are spent reviewing the child's history; examining the patient; ordering physical, occupational, and speech-language therapies; obtaining a consultation for possible hyperbaric oxygen therapy; and explaining management plans to the parents.	**99306** (initial nursing facility care, per day requiring a comprehensive history; comprehensive examination; and MDM of high complexity or 45 minutes are spent at the bedside and on the patient's facility floor or unit)
The pediatrician conducts an established patient nursing facility visit to follow the child's progress since the last visit and orders changes to the plan of care based on reports from therapists and clinical staff of the facility. Detailed interval history, detailed examination, and moderate-complexity MDM are documented.	**99309** (subsequent nursing facility care, per day requiring a detailed interval history; detailed examination; and MDM of moderate complexity or 25 minutes are spent at the bedside and on the patient's facility floor or unit)
The pediatrician performs an annual assessment of the child, whose stay in the nursing facility has lasted 1 year. Documentation supports a detailed history, comprehensive examination, and MDM of moderate complexity.	**99318** (annual nursing facility assessment, requiring a detailed interval history; a comprehensive examination; and MDM of low to moderate complexity and 30 minutes are spent at the bedside and on the patient's facility floor or unit)
The pediatrician spends 45 minutes in discharge management activities to order home health and outpatient therapies for the child, who can now be cared for in the parent's home.	**99316** (nursing facility discharge day management; >30 minutes)

Abbreviation: MDM, medical decision-making.

Table 9-7. Nursing Facility Place of Service Codes	
Place of Service Code	**Description**
31	A facility which primarily provides inpatient skilled nursing care and related services to patients who require medical, nursing, or rehabilitative services but does not provide the level of care or treatment available in a hospital
32	A facility which primarily provides to residents skilled nursing care and related services for the rehabilitation of injured, disabled, or sick persons, or, on a regular basis, health-related care services above the level of custodial care to other than individuals with intellectual disabilities

Initial Nursing Facility Care (99304–99306)

- Services are reported for a new or an established patient.
- The level of service reported is dependent on performance and documentation of the 3 key components (ie, history, physical examination, and MDM) or time if more than 50% of the floor or unit time is spent in counseling and/or care coordination (**Table 9-8**).
- The nursing facility care level of service reported by the admitting physician should include services related to the admission the physician provided in the other sites of service (eg, hospital emergency department, physician's office) on the same date.
  - Do not separately report E/M services performed in other sites of service by the same physician or physicians of the same specialty and same group practice on the same date.
  - *Exception:* When a patient is discharged from hospital inpatient or observation status on the same date of nursing facility admission or readmission, hospital discharge services (**99238**, **99239**, or **99217**) should be reported in addition to the initial nursing facility care. (For a patient admitted and discharged from observation or inpatient status on the same date, see codes **99234–99236**.)
- For nursing facility care discharge, see codes **99315** and **99316** (discussed later in this chapter).
- Prolonged service provided in conjunction with a face-to-face nursing facility service is reported with codes **99356** and **99357**. For more information on these codes, see **Chapter 16**, Noncritical Hospital Evaluation and Management Services.

Table 9-8. Initial Nursing Facility Care: New or Established Patient

Key Components (For a description of key components, see Table 9-1.)

3 of 3 key components must be performed to at least the degree specified for each code.

CPT Code/Time[a]	Medical Decision-making	History[b]	Examination[c]
99304 25 min	Straightforward or low PP: Usually low severity	HPI: ≥4 or 3 CC; ROS: 2–9; PFSH: 1/3	2–7 detailed
99305 35 min	Moderate complexity PP: Usually moderate severity	HPI: ≥4 or 3 CC; ROS: ≥10; PFSH: 3/3	≥8 body areas/systems
99306 45 min	High complexity PP: Usually high severity	HPI: ≥4 or 3 CC; ROS: ≥10; PFSH: 3/3	≥8 body areas/systems

Abbreviations: CC, chronic condition; CPT, *Current Procedural Terminology;* HPI, history of present illness; PFSH, past, family, and social history; PP, presenting problem; ROS, review of systems.

[a] Typical time is an average and represents a range of times that may be higher or lower depending on clinical circumstances. The presenting problem is considered to be a contributory factor and does not need to be present to the degree specified.

[b] A chief complaint is required for all levels of history.

[c] Number of body areas or organ systems examined; see **Table 9-1** for details.

Subsequent Nursing Facility Care (99307–99310)

- Codes are used to report services provided to residents of nursing facilities who do not require a comprehensive assessment and/or who have not had a major, permanent change of status.
- Code selection is based on the performance and documentation of 2 of the 3 key components or time if more than 50% of the floor or unit time is spent in counseling and/or coordination of care (**Table 9-9**).
- All levels of service include reviewing the medical record and results of diagnostic studies, noting changes in the resident's status and response to management since the last visit, and reviewing and signing orders.
- An interval history, not requiring past, family, or social history, is used in selecting the level of history.

Table 9-9. Subsequent Nursing Facility Care

Key Components (For a description of key components, see Table 9-1.)

2 of 3 key components must be performed to at least the degree specified for each code. Some payers may require medical decision-making as 1 of the 2 components performed and documented.

CPT Code/Time[a]	Medical Decision-making	History[b]	Examination[c]
99307 10 min	Straightforward PP: Usually stable, recovering, or improving	HPI: 1–3; ROS: 0; PFSH: 0	1 body area/system
99308 15 min	Low complexity PP: Usually responding inadequately to therapy or minor complication	HPI: 1–3; ROS: 1; PFSH: 0	2–7 limited
99309 25 min	Moderate complexity PP: Usually patient develops significant complication or new problem.	HPI: ≥4 or 3 CC; ROS: 2–9; PFSH: 0	2–7 detailed
99310 35 min	High complexity PP: Usually patient is unstable or has a new problem requiring immediate attention.	HPI: ≥4 or 3 CC; ROS: ≥10; PFSH: 0	≥8 body areas/systems

Abbreviations: CC, chronic condition; CPT, *Current Procedural Terminology;* HPI, history of present illness; PFSH, past, family, and social history; PP, presenting problem; ROS, review of systems.

[a] Typical time is an average and represents a range of times that may be higher or lower depending on clinical circumstances. The presenting problem is considered to be a contributory factor and does not need to be present to the degree specified.

[b] A chief complaint is required for all levels of history.

[c] Number of body areas or organ systems examined; see **Table 9-1** for details.

Nursing Facility Discharge Services (99315, 99316)

99315   Nursing facility discharge day management; 30 minutes or less
99316   more than 30 minutes

- The nursing facility discharge day management codes are used to report the total time spent by a physician for the final nursing facility discharge of a patient, even if the time spent by the physician on that date is not continuous.
- The codes include, as appropriate, final patient examination and discussion of the nursing facility stay. Instructions are given to all relevant caregivers for continuing care, preparation of discharge records, prescriptions, and referral forms.
- If the work of performing the discharge management is more than 30 minutes, the total time must be documented in the medical record.

Annual Nursing Facility Assessment (99318)

Code **99318** is used to report a comprehensive annual assessment that includes a detailed interval history, comprehensive physical examination, and minimum data set or resident assessment instrument evaluation. The patient's and family's goals for care and preferences for medical interventions are assessed, including, if applicable, reassessment of advance directives and updates of contact information for surrogate decision-makers. **Table 9-10** describes the 3 key components for code **99318**.

Table 9-10. Annual Nursing Facility Assessment

Key Components (For a description of key components, see Table 9-1.)
3 of 3 key components must be performed to at least the degree specified under the code.

CPT Code/Time[a]	Medical Decision-making	History[b]	Examination[c]
99318 30 min	Low to moderate complexity PP: Usually stable, recovering, or improving	HPI: ≥4 or 3 CC; ROS: 2–9; PFSH: 0	≥8 body areas/systems

Abbreviations: CC, chronic condition; CPT, *Current Procedural Terminology*; HPI, history of present illness; PFSH, past, family, and social history; PP, presenting problem; ROS, review of systems.

[a] Typical time is an average and represents a range of times that may be higher or lower depending on clinical circumstances. The presenting problem is considered to be a contributory factor and does not need to be present to the degree specified.
[b] A chief complaint is required for all levels of history.
[c] Number of body areas or organ systems examined; see **Table 9-1** for details.

Prolonged Services

Prolonged Service With Direct Patient Contact (99354–99357)

+★**99354**   Prolonged service(s) in the outpatient setting requiring direct patient contact beyond the time of the usual service; first hour

+★**99355**   each additional 30 minutes

+**99356**   Prolonged service in the inpatient or observation setting, requiring unit/floor time beyond the usual service; first hour

+**99357**   each additional 30 minutes

Prolonged service codes **99354** and **99355** are used to report 30 minutes or more of a physician's or QHP's prolonged face-to-face E/M service provided on the same date as designated E/M services that have a typical or designated time published in *CPT* or for prolonged service in conjunction with psychotherapy of 60 minutes or more (**90837**). Codes **99354** and **99355** are reported for prolonged service in conjunction with office or other outpatient consultations and E/M services provided in a patient home or a domiciliary or rest home.

Prolonged service codes **99356** and **99357** are used to report 30 minutes or more of a physician's or QHP's prolonged unit/floor time of an E/M service provided on the same date as nursing facility services. See **Chapter 16** for more information on these codes.

Prolonged Service Without Direct Patient Contact (99358, 99359)

99358   Prolonged evaluation and management service before and/or after direct patient care; first hour

+99359   each additional 30 minutes (Use in conjunction with code 99358.)

Prolonged service without direct patient contact (ie, non–face-to-face) is reported when a physician provides prolonged service that does not involve face-to-face care. The prolonged service must relate to a service and patient where direct (face-to-face) patient care has occurred or will occur and to ongoing patient management.

Only time spent by a physician or other QHP may be counted toward the time of prolonged service. Prolonged service of less than 30 minutes on a given date is not separately reported. Report code 99359 for 15 or more minutes beyond the first hour or the last full 30-minute period of prolonged service. See **Chapter 12**, Outpatient Management of Chronic and Complex Conditions, for more information and a coding example.

Example

➤ **A physician provides an office or other outpatient consultation to a patient to evaluate if surgery is indicated.** After the consultation, the physician requests records from a prior surgery. The following day, the physician spends 30 minutes reviewing the old records, plans a surgical approach, and speaks to the referring physician about perioperative management. The total time of service is 45 minutes. The physician reports code 99358 for the first hour of prolonged service (reported for services of 30 minutes or more).

     Teaching Point: Payers may or may not allow payment for codes 99358 and 99359. Code 99359 may be reported for the first and each additional 30 minutes of service time, including a period of 15 minutes or more beyond the first hour or beyond the last 30-minute period.

Critical Care (99291, 99292)

Regardless of the patient's age, critical care services provided in outpatient settings are reported with hourly critical care codes (99291, 99292).

> **See Chapter 18 for reporting guidelines for critical care services.**

If the same patient requires outpatient and inpatient critical care services on the same day, the physician or a physician of the same group and specialty would report his or her services based on where the services were provided as well as the patient's age. Refer to **Figure 9-1** for information on coding when critical care occurs in the outpatient setting.

Examples

➤ **A physician receives an urgent request to evaluate a 13-year-old girl in a nursing facility.** The patient was admitted to the nursing facility for long-term care after incurring multiple traumas in a car accident. The patient has developed a respiratory illness and has become increasingly short of breath following coughing spells. During the examination, the patient goes into respiratory failure with hypoxia, and her vital signs are deteriorating. The physician initiates critical care. An ambulance is called, and the physician continues critical care services until the transport team accepts care of the patient. The total time for critical care services provided by the physician was 50 minutes. The physician provides no further care to the patient and reports outpatient critical care services with a diagnosis of acute respiratory failure. Documentation includes the critical nature of the patient's condition, the care provided, and the total time spent in critical care dedicated to this patient.

ICD-10-CM	CPT
J96.01 (acute respiratory failure with hypoxia)	99291 (critical care, first 30–74 minutes)

     Teaching Point: If the same physician or physician of the same specialty and group practice provided outpatient and inpatient critical care services on the same calendar date and the total critical care time was 75 minutes or more, code 99292 would be reported with 1 unit for each block of time of up to 30 minutes beyond the first 74 minutes.

Chapter 9. Consultation, Residential, and Non–face-to-face Evaluation and Management Services

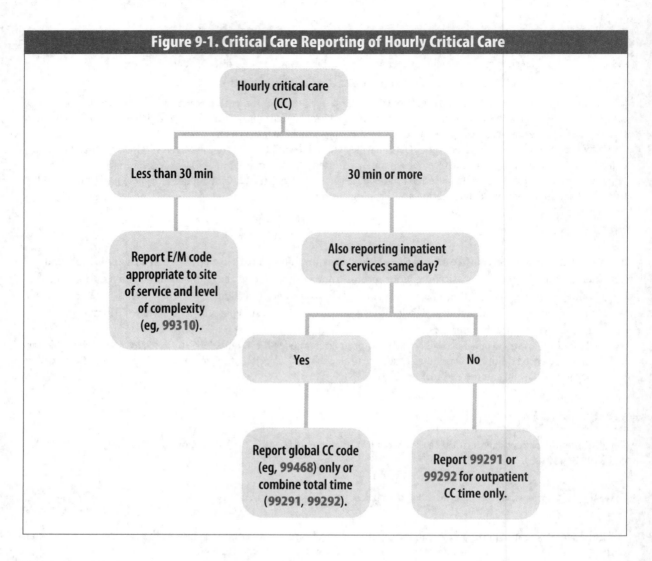

Figure 9-1. Critical Care Reporting of Hourly Critical Care

Resources

Consultations

American Academy of Pediatrics position on Medicare consultation policy (www.aap.org/cfp)

"Consultations: Aligning With Payer Guidelines (Online Exclusive)," January 2018 *AAP Pediatric Coding Newsletter*™ (https://coding.solutions.aap.org/article.aspx?articleid=2667610; subscription required)

Non–face-to-face Services

"General Documentation Requirements for Digital and Telephone Evaluation and Management Services," December 2020 *AAP Pediatric Coding Newsletter* (https://coding.solutions.aap.org/article.aspx?articleid=2765248; subscription required)

Special Services

"Coding for Special Services In and Out of the Office," May 2018 *AAP Pediatric Coding Newsletter* (https://coding.solutions.aap.org/article.aspx?articleid=2679118; subscription required)

Test Your Knowledge!

1. **Which of the following is true for outpatient consultation services 99241–99245?**
   a. Codes may be selected based on 2 of 3 key components.
   b. Codes **99241–99245** may be selected based on typical time when more than 50% of the physician's face-to-face time is spent in counseling and/or coordination of care.
   c. Codes distinguish new or established patients.
   d. Codes **99241–99245** may be selected based on the physician's total time on the date of service.

2. **True or false? Services provided to a patient in a group home are reported as home visits (99341–99350).**
   a. True
   b. False

3. **Which is of the following is reported as a telephone evaluation and management (E/M) service?**
   a. A physician calls a patient's parents to provide laboratory results.
   b. A new patient's parents request a telephone service and the physician spends more than 5 minutes providing the service to a patient.
   c. A physician spends at least 5 minutes speaking to an established patient who requested a telephone service for a new problem unrelated to and not resulting in any face-to-face visit.
   d. A physician's clinical staff speak to a patient's mother to deliver instructions from the physician.

4. **Which of the following is true of online digital E/M services?**
   a. Online digital E/M services are synonymous with telemedicine services.
   b. Codes **99421–99423** include a physician's time spent within a calendar week.
   c. Online digital E/M services by a nurse practitioner are reported with codes **98970–98972**.
   d. Time of online digital E/M services begins with a physician's personal review of the patient's initial inquiry.

5. **How is time spent providing critical care services reported in an outpatient setting?**
   a. Codes include all time spent on the date of the encounter.
   b. Code **99291** includes the first 30 to 74 minutes, and code **99292** is reported for each additional period of up to 30 minutes.
   c. Code **99291** includes the first 30 to 60 minutes, and code **99292** is reported for each additional hour.
   d. One unit of code **99291** is reported for at least 74 minutes of critical care services, and each additional 30-minute period is reported with code **99292**.

CHAPTER 10

Surgery, Infusion, and Sedation in the Outpatient Setting

Contents

Surgical Package Rules 229
   Medicare Surgical Package Definition 229
   Significant Evaluation and Management Service and Procedure 230
   Reporting Postoperative Care 231
   Supplies and Materials 232
   Reporting Terminated Procedures 232
Common Pediatric Procedures 232
   Minor Procedures That Do Not Have a Code 232
   Common Procedure Values and Global Days 232
Integumentary Procedures 234
   Incision and Drainage 234
   Removal of Skin Tags and Congenital Accessory Digits 234
   Destruction of Benign Lesions (eg, Warts) 234
   Chemical Cauterization of Granulation Tissue 234
   Laceration Repairs 235
      Suture Removal 237
   Other Repairs 237
   Burn Care 238
Removal of Foreign Bodies 238
   Integumentary Foreign Bodies 238
   Musculoskeletal Foreign Bodies 239
   Foreign Bodies of Other Body Sites 239
Fracture and/or Dislocation Care 240
   Fracture and Dislocation Care Codes 240
   Casts/Strapping/Splints 241
   Supplies 242
Ear, Nose, and Throat Procedures 243
   Control of Nasal Hemorrhage 243
   Removal of Impacted Cerumen 243
Digestive System Procedures 245
   Incision in Lingual Frenulum 245
   Gastrostomy Tube Replacement 246
Genitourinary System Procedures 246
   Urinary Catheterization 246
   Lysis/Excision of Labial or Penile Adhesions 246
   Newborn Circumcision 247
Hydration, Injections, and Infusions 247
   Subcutaneous or Intramuscular Injection (Therapeutic, Prophylactic, and Diagnostic) 247
   Hydration and Infusions 249
      Hydration 249
      Intra-arterial and Intravenous Push Injections 249
      Therapeutic, Prophylactic, and Diagnostic Infusions 250
      Initial Infusion 250
      Sequential Infusion 251
      Concurrent Infusion 251
      Other Injection and Infusion Services 251
   Chemotherapy and Other Highly Complex Drug/Biologic Agent Administration 252
Moderate Sedation 252
Resources 255
Test Your Knowledge! 256

Surgical Package Rules

Current Procedural Terminology (*CPT*®) surgical codes (**10004–69990**) are *packaged* or *global* codes. To understand documentation and coding of procedural services, it is necessary to know what is included in each service from a coding and payment perspective. *CPT* directs that each procedure code represents a "surgical package" of service components. These include

- Evaluation and management (E/M) services subsequent to the decision for surgery on the day before and/or day of surgery (including the history and physical examination)
- Local or topical anesthesia, including metacarpal, metatarsal, and/or digital block
- Immediate postoperative care
- Writing orders
- Evaluation of the patient in the recovery area
- Typical postoperative follow-up care

Using the *CPT* definition of the surgical package, relative value units (RVUs) are assigned to each procedure based on the typical preoperative, intraoperative, and postoperative physician work; practice expense (eg, procedure room, instruments, supplies, support staff); and professional liability. Payers that use RVUs to calculate payments will typically not pay separately for any components of the surgical package.

> The relative value units assigned to procedures include the typically used supplies under the practice expense component. Know your payer policies on this.

Medicare Surgical Package Definition

Most state Medicaid programs follow the Medicare definition of the surgical package. The Medicare definition differs from that of *CPT*.

- Medicare defines procedures as *minor* (procedures assigned a 0- or 10-day global period or endoscopies) or *major* (procedures assigned a 90-day global period). (**Table 10-1** includes global periods for common pediatric procedures.) *The day of surgery is day 0 (zero); the postoperative period begins the next day.*

> Throughout this chapter, when an assigned global period is noted, this refers to the period assigned in the Medicare Physician Fee Schedule (MPFS). While most payers use the MPFS, individual payers may assign different global periods.

- For minor procedures, the E/M visit on the date of the procedure is considered a routine part of the procedure *regardless of whether it is prior or subsequent to the decision for surgery*. In these cases, modifier **57** (decision for surgery) is not recognized.
- Medicare states an E/M code may be reported on the same day as a minor surgical procedure only when a significant, separately identifiable E/M service is performed and with modifier **25** appended to the E/M code. *CPT* does not specifically include the initial E/M service prior to a minor procedure when the decision for surgery occurs at the visit.
- *CPT* does not include care related to surgical complications in the surgical package. Medicare considers care related to complications following surgery to be included in the surgical package unless a return to the operating room is necessary.
- Global periods and minor or major surgery are not defined in *CPT*. Global periods are defined in the Medicare Physician Fee Schedule (MPFS). Although other payers can assign different global periods, most follow the MPFS.
- The RVUs and global period assigned to each service can be found in the current MPFS at www.cms.gov/medicare/medicare-fee-for-service-payment/physicianfeesched.

> Learn more about the Resource-Based Relative Value Scale in Chapter 4.

Chapter 10. Surgery, Infusion, and Sedation in the Outpatient Setting

Table 10-1. The Medicare Surgical Package			
Global Periods	**0-Day Global Surgeries**	**10-Day Global Surgeries**	**90-Day Global Surgeries**
Services before the date of surgery	Not included		All related services 1 day before surgery if after decision for surgery
Services on the date of procedure	E/M services typically included regardless of when decision for surgery is made		All related services except E/M services at which decision for surgery is made
Postoperative services	Typical postoperative care on the same date	All related care on date of service and 10 days following	All related care on date of service and 90 days following, including care for complications that does not require a return to the OR

Abbreviations: E/M, evaluation and management; OR, operating room.

Most office and outpatient clinic procedures will have 0- or 10-day global periods. Exceptions are certain services such as care of fractures (discussed later in this chapter).

The day of surgery is day 0 (zero) of the global period; the postoperative period begins the next day.

Significant Evaluation and Management Service and Procedure

The Medicare Resource-Based Relative Value Scale is used by most private payers and Medicaid plans to determine RVUs and global periods for services. Under this payment methodology, procedural services include some preservice and postservice E/M by the performing physician. Payer edits, such as the National Correct Coding Initiative (NCCI) edits used by Medicare, Medicaid, and many other payers, also bundle E/M services with certain procedures.

For minor procedures, separate payment for a significant, separately identifiable E/M service is allowed when modifier **25** is appended to the E/M code. However, care should be taken to use modifier **25** only when documentation supports a significant and separately identifiable E/M service.

For major procedures (typically 90-day global period), modifier **57** may be appended when the decision for surgery or a procedure is made during the E/M service on the same date as the procedure. Documentation should clearly show E/M of the problem resulting in the initial decision to perform the related procedure.

Coding Conundrum: Procedure, or Evaluation and Management and Procedure?

The differences in the Centers for Medicare & Medicaid Services (CMS) and *Current Procedural Terminology* (*CPT*) surgical package guidelines may lead to confusion. Try to answer the following questions when determining if you should report a procedure alone or a procedure with an evaluation and management (E/M) service:

- Did you address a problem or condition prior to deciding to perform the procedure (above and beyond the usual preoperative care associated with the procedure) or a significant and separately identifiable problem? If yes, report an E/M service and procedure.
- Does the medical record documentation clearly support the performance of a medically necessary E/M service (and meet code descriptor requirements), the procedure (procedure note), the clinical indications for both, and the decision to perform the surgery? If yes, report an E/M service and procedure.
- Was the purpose of the visit for the procedure only (eg, decision for surgery made at an earlier visit)? If yes, do not report an E/M service.
- Does the payer follow the *CPT* or CMS guidelines for reporting surgical procedures? If the focus of an E/M service is related to the procedure, the history and physical examination are part of preoperative service and only the surgical procedure should be reported.

Example

➤ **A physician sees a patient who returns for a previously planned removal of impacted cerumen from the left ear.**
On examination, the physician notes and documents that the patient has a blackhead on the left earlobe. Documentation includes notation of patient/caregiver consent, procedure including instrumentation used to remove impacted cerumen, patient tolerance, outcome, and post-procedural examination finding (eg, hearing improved).

International Classification of Diseases, 10th Revision, Clinical Modification (ICD-10-CM)	CPT
H61.22 (impacted cerumen, left ear)	**69210** (removal impacted cerumen requiring instrumentation, unilateral)

Teaching Point: Although the physician noted a blackhead, this did not require or affect patient care treatment or management and does not support a significant and separately identifiable E/M service beyond the preservice/postservice work of the procedure that was provided or documented.

Reporting Postoperative Care

- Report *CPT* code **99024** (postoperative follow-up visit) for follow-up care provided during the global surgery period. No RVUs are assigned to **99024**, as the RVUs were included in the total value of the related procedure.
  - Reporting code **99024** allows a practice to track the number of visits performed during the postoperative period of specific procedures, calculate office overhead expenses (eg, supplies, staff, physician time) associated with the procedure, and potentially use the data to negotiate higher payment rates.
  - Payment for postoperative care is included as part of the procedure. Payers track the postoperative care provided.
  - If a physician is not providing or reporting the postoperative care typically performed for a procedure, payers may reduce payment for the surgical service.

> Payment of a surgical procedure may be reduced if the physician does not report code **99024**. See an example of **99024** in the Fracture and/or Dislocation Care section later in this chapter.

- When the physician who performed a procedure provides an unrelated E/M service during the postoperative period, modifier **24** (unrelated E/M service by the same physician during a postoperative period) should be appended to the E/M service code.
- When a physician *other than the surgeon* provides unrelated services to a patient during the postoperative period, the services are reported without a modifier. Despite the use of different National Provider Identifiers and diagnosis codes, some payers with assigned follow-up surgical periods will deny the service. The claim should be appealed for payment with a letter advising the payer that the service was unrelated to surgical care.

Example

➤ **A 4-year-old patient returns 8 days after removal of a foreign body from his right foot (10120 RT) with complaint of rhinorrhea and sore throat.** The physician diagnoses seasonal allergic rhinitis and acute pharyngitis. The physician also rechecks the wound on the right foot, which is healing as expected.

ICD-10-CM	CPT
J30.2 (other season allergic rhinitis) **J02.9** (acute pharyngitis, unspecified) **S90.851D** (superficial foreign body, right foot, subsequent encounter)	**99213 24**

Teaching Point: Modifier **24** is reported to identify that the service provided was unrelated to the prior procedure. The medical decision-making (MDM) of the E/M service was low based on a low number and complexity of problems addressed (otitis media, pharyngitis), assessment requiring an independent historian, and minimal to low risk. The evaluation of the healing wound during the postoperative period is not included in determining the level of service for the encounter because it is included in postoperative care when provided during the 10-day global period.

> See Chapter 2 for more information on modifiers.

Chapter 10. Surgery, Infusion, and Sedation in the Outpatient Setting

Supplies and Materials

99070   Supplies and materials provided by the physician over and above those usually included with the office visit or other services rendered

- Items such as elastic wraps, clavicle splints, or circumcision and suturing trays may be reported with this code. Remember that some supplies (eg, suturing trays, circumcision trays) may be included with the surgical procedure if the payer uses RVUs as its basis for payment.
- Only the supplies purchased in an office-based practice may be reported.

> If reporting code 99070, identify the supplies or materials on the claim form and be prepared to submit an invoice.

- Some payers will require the use of Healthcare Common Procedure Coding System (HCPCS) codes. More specific HCPCS codes are available for a number of supplies (eg, codes **Q4001–Q4051** for cast and splint supplies). Use HCPCS codes when they are more specific.

> For more information on Healthcare Common Procedure Coding System codes, see Chapter 1.

Reporting Terminated Procedures

When a procedure is started but cannot be completed due to extenuating circumstances, physicians should consider the individual situation, including the reason for termination of the procedure and the amount of work that was performed, when determining how to report the service rendered.

 When a procedure was performed but not entirely successful (eg, portion of foreign body removed), it may be appropriate to report the procedure code that represents the work performed without modification.

- Only report reduced services (modifier **52**) or discontinued procedure (modifier **53**) when the service was significantly reduced from the typical service.
- If the work performed prior to discontinuation was insignificant, it may be appropriate to not report the procedure. If you choose to not report the procedure, consider whether the level of a related E/M service was increased due to the complexity of MDM associated with the attempted procedure, any complicating factors, and the revised management or treatment plan.

> See an example of a discontinued service later in this chapter in the Removal of Impacted Cerumen section.

Common Pediatric Procedures

Minor Procedures That Do Not Have a Code

Some minor procedures are considered inherent to an E/M code or do not have separate *CPT* codes. However, any supplies used may be reported. The following procedures are included in an E/M service:

- Insertion or removal of an ear wick
- Removal of *nonimpacted* cerumen from the ear
- Nasal aspiration
- Nasogastric tube insertion without fluoroscopic guidance
- Removal of an umbilical clamp
- Removal of foreign bodies from skin that do not require an incision
- Puncture of abscess without aspiration
- Wound closure with adhesive strips only (eg, Steri-Strips, butterfly bandages)
- The use of fluorescein dye and a Wood lamp to examine for a corneal abrasion or foreign body of the eye

Common Procedure Values and Global Days

For other procedural services, verify separate reporting through your procedural coding reference. There is value in capturing the procedural services that are distinct from E/M services.

Example

➤ **A physician removes a foreign body from a child's nose.** If the MDM for the office visit supports code **99213** (level 3 established patient office E/M), the E/M service was assigned 2.65 total non-facility RVUs in 2021, whereas code **30300** (foreign body removal from nose) was assigned 6.06 non-facility RVUs in 2021.

Both services are reported only if a significant, separately identifiable E/M service, beyond the preservice work of the foreign body removal, is provided.

Table 10-2 details the number of global days for each of the commonly reported office procedures.

Table 10-2. Common Office Procedures and Global Days			
CPT Code	**Description**[a]	**Global Period (d)**	**Total Non-facility RVUs (2021)**
Procedures Assigned a 0-day Global Period			
12001, 12011	Laceration repair, simple <2.5 cm	0	2.76, 3.34
16000, 16020	Burn care	0	2.18, 2.50
17250	Chemical cautery	0	2.63
30901	Nosebleed cautery/packing	0	4.63
51701, 51702	Bladder catheterization	0	1.34, 1.87
54150	Circumcision	0	4.49
Procedures Assigned a 10-day Global Period			
10060, 10061	Drainage of skin abscess	10	3.62, 6.21
10120, 10121	FB removal, SQ	10	4.50, 7.98
11200	Removal of skin tags	10	2.63
11760	Repair of nail bed	10	5.74
12031, 12041, 12051	Laceration repair, intermediate <2.5 cm	10	7.79, 7.82, 8.37
17110, 17111	Destruction benign lesions (eg, warts)	10	3.33, 3.90
24640	Treatment elbow dislocation (nursemaid)	10	3.04
28190	FB removal, foot, subcutaneous (above fascia)	10	7.44
30300	Removal intranasal FB, office	10	6.06
41010	Incision in lingual frenulum	10	6.53
Procedures Assigned a 90-day Global Period			
23500	Treatment of clavicle fracture	90	6.60
28490	Treatment big toe fracture (closed)	90	4.15

Abbreviations: *CPT, Current Procedural Terminology*; FB, foreign body; RVU, relative value unit; SQ, subcutaneous.

[a] Descriptors are abbreviated. Please see your 2022 coding reference for full descriptors and code selection.

- Remember that when reporting any procedures containing 0, 10, or 90 global days, modifier **25** or **57** is required on any separately identifiable E/M service done on the same day (or, in some instances, the previous day prior to a planned major surgery).
- Those E/M services that are unrelated to the procedure that take place within the code's 10- or 90-day global period will require modifier **24**.

Integumentary Procedures

Incision and Drainage

10060   Incision and drainage of abscess (eg, carbuncle, suppurative hidradenitis, cutaneous or subcutaneous abscess, cyst, furuncle, or paronychia); simple or single

10061   complicated or multiple

- The global period for codes **10060** and **10061** is 10 days.
- *CPT* does not provide differentiation between simple and complicated incision and drainage (I&D) and leaves code selection to the physician's judgment.
- The simple I&D procedure typically involves local anesthesia, an incision, expression of purulent drainage, obtaining a culture, irrigation, completely opening the cavity, and packing/dressing the wound.
- Complex I&D often typically involves a deeper incision, breakdown of multiple loculations, placement of a drain, and/or debridement of the cavity.
- The difference in RVUs for **10060** (3.62 total non-facility) and **10061** (6.21 total non-facility) indicates the significant additional work and practice expense associated with complicated or multiple I&D procedures.

Example

➤ **A 12-year-old presents with an abscess on his right lower leg.** The decision is made to perform I&D. The physician documents administration of local anesthetic, incision of skin above the abscess, and expression of purulent material. The wound was irrigated and packed. The patient will return in 3 days for reevaluation.

    Code **10060** is reported for the procedure. All related visits (eg, follow-up visit to recheck the wound) within the 10 days following the date of surgery may be reported with code **99024** and no charge.

Removal of Skin Tags and Congenital Accessory Digits

11200   Removal of skin tags, multiple fibrocutaneous tags, any area; up to and including 15 lesions

    A 10-day global period applies.

    Code **11200** is used to report the removal of a sixth digit from a newborn. It is equivalent to a skin tag and would not be assigned the code for an actual digit removal. The *ICD-10-CM* codes for accessory digits would be **Q69.0**, accessory fingers; **Q69.1**, accessory thumb; **Q69.2**, accessory toes; or **Q69.9**, unspecified. A 10-day global period applies under the MPFS.

Destruction of Benign Lesions (eg, Warts)

17110   Destruction (eg, laser surgery, electrosurgery, cryosurgery, chemosurgery, surgical curettement) of benign lesions other than skin tags or cutaneous vascular proliferative lesions; up to 14 lesions

17111   15 or more lesions

    A 10-day global period applies to codes **17110** and **17111**.

    Report destruction of common or plantar warts, flat warts, or molluscum contagiosum with code **17110** or **17111** (with 1 unit of service), depending on the number of lesions removed. Do not report both **17110** and **17111** because they are mutually exclusive. Report *ICD-10-CM* using code **B08.1** for molluscum contagiosum, **B07.8** for common warts, or **B07.0** for plantar warts.

Chemical Cauterization of Granulation Tissue

17250   Chemical cauterization of granulation tissue (ie, proud flesh)

    A 0-day global period applies. If reporting a significant and separately identifiable E/M service on the date, append modifier **25** to the E/M code reported.

    Code **17250** is appropriately reported for cauterization of an umbilical granuloma. Do not report **17250** with removal or excision codes for the same lesion, for achieving wound hemostasis, or in conjunction with active wound care management.

Example

➤ **A 2-week-old presents for her well-baby check.** On examination, a moderate-sized umbilical granuloma is noted. The physician takes a very brief history and decides to cauterize. The routine well-baby check is completed in addition to cauterization of the umbilical granuloma.

ICD-10-CM	CPT
Z00.121 (encounter for routine child health examination with abnormal findings)	99391 25
P83.81 (umbilical granuloma)	17250

Teaching Point: Preservice work includes explanation of the procedure, obtaining informed consent, positioning and draping, preparing the site, and scrubbing in. Post-service work includes discussing follow-up care with parents and/or caregivers. Supplies and equipment, such as silver nitrate and an applicator, are included in the value assigned to the code when reporting to payers using RVUs. This service has a 0-day global period.

Laceration Repairs

12001–12018 Simple repair
12031–12057 Intermediate repair
13100–13160 Complex repair

- Categories of difficulty of wound repairs are described as
  - *Simple:* Superficial wound and/or subcutaneous wound requiring a simple single-layer closure or tissue adhesives. A 0-day global period applies. *When performed, local or topical anesthesia and hemostasis are not reported separately.*
  - *Intermediate:* Includes the repair of wounds that, in addition to the requirements for simple repair, require layered closure of 1 or more of the deeper layers of subcutaneous tissue and superficial (non-muscle) fascia, in addition to skin (epidermal and dermal) closure. Intermediate repair includes limited undermining (defined as a distance less than the maximum width of the defect, measured perpendicular to the closure line, along at least 1 entire edge of the defect). A 10-day global period applies.

> **Single-layer closure of heavily contaminated wounds that require extensive cleaning or removal of particulate matter also constitutes intermediate repair.**

  - *Complex:* Includes the repair of wounds that, in addition to the requirements for intermediate repair, require at least 1 of the following: exposure of bone, cartilage, tendon, or named neurovascular structure; debridement of wound edges (eg, traumatic lacerations or avulsions); extensive undermining (defined as distance equal to or greater than the maximum width of the defect, measured perpendicular to the closure line, along at least 1 entire edge of the defect); involvement of free margins of helical rim, vermilion border, or nostril rim; or placement of retention sutures. Necessary preparation includes creation of a limited defect for repairs or the debridement of complicated lacerations or avulsions. A 10-day global applies to most complex wound repairs. Late wound closure (**13160**) has a 90-day global period.

> **Complex repair does not include excision of benign (11400–11446) or malignant (11600–11646) lesions, excisional preparation of a wound bed (15002–15005), or debridement of an open fracture or open dislocation.**

- Codes **12001–13160** are used to report wound closure using sutures, staples, or tissue adhesives (eg, Dermabond), singly or in combination with adhesive strips.
- Wound closure using chemical cauterization, electrocauterization, or adhesive strips (eg, Steri-Strips, butterfly bandages) only is considered inherent to the E/M service. However, the supplies (eg, Steri-Strips, butterfly bandages) may be reported separately using code **99070** (supplies and materials) or **A4450** (tape, non-waterproof, per 18 sq in). There are no specific HCPCS codes for Steri-Strips or butterfly bandages.
- Some payers may accept HCPCS code **G0168** (wound closure using tissue adhesive[s]) in lieu of simple repair codes (eg, **12001**, **12011**).

- Codes are reported based on the difficulty of the repair, measured length of the wound, and the location. To report wound repair, measure the length of the repaired wound(s) in centimeters.
  - If multiple wounds belong to the same category of difficulty and location, add the lengths and report with a single code.
  - If multiple wounds do not belong in the same category, report each repair separately with the more complicated repair reported as the primary procedure and the less complicated repair reported as the secondary procedure. Modifier 51 (multiple procedures) should be appended to the secondary code(s).
  - Simple ligation of vessels is considered as part of the wound closure.
- Wound debridement and/or cleaning and the provision of topical or injected local anesthesia are included in the wound repair code.
  - Debridement is considered a separate procedure only when gross contamination requires prolonged cleaning, excessive amounts of devitalized tissue are removed, or debridement is performed without immediate primary closure.
  - To report extensive tissue debridement, see codes 11042–11047 for selective debridement of subcutaneous, muscle, fascial tissues, and/or bone (includes debridement of dermis and epidermis when performed) or 97597 and 97598 for debridement of skin, epidermis, and/or dermis.

Know Your A, D, S Seventh Characters!

International Classification of Diseases, 10th Revision, Clinical Modification seventh characters A, D, and S define an encounter type for injuries and certain other diagnoses. Here are tips for remembering which character to use.

- **A**: active management of the initial injury or complications
- **D**: during healing of an injury that does not require active management (eg, routine follow-up, suture removal)
- **S**: scars and other sequela (effects of an injury) (Always report the sequela code before the injury code when the service is directed to the sequela. Injury codes with seventh character S are never the first-listed diagnosis.)

Seventh characters are also appended to codes for external cause of injury (eg, tripping).

Examples

➤ **A 10-year-old sustained a 1.5-cm laceration on his left knee requiring a simple (single layer) repair after a fall from playground equipment.**

ICD-10-CM	CPT
S81.012A (laceration without foreign body left knee, initial encounter) W09.8XXA (fall on or from other playground equipment, initial encounter) Y92.838 (other recreation area)	12001 (simple repair of superficial wounds of scalp, neck, axillae, external genitalia, trunk and/or extremities [including hands and feet]; 2.5 cm or less)

Teaching Point: Simple repair includes only the care on the date of the repair (0-day global period). Follow-up E/M visits are separately reported and do not require a modifier.

➤ **A 10-year-old fell from playground equipment and sustained a 1.5-cm laceration on his left knee and a 1.5-cm laceration on his left forearm. Each laceration required an intermediate repair.**

ICD-10-CM	CPT
S81.012A (laceration without foreign body left knee, initial encounter) S51.812A (laceration of left forearm without foreign body, initial encounter) W09.8XXA Y92.838	12032 (intermediate repair, extremities, 2.6–7.5 cm)

Teaching Point: The measurement of both wounds (3 cm) is between 2.6 and 7.5 cm, both wounds are in the same family of anatomical sites, and both require the same level of repair. If the patient returns for wound follow-up within the 10 days following the date of repair, code 99024 (postoperative follow-up visit) is reported for the encounter because intermediate repair has a 10-day global period. There is no separate charge for care within the global period.

Suture Removal

The Medicare global surgery period for *CPT* codes **12001–12018** (simple repair of superficial wound) is 0 days, meaning payment includes the procedure or service plus any associated care provided on the same day of service. Therefore, practices may report a separate E/M service for removal of sutures placed in the office.

The Medicare global surgery period for intermediate (**12031–12057**) and complex (**13100–13153**) wound repairs is 10 days. Payment includes the procedure or service plus any associated follow-up care for a period of 10 days. Therefore, the charge for the procedure already includes suture removal by the same physician or a physician of the same group and specialty as part of the global surgical package.

When sutures are removed by another physician with a different tax identification number, an E/M office visit code may be reported for the suture removal. Some payers may allow reporting of HCPCS code **S0630**. Code **S0630** is for removal of sutures by a physician other than the physician who originally closed the wound. **S** codes are HCPCS Level II codes, designated by the Centers for Medicare & Medicaid Services and recognized by national BlueCross BlueShield payers, but coverage is on a payer-by-payer basis.

For aftercare of an injury, assign the acute injury code with the seventh character **D** (subsequent encounter). *ICD-10-CM* code **Z48.02** (encounter for removal of sutures) *is not reported* for removal of sutures previously placed to repair an injury but may be reported when removal of sutures is unrelated to care for an injury (eg, removal of sutures from a surgical incision).

Examples

➤ **An 8-year-old sustained a 0.5-cm laceration on her forehead.** The wound on her face requires a simple repair. She is seen in follow-up 7 days later. The wound is clean, and sutures are removed.

Visit	*ICD-10-CM*	*CPT*
Initial visit	**S01.81XA** (laceration without foreign body of other part of head, initial encounter)	**12011** (simple repair of the facial laceration 2.5 cm or less)
Follow-up visit	**S01.81XD** (laceration without foreign body of other part of head, subsequent encounter)	**99212** (problem-focused E/M visit, office or outpatient)

Teaching Point: The seventh character **D** (ie, **S01.81XD**) is reported for encounters after the patient has received active treatment of the condition and is receiving routine care for the condition during the healing or recovery phase. Simple laceration repair has a 0-day global period, so any medically necessary follow-up care is separately reported.

➤ **A 3-year-old with 5 sutures placed in the emergency department (ED) presents at her pediatrician's office for suture removal.** The child is uncooperative and 2 clinical staff members are required to assist the pediatrician in removing the sutures. The physician's total time devoted to the patient's care on the date of service is 25 minutes.

ICD-10-CM	*CPT*
Appropriate code for injury with seventh character **D** (eg, **S51.812D**, laceration of left forearm without foreign body, subsequent encounter)	**S0630** (removal of sutures by a physician other than the physician who originally closed the wound), or **99213** (established patient E/M 20–29 minutes) based on the physician's total time

Teaching Point: The office and other outpatient E/M codes may be reported based on the physician or other qualified health care professional's (QHP's) total time on the date of the encounter. Do not include time of clinical staff.

Other Repairs

Code **11760** (repair of nail bed) is reported when part or all of the nail plate is lifted and a laceration of the nail bed is repaired. A 10-day global period applies.

Report code **40650** (repair of lip, full-thickness, vermilion only) when a laceration of the full thickness of the lip and vermilion is repaired. A 90-day global period applies to this service. For less than full-thickness repair, see codes for repair of skin. For repair of a laceration that crosses the vermilion border, see codes **40652** (up to half vertical height) and **40654** (over half of vertical height).

Laceration repairs of the tongue (**41250–41252**) are reported based on size and location (eg, repair of laceration 2.5 cm or less, anterior two-thirds of the tongue is reported using code **41250**). These codes are assigned a 10-day global period.

> **Please see Chapter 19 for discussion of coding for negative pressure wound therapy (97605 and 97606 or 97607 and 97608.)**

Burn Care

CPT code **16000** (initial treatment, first-degree burn, where no more than local treatment is required) is reported when initial treatment is performed for the symptomatic relief of a first-degree burn that is characterized by erythema and tenderness.

16020 Dressings and/or debridement of partial-thickness burns, initial or subsequent; small or less than 5% total body (eg, finger)

A 0-day global period applies.

Code **16020**

- Is used to report treatment of burns with dressings and/or debridement of small partial-thickness burns (second degree), whether initial or subsequent.
- An E/M visit with modifier **25** appended may be reported if a significant, separately identifiable E/M service is clinically indicated, performed, and documented in addition to the burn care.

> **See Chapter 19 for coding of larger partial-thickness or full-thickness burns.**

Examples

➤ **A 9-year-old complaining of sunburn on her shoulders is seen by the physician.** There is redness and tenderness, but no blistering. Topical treatment is applied and an over-the-counter treatment for the first-degree burn is ordered.

ICD-10-CM	CPT
L55.0 (first-degree sunburn)	**16000** (first-degree burn requiring local treatment)

➤ **A 4-year-old is seen in the office after sustaining a burn on the first finger of her right hand from touching a hot pan.** The area is red and blistered. Following examination by the physician, the finger is treated with a topical cream and bandaged.

ICD-10-CM	CPT
T23.221A (second-degree burn of single finger, initial encounter) **X15.3XXA** (contact with other heat and hot saucepan or skillet, initial encounter)	**16020**

Teaching Point: External cause of injury codes such as **X15.3XXA** are used to report the source, place, and/or intent of a burn injury. These codes are only required when state regulations mandate reporting cause of injury (typically applies to ED services). However, it is appropriate to report external cause of injury codes when the cause is known.

Removal of Foreign Bodies

Integumentary Foreign Bodies

10120 Incision and removal of foreign body, subcutaneous tissues; simple
10121 complex

A 10-day global period applies.

Incision and removal of a foreign body from within the subcutaneous tissues above the fascia is reported with a code from the integumentary system regardless of the site (eg, hand, foot).

Do not report codes **10120** or **10121** when a foreign body is removed using forceps alone with no incision. Instead, report an E/M service. Incising of the skin can be accomplished by a scalpel or other instrument needed to break open the skin.

The removal of an embedded earring requiring an incision would be reported with code **10120** or **10121**, depending on the complexity of the procedure required to remove it. If the earring is removed by wiggling it out or another method that does not require incision, this work is included in the E/M service.

- Code **10120** includes the removal of splinters or ticks when the physician has to "break open" or incise the skin to retrieve the foreign body.
- Code **10121** is used to report the complicated removal of a foreign body by incision.

The physician determines whether the procedure is simple or complex, but the significant difference in physician work RVUs for the procedures may be used as an indicator of the difference—1.22 for **10120** versus 2.74 for **10121**. Clearly, a procedure described by code **10121** would involve double the time and effort of the simple procedure. *CPT* does not provide examples of simple versus complex procedures.

- A complex removal may require extended exploration and removal of multiple foreign bodies (eg, pieces of glass), use of imaging to help locate the foreign body, or removal that is complicated by the anatomical site of the foreign body (eg, area that is not easily seen) and will have a greater intensity of physician work.

Musculoskeletal Foreign Bodies

Musculoskeletal codes are reported when a foreign body is removed from *within the fascia, subfascial, or muscle.* Always check the *CPT* index to ensure you are reporting the most accurate code.

Codes in the musculoskeletal system are not reported for removal of foreign bodies within the skin and subcutaneous fat. Examples of codes for removal of foreign bodies within the musculoskeletal system are

- *Foot:* For foreign body removal *from within the fascia, subfascial, or muscle,* code **28190** (10-day global period) is used to report the removal of a subcutaneous foreign body from the foot; code **28192** (90-day global period) is used to report removal of a foreign body from the deep tissue of the foot.
- *Upper arm or elbow:* Report removal of foreign bodies of the upper arm or elbow area from subcutaneous tissues within the fascia with **24200** (10-day global period) or from deep, below the fascia, or in the muscle with **24201** (90-day global period).

> An object that is unintentionally placed (eg, trauma, ingestion) is considered a foreign body. An object intentionally placed by a physician or other qualified health care professional for any purpose (eg, diagnostic, therapeutic) is considered an implant. A broken or misplaced implant is a foreign body for coding purposes.

Foreign Bodies of Other Body Sites

CPT includes codes for reporting removal of foreign bodies from many different body sites. **Table 10-3** summarizes foreign body removal services from areas other than skin or muscle.

Table 10-3. Codes for Removal of Foreign Bodies Other Than From Skin or Muscle	
Site	**Code(s)**
Anal foreign body or fecal impaction	Use appropriate E/M code or **45999** (unlisted procedure, rectum) or if removed under anesthesia (**45915**, more than local anesthesia).
External auditory canal	**69200** (removal foreign body from external auditory canal; without general anesthesia) (For removal of impacted cerumen, see discussion in this chapter.)
Eye	**65205** (removal of foreign body, external eye; conjunctival superficial) **65220** (removal of foreign body, external eye; corneal, without slit lamp)
Nose	**30300** (removal of intranasal foreign bodies when performed in the office) **30310** (removal of intranasal foreign bodies under general anesthesia)
Vagina	Use appropriate E/M code or **58999** (unlisted procedure, female genital system) or if removed under anesthesia (**57415**, more than local anesthesia).
Abbreviation: E/M, evaluation and management.	

Fracture and/or Dislocation Care

New in 2022

Code 21310 (closed treatment of nasal bone fracture without manipulation) has been deleted. Closed treatment of a nasal bone fracture without manipulation or stabilization is reported with an evaluation and management code (eg, 99283, 99213) based on the site of service. Codes 21315 and 21320 are also revised to indicate that manipulation is required for these services.

▲ 21315   Closed treatment of nasal bone fracture with manipulation; without stabilization
▲ 21320   with stabilization

Fracture and Dislocation Care Codes

Fracture and dislocation care codes are reported for care that is intended to begin the course of treatment of the injury. If a physician or QHP provides casting or strapping only for stabilization pending restorative treatment by another physician or QHP, see codes 29000–29799 and discussion later in this section. A significant, separately identifiable E/M service to diagnose and manage the injury is separately reported.

Most fracture and dislocation care codes include a 90-day period of follow-up care under the Medicare global package. Modifiers are required when one physician or QHP provides initial care of a fracture or dislocation (eg, closed treatment of a fracture without manipulation in the ED) and another physician or QHP provides follow-up care.

- When a patient presents for follow-up care after initial fracture care is provided in another setting (eg, ED, urgent care), it is necessary to determine if the provider of initial fracture care reported a code for fracture care with modifier **54** (surgical care only) or only reported casting/strapping for the initial care.
- If initial fracture care has been reported with modifier **54**, the physician providing continued fracture care reports the fracture care code with modifier **55** (postoperative care only) appended.

Codes for fracture/dislocation care
- Are listed by anatomical location.
- Are provided (in most cases) for closed or open treatment, with or without manipulation, and with or without internal fixation.
- Include the initial casting, splinting, or strapping.
- Do not include radiographs or E/M to determine the extent of injury and treatment options.

Fractures most commonly seen in a primary care pediatric practice include closed fractures (ie, skin is intact on presentation), and treatment is typically closed (ie, fracture site is not surgically opened) without manipulation (an exception is treatment of nursemaid elbow).
- *Clavicular fracture:* Report closed treatment without manipulation with code **23500**.
- *Nursemaid elbow:* Report closed treatment of radial head subluxation (nursemaid elbow) with manipulation with code **24640**. (This code has a 10-day global period.)
- *Radial fracture:* Report code **25500** for closed treatment of radial shaft fracture without manipulation and **25600** for closed treatment of distal radius fracture without manipulation.
- *Phalanx fracture:* Closed treatment of a proximal or middle phalanx, finger, or thumb (each) without manipulation is reported with code **26720**. Closed treatment of a distal phalangeal fracture (each) without manipulation is reported with code **26750**.
- *Great toe fracture:* Code **28490** is reported for the closed treatment of a fracture of the great toe, phalanx, or phalanges without manipulation.
- *Metatarsal fracture:* Report code **28470** for closed treatment of a metatarsal fracture without manipulation.
- *Lesser toe fracture:* Closed treatment of fracture, phalanx, or phalanges, other than great toe without manipulation, is coded with **28510**.

Tip: Unrelated services that are provided during the global surgery period by the same physician (or physician of the same group and specialty) may be reported. Modifier **24** would be appended to an unrelated E/M service.

Fractures not specified as displaced or non-displaced are reported with an *International Classification of Diseases, 10th Revision, Clinical Modification* code for a displaced fracture. Fractures not specified as open or closed are reported with a code for a closed fracture.

Examples

➤ **An urgent care physician performs and documents a comprehensive evaluation on a child to assess for injuries following an unwitnessed fall from the stairs in her home. The child is diagnosed with a fracture of the shaft of the left clavicle and received closed treatment without manipulation.**

ICD-10-CM	CPT
S42.022A (displaced fracture shaft of clavicle, closed, initial encounter) **W10.9XXA** (fall [on] [from] unspecified stairs and steps, initial encounter)	**99202–99205 57**
S42.022A **W10.9XXA**	**23500** (closed treatment clavicle fracture without manipulation)

Teaching Point: Because code **23500** is assigned a 90-day global period in the MPFS and is placed in the surgery section of *CPT,* many payers may require modifier **57** (decision for surgery) appended to the E/M code. Individual payers may have different policies.

➤ **A physician evaluates a 22-month-old girl (established patient) whose parents report that she will not move her left arm after falling on steps while holding her father's hand.** After obtaining history and physical examination to rule out other injuries, the physician diagnoses subluxation of the radial head that is reduced by manipulation. Reassessment after 10 minutes shows the child uses both arms now when presented with a balloon. The parents are counseled about potential for recurrent injury and avoidance. Follow-up will be at previously scheduled 2-year-old visit unless otherwise indicated.

ICD-10-CM	CPT
S53.032A (nursemaid's elbow, left, initial encounter) **W10.9XXA** (fall [on] [from] unspecified stairs and steps, initial encounter)	**99213 25** (low-complexity MDM—acute uncomplicated injury with assessment requiring an independent historian and low risk of morbidity) **24640** (closed treatment of radial head subluxation in child, nursemaid elbow, with manipulation)

Teaching Point: The physician provided a significant and separately identifiable E/M service to evaluate extent of injury in addition to treatment of nursemaid elbow. Modifier **25** is required by most payers to indicate the E/M service was significant and separately identifiable from the preservice work of the minor procedure (eg, 10-day global period) performed on the same date of service.

Casts/Strapping/Splints

- Codes for the application of casts, splints, or strapping (**29000–29590**) are reported only when they are replacements for the initial application *or performed as part of the initial E/M visit and fracture care is not reported.*
- Codes **29000–29590** cannot be reported for the initial (first) application when a fracture or dislocation care code is reported because they are included as part of the global surgery package.

  The following codes are commonly used when treating a fracture or dislocation:
- Application of splints
  - Short arm splint (forearm to hand): static (**29125**); dynamic (**29126**)
  - Finger splint: static (**29130**); dynamic (**29131**)
  - Short leg splint (calf to foot): **29515**
- Strapping
  - Shoulder: **29240**
  - Elbow or wrist: **29260**

Chapter 10. Surgery, Infusion, and Sedation in the Outpatient Setting

Example

➤ **An established adolescent patient returns to a physician for follow-up on an injury to the left wrist.** The patient was previously examined and a cast applied for a presumed scaphoid fracture (ie, diagnosed based on examination findings) that was not found on x-ray. The service was reported with code **25622** (closed treatment of carpal scaphoid [navicular] fracture; without manipulation) The diagnosis documented at the first visit was initial encounter for unspecified scaphoid fracture of the left wrist (**S62.001A**) due to tripping while playing soccer with friends at a soccer field. The initial cast is removed and a 3-view radiograph of the wrist is ordered and performed in the office. The physician interprets the radiograph, which now shows a fracture of the middle third (waist) of the left proximal scaphoid. The physician applies a replacement thumb spica cast. The patient will return in 4 weeks for reevaluation.

ICD-10-CM	CPT
S62.025D (nondisplaced fracture of middle third of navicular [scaphoid] bone of left wrist, subsequent encounter for fracture with routine healing) **W01.0XXD** (fall on same level from slipping, tripping and stumbling without subsequent striking against object, subsequent encounter)	**99024** (postoperative follow-up visit) **29085 58** (application cast; hand and lower forearm [gauntlet]) **Q4013** (cast supplies, gauntlet cast [includes lower forearm and hand], adult [11 years +], plaster) or **Q4014** (same but fiberglass) **73110** (radiologic examination, wrist; complete, minimum of 3 views)

Teaching Point: Code **25622** is assigned a 90-day global period by most payers. The physician reports codes for follow-up during the global period (**99024**), radiograph, and application of the replacement cast. Diagnosis codes include the seventh character **D** to report subsequent care of this fracture, although a more specific diagnosis is now confirmed. Inclusion of codes for external cause of injury, although not required, may provide information that facilitates timely payment. Modifier **58** (staged or related procedure) is appended to **29085**, as the service is related to the procedure performed by the same physician at the previous encounter.

Cast supplies are separately reported with either *CPT* code **99070** (supplies and materials [except spectacles], provided by the physician or other QHP over and above those usually included with the office visit or other services rendered) or, as shown here, more specific HCPCS codes.

If the initial care of the fracture had included only application of a splint to stabilize and protect the injury until a definitive diagnosis could be confirmed, codes for an E/M service and application of a splint would have been appropriate in lieu of fracture care. In that case, the return visit at which the fracture was diagnosed would be initial fracture care and code **25622** would be reported for this encounter in lieu of **99024** and **29085**.

When reporting codes for radiographs, documentation should include a report of the indication for the test, number of views, findings, and, when applicable, comparison to previous radiographs.

- Do not report a charge for interpretation and report when reviewing images that have been previously interpreted (eg, by a radiologist).
- The independent review of previously interpreted images is included in an evaluation and management service or follow-up during the global period of a service.

Supplies

- Supplies associated with fracture care may be billed with every application, including the initial casting, splinting, or strapping performed in association with the global surgery procedure code when the service is performed in the private office setting.
- HCPCS codes **A4580**, **A4590**, and **Q4001–Q4051** may be reported for cast supplies; codes **E1800–E1841** may be reported for splints. Check with your major payers and/or review their payment policies for reporting these supplies.
- HCPCS codes are accepted by many Medicaid and commercial payers and are very specific to the age of the patient and type of supply and/or material.
- A description of supplies may be required when reporting special supplies code **99070**.

- The following codes are commonly used:

99070	Supplies and materials (except spectacles)
A4565	Slings
A4570	Splint
L3650–L3678	Clavicle splints
Q4001–Q4051	Cast and splint supplies
S8450–S8452	Splint, prefabricated for finger, wrist, ankle, or elbow

Ear, Nose, and Throat Procedures

Control of Nasal Hemorrhage

30901	Control nasal hemorrhage, anterior, simple (cautery or packing)
30903	Control nasal hemorrhage, anterior, complex (extensive cautery and/or packing) any method

A 0-day global period applies.

- If performing cautery or packing on both sides, report **30901** with modifier **50**.
- If bleeding is controlled with manual pressure or placement of a nasal clamp (clip), only the appropriate level of E/M service is reported.

Do not report **30901** when packing is placed short-term to administer medication (eg, insertion of medicated gauze into the nostrils) and not to serve a hemostatic and/or tamponade role following the encounter. Illumination and instrumentation (eg, suction, nasal speculum, forceps) are typically required for placement of packing to control nasal hemorrhage.

Example

➤ **A 7-year-old established patient presents with a facial injury sustained when he tripped and fell at school.** Part of his face hit the pavement, causing mild bruising on his nose and a significant nosebleed. The patient did not experience headache, vomiting, or loss of consciousness. Medical history was negative for a bleeding disorder, and family history was negative for a bleeding disorder within the family.

The patient had minimal abrasion and ecchymosis on the tip of the nose, with no pain on palpation over the bridge of the nose and cheeks. The septum was not deviated, and no hematoma was present. There was a moderate amount of crusted blood from the left naris, and small bleed medially of the left naris was visible. The remainder of the examination was normal. The decision was made to cauterize with silver nitrate and result of cautery was satisfactory.

ICD-10-CM	*CPT*
R04.0 (epistaxis) **S00.31XA** (abrasion of nose) **W01.0XXA** (fall on same level from slipping, tripping and stumbling without subsequent striking against object, initial encounter) **Y92.480** (sidewalk as the place of occurrence of the external cause) **Y93.01** (activity walking, marching, and hiking)	**99213 25** (MDM of low complexity—acute uncomplicated injury with low risk of morbidity from treatment) **30901**

Teaching Point: The physician provided a significant and separately identifiable E/M service to evaluate extent of injury in addition to treatment of the nosebleed. Only 4 diagnosis codes may be linked to each procedure code on the claim. However, it is appropriate to include all diagnoses on the claim.

Removal of Impacted Cerumen

69209	Removal of impacted cerumen using irrigation/lavage, unilateral
69210	Removal of impacted cerumen requiring instrumentation, unilateral

A 0-day global period applies.

Chapter 10. Surgery, Infusion, and Sedation in the Outpatient Setting

Modifier **25** should be appended to the significant, separately identifiable E/M service (eg, **99213**) provided on the same date as removal of impacted cerumen based on NCCI edits. Payers that use NCCI edits may deny the E/M service when submitted without modifier **25**.

Code **69209** is used to report removal of impacted cerumen by ear wash without direct visualization and instrumentation. This service may be provided by clinical staff under supervision by a physician or other QHP.

- *Do not report* **69209** for removal of cerumen that is not impacted.
- This code is intended to capture the practice expense associated with the service and is not valued to include physician work.
- Separately report any significant and separately identifiable E/M service provided by a physician or other QHP on the same date (modifier **25** may be appended to the E/M code when required by payers).
- For a bilateral procedure, report **69209** with modifier **50**.
- Do not report **69209** in conjunction with **69210** when performed on the same ear (modifiers **LT** and **RT** may be used to identify contralateral procedures).

Code **69210** is *only* reported when the physician or QHP, under direct visualization, removes impacted cerumen using, at a minimum, an otoscope and instruments such as wax curettes or by using an operating microscope and suction plus specific ear instruments (eg, cup forceps, right angles).

- Medical record documentation must support that the cerumen was impacted and removed by the physician and include a description of what equipment and method were used to perform the procedure. Visualization of the impacted cerumen should also be documented.
- Report code **69210** with modifier **50** when bilateral procedures are performed.
- Removal of cerumen that is not impacted is included in an E/M code regardless of how it is removed.
- National Correct Coding Initiative edits bundle impacted cerumen removal (**69209**, **69210**) with some hearing assessments (eg, tympanometry [**92567**]). There is no modifier to override this edit.

Note: Medicare does not recognize modifier **50** when reported with code **69210** (impacted cerumen removal); therefore, those payers that follow Medicare payment policy will not recognize it and may deny the claim outright. Check with your payers.

Coding Conundrum: Unsuccessful Removal of Impacted Cerumen

If a physician or other qualified health care professional attempts to remove impacted cerumen but finds the impaction too hard for safe removal, what code is reported for the attempt? The answer depends on the individual situation, including the amount of work that was performed and whether another procedure was successful.

If the portion of the procedure completed required insignificant work and practice expense (eg, staff time), report only the services completed on that date (eg, evaluation and management).

If the patient is instructed to use softening drops and return later for removal, consider whether the effort and practice expense were sufficient to justify reporting the removal with reduced services modifier **52**.

If the procedure was discontinued after significant effort and practice expense due to extenuating circumstances or concerns that the procedure may threaten the patient's well-being, report the procedure code with modifier **53** (discontinued procedure).

If, after attempted removal by a physician is discontinued, softening drops are administered in the office and clinical staff perform removal of the impaction by lavage (**69209**), report only the completed procedure.

Examples

➤ **A physician orders removal of impacted cerumen from the right ear by lavage.** Clinical staff perform the lavage, removing the impacted cerumen. Because the child is uncooperative, the procedure takes 10 minutes.

ICD-10-CM	CPT
H61.21 (impacted cerumen, right ear)	**99202–99215 25** (Report if appropriate and use modifier **25** if required by payer.)
	69209 RT (**RT** indicates right ear.)

Teaching Point: This procedure was unilateral. If it were bilateral, modifier **50** would be appended to code **69209**. The anatomical modifier **RT** (right) is informational and typically does not affect payment. The extended time of service alone is not sufficient to support reporting increased procedural service (ie, modifier **22**).

➤ **Physician documents, "Impacted cerumen removed from both ears using an otoscope and curette," in a patient with complaint of decreased hearing.** Following the procedure, the patient's hearing is assessed as normal.

ICD-10-CM	CPT
H61.23 (impacted cerumen, bilateral)	**99202–99215 25** (Report if appropriate and use modifier **25** if required by payer.)
	69210 50 (bilateral removal of impacted cerumen using instrumentation)

Teaching Point: Unless a payer instructs otherwise, modifier **50** is appended to **69210** to indicate a bilateral procedure. An E/M service is reported only if significant and separately identifiable. If selecting an E/M code based on time, do not include time spent performing the procedure.

Digestive System Procedures

Incision in Lingual Frenulum

41010   Incision in the lingual frenum to free the tongue

A 10-day global period applies.

Note that code **41115** (excision of lingual frenum) is not appropriate when an incisional release of tongue-tie is performed rather than excision (removal) of the frenum.

Example

➤ **A 14-day-old is seen for feeding difficulty caused by ankyloglossia.** The physician documents obtaining informed consent, positioning and restraining of the neonate, and gentle lifting of the tongue with a sterile, grooved retractor to expose the frenulum. The frenulum, adjacent to the ventral aspect of the tongue, is divided by 2 to 3 mm using sterile scissors. Afterward, the newborn is immediately returned to his mother for comfort and feeding. The latch appears improved. After feeding, the neonate is reevaluated with no evidence of complications. Code **41010** is reported for the procedure.

ICD-10-CM	CPT
Q38.1 (congenital ankyloglossia) **P92.5** (neonatal difficulty in feeding at breast)	**41010**

Teaching Point: If a significant and separately identifiable E/M service was provided in addition to the preservice work of the procedure, modifier **25** would be appended to the appropriate E/M code. Any related visit within the 10 days following the procedure may be reported (with no charge) with code **99024**. An unrelated E/M service within

Chapter 10. Surgery, Infusion, and Sedation in the Outpatient Setting

10 days following the procedure may be reported with modifier **24** (unrelated E/M service by the same physician or QHP during a postoperative period). When reporting modifier **24**, the diagnosis code(s) reported should be indicative of an unrelated service.

Gastrostomy Tube Replacement

43762   Replacement of gastrostomy tube, percutaneous, includes removal, when performed, without imaging or endoscopic guidance; not requiring revision of gastrostomy tract

43763   requiring revision of gastrostomy tract

A 0-day global period is assigned.

- To report gastrostomy tube change without imaging or endoscopic guidance, see codes **43762** and **43763**.
- See codes **49450** and **43246** for placement with imaging or endoscopic guidance.
- A significant, separately identifiable E/M service on the same date may be reported with modifier **25** appended to the E/M code (eg, **99213 25**).
- An E/M service should not be reported when the encounter is solely for replacement of the gastrostomy tube.
- Codes **43762** and **43763** include the gastrostomy tube kit.

Genitourinary System Procedures

Urinary Catheterization

51701   Urinary catheterization, straight

51702   Urinary catheterization, temporary

A 0-day global period applies.

- Code **51701** is reported when a non-indwelling bladder catheter (straight catheterization) is inserted (eg, for residual urine, for a urine culture collection).
- Code **51702** is reported when a temporary indwelling bladder catheter is inserted (ie, Foley).

> **Report code 51701** when you insert a urinary catheter to collect a clean-catch urine specimen, after which the catheter is removed.

Lysis/Excision of Labial or Penile Adhesions

If lysis of labial or penile adhesions is performed by the application of manual pressure without the use of an instrument to cut the adhesions, it would be considered part of the E/M visit and not reported separately.

54450   Foreskin manipulation including lysis of preputial adhesions and stretching

A 0-day global period is assigned.

Code **54450** does not require general anesthesia.

- 2.00 total RVUs are assigned when performed in a non-facility setting (eg, office).
- This procedure is performed on the uncircumcised foreskin and the head of the penis. Adhesions are broken by stretching the foreskin back over the head of the penis onto the shaft or by inserting a clamp between the foreskin and the head of the penis and spreading the jaws of the clamp.

54162   Lysis or excision of penile post-circumcision adhesions

This service includes a 10-day global surgery period.

Code **54162** is only reported when lysis is performed under general anesthesia or regional block, with an instrument, and under sterile conditions.

- This code has 7.67 total RVUs when performed in a non-facility setting (eg, office).
- If post-circumcision adhesions are manually broken during the postoperative period by the physician or physician of the same group and specialty who performed the procedure, it would be considered part of the global surgical package.
- Report the service with *ICD-10-CM* code **N47.0**, adherent prepuce in a newborn, or **N47.5**, adhesions of prepuce and glans penis (patients older than 28 days).

56441   Lysis of labial adhesions

This procedure also includes a Medicare 10-day global surgery period.

Code **56441** is performed by using a blunt instrument or scissors under general or local anesthesia.

- The total RVUs for this procedure in a non-facility setting are 5.24.
- *ICD-10-CM* code **Q52.5** (fusion of labia) would be reported with *CPT* code **56441**.
- When provided without anesthesia, modifier **52** may be appended to indicate reduced services. Payer guidance may vary in regard to use of modifier **52**.

Newborn Circumcision

When circumcisions are performed in the office

- If a payer does not base payment on a global surgical package, a supply code for the surgical tray can be reported with code **99070**. The description of the supply (circumcision tray) would need to be included on the claim form.
- Anesthetic creams (eutectic mixture of local anesthetics) are included in the circumcision code itself and should not be reported unless a third-party payer pays separately for topical anesthetic agents. In that case, they would be reported with code **99070**.

54150 Circumcision, using clamp or other device with regional dorsal penile or ring block

- If the circumcision using a clamp or other device is performed without dorsal penile or ring block, append modifier **52** (reduced services) to **54150**.
- 4.49 total non-facility RVUs and a Medicare global period of 0 (zero) are assigned to code **54150**.
  — When an E/M service (eg, well-baby visit) is provided on the same date, append modifier **25** to the E/M code.
  — Link the appropriate *ICD-10-CM* code (eg, **Z00.110**, health check for newborn under 8 days old) to the E/M service and link *ICD-10-CM* code **Z41.2** (encounter for routine and ritual male circumcision) to the circumcision code.

54160 Circumcision, surgical excision other than clamp, device, or dorsal slit; neonate (28 days of age or less)
54161 older than 28 days

Medicare assigns a global period of 10 days to codes **54160** and **54161**. Services described by **54160** and **54161** are often provided in facility settings.

See Chapter 15 for information on reporting circumcision in a facility setting.

Hydration, Injections, and Infusions

Services included as inherent to an infusion or injection are the use of local anesthesia, starting the intravenous (IV) line, access to indwelling IV lines or a subcutaneous catheter or port, flushing lines at the conclusion of an infusion or between infusions, standard tubing, syringes and supplies, and preparation of chemotherapy agents.

These services are not assigned a global period.

- These codes are intended for reporting by the physician or other QHP in an office setting. They are not reported by a physician or other QHP when performed in a facility setting because the physician work associated with these procedures involves only affirmation of the treatment plan and direct supervision of the staff performing the services.
- If a significant, separately identifiable E/M service is performed, the appropriate code may be reported with modifier **25** appended. The diagnosis may be the same for the E/M service and codes **96360–96379**.

Documentation of medications administered in the outpatient pediatric practice should include

- **Order for medication**
- **Date and time of administration (include start/stop times for timed procedures)**
- **Medication, manufacturer, lot number, and expiration date**
- **Dose**
- **Route (eg, intramuscular) and site of administration (eg, left deltoid)**
- **Observations (eg, held by mother, no sign of adverse reaction after 5 minutes)**
- **Signature and credentials of individual administering medication**

Subcutaneous or Intramuscular Injection (Therapeutic, Prophylactic, and Diagnostic)

96372 Therapeutic, prophylactic, or diagnostic injection (specify substance or drug); subcutaneous or intramuscular

Report code **96372** for the administration of a diagnostic, prophylactic, or therapeutic (eg, antibiotic) subcutaneous or intramuscular (IM) injection. Do not report for the administration of a purified protein derivative test.

For administration of immunizations, see discussion of codes 90460, 90461, and 90471–90474 in Chapter 8.

Examples

➤ **A 2-year-old established patient presents with moderate symptoms of croup that began last evening and worsened during the night.** After obtaining history and performing an examination, the physician recommends injection of dexamethasone sodium phosphate. A 7-mg dose of dexamethasone sodium phosphate is administered by IM injection. The child is observed for reaction and released to home with instructions and precautions.

ICD-10-CM	CPT
J05.0 (acute obstructive laryngitis [croup])	99213 25 (established patient E/M with low MDM) 96372 (IM injection) J1100 × 7 units (injection, dexamethasone sodium phosphate per 1 mg)

Teaching Point: The medication is reported with HCPCS code J1100, which indicates the unit of measure for reporting is 1 mg. Because 7 mg were administered, 7 units of service are reported. Also report the appropriate National Drug Code (NDC) and units.

See Chapter 1 for more information on National Drug Codes.

The E/M service included addressing an acute uncomplicated illness with prescription drug management, supporting code 99213. (Although prescription drug management supports moderate MDM and code 99214, neither the number and complexity of problems addressed nor the data to be reviewed and analyzed support this level. Two of 3 elements of MDM must meet the requirements for a level of MDM.) Modifier 25 must be appended to the E/M service code to indicate the significant, separately identifiable E/M service on the date of the injection for payers that use NCCI edits.

➤ **A 2-year-old girl presents with a fever (39.4°C [103.0°F]). Her mother states the girl has been tugging at her right ear for 2 days.** An expanded problem-focused history and examination are completed. When the doctor examines the ears, he notices that the right middle ear is very inflamed (pus is present) and the child is extremely uncomfortable. The child's mother states that it is very difficult to get her daughter to swallow medicine rather than spit it out. The doctor decides to administer a single injection of ceftriaxone sodium 600 mg to the child. The final diagnosis is right acute suppurative otitis media without rupture of eardrum. Medical decision-making is moderate.

ICD-10-CM	CPT
H66.001 (acute suppurative otitis media without spontaneous rupture of ear drum, right ear) R50.81 (fever in conditions classified elsewhere)	99213 25 (established patient level E/M with low MDM—acute uncomplicated problem with prescription drug management) 96372 (IM injection) J0696 × 3 units (injection, ceftriaxone sodium, per 250 mg)

Teaching Point: The medication is reported with HCPCS code J0696, which indicates the unit of measure for reporting is 250 mg. Because 600 mg was administered, 3 units are reported per Medicare guidelines. However, if the payer accepts actual dosage, 2.4 units (2 units for the first two 250 mg of the medication and 0.4 units for the last 100 mg) would be reported rather than 3 units. Report also the appropriate NDC.

If the patient were scheduled for a series of injections of the same antibiotic over several days, report only the services rendered (eg, 96372 and J0696) each day (ie, do not report an E/M unless there is clinical indication for a significant and separately identifiable E/M service).

Modifier 25 must be appended to the E/M service code (99213) to indicate the significant, separately identifiable E/M service on the date of the injection for payers that use NCCI edits.

Chapter 10. Surgery, Infusion, and Sedation in the Outpatient Setting

Hydration and Infusions

Hydration and infusion codes are reported based on the time when medication administration begins to the end of administration. Time must be documented.

When reporting multiple infusions on the same date, physicians select an initial service based on the service that is the primary reason for infusion services on that date.

Example

➤ **A patient receives infusion of a medication and a separate infusion of hydration fluid.** The physician determines whether the therapeutic infusion or the hydration was the primary service and selects the appropriate initial service code. The other service is reported with a code for sequential or subsequent administration.

Hydration

Codes **96360** (IV infusion, hydration; initial, 31 minutes to 1 hour) and **96361** (each additional hour)

- Are intended to report IV hydration infusion using prepackaged fluid and/or electrolyte solutions (eg, physiologic [normal] saline solution, D_5-0.45% physiologic saline solution with potassium).
- **96360** may be reported for hydration infusion lasting more than 31 minutes and up to 1 hour.
- **96361** is reported for each additional hour of hydration infusion and for a final interval of greater than 30 minutes beyond the last hour reported.

Code **96361** is reported if an IV hydration infusion is provided secondary or subsequent to a therapeutic, prophylactic, or diagnostic infusion and administered through the same IV access.

- Typically require direct physician supervision for purposes of consent, safety oversight, or supervision of staff with little special handling for preparation or disposal of materials.
- Do not typically require advanced training of staff because there usually is little risk involved and little patient monitoring required.
- Are reported based on the actual time over which the infusion is administered and do not include the time spent starting the IV and monitoring the patient after infusion.
- Medical record documentation must support the service reported.
- Are not reported when IV infusions are 30 minutes or less.
- Are not used to report infusion of drugs or other substances; nor are they reported when hydration is incidental to non-chemotherapeutic/diagnostic or chemotherapeutic services.

Intra-arterial and Intravenous Push Injections

96373	Therapeutic, prophylactic, or diagnostic injection (specify substance or drug); intra-arterial
96374	intravenous push, single or initial substance/drug
+96375	each additional sequential intravenous push of a new substance/drug (List separately in addition to **96365**, **96374**, **96409**, or **96413**)

- Each drug administered is reported separately with the appropriate infusion code.
- Report code **96373** for an initial intra-arterial injection and **96374** for an initial injection administered by IV push.
- Codes **96374** and **96375** are only used when the health care professional administering the substance or drug is in constant attendance during the administration *and* must observe the patient. The IV push must be less than 15 minutes.

> Short infusions of less than 15 minutes are reported as a push (eg, **96374**).

- Sequential IV push of a new substance or drug is reported with add-on code **96375**.
- Code **96375** may be reported in addition to codes for IV infusion (**96365**), initial IV push (**96374**), or chemotherapy administration (**96409**, **96413**).
- Additional sequential IV push of the same substance or drug (**96376**) is not reported for services provided in the physician office (ie, is reported only by a facility).

Therapeutic, Prophylactic, and Diagnostic Infusions

96365	Intravenous infusion, for therapy, prophylaxis, or diagnosis (specify substance or drug); initial, up to 1 hour
+96366	each additional hour (List separately in addition to **96365** or **96367**.)
+96367	additional sequential infusion of a new drug/substance, up to 1 hour (List separately in addition to **96365**, **96374**, **96409**, **96413**.)
+96368	concurrent infusion (List separately in addition to **96365**, **96366**, or chemotherapy services **96413**, **96415**, or **96416**.)

Table 10-4 lists primary and additional IV infusion and IV push codes. See the table notes for additional instructions on reporting multiple services.

Codes **96365–96368**

● Are for infusions for the purpose of administering drugs or substances.

Table 10-4. Primary and Additional Intravenous Infusion Codes[a]

For all services, you must specify the substance or drug administered.

Service (Select the primary reason for encounter irrespective of order of infusion services.)[b]	IV Infusion, for Therapy, Prophylaxis, or Diagnosis	Subcutaneous Infusion for Therapy or Prophylaxis[b]	Therapeutic, Prophylactic, or Diagnostic Injection IV Push
Initial service, up to 1 h	**96365** (16 min–1 h)	**96369** (16 min–1 h)	**96374** (IV push or infusion ≤15 min)
Each additional hour (>30 min) of *same substance or drug*	**+96366**[c] (List separately in addition to **96365**, **96367**)	**+96370** (Use **96370** in conjunction with **96369**.)	
Additional sequential infusion of *new substance or drug*	**+96367**[c]	**+96371** (additional pump setup with new subcutaneous infusion site[s])	**+96367**
Sequential IV push of a *new substance/drug*	**+96375**		**+96375**
Concurrent infusion	**+96368** (Report only once per date of service.)		

Abbreviation: IV, intravenous.

[a] If IV infusion for hydration of longer than 30 minutes is provided in addition to a therapeutic infusion service (**96360**, **96365**, **96374**) through the same IV access, report **+96361** in addition to **96365** or **96374**.

[b] Includes pump setup and establishment of infusion site(s). Use **96369** and **96371** only once per encounter.

[c] Report **96367** only once per sequential infusion of same infusate mix. Report **96366** for each additional hour (includes final time unit of 31 minutes or more) beyond the first hour of the service reported with **96367**.

● Typically require direct physician supervision and special attention to prepare, calculate dose, and dispose of materials.
● If fluid infusions are used to administer the drug(s), they are considered incidental hydration and are not reported. Each drug administered is reported separately with the appropriate infusion code.
● Short infusions of less than 15 minutes are reported as a push (eg, **96374**).
● Only 1 initial service code (eg, **96365**) should be reported unless the protocol or patient condition requires that 2 separate IV sites must be used. A second IV site access is also reported using the initial service code with modifier **59** appended (eg, **96365**, **96365 59**).
● Subcutaneous infusion is reported with codes **96369–96371** (see **Table 10-4**).

When services are performed in the physician's office, report as follows:

Initial Infusion

Report the code that best describes the key or primary reason for the service regardless of the order in which the infusions or injections occur. Only 1 initial service code (eg, **96365**) should be reported unless the protocol or patient condition requires using 2 separate IV sites. The difference in time and effort in providing this second IV site access is also reported using the initial service code with modifier **59**, distinct procedural service, appended (eg, **96365**, **96365 59**).

Coding Conundrum: Multiple and Concurrent Infusions or Injections

When administering multiple infusions, injections, or combinations, only 1 "initial" service code should be reported for a given date, unless protocol requires that 2 separate intravenous (IV) sites must be used.

- Do not report a second initial service on the same date due to an IV line requiring a restart, an IV rate not being able to be reached without 2 lines, or a need to access a port of a multi-lumen catheter.
- If an injection or infusion is of a subsequent or concurrent nature, even if it is the first such service within that group of services, a subsequent or concurrent code from the appropriate section should be reported. For example, the first IV push given subsequent to an initial 1-hour infusion is reported using a subsequent IV push code.

Sequential Infusion

This is an infusion or IV push of a new substance or drug following a primary or initial service. For example, if an IV push was performed through the same IV access subsequent to an IV infusion for therapy, the appropriate codes to report would be **96365** and **96375**. If an IV push was performed through a different IV access route, the services would be reported using codes **96365** and **96374**. Sequential infusions are reported only 1 time for the same infusate. However, if additional hours were required for the infusion, the appropriate "each additional hour" add-on code would be reported. Different infusates can be reported using the same code as the original sequential code. Hydration may not be reported concurrently with any other service. All sequential services require that there be a new substance or drug; only a facility may report a sequential IV push of the same drug using **96376**.

Concurrent Infusion

This is an infusion of a new substance or drug infused at the same time as another drug or substance. This is not time-based and is only reported once per day regardless of whether a new drug or substance is administered concurrently. Hydration may not be reported concurrently with any other service. A separate subsequent concurrent administration of another new drug or substance (the third substance or drug) is not reported.

Example

➤ **A 3-year-old established patient is seen with a complaint of vomiting and fever for the past 24 hours.** She has refused all food and liquids and last voided 12 hours prior to the visit. A detailed history and physical examination with moderate-level MDM are performed. Her diagnosis is bilateral acute suppurative otitis media with fever and dehydration. Intravenous fluids are initiated with physiologic (normal) saline solution, and IV ceftriaxone (750 mg) is infused over 30 minutes for her otitis media. After 1 hour and 45 minutes of IV hydration, she urinates, begins tolerating liquids, and is released to home.

ICD-10-CM	CPT
E86.0 (dehydration)	**99214 25** (established patient office E/M)
H66.003 (acute suppurative otitis media without spontaneous rupture of ear drum, bilateral)	**96365** (IV infusion, for therapy)
	96361 (IV infusion, hydration, each additional hour)
R11.10 (vomiting)	**J0696** × 3 units (ceftriaxone sodium, per 250 mg)
R50.81 (fever in conditions classified elsewhere)	**J7030** (infusion, normal saline solution, 1,000 cc)

Teaching Point: Link the appropriate diagnosis code to each procedure (eg, code **H66.003** is linked to code **J0696**). If required by the payer, the medication and infusion solution may need to be reported with the NDC. The fluid used to administer ceftriaxone is not reported because it is considered incidental hydration.

Other Injection and Infusion Services

96523   Irrigation of implanted venous access device for drug delivery systems

Code **96523** is used to report irrigation required for implanted venous access devices for drug delivery systems when services are provided on a separate day from the injection or infusion service. Do not report **96523** in conjunction with other services.

●=New code   ▲=Revised code   #=Re-sequenced code   +=Add-on code   ★=Telemedicine

Chemotherapy and Other Highly Complex Drug/Biologic Agent Administration

Codes **96401–96549** are reported for chemotherapy administration. *CPT* defines *chemotherapy administration* as parenteral administration of non-radionuclide antineoplastic drugs, antineoplastic agents provided for treatment of non-cancer diagnoses and to substances such as certain monoclonal antibody agents, and other biologic response modifiers.

Example

➤ **A patient with severe persistent asthma is receiving injections of omalizumab 225 mg every 2 weeks.** The patient presents for administration of the medication. The medication is divided and injected at 2 different sites, as only 150 mg may be injected to a single site. The diagnosis code reported is **J45.50** (severe persistent asthma). Omalizumab injection is reported as a chemotherapy administration of monoclonal antibody (**96401**) with only 1 unit of service *unless prohibited by payer policy.* Omalizumab is provided in 150-mg single-use vials with an NDC of 50242-040-62. The NDC on the claim must contain 11 digits using the 5-4-2 format (ie, 50242-0040-62). HCPCS code **J2357** (injection, omalizumab, 5 mg) is used to report the medication supplied by the physician practice. The following sample claim form illustrates reporting for this example:

Claim Form Sample National Drug Code											
21. Diagnosis or nature of illness or injury (Relate A–L to service line below 24E) A.J45.50	B.		C.	D.		ICD Ind. 0					
24. A. Dates of service	B. Place of service	C. EMG	D. Procedures, services or supplies CPT/HCPCS	Modifier	E. Diagnosis Pointer	F. Charges	G. Days or units	H. EPSDT	I. ID Qual	J. Rendering Provider #	
1/1/2022–1/1/2022	11		96401		A	$$$	1		NPI	NPI No.	
N450242004062 UN2											
1/1/2022–1/1/2022	11		J2357		A	$$$	45		NPI	NPI No.	

Abbreviations: *CPT, Current Procedural Terminology*; EMG, emergency; EPSDT, Early and Periodic Screening, Diagnostic, and Treatment; HCPCS, Healthcare Common Procedure Coding System; *ICD, International Classification of Diseases*; NPI, National Provider Identifier.

Teaching Point: Check payer policies before reporting administration of omalizumab and other highly complex drug/biologic agents. *CPT* instructs that administration of certain monoclonal antibody agents may be reported with code **96401**. However, not all payers accept code **96401** for administration of omalizumab. Some payers limit reporting to code **96372** (subcutaneous or IM injection) and/or allow only 1 administration code despite requirements to administer by 2 or more separate injections.

The HCPCS codes and NDCs for the omalizumab are included on the claim with units based on the HCPCS code descriptor (225-mg dose/5-mg HCPCS unit = 45 units) and NDC quantity (payers may require NDC units per vial—UN2 or per gram—GR0.225) to identify the substance administered. Some payers allow reporting of the full amount of single-dose vials when only a portion of the medication is provided to a patient to account for drug waste. Report units for the full single-dose vial only as instructed by payer policy.

Moderate Sedation

Moderate sedation codes **99151–99153** and **99155–99157** are used for reporting moderate sedation when intraservice time is 10 minutes or more. **Table 10-5** contains sedation codes and descriptors.

Codes for moderate sedation are not assigned a global period.

Moderate sedation is a drug-induced depression of consciousness.

- No interventions are required to maintain cardiovascular functions or a patent airway, and spontaneous ventilation is adequate.
- Moderate sedation codes are not used to report administration of medications for pain control, minimal sedation (anxiolysis), deep sedation, or monitored anesthesia care (**00100–01999**).
- Moderate sedation provided and reported by the same physician or QHP who is performing the diagnostic or therapeutic service requires the presence of an independent trained observer.

An *independent trained observer* is an individual qualified to monitor the patient during the procedure but who has no other duties (eg, assisting at surgery) during the procedure.

- Alternatively, a physician or QHP other than the person performing the diagnostic or therapeutic service may provide and report moderate sedation services.
- Codes **99151–99157** are distinguished by service provider, patient age, and time spent (see **Table 10-5**).

Table 10-5. Moderate Sedation		
Moderate Sedation	**Intraservice Time**	
	First 15 min (10–22 min)	**Each Additional 15 min and Last 8–22 min**
Moderate sedation services provided by the same physician or other qualified health care professional performing the diagnostic or therapeutic service that the sedation supports, requiring the presence of an independent trained observer to assist in the monitoring of the patient's level of consciousness and physiological status; initial 15 minutes of intra-service time, patient younger than 5 years of age	99151	+**99153** (report only in addition to **99151** or **99152**)
5 years or older	99152	+**99153**
Moderate sedation services (other than those services described by codes **00100– 01999**) provided by a physician other than the health care professional performing the diagnostic or therapeutic service that the sedation supports; younger than 5 years	99155	+**99157** (report only in addition to **99155** or **99156**)
5 years or older	99156	+**99157**

Codes **99151–99153** are reported when

- The administration of moderate sedation is provided by the physician who is simultaneously performing a procedure (eg, fracture reduction, vessel cutdown, central line placement, wound repair).
- An independent trained observer is present to assist the physician in the monitoring of the patient during the procedure or diagnostic service.

Codes **99155–99157** are reported when

- A second physician or QHP other than the health care professional performing the diagnostic or therapeutic services provides moderate sedation.

Codes **99153** and **99157** are reported for each additional 15 minutes of intraservice time. The midpoint between the end of the previous 15-minute period must be passed to report an additional unit of intraservice time (ie, intraservice time must continue for at least 8 minutes beyond the last full 15 minutes of intraservice time).

- Codes are selected based on intraservice time. Intraservice time
  - Begins with the administration of the sedating agent(s)
  - Ends when the procedure is completed, the patient is stable for recovery status, and the physician or other QHP providing the sedation ends personal continuous face-to-face time with the patient
  - Includes ordering and/or administering the initial and subsequent doses of sedating agents
  - Requires continuous face-to-face attendance of the physician or other QHP
  - Requires monitoring patient response to the sedating agents, including
    - Periodic assessment of the patient
    - Further administration of agent(s) as needed to maintain sedation
    - Monitoring of oxygen saturation, heart rate, and blood pressure
- Moderate sedation service of less than 10 minutes of intraservice time is not separately reported.
- Preserve work of moderate sedation services *is not separately reported* and is not included in intraservice time. Preserve work includes
  - Assessment of the patient's past medical and surgical history with particular emphasis on cardiovascular, pulmonary, airway, or neurologic conditions
  - Review of the patient's previous experiences with anesthesia and/or sedation
  - Family history of sedation complications
  - Summary of the patient's present medication list
  - Drug allergy and intolerance history
  - Focused physical examination of the patient, with emphasis on
    - Mouth, jaw, oropharynx, neck, and airway for Mallampati score assessment
    - Chest and lungs
    - Heart and circulation
    - Vital signs, including heart rate, respiratory rate, blood pressure, and oxygenation, with end-tidal carbon dioxide when indicated

Chapter 10. Surgery, Infusion, and Sedation in the Outpatient Setting

> **Do not report a separate evaluation and management service for preservice or post-service work associated with moderate sedation.**

— Review of any pre-sedation diagnostic tests
— Completion of a pre-sedation assessment form (with American Society of Anesthesiologists physical status classification)
— Patient informed consent
— Immediate pre-sedation assessment prior to first sedating doses
— Initiation of IV access and fluids to maintain patency

- Do not separately report or include the time of post-service work in the intraservice time. Post-service work of moderate sedation includes
  — Assessment of the patient's vital signs, level of consciousness, and neurologic, cardiovascular, and pulmonary stability in the post-sedation recovery period
  — Assessment of patient's readiness for discharge following the procedure
  — Preparation of documentation for sedation service
  — Communication with family or caregiver about sedation service
- Oxygen saturation (**94760–94762**) cannot be reported separately.

> **Documentation of moderate sedation services must include all of the following:**
> - **The description of the procedure**
> - **Name and dosage(s) of the sedation agent(s)**
> - **Route of administration of the sedation agent(s) and who administered the agent (physician or independent observer)**
> - **The ongoing assessment of the child's level of consciousness and physiological status (eg, heart rate, oxygen saturation levels) during and after the procedure**
> - **The presence, name, and title of the independent observer or performing physician or other qualified health care professional**
> - **Total time from administration of the sedation agent(s) (start time) until the physician's face-to-face service is no longer required (end time)**

Examples

➤ **A 3-year-old requires incision and removal of a piece of glass from a puncture wound of the right foot.** Moderate sedation is required and is performed by the Pediatric Advanced Life Support–trained physician with an independent trained observer who has been trained in pediatric basic life support. The physician supervises the administration of the sedating agent and assesses the child until an effective, safe level of sedation is achieved and continues to assess the child's level of consciousness and physiological status while also performing the procedure. The procedure takes a total of 28 minutes from the time of administration of the agent until the physician completes the procedure and determines the child is stable and face-to-face physician time is no longer required.

ICD-10-CM	CPT
S91.341A (puncture wound with foreign body, right foot) Codes for external cause, activity, and place of injury are reported when documented.	**10121** (incision and removal of foreign body, subcutaneous tissues; complicated) **99151** (moderate [conscious] sedation, patient younger than 5 years, first 15 minutes) **+99153** (moderate [conscious] sedation, each additional 15 minutes of intraservice time)

Teaching Point: If a medically necessary, significant, and separately identifiable E/M service had also been performed, an E/M visit with modifier **25** appended could be reported. The agent itself should also be reported.

➤ **Same patient as previous example, except moderate sedation is performed by the Pediatric Advanced Life Support–trained physician while another physician performs the procedure.** The procedure, from the time of administration of the agent until the repair is complete and the child is stable and no longer requires face-to-face physician time, takes a total of 28 minutes.

ICD-10-CM	CPT
S91.341A (puncture wound with foreign body, right foot) Codes for external cause, activity, and place of injury are reported when documented.	The physician repairing the wound reports **10121** (incision and removal of foreign body, subcutaneous tissues; complicated)
	The physician performing moderate sedation reports **99155** (moderate [conscious] sedation, patient younger than 5 years, first 15 minutes) **+99157** (moderate [conscious] sedation, each additional 15 minutes of intraservice time)

Teaching Point: Each physician reports the service provided. The time of moderate sedation used in code selection is only the intraservice time.

Resources

Fracture Care

"Initial Fracture Care: Musculoskeletal or Evaluation and Management," February 2021 *AAP Pediatric Coding Newsletter˜* (https://coding. solutions.aap.org/article.aspx?articleid=2765276; subscription required)

Global Periods and Relative Value Units

Medicare Physician Fee Schedule (www.cms.gov/medicare/medicare-fee-for-service-payment/physicianfeesched)

"The Surgical Package and Related Services," May 2018 *AAP Pediatric Coding Newsletter* (https://coding.solutions.aap.org/article. aspx?articleid=2679119; subscription required)

Integumentary Repair

"You Code It! Integumentary Repair" and "You Code It! Answers: Integumentary Repair," April 2020 *AAP Pediatric Coding Newsletter* (https://coding.solutions.aap.org/article.aspx?articleid=2763375 and https://coding.solutions.aap.org/article.aspx?articleid=2763378; subscription required)

Modifiers

"Modifier **25**: Documenting and Reporting Significant, Separately Identifiable Services," June 2020 *AAP Pediatric Coding Newsletter* (https://coding.solutions.aap.org/article.aspx?articleid=2765187; subscription required)

"Coding Challenge: Modifiers and Procedural Services (Online Exclusive)," May 2018 *AAP Pediatric Coding Newsletter* (https://coding. solutions.aap.org/article.aspx?articleid=2679120; subscription required)

Reduced or Discontinued Procedures

"Reporting Terminated Procedural Services," November 2014 *AAP Pediatric Coding Newsletter* (https://coding.solutions.aap.org/article. aspx?articleid=1921435; subscription required)

Suture Removal

"You Code It! Removal of Sutures," March 2018 *AAP Pediatric Coding Newsletter* (https://coding.solutions.aap.org/article. aspx?articleid=2673748; subscription required)

Test Your Knowledge!

1. **How is an unrelated evaluation and management (E/M) service provided during the global surgical period reported?**
   a. The appropriate E/M code appended with modifier **24**
   b. The appropriate E/M code appended with modifier **25**
   c. **99214**
   d. **99204**

2. **What global period is assigned to simple skin wound repair?**
   a. Zero (0) days
   b. 10 days
   c. 90 days
   d. The concept of global period does not apply to wound repairs.

3. **Layered closure of 1 or more of the deeper layers of subcutaneous tissue and superficial (non-muscle) fascia is what type of repair?**
   a. Complicated
   b. Simple
   c. Intermediate
   d. Complex

4. **Which codes describe infusion using prepackaged fluid and/or electrolyte solutions?**
   a. None; this service is included in a related E/M service.
   b. **96365, 96366**
   c. **96360, 96361**
   d. **96372**

5. **How many units of service are linked to code 96372 for an intramuscular injection of 7 mg of dexamethasone sodium phosphate?**
   a. 2
   b. 1
   c. 7
   d. 70

||||||

Common Non-facility Testing and Therapeutic Services

||||||

Contents

Interpretation and Report 261

Professional and Technical Components 261

Supplies and Medications.. 262
   Supplies and Materials 262
   Medications 262

Blood Sampling for Diagnostic Study 262
   Venipuncture 262
   Arterial Puncture 265

Pathology and Laboratory Procedures.. 265
   Clinical Laboratory Improvement Amendments–Waived Tests.. 265
   General Guidance for Reporting Laboratory Services.. 265
      Laboratory Panel Coding 266
      Direct Optical Observation 266
      Cultures 266
      Proprietary Laboratory Analysis and Multianalyte Assays With Algorithmic Analyses........................... 266

Laboratory Tests Frequently Performed in the Office 267
   Coronavirus (SARS-CoV-2) Testing... 267
      SARS-CoV-2 Infection Testing... 267
      Combination Testing for SARS-CoV-2 and Other Infectious Agent(s)... 267
      SARS-CoV-2 Antibody Testing 268
   Urinalysis 269
   Urine Pregnancy Test.. 269
   Glucose Tests 269
   Hematology 269
   Influenza—Point-of-Care Testing... 269
   Lead Testing... 270
   Mononucleosis—Heterophile Antibodies Screening.. 270
   Papanicolaou Tests 270
   Presumptive Drug Tests... 271
   Respiratory Syncytial Virus Test 271
   Serum and Transcutaneous Bilirubin Testing.. 271
   Streptococcal Test.. 271
   Testing Stool for Occult Blood... 271
   Tuberculosis Skin Test (Mantoux) 272
   Zika Virus Testing 272

Respiratory Function Tests and Treatments 272
   Pulmonary Function Tests... 272
   Inhalation Treatment 273
   Nebulizer Demonstration or Evaluation 273
   Car Seat/Bed Testing 274

Allergy and Clinical Immunology 275
   Allergy Testing... 275
   Allergen Immunotherapy 276
      Preparation and Provision of Extract Only 276
      Administration of Extract Only 277
      Combined Provision of Allergenic Extract With Administration 277
   Epinephrine Auto-injector Administration.. 278
   Immunoglobulins.. 278

Hearing Screening and Other Audiological Function Testing Codes 278

Emotional/Behavioral Assessment 280

Radiology Services 280

    Imaging Guidance 281

    Abdominal Radiographs 281

    Chest Radiographs 281

    Hip Radiographs 281

    Total Spine Radiographs 281

Administrative Services and Supplies 282

    Administrative Services 282

    Physician Group Education Services 282

Resources 282

Test Your Knowledge! 283

Chapter 11. Common Non-facility Testing and Therapeutic Services

This chapter includes discussion of codes for some of the most common tests and therapeutic services performed in physician offices and outpatient clinics.

Interpretation and Report

Many tests include recording of results and a report with interpretation. *Current Procedural Terminology* (*CPT*®) instructs

- *Results* are the technical component of a service. Testing leads to results; results lead to interpretation.
- *Reports* are the work product of the interpretation of test results.
- Certain procedures or services described in *CPT* involve a technical component (eg, tests), which produces results (eg, data, images, slides). For clinical use, some of these results require interpretation. Some *CPT* descriptors specifically require interpretation and reporting to report that code.

Pediatricians performing services that include an interpretation of results should become familiar with the types of reports typical for each test (eg, typical report produced for the interpretation of electrocardiogram [ECG] tracings). A report generated by an automated system is not typically sufficient to support reporting a service described as "with interpretation and report."

Professional and Technical Components

26   Professional component: When the physician or other qualified health care professional is reporting only the professional component of a service, append modifier **26** to the procedure code.

TC   Technical component: When reporting only the technical component of a service, append modifier **TC** to the procedure code.

Certain procedures (eg, ECGs, radiographs, surgical diagnostic tests) include a professional and technical component. Modifiers are used to indicate that either the professional or technical component was performed, but not both.

> When the physician owns the equipment and is performing the technical and professional services, a modifier should not be appended to the code.

- The *professional component* includes the physician work (eg, interpretation of the test, written report).
- If a physician is performing a service or procedure with equipment owned by a facility or another entity and the codes are written as a global service, services are reported with modifier **26** (professional component).
- The *technical component* includes the costs associated with providing the service (eg, equipment, salaries of technical personnel, supplies, facility expense).

    CPT does not include a modifier for reporting the technical component. However, most payers recognize Healthcare Common Procedure Coding System (HCPCS) modifier **TC**. Facilities or an office providing use of its equipment would only report the same service using modifier **TC**.

- Some codes were developed to distinguish between the technical and professional components (eg, routine ECG codes **93000–93010**); however, many do not.

No modifier is appended when the code descriptor for the service identifies whether the professional, technical, or global service is being reported.

Examples

➤ **A physician orders a 2-view chest radiograph on a child.** The child is sent to a neighboring physician's office (or outpatient department) for the radiograph (without interpretation). The films are then brought back to the office and the pediatrician interprets them and creates a report of the findings.

     Physician: **71046 26** (radiologic examination, chest; 2 views)
     Neighboring physician's office: **71046 TC**

➤ **A physician orders a 12-lead ECG on an adolescent patient.** The patient is sent to another office that has an ECG machine to perform the ECG. The tracings are taken back to the pediatrician for review and written interpretation and report.

     Physician: **93010** (routine ECG with at least 12 leads; interpretation and report only)
     Other office: **93005** (routine ECG with at least 12 leads; tracing only, without interpretation and report)

Modifiers **26** and **TC** are not appended because the codes designate the professional and technical components.

Do not separately report review of another physician's interpretation and report or personal review of the tracing that has been interpreted by another physician. However, these activities contribute to the medical decision-making for any related evaluation and management (E/M) service.

When interpreting an ECG at a location remote from the site of the tracing, follow payer guidelines for reporting. The place of service for remote interpretation and report is typically the site where the technical component of the test was performed (eg, outpatient hospital). Payer guidelines may vary.

Supplies and Medications

Supplies and Materials

99070   Supplies and materials provided by the physician over and above those usually included with the office visit or other services rendered

The relative value units (RVUs) assigned to testing services include the value of supplies (eg, masks, tubing, gauze, needles) that are typically required for each service.

> If reporting code 99070, identify the supplies or materials on the claim form and be prepared to submit an invoice.

- Supplies should be separately reported when a payer does not use a payment methodology based on the RVUs assigned to each code under the Medicare Physician Fee Schedule (MPFS). However, most payers today use a payment method based on RVUs and do not provide separate payment for supplies.
- Items such as elastic wraps, clavicle splints, or circumcision and suturing trays may be reported with this code. Remember that some supplies (eg, suturing trays, circumcision trays) may be included with the surgical procedure if the payer uses the Resource-Based Relative Value Scale as its basis for payment.
- Only the supplies purchased in an office-based practice may be reported.
- Some payers will require the use of HCPCS codes. HCPCS codes are available for a number of supplies (eg, codes Q4001–Q4051 for cast and splint supplies). Use HCPCS codes when they are more specific than code 99070.

Medications

Medications used in testing or treatment (eg, albuterol) are not included in the value of service and are separately reported using HCPCS codes (eg, J7613, albuterol, inhalation solution, US Food and Drug Administration [FDA]-approved final product, noncompounded, administered through durable medical equipment [DME], unit dose, 1 mg).

See Table 11-1 for a list of the most commonly used HCPCS J codes.

- The practice must have incurred a cost for the medication reported.
- Most payers do not cover services reported with nonspecific codes.
- Check with payers to determine if they accept these HCPCS codes or if they require reporting with code 99070.
- Drugs are listed with a base dosage. When the dosage exceeds the amount listed, report additional units for the total dosage administered.
- Some payers require use of the National Drug Code (NDC) instead of or in addition to J codes. The NDC should always be reported in addition to code 99070 or J3490 (unclassified drug). You can find a list of NDCs at www.fda.gov/drugs/drug-approvals-and-databases/national-drug-code-directory.

> For more information on National Drug Codes, see Chapter 1.

Blood Sampling for Diagnostic Study

Collection of blood samples for testing (eg, venipuncture) in a physician practice is reported regardless of whether the laboratory test is performed in the office or at an outside facility.

Venipuncture

36400   Venipuncture, younger than age 3 years, necessitating the skill of a physician or other qualified health care professional, not to be used for routine venipuncture; femoral or jugular vein

Table 11-1. Common Healthcare Common Procedure Coding System Codes

Inhalation Solution	Brand Name(s)[a]	J Code	Administration
Albuterol, inhalation solution, FDA-approved final product, noncompounded, administered through DME, concentrated form, 1 mg	Proventil, Ventolin	J7611	94640 or 94644 (for first hour)
Albuterol, inhalation solution, FDA-approved final product, noncompounded, administered through DME, unit dose, 1 mg	AccuNeb, Proventil, Ventolin	J7613	94640 or 94644 (for first hour)
Albuterol, up to 2.5 mg, and ipratropium bromide, up to 0.5 mg, FDA-approved final product, noncompounded, administered through DME	Albuterol, DuoNeb, ipratropium bromide	J7620	94640 or 94644 (for first hour)
Budesonide, inhalation solution, FDA-approved final product, noncompounded, administered through DME, unit dose form, up to 0.5 mg	Pulmicort	J7626	94640 or 94644 (for first hour)
Budesonide, inhalation solution, compounded product, administered through DME, unit dose form, up to 0.5 mg	Pulmicort Respules	J7627	94640 or 94644 (for first hour)
Levalbuterol, inhalation solution, FDA-approved final product, noncompounded, administered through DME, concentrated form, 0.5 mg	Xopenex	J7612	94640 or 94644 (for first hour)
Levalbuterol, inhalation solution, FDA-approved final product, noncompounded, administered through DME, unit dose, 0.5 mg	Xopenex	J7614	94640 or 94644 (for first hour)
Levalbuterol, inhalation solution, compounded, administered through DME, unit dose, 0.5 mg	Levalbuterol hydrochloride	J7615	94640 or 94644 (for first hour)
Injection	**Brand Name(s)[a]**	**J Code**	**Administration**
Ampicillin, 500 mg	Omnipen-N, Totacillin-N	J0290	96372 (IM) (IV)[b]
Atropine sulfate, 0.01 mg	Atropen	J0461	96372
Betamethasone acetate, 3 mg, and betamethasone sodium phosphate, 3 mg	Celestone Soluspan	J0702	96372
Ceftriaxone, per 250 mg	Rocephin	J0696	96372 (IM) (IV)[b]
Cefotaxime, per gram	Claforan	J0698	96372 (IM) (IV)[b]
Dexamethasone acetate, 1 mg	Decadron-LA	J1094	96372
Dexamethasone sodium phosphate, 1 mg	Decadron	J1100	96372 (IM) (IV)[b]
Diphenhydramine hydrochloride, up to 50 mg	Benadryl	J1200	96372
Epinephrine, 0.1 mg	Adrenalin chloride, Sus-Phrine	J0171	96372
Gentamicin, up to 80 mg	Garamycin	J1580	96372 (IM) (IV)[b]
Glucagon, per 1 mg	GlucaGen	J1610	96374
Heparin sodium (heparin lock flush), per 10 units	Hep-Lock	J1642	96374
Hydrocortisone sodium succinate, up to 100 mg	Solu-Cortef	J1720	96374
Immunoglobulin, IM, 1 cc Immunoglobulin, IM, >10 cc	Gammar Gamastan	J1460 J1560	96372
Immunoglobulin, 500 mg	Gammagard S/D IV	J1566	96374
Penicillin G benzathine and penicillin G procaine, 100,000 units	Bicillin C-R	J0558	96372

● =New code ▲ =Revised code # =Re-sequenced code + =Add-on code ★ =Telemedicine

Table 11-1 (*continued*)

Injection (*continued*)	Brand Name(s)ᵃ	J Code	Administration
Penicillin G benzathine, 100,000 units	Bicillin L-A	J0561	96372
Phenytoin sodium, per 50 mg	Dilantin	J1165	96374
Promethazine hydrochloride, up to 50 mg	Phenergan	J2550	96372
Other	**Brand Nameᵃ**	**J Code**	**Administration**
Antiemetic drug, rectal/suppository, not otherwise specified	Phenergan	J8498	None
Dexamethasone, oral, 0.25 mg	Decadron	J8540	None
Prednisolone, oral, 5 mg	Delta-Cortef	J7510	None
Prednisone, immediate release or delayed release, oral, 1 mg	Rayos	J7512	None

Abbreviations: DME, durable medical equipment; FDA, US Food and Drug Administration; IM, intramuscular; IV, intravenous.

ᵃ Brand names are furnished for identification purposes only. No endorsement of the manufacturers or products is implied.

ᵇ For IV administration codes, see **Table 10-4.**

The 2022 Healthcare Common Procedure Coding System codes were released subsequent to the publication of this book. Refer to www.aap.org/cfp for updates.

36405	scalp vein
36406	other vein
36410	Venipuncture, age 3 years or older, necessitating the skill of a physician or other qualified health care professional (separate procedure), for diagnostic or therapeutic purposes (not to be used for routine venipuncture)
36415	Collection of venous blood by venipuncture
36416	Collection of capillary blood specimen (eg, finger, heel, ear stick)
36591	Collection of blood specimen from a completely implantable venous access device

Codes **36415** and **36416** are used for children of any age when the physician is not needed to perform the procedure. Code **36416** is considered bundled under the MPFS and, therefore, not separately payable. Some payers may follow this bundling practice.

- When a physician's skill is required to perform venipuncture (eg, access is too difficult for other staff to attain) on a child younger than 3 years, codes **36400–36406** are reported based on the anatomical site of the venipuncture as follows:
  - **36400** (femoral or jugular vein)
  - **36405** (scalp vein)
  - **36406** (another vein)
- When a physician's skill is required to perform venipuncture on a child 3 years and older, code **36410** is reported.

> If the physician performs the venipuncture as a convenience or because staff is not trained in the procedure, code **36415** is reported because the physician's skill was not required.

Although typically not required, some payers will require that modifier **25** be appended to the E/M code if an E/M service is reported on the same day of service.

- It is not appropriate to report *CPT* code **99211** (nurse visit) along with code **36415** if the nurse only collects the blood specimen and no medically necessary and separately identifiable E/M service is provided.
- Code **36591** (collection of blood specimen from a completely implantable venous access device) is reported only when in conjunction with a laboratory service.

> See Chapter 19 for discussion of arterial catheterization.

Arterial Puncture

36600   Arterial puncture, withdrawal of blood for diagnosis

Arterial puncture (eg, radial artery) with withdrawal of blood for diagnosis is reported with code **36600**.

> **Specimen collection (eg, nasal or oral swab, urine collection), other than blood sampling, is typically not separately reported. Follow payer guidelines when exceptions are made for specimen collection as occurred during the public health emergency due to COVID-19.**

Pathology and Laboratory Procedures

CPT laboratory codes may either be generic for a particular analyte that is independent of testing method or have a specific *CPT* code, depending on the method used for the particular analysis.

Clinical Laboratory Improvement Amendments–Waived Tests

The Clinical Laboratory Improvement Amendments (CLIA) establish quality standards for all laboratory testing to ensure the accuracy, reliability, and timeliness of patient test results regardless of where the test was performed.

- A *laboratory* is defined as any facility that performs laboratory testing on specimens derived from humans for the purpose of providing information for the diagnosis, prevention, and treatment of disease or impairment or assessment of health.
- The term *CLIA waived* refers to simple laboratory examinations and procedures that have an insignificant risk of an erroneous result. One typical test that is CLIA waived is urinalysis without microscopy (**81002**). Other tests require higher levels of CLIA certification (eg, provider-performed microscopy).
  - Payers may require a practice's current CLIA certificate number on claims.
  - Some codes represent both CLIA-waived and higher complexity test systems.

Not Sure How a Test Is Categorized?
See the US Food and Drug Administration Clinical Laboratory Improvement Amendments database at www.accessdata.fda.gov/scripts/cdrh/cfdocs/cfCLIA/search.cfm that includes tests of all categories by test system, manufacturer, or analyte. If your practice provides only waived test systems and analytes, see www.accessdata.fda.gov/scripts/cdrh/cfdocs/cfClia/analyteswaived.cfm.

- Laboratories and physician offices performing waived tests may need to append modifier **QW** to the *CPT* code for CLIA-waived procedures. The use of modifier **QW** is payer specific.

  Only a small number of CLIA-waived tests are exempt from the use of modifier **QW** (eg, **81002**, non-automated urinalysis without microscopy; **81025**, urine pregnancy test; **82272**, occult blood by peroxidase for other than colorectal neoplasm screening).

General Guidance for Reporting Laboratory Services

- A test performed in the office's laboratory should be billed by using the appropriate laboratory code and, if performed, the appropriate blood collection code (**36400–36416**).
- Link the appropriate diagnosis code to the laboratory procedure and/or venipuncture and handling fee. The diagnosis must support the medical necessity or reason for the test or service.
- If the *only service* provided is a urinalysis or the obtainment of a blood specimen, only the laboratory test and/or venipuncture or capillary finger stick is reported.
  - It is not appropriate to report a nurse visit (**99211**) in these cases.
  - If a medically necessary nursing E/M service is performed in compliance with payer guidelines (eg, incident to a physician's service) on the same date as venipuncture, append modifier **25** to code **99211**.
- Do not report any laboratory test that is *not performed* in the office (eg, thyroid function, laboratory panels, phenylketonuria). Instead, report the appropriate blood-drawing code (**36415** or **36416**), when applicable, and handling fee code (**99000**).

  Exception: Follow state regulations and payer policies for physician billing of laboratory services performed by an outside laboratory. Generally, if the laboratory bills the pediatrician for the test, bill the patient by using the appropriate laboratory analysis code with modifier **90** to indicate that the procedure was performed in an outside laboratory.

Example

➤ **The physician orders a laboratory test requiring a blood sample, and the nurse obtains the blood via venipuncture.** The specimen is sent to an outside laboratory for processing.

Only the venipuncture (**36415**) and handling fee (**99000**) would be reported in addition to the E/M service and other procedures performed on that day.

Laboratory Panel Coding

All laboratory test panels in *CPT* were specifically developed for coding purposes only and should not be interpreted as clinical parameters. (See codes **80047–80076** for a component listing of these panels.) For example, the lipid panel (**80061**) includes total cholesterol (**82465**), high-density lipoprotein cholesterol (**83718**), and triglycerides (**84478**). Any additional tests performed can be coded separately from the panel code. *Do not unbundle individual laboratory tests if a laboratory panel code is available.*

Direct Optical Observation

Direct optical (ie, visual) observation is a testing platform that provides a result (ie, positive or negative) by producing a signal on the reaction chamber (eg, test strip with colored bands) that can be interpreted visually (eg, point-of-care influenza testing). (See codes **87804** [influenza], **87807** [respiratory syncytial virus], and **87880** [group A streptococcus].)

Per *CPT*, when reporting tests using direct optical observation, the number of results (eg, 2 results—positive for influenza A and negative for influenza B) determines the units of service reported.

A test for coronavirus (SARS-CoV-2) by direct optical observation is discussed in the SARS-CoV-2 Infection Testing section later in this chapter.

Cultures

- Use code **87086** (culture, bacterial; quantitative colony count, urine) once per encounter for urine culture to determine the approximate number of bacteria present per milliliter of urine.
- Use of a commercial kit with defined media to identify isolates in a positive urine culture is reported with **87088** (culture, bacterial; quantitative colony count, urine with isolation and presumptive identification of each isolate).
- Code **81007** (urinalysis; bacteriuria screen, except by culture or dipstick) (CLIA waived) can be used for a bacteriuria screen by non-culture technique using a commercial kit. The type of commercial kit must be specified.
- Code **87070** (culture, bacterial; any other source except urine, blood, or stool) is reported for throat cultures.
- Use code **87045** to report culture, bacteria of the stool, aerobic, with isolation and preliminary examination (eg, Kligler [triple sugar] iron agar, lysine iron agar) for *Salmonella* and *Shigella* species. Additional pathogens are reported with code **87046** with 1 unit per plate.
- Culture, presumptive pathogenic organisms, screening only (**87081**), is reported for testing for a specific organism (eg, *Streptococcus*).
- Report services with the symptoms (eg, dysuria) or the confirmed diagnosis (eg, urinary tract infection).

Proprietary Laboratory Analysis and Multianalyte Assays With Algorithmic Analyses

To report testing using a proprietary laboratory analysis (PLA) or multianalyte assays with algorithmic analyses (MAAA), see Appendix O in your *CPT* reference and, for quarterly code updates, www.ama-assn.org/practice-management/cpt/cpt-pla-codes. Code selection for PLA and MAAA codes is based on the analysis performed and the proprietary name of the test. **Table 11-2** exemplifies how PLA and MAAA codes are listed in Appendix O.

Table 11-2. Example of Appendix O Proprietary Laboratory Analysis Code List

Test Name	Code	Code Descriptor
ePlex Respiratory Pathogen Panel 2, GenMark Dx, GenMark Diagnostics, Inc	0225U	Infectious disease (bacterial or viral respiratory tract infection), pathogen-specific DNA and RNA, 21 targets, including severe acute respiratory syndrome coronavirus 2 (SARS-CoV-2), amplified probe technique, including multiplex reverse transcription for RNA targets, each analyte reported as detected or not detected

Laboratory Tests Frequently Performed in the Office

Coronavirus (SARS-CoV-2) Testing

The coronavirus pandemic was ongoing at the time this publication was written. Because the frequency at which we will see this virus is unclear, the codes for testing will be included until they are no longer needed. Related tests include those to detect the virus and those to detect antibodies to the virus as available at time of publication.

Some tests for SARS-CoV-2 are designated as CLIA waived under an Emergency Use Authorization. It is advisable to verify the current classification of a test before purchase.

> During the public health emergency (PHE) due to COVID-19, some payers specifically instruct that code 99211 be reported when clinical staff assess a patient for COVID-19 exposure or symptoms and collect a specimen to test for COVID-19 (without requirement for continuing a physician's plan of care for an established problem). Payer policies may change during or after the PHE, so individual payer guidance should be verified.

SARS-CoV-2 Infection Testing

When multiple specimens are collected (eg, nasopharyngeal and oropharyngeal swabs), verify payer instructions for reporting separate assays on each specimen (eg, report **87635** and **87635 59**).

87635	Infectious agent detection by nucleic acid (DNA or RNA); severe acute respiratory syndrome coronavirus 2 (SARS-CoV-2) (Coronavirus disease [COVID-19]), amplified probe technique
▲87426	Infectious agent antigen detection by immunoassay technique (eg, enzyme immunoassay [EIA], enzyme-linked immunosorbent assay [ELISA], fluorescence immunoassay [FIA], immunochemiluminometric assay [IMCA]), qualitative or semiquantitative; severe acute respiratory syndrome coronavirus (eg, SARS-CoV, SARS-CoV-2 [COVID-19]) (CLIA-waived)
#●87811	Infectious agent antigen detection by immunoassay with direct optical (ie, visual) observation; severe acute respiratory syndrome coronavirus 2 (SARS-CoV-2) (Coronavirus disease [COVID-19]) (CLIA-waived)

See also HCPCS codes **U0001–U0004**, which may be used to identify tests developed by the Centers for Disease Control and Prevention and/or performed via high-throughput technologies.

Combination Testing for SARS-CoV-2 and Other Infectious Agent(s)

To distinctly report testing for SARS-CoV-2 infection (COVID-19) in combination with other seasonal respiratory infections, *CPT* includes distinct combination codes for these services. Do not report **87631–87633**, infectious agent detection by nucleic acid (DNA or RNA); respiratory virus (eg, adenovirus, influenza virus, coronavirus, metapneumovirus, parainfluenza virus, respiratory syncytial virus, rhinovirus) (reported by number of targets).

#●87428	Infectious agent antigen detection by immunoassay technique (eg, enzyme immunoassay [EIA], enzyme-linked immunosorbent assay [ELISA], fluorescence immunoassay [FIA], immunochemiluminometric assay [IMCA]), qualitative or semiquantitative; severe acute respiratory syndrome coronavirus (eg, SARS-CoV, SARS-CoV-2 [COVID-19]) and influenza virus types A and B
●87636	Infectious agent detection by nucleic acid (DNA or RNA); severe acute respiratory syndrome coronavirus 2 (SARS-CoV-2) (Coronavirus disease [COVID-19]) and influenza virus types A and B, multiplex amplified probe technique
●87637	Infectious agent detection by nucleic acid (DNA or RNA); severe acute respiratory syndrome coronavirus 2 (SARS-CoV-2) (Coronavirus disease [COVID-19]), influenza virus types A and B, and respiratory syncytial virus, multiplex amplified probe technique

Proprietary laboratory analysis codes for detecting SARS-CoV-2 in addition to other pathogens include the following. The specific test name follows the code descriptor. Remember that both the code descriptor and the proprietary name must match the test performed.

0202U	Infectious disease (bacterial or viral respiratory tract infection), pathogen-specific nucleic acid (DNA or RNA), 22 targets including severe acute respiratory syndrome coronavirus 2 (SARS-CoV-2), qualitative RT-PCR, nasopharyngeal swab, each pathogen reported as detected or not detected (BioFire Respiratory Panel 2.1 [RP2.1], BioFire Diagnostics, BioFire Diagnostics, LLC)

0223U Infectious disease (bacterial or viral respiratory tract infection), pathogen-specific nucleic acid (DNA or RNA), 22 targets including severe acute respiratory syndrome coronavirus 2 (SARS-CoV-2), qualitative RT-PCR, nasopharyngeal swab, each pathogen reported as detected or not detected (QIAstat-Dx Respiratory SARS-CoV-2 Panel, QIAGEN Sciences, QIAGEN GMbH)

0225U Infectious disease (bacterial or viral respiratory tract infection), pathogen-specific DNA and RNA, 21 targets, including severe acute respiratory syndrome coronavirus 2 (SARS-CoV-2), amplified probe technique, including multiplex reverse transcription for RNA targets, each analyte reported as detected or not detected (ePlex Respiratory Pathogen Panel 2, GenMark Dx, GenMark Diagnostics, Inc)

0240U Infectious disease (viral respiratory tract infection), pathogen-specific RNA, 3 targets (severe acute respiratory syndrome coronavirus 2 [SARS-CoV-2], influenza A, influenza B), upper respiratory specimen, each pathogen reported as detected or not detected (Xpert Xpress SARS-CoV-2/Flu/RSV [SARS-CoV-2 & Flu targets only], Cepheid)

0241U Infectious disease (viral respiratory tract infection), pathogen-specific RNA, 4 targets (severe acute respiratory syndrome coronavirus 2 [SARS-CoV-2], influenza A, influenza B, respiratory syncytial virus [RSV]), upper respiratory specimen, each pathogen reported as detected or not detected (Xpert Xpress SARS-CoV-2/Flu/RSV [all targets], Cepheid)

> It is important to note that the same cartridge is used for the assay performed with respiratory syncytial virus (RSV) analysis (0241U) or without RSV analysis (0240U), and the code selection is differentiated by the number of targets tested.

SARS-CoV-2 Antibody Testing

Testing for antibodies produced in response to COVID-19 may be performed to identify antibodies to SARS-CoV-2 (eg, 86328, 86413) or to determine whether the antibodies present can block the infection (86408, 86409; 0226U).

86328 Immunoassay for infectious agent antibody(ies), qualitative or semi-quantitative, single step method (eg, reagent strip); severe acute respiratory syndrome coronavirus 2 (SARS-CoV-2) (Coronavirus disease [COVID-19])

> Code 86328 is reported with 1 unit per reagent strip regardless of the number of antibodies evaluated and reported.

86413 Severe acute respiratory syndrome coronavirus 2 (SARS-CoV-2) (Coronavirus disease [COVID-19]) antibody, quantitative

86769 Antibody; severe acute respiratory syndrome coronavirus 2 (SARS-CoV-2) (Coronavirus disease [COVID-19])

> When 2 distinct analyses are performed (eg, immunoglobulins G and M), report codes 86769 and 86769 59.

0224U Antibody, severe acute respiratory syndrome coronavirus 2 (SARS-CoV-2) (Coronavirus disease [COVID-19]), includes titer(s), when performed (COVID-19 Antibody Test, Mt Sinai, Mount Sinai Laboratory)

Neutralizing antibody tests determine whether antibodies in a patient specimen can directly block the infection of cells expressing the viral entry receptor on their surface. Screening for neutralizing antibodies to COVID-19 is reported with 86408. Measurement of the level of neutralizing activity of COVID-19 antibodies is reported with 86409.

#●86408 Neutralizing antibody, severe acute respiratory syndrome coronavirus 2 (SARS-CoV-2) (Coronavirus disease [COVID-19]); screen

#●86409 Neutralizing antibody, severe acute respiratory syndrome coronavirus 2 (SARS-CoV-2) (Coronavirus disease [COVID-19]); titer

●0226U Surrogate viral neutralization test (sVNT), severe acute respiratory syndrome coronavirus 2 (SARS-CoV-2) (Coronavirus disease [COVID-19]), ELISA, plasma, serum (Tru-Immune, Ethos Laboratories, GenScript USA Inc)

Urinalysis

81000	Urinalysis, by dipstick or tablet reagent for bilirubin, glucose, hemoglobin, ketones, leukocytes, nitrite, pH, protein, specific gravity, urobilinogen, any number of these constituents; nonautomated, with microscopy
81001	as per **81000** with microscopy, but automated
81002	as per **81000** but without microscopy (CLIA waived)
81003	as per **81000** but without microscopy, automated (CLIA waived)

It is important to report the correct code for the urinalysis test performed.

- Code **81000** is reported when the results are shown as color changes for multiple analytes (eg, ketones, specific gravity) that are compared against a standardized chart (nonautomated) and when microscopy (in a second step, the urine is centrifuged and examined under microscope) is performed.

- Code **81002** is reported if the test results are obtained by the same method but a microscopic examination is not performed.

- Codes **81001** and **81003** are reported for urinalysis performed by a processor that reads the results (automated).

For urinalysis, infectious agent detection, semiquantitative analysis of volatile compounds, use code **81099**.

Urine Pregnancy Test

81025	Urine pregnancy test, by visual color comparison method (CLIA waived)

Report code **81025** with *International Classification of Diseases, 10th Revision, Clinical Modification* (*ICD-10-CM*) codes **Z32.00–Z32.02**, depending on the findings of the test (ie, unconfirmed result, positive result, or negative result).

Glucose Tests

82947	Glucose, quantitative, blood (without a reagent strip) (CLIA waived)
82948	blood, reagent strip
82951	Glucose tolerance test (GTT), 3 specimens (CLIA waived)
82952	each additional beyond 3 specimens (CLIA waived)
82962	Glucose, blood by glucose monitoring device(s) cleared by the FDA specifically for home use (CLIA waived)
83036	Hemoglobin; glycosylated (A_{1c}) (CLIA waived)
83037	Hemoglobin; glycosylated (A_{1c}) by device cleared by FDA for home use (CLIA waived)

Report code **83037** for in-office hemoglobin A_{1c} measurement using a device that is cleared by the FDA for home use. This test is not limited to use in a patient's home.

Code **82962** describes the method when whole blood is obtained (usually by finger-stick device) and assayed by glucose oxidase, hexokinase, or electrochemical methods and spectrophotometry using a small portable device designed for home blood glucose monitoring. The devices are also used in physician offices, during home visits, or in clinics.

Continuous glucose monitoring is reported with codes **95249–95251** (see discussion later in this chapter).

Hematology

85013	Spun microhematocrit (CLIA waived)
85018	Hemoglobin (CLIA waived)
85025–85027	Complete blood cell count, automated (**85025** is CLIA waived.)
88738	Hemoglobin (Hgb), quantitative, transcutaneous

If using a complete blood cell count (CBC) machine to perform only a hemoglobin test, follow these guidelines.

- If the CBC result is normal, only the hemoglobin may be reported because that was the medically necessary test ordered.

- If the CBC reveals an abnormality and it is addressed during the course of the visit, the CBC result may be reported. The abnormality would be linked to the procedure, and the medical record would need to include documentation for the ordering of the test and to support the medical necessity of the procedure.

Influenza—Point-of-Care Testing

87502	Infectious agent detection by nucleic acid (DNA or RNA); influenza virus, for multiple types or sub-types, includes multiplex reverse transcription, when performed, and multiplex amplified probe technique, first 2 types or sub-types (CLIA waived)

● =New code   ▲ =Revised code   # =Re-sequenced code   + =Add-on code   ★ =Telemedicine

▲87804   Infectious agent antigen detection by immunoassay with direct optical (ie, visual) observation; influenza (CLIA waived)

> **Code 87502 describes a test that already takes into account the first 2 types or subtypes; therefore, do not report multiple units of code 87502 for the separate testing of influenza A and B.**

- Code **87804** may be reported twice with modifier **59** appended to the second code when tests performed separately detect the influenza A and B antigen, providing 2 distinct results. This applies whether the test kit uses 1 or 2 analytic chambers to deliver 2 distinct results.
  — Check with payers; some do not recognize modifier **59** and may require reporting with 2 units of service and no modifier.
  — Some payers (eg, Medicaid plans) may limit units reported to the number of separate test kits used rather than following *CPT* instruction.

   See also the Combination Testing for SARS-CoV-2 and Other Infectious Agent(s) section earlier in this chapter for a discussion of codes as related to combination testing of COVID-19 and other respiratory illnesses, including influenza.

Lead Testing

83655   Lead, quantitative analysis (CLIA waived)

- This test does not specify the specimen source or the method of testing. Alternative tests sometimes (although rarely) used for lead screening are **82135** (aminolevulinic acid, delta), **84202** (protoporphyrin, red blood cell count, quantitative), and **84203** (protoporphyrin, red blood cell count, screen).
- Some states provide lead testing at no cost to patients covered under the Medicaid Early and Periodic Screening, Diagnostic, and Treatment program. Check your state Medicaid requirements for reporting this service.
- Report *ICD-10-CM* code **Z13.88** (encounter for screening for disorder due to exposure to contaminants) when performing lead screening. Some payers require **Z77.011**, contact with and (suspected) exposure to lead, in lieu of **Z13.88**.

> *International Classification of Diseases, 10th Revision, Clinical Modification* **allows separate reporting of special screening examinations (codes in categories Z11–Z13) in addition to the codes for routine child health examinations (eg, Z00.121, Z00.129) when these codes provide additional information. A screening code is not necessary if the screening is inherent to a routine examination.**

Mononucleosis—Heterophile Antibodies Screening

86308   Heterophile antibodies; screening (CLIA waived)

   This code may be appropriate for rapid mononucleosis screening.

Papanicolaou Tests

- The laboratory performing the cytology and interpretation reports Papanicolaou (Pap) tests with codes **88141–88155**, **88164–88167**, or **88174** and **88175**.
- Obtaining a Pap test specimen is inherent to the physical examination performed during a preventive medicine visit or a problem-oriented office visit.
- Medicare does require reporting HCPCS code **Q0091** (screening Papanicolaou, obtaining, preparing, and conveyance of cervical and vaginal smear to laboratory) in addition to the E/M service for preventive medicine and problem-oriented office visits.
  — Some state Medicaid programs and commercial payers may also recognize obtaining a Pap test as a separate service.
  — Code **Q0091** cannot be reported when a patient must return for a repeat Pap test due to inadequate initial sampling.
  — If not reporting **Q0091**, a handling fee (**99000**) can be reported in addition to an E/M service if the Pap test was obtained and sent to a laboratory.
- The appropriate *ICD-10-CM* code to link to the E/M code or code **Q0091** is either **Z01.411** (encounter for gynecological examination [general] [routine] with abnormal findings) or **Z01.419** (encounter for gynecological examination [general] [routine] without abnormal findings).
- For screening cervical Pap test not part of a gynecologic examination, report *ICD-10-CM* code **Z12.4** (encounter for screening for malignant neoplasm of cervix).
- For high-risk patients, you may also report secondary diagnosis codes to indicate personal history of other medical treatment (**Z92.89**) or other contact with and (suspected) exposures hazardous to health (**Z77.9**).

Presumptive Drug Tests

#80305   Drug test(s), presumptive, any number of drug classes, any number of devices or procedures; capable of being read by direct optical observation only (eg, utilizing immunoassay [eg, dipsticks, cups, cards, or cartridges]); includes sample validation when performed, per date of service (CLIA waived)

#80306   read by instrument assisted direct optical observation (eg, utilizing immunoassay [eg, dipsticks, cups, cards, or cartridges]); includes sample validation when performed, per date of service

#80307   by instrument chemistry analyzers (eg, utilizing immunoassay [eg, EIA, ELISA, EMIT, FPIA, IA, KIMS, RIA]), chromatography (eg, GC, HPLC), and mass spectrometry either with or without chromatography (eg, DART, DESI, GC-MS, GC-MS/MS, LC-MS, LC-MS/MS, LDTD, MALDI, TOF); includes sample validation when performed, per date of service

- Presumptive drug class screening includes all drugs and drug classes performed by the respective methodology (eg, dipstick kit with direct optical observation) on a single date of service. Sample validation is included in presumptive drug screening service.
- Venipuncture to obtain samples for drug testing may be separately reportable with code **36415** (collection of venous blood by venipuncture).
- When testing is performed with a method using direct optical observation to determine the result, code **80305** is reported. Tests that have a waived status under CLIA may be reported with modifier **QW** (waived test).
- When a reader is used to determine the result of testing (eg, a dipstick is inserted into a machine that determines the final reading), code **80306** is reported.
- Testing that uses a chemistry analyzer or more effort than tests represented by codes **80305** and **80306** is reported with code **80307**.

Respiratory Syncytial Virus Test

87634   Infectious agent detection by nucleic acid (DNA or RNA); respiratory syncytial virus, amplified probe technique

▲87807   Infectious agent antigen detection by immunoassay with direct optical (ie, visual) observation; respiratory syncytial virus (CLIA waived)

For assays that include respiratory syncytial virus (RSV) with additional respiratory viruses, see **87631–87633**. Tests reported with codes **87631** and **87633** are CLIA waived. Append modifier **QW** if required. See also the Combination Testing for SARS-CoV-2 and Other Infectious Agent(s) section earlier in this chapter for a discussion of codes as related to tests for combinations of respiratory infectious agents, including SARS-CoV-2, influenzavirus, and RSV.

Serum and Transcutaneous Bilirubin Testing

82247   Total bilirubin (CLIA waived)

82248   Direct bilirubin

88720   Transcutaneous total bilirubin

Streptococcal Test

▲87880   Infectious agent antigen detection by immunoassay with direct optical (ie, visual) observation; streptococcus group A (CLIA waived)

87651   Infectious agent detection by nucleic acid (DNA or RNA); streptococcus, group A, amplified probe technique (CLIA waived)

87081   Culture, presumptive pathogenic organisms, screening only

▲87430   Enzyme immunoassay, qualitative, streptococcus group A

- Report the code based on the test method rather than on the site of specimen collection.
- Culture plates using sheep blood agar with bacitracin disks should be coded with **87081**.

Testing Stool for Occult Blood

82272   Blood, occult, by peroxidase activity (eg, guaiac), qualitative, feces, 1–3 simultaneous determinations, performed for other than colorectal neoplasm screening (CLIA waived)

- Code **82272** is reported when a single sample is obtained from a digital rectal examination or a multi-test card is returned from the patient and is tested for blood. Report **82272** with 1 unit when up to 3 cards are returned.

Chapter 11. Common Non-facility Testing and Therapeutic Services

Tuberculosis Skin Test (Mantoux)

86580   Tuberculosis, intradermal

- This test is exempt from CLIA requirements.
- The tuberculosis (TB) skin test (Mantoux) using the intradermal administration of purified protein derivative (PPD) is the recommended diagnostic skin test for TB.
  - This is not the BCG TB vaccine.
  - The American Academy of Pediatrics (AAP) supports the use of the Mantoux test (TB, intradermal) for TB screening when appropriate
- A separate administration code *is not reported* when the PPD is placed.
- Code **99211** is the appropriate code to report the reading of a PPD test when that is the only reason for the encounter.

  The appropriate *ICD-10-CM* code is **Z11.1** (encounter for screening for respiratory TB). In the case of a positive test result when the physician sees the patient, the complexity may lead to a higher-level code.
- Because risk-based testing is recommended for pediatric patients, an E/M service to evaluate the need for testing may be indicated when testing is requested by a third party (eg, school, employer).
- If TB testing by cell-mediated immunity antigen response measurement, gamma interferon (**86480**) is ordered, and a specimen obtained, venipuncture (**36415**) may be separately reported.

Zika Virus Testing

86794   Zika virus, IgM
87662   Zika virus, amplified probe technique

- The amplified probe technique (**87662**) is used when potential exposure occurred 2 weeks or more prior to testing.
- The IgM test described by code **86794** is used when suspected patient exposure to the Zika virus was less than 2 weeks before testing.

Respiratory Function Tests and Treatments

Pulmonary Function Tests

National Correct Coding Initiative (NCCI) edits exist between office-based E/M services and all pulmonology services (**94010–94799**). Append modifier **25** to the E/M service code as appropriate when reporting a pulmonology service on the same claim.

> There is no code for peak flow analysis or oxygen administration. These services are considered part of the evaluation and management service and/or a component of pulmonary function testing.

- Codes include laboratory procedure(s) and interpretation of test results. If a separately identifiable E/M service is performed, the appropriate E/M service code may also be reported.
- When spirometry (**94010**) is performed before and after administration of a bronchodilator, report only code **94060** (bronchodilation responsiveness, spirometry as in **94010**, pre- and post-bronchodilator administration).
  - Code **94640** (nebulizer treatment) is inherent to (ie, included as part of) code **94060**. When an additional nebulizer treatment is performed as a distinct separate procedure on the same date as **94060**, NCCI edits allow use of a modifier (eg, **94640 59**), when applicable.
  - Relative value units assigned to codes include typical supplies (eg, masks, tubing). Report codes for supplies only if the payer does not use an RVU payment methodology.
  - Medication is separately reported with the appropriate HCPCS code (eg, **J7613**, albuterol, inhalation solution, FDA-approved final product, noncompounded, administered through DME, unit dose, 1 mg).
- Measurement of vital capacity (**94150**) is a component of spirometry and is only reported when performed alone.
- Measurement of spirometric forced expiratory flows in an infant or child through 2 years of age is reported with code **94011**.
- Code **94012** is used to report measurement of bronchodilation spirometric forced expiratory flows (before and after bronchodilator) in an infant or child.
- Code **94013** is used to report measurement of lung volumes (eg, functional residual capacity, expiratory reserve volume, forced vital capacity) in an infant or child through 2 years of age.

> *Current Procedural Terminology* guidelines allow reporting pulse oximetry (**94760, 94761**), but health plans using the Medicare Physician Fee Schedule will pay only if no other service is paid to the same physician on the same date (ie, some plans consider this an examination component similar to determining blood pressure).

- Pulmonary stress testing (**94618**) includes measurement of heart rate, oximetry, and oxygen titration, when performed. If spirometry is performed prior to and following a pulmonary stress test, separately report 2 units of spirometry (**94010**).

Inhalation Treatment

94640   Pressurized or nonpressurized inhalation treatment for acute airway obstruction for therapeutic purposes and/or for diagnostic purposes such as sputum induction with an aerosol generator, nebulizer, metered dose inhaler (MDI) or intermittent positive pressure breathing (IPPB) device

94644   Continuous inhalation treatment with aerosol medication for acute airway obstruction; first hour (For services of less than 1 hour, use **94640**)

+94645   each additional hour (List separately in addition to code for primary procedure)

   Report **94640**

- When treatment such as aerosol generator, nebulizer, MDI, or IPPB device is administered.
- With modifier **76** (repeat procedure) with the number of units when more than 1 treatment is given on a date of service. Some payers require reporting with the number of units only and no modifier. Follow payer guidelines for reporting these services.
- When any treatment of less than 30 minutes is performed.

> *Current Procedural Terminology* code **94060** includes spirometry and pre- and post-bronchodilation. Report only **94060** when **94010** and/or **94640** is a component of the **94060** service.

   Current NCCI edit policy does not allow reporting code **94640** more than once per patient encounter. The AAP is working with NCCI edit staff to change this policy.

   Report codes **94644** and **94645** when

- A treatment lasts 31 minutes or longer.
- The total time spent in the provision of continuous inhalation treatments is documented in the medical record.

   Codes **94644** and **94645** are not reported by physicians when services are provided in a facility setting because no physician work value is assigned to these codes.

Nebulizer Demonstration or Evaluation

94664   Demonstration and/or evaluation of patient utilization of an aerosol generator, nebulizer, metered dose inhaler or IPPB device

- Code **94664** is reported only once per date of service.
- Report code **94664** (demonstration and/or evaluation of patient utilization of an aerosol generator, nebulizer, MDI, or IPPB device) when an initial or subsequent demonstration and/or evaluation is performed and documented.
- Physicians providing nebulizer instruction in conjunction with an E/M service may include the time of nebulizer instruction in the time of counseling and/or coordination of care or the total physician time on the date of an office E/M service (**99202–99205, 99212–99215**) in lieu of reporting **94664**. No physician work is attributed to code **94664**.

   When the physician or nurse (of the same group and specialty) performs demonstration and/or evaluation of patient use of a device such as an MDI (**94664**) on the same day as a nebulizer treatment (**94640**), modifier **59** (distinct procedural service) should be appended to code **94664** to indicate to the payer that the services were separate and distinct and that both were clinically indicated.

- Per the Medicaid NCCI manual, the demonstration and/or evaluation described by code **94664** is included in code **94640** if the same device (eg, aerosol generator) is used for both services. The NCCI edits pair code **94664** with **94640** but allow an override of the edit with modifier **59** when both services are indicated (eg, treatment via nebulizer and teaching for MDI). However, some payers may not allow the use of modifier **59** in this instance if the 2 services did not occur at separate encounters. Check with your Medicaid payers.

Modifier **25** should be appended to an E/M service code reported on the same date to signify a separately identifiable service. All services must be documented in the medical record as significant, separately identifiable, and medically necessary.

Examples

➤ **A 6-year-old established patient with asthma arrives to the office in acute asthma exacerbation.** Pulse oximetry is performed and indicative of moderate asthma exacerbation. One nebulizer treatment is given via a small-volume nebulizer. Physical examination after first treatment shows decreased wheezing and work of breathing. Pulse oximetry is remeasured and normal. An asthma control test is completed, scored, and documented. An order is written for continuing treatments at home, evaluation and education in use of MDI, and return to the office as needed. The nurse documents her evaluation of use and education for home use of the MDI. Later the same day, the patient returns, again in acute exacerbation. A second nebulizer treatment is given by a small-volume nebulizer. Physical examination after the second treatment shows no improvement and the patient is borderline hypoxic on second pulse oxygen measurement. He is sent to the hospital to be admitted to observation by a hospitalist. Diagnosis is acute exacerbation of mild persistent asthma with hypoxemia.

ICD-10-CM	**J45.31** (mild persistent asthma with acute exacerbation) **R09.02** (hypoxemia)
CPT	**99214** or **99215 25** (office/outpatient E/M, established patient) **94640** × 1, **94640 76** × 1 unit (nebulizer treatments) **96160** (administration of asthma control test) **94664 59** (MDI demonstration) Medication (appropriate HCPCS code; see examples in **Table 11-1**) **94761** (pulse oximetry, multiple determinations)

Teaching Point: Modifier **59** appended to **94664** indicates the MDI demonstration is reported in addition to nebulizer treatments provided via a different device. Physicians should also report any medications provided at the expense of the practice. HCPCS codes describe medications such as albuterol. (See HCPCS codes listed in **Table 11-1**.) The documented severity of the exacerbation in combination with a decision about hospital admission will support either **99214** (less than severe exacerbation) or **99215** (severe exacerbation).

Car Seat/Bed Testing

94780   Car seat/bed testing for airway integrity, for infants through 12 months of age, with continual clinical staff observation and continuous recording of pulse oximetry, heart rate and respiratory rate, with interpretation and report; 60 minutes

+94781   each additional full 30 minutes (List separately in addition to **94780**.)

To report codes **94780** and **94781**, the following conditions must be met:

- The patient must be an infant (12 months or younger). Reassessment after the patient is 29 days or older may be necessary.
- Continual clinical staff observation with continuous recording of pulse oximetry, heart rate, and respiratory rate is required.
- Vital signs and observations must be reviewed and interpreted and a written report generated by the physician.
- Codes are reported based on the total observation time spent and documented.
- If less than 60 minutes is spent in the procedure, code **94780** may not be reported.
- Each additional full 30 minutes (ie, not less than 90 minutes total) is reported with code **94781**.
- A significant, separately identifiable office or other outpatient E/M service [eg, **99213 25**]) may be reported on the same data as car seat/bed testing, when provided.

Example

➤ **A male neonate born at 34 weeks' gestation was released from the hospital 2 weeks ago with instructions to the parents to use only a car bed when transporting him until the pediatrician retests and determines that the neonate can safely ride in a car seat.** The newborn is seen in the outpatient clinic for a preventive medicine visit, and car seat testing is conducted for a period of 1 hour and 45 minutes. The physician reviews and interprets the nurse's records of pulse oximetry, heart and respiratory rates, and observations during the testing period. The interpretation is documented in a formal report and plan of care clearing the neonate to begin use of a rear-facing car seat. The plan of care is discussed with the parents, who also receive further instruction on appropriate use of the car seat.

ICD-10-CM	Codes for conditions of the newborn and **P07.37** (preterm newborn, gestational age 34 completed weeks)
CPT	**94780** (car seat/bed testing; first 60 minutes) **94781** (each additional full 30 minutes)

Teaching Point: In this scenario, a total of 105 minutes of testing was conducted. This would be reported with 1 unit of code **94780** for the initial 60 minutes of testing and 1 unit of code **94781** for the last 45 minutes (only 1 full period of 30 minutes beyond the first 60 minutes was performed). The 15 minutes beyond the last full 30-minute period are not separately reported. An associated preventive E/M service with modifier **25** would be separately reportable.

Allergy and Clinical Immunology

Allergy Testing

95004   Percutaneous tests (scratch, puncture, prick) with allergenic extracts, immediate type reaction, including test interpretation and report, specify number of tests

95017   Allergy testing, any combination of percutaneous (scratch, puncture, prick) and intracutaneous (intradermal), sequential and incremental, with venoms, immediate type reaction, including test interpretation and report, specify number of tests

95018   Allergy testing, any combination of percutaneous (scratch, puncture, prick) and intracutaneous (intradermal), sequential and incremental, with drugs or biologicals, immediate type reaction, including test interpretation and report, specify number of tests

95024   Intracutaneous (intradermal) tests with allergenic extracts, immediate type reaction, including test interpretation and report, specify number of tests

95027   Intracutaneous (intradermal) tests, sequential and incremental, with allergenic extracts for airborne allergens, immediate type reaction, including test interpretation and report, specify number of tests

95028   Intracutaneous (intradermal) tests with allergenic extracts, delayed type reaction, including reading, specify number of tests

- *CPT* codes for allergy testing are reported by type of test.
  - Percutaneous, immediate type reaction (**95004**)
  - Intracutaneous (intradermal) with immediate (**95024**, **95027**) or delayed type reaction (**95028**)
  - Any combination of percutaneous and intracutaneous, sequential and incremental tests with venoms (**95017**) or with drugs or biologicals (**95018**)
- Specification of the number of tests applied is required for accurate reporting of the units of service provided. Medicaid NCCI edits do not allow inclusion of positive or negative controls in the number of tests reported.
- Codes **95004**, **95017**, **95018**, **95024**, and **95027** include test interpretation and report. Code **95028** includes reading.

An E/M service should not be reported for interpretation and report. However, if a significant, separately identifiable E/M service is performed and documented, it may be reported with modifier **25** appended to the appropriate E/M code.

Example

➤ **A patient with seasonal allergies undergoes percutaneous testing with 24 allergenic extracts.** A clinician administers the extracts per the physician's order and monitors the patient for signs of reaction. For each extract administered, the reaction (eg, size of wheal) or lack of reaction is noted. The physician interprets the test and creates a report of the findings.

The physician reports code **95004** with 24 units of service. If a significant E/M service is provided on the same date and is separately identifiable in the documentation from the preservice and post-service work of the testing (eg, interpretation and report), append modifier **25** to the code for the E/M service provided.

See "Allergy Skin Testing: Codes, Unit Counts, and Tips for Reporting" in the February 2020 *AAP Pediatric Coding Newsletter*™ for more information (https://coding.solutions.aap.org/article.aspx?articleid=2759685; subscription required).

- Patch and photo patch testing are reported with code **95044–95056**.
- Specific challenge testing (**95060–95079**) is coded according to target organ (eg, ophthalmic mucous membrane, nasal, inhalation bronchial challenges without pulmonary function testing, ingestion).
- Nasal cytology, a test for allergy-type cells (eosinophils) or infection-type cells (neutrophils) on a nasal scraping, is reported with code **89190**.
- Nitric oxide expired gas determination is reported with code **95012**. Nitric oxide determination by spectroscopy should be reported with code **94799**.

Allergen Immunotherapy

Codes for allergen immunotherapy are reported based on the service provided: preparation and provision of allergen extract only, administration only, or combined provision and administration.

An appropriate office or outpatient code may be reported with allergen immunotherapy codes. Modifier **25** is appended to the E/M service when it is performed and documented.

Preparation and Provision of Extract Only

95144	Professional services for the supervision of the preparation and provision of antigens for allergen immunotherapy, single-dose vials(s) (specify number of vials)
95145	Professional services for the supervision of the preparation and provision of antigens for allergy immunotherapy (specify number of doses); single stinging insect venom
95146	2 stinging insect venoms
95147	3 stinging insect venoms
95148	4 stinging insect venoms
95149	5 stinging insect venoms
95165	Professional services for the supervision of preparation and provision of antigens for allergen immunotherapy; single or multiple antigens (specify number of doses)
95170	Professional services for the supervision of preparation and provision of antigens for allergen immunotherapy; whole body extract of biting insect or other arthropod (specify number of doses)

- Codes **95144–95170** are used to report preparation and provision of antigens for allergen immunotherapy without administration of the allergenic extract.
  - Codes **95144–95170** describe the preparation of the antigen, the antigen extract itself, the physician's assessment and determination of the concentration and volume to use based on the patient's history and results of previous skin testing, and the prospective planned schedule of administration of the extract.
  - The number vials must be specified when reporting code **95144**.
  - Report codes **95145–95170** based on the *number of doses* (eg, preparation of 2 vials that will provide 20 doses of extract containing 4 insect venoms is reported with code **95148** and 20 units of service).
  - Services may be reported at the time the allergenic extract is prepared because injections occur on later dates (prospectively planned) or may not occur at all.
  - Administration of the allergenic extract is not included.
- Report **95146–95149** for preparation of extracts containing more than 1 single stinging venom (eg, code **95146** is reported for 2; code **95147** is reported for 3).

National Correct Coding Initiative Immunotherapy Edits

The Medicaid National Correct Coding Initiative (NCCI) manual instructs that for purposes of reporting units of service for antigen preparation (ie, *Current Procedural Terminology* codes 95145–95170), the physician reports "number of doses." The NCCI program defines a dose for reporting purposes as 1 mL. Thus, if a physician prepares a 10-mL vial of antigen, the physician may only report a maximum of 10 UOS for that vial even if the number of actual administered doses is greater than 10. Verify payer policies on units of service before reporting.

Administration of Extract Only

95115   Professional services for allergen immunotherapy not including provision of allergenic extracts; single injection

95117   2 or more injections

Either code **95115** or **95117** (not both) are used to report administration of the allergenic extract only. Report based on the number of injections when another health care professional (eg, the patient's allergist) has prepared and supplied the allergenic extract or when a physician (usually an allergist) administers the prospectively prepared extract (ie, prepared with the intent to administer on a planned schedule).

Example

➤ **The pediatrician administers 3 injections of allergen extract for a patient with allergic rhinitis due to pollen.** The extract was prepared and supplied by an allergist.

The pediatrician will report code **95117** with *ICD-10-CM* code **J30.1**.

Combined Provision of Allergenic Extract With Administration

Current Procedural Terminology (*CPT*) recommends codes 95120–95134 be reported only when specifically required by the payer. These codes are not assigned relative value units in the Medicare Physician Fee Schedule that many payers use as a basis for physician payment. The Centers for Medicare & Medicaid Services (CMS) Medicare program will only accept codes 95115, 95117, and 95144–95170 and will not allow payment for codes 95120–95134. State Medicaid and commercial payers may follow the CMS Medicare guidelines or may have their own established guidelines. Therefore, before reporting these services, research the reporting policies of your major payers.

See your *CPT* code manual or other code reference for full code descriptors for 95120–95134.

- Codes **95120–95134** are reported when the entire service of preparing, providing, and administering (injection) allergenic extract is performed at 1 patient encounter.
- Codes **95131–95134** are reported for extracts containing more than 1 single stinging insect venom.
- Codes **95115** and **95117** *cannot* be reported with codes **95120–95134**.
- Codes **95120** and **95125** are reported based on the number of injections administered (ie, a single injection or ≥2 injections).
- Codes **95130–95134** are reported per injection. Therefore, if 2 separate injections of 2 stinging insect venoms (eg, wasp and bee) are provided, code **95131** would be reported 2 times.
- For rapid desensitization per hour, see code **95180**.

Example

➤ **An allergist prepares a 10-dose vial of allergen extract and administers 1 dose at the time of the visit (allergenic extract was prepared with the intent to administer on a planned schedule).**

The allergist will report code **95165** with 10 units of service and **95115** with 1 unit of service and the specific diagnosis code. Allergic rhinitis due to pollen would be reported with *ICD-10-CM* code **J30.1** or, if due to food, code **J30.5**. Alternately, code **95120** would describe provision of allergenic extract and a single injection if required by a payer.

Epinephrine Auto-injector Administration

Administration of epinephrine via an epinephrine auto-injector in the office or other outpatient setting is reported with code **96372** (therapeutic, prophylactic, or diagnostic injection [specify substance or drug]; subcutaneous or intramuscular). Follow payer guidance for reporting an epinephrine injector kit furnished by the practice.

- Many payers require submission of code **J0171** (injection, adrenalin, epinephrine, 0.1 mg) with 1 unit for 1 injection.

Example

➤ **The patient has a reaction to the allergenic extract.** The physician injects epinephrine by using an auto-injector device (eg, EpiPen Jr, Adrenaclick) supplied by the physician.

The injection using an auto-injection device would be reported as an intramuscular injection with code **96372**. The HCPCS table of drugs references the epinephrine injectors to code **J0171**. It is advisable to include the product NDC and NDC units to specify the exact product and dose provided.

Immunoglobulins

> Note: This information does not apply to immunization services. See Chapter 8.

When reporting codes **90281–90399**, remember that they are only for the cost of the immunoglobulin and the appropriate separate administration code should also be reported (eg, **96372**, **96374**).

- A significant, separately identifiable E/M service performed during the same visit may also be billed if indicated.
- *ICD-10-CM* diagnosis codes to support immunoglobulin services include codes from categories **D80–D84** for certain disorders involving the immune mechanism or codes for specific conditions, such as mucocutaneous lymph node syndrome (**M30.3**).

Example

➤ **An infant requires administration of 150 mg of palivizumab for preventing serious lower respiratory tract disease caused by RSV.** A clinical staff member administers the immunoglobulin under direct physician supervision. Two single-dose vials (one 100-mg and one 50-mg) are administered. The supervising physician reports

96372	(intramuscular injection)
90378 KP × 2	(RSV, monoclonal antibody, recombinant, for intramuscular use, 50 mg, each)
90378 KQ × 1 unit	(additional 50 mg single-dose vial)

The appropriate number of units reported for the dose of the RSV monoclonal antibody given is 1 unit per 50 mg (eg, 3 units for 150 mg). The NDC for each vial should be included on claims for most payers requiring submission on separate claim lines. Modifiers **KP** (first drug of a multiple drug unit dose formulation) and **KQ** (second drug of a multiple drug unit dose formulation) may be required when you are reporting the doses of *a single drug* supplied in a unit dose formulation when the total dose is greater than the amount supplied in a single-dose vial or container. Review individual payer policies for reporting these services.

See Chapter 1 for more information on reporting National Drug Codes.

Hearing Screening and Other Audiological Function Testing Codes

(For central auditory function evaluation, see **92620**, **92621**.*)*

Audiometric tests require the use of calibrated electronic equipment, recording of results, and a written report with interpretation (eg, chart of hertz and decibels with pass/fail result for each ear tested and overall pass/fail result). Services include testing of both ears. If the test is applied to 1 ear only, modifier **52** (reduced services) must be appended to the code.

> Medicaid plans may offer physician resources providing hearing screening/testing coverage information and documentation forms/requirements.

- Code **92551** (screening test, pure tone, air only) is used when earphones are placed on the patient and the patient is asked to respond to tones of different pitches and intensities. This is a limited study to identify the presence or absence of a potential hearing problem. Code **92551** is not used to report hearing screenings performed on newborns and infants.

> Report hearing tests conducted following a failed hearing screening with *International Classification of Diseases, 10th Revision, Clinical Modification* code **Z01.110** if results are normal. If findings are atypical, report code **Z01.118** and a code to identify the abnormality.

- Code **92552** (full pure tone audiometric assessment) is used when earphones are placed on the patient and the patient is asked to respond to tones of different pitches and intensities. The threshold, which is the lowest intensity of the tone that the patient can hear 50% of the time, is recorded for a number of frequencies.
- Air and bone thresholds (**92553**) may be obtained and compared to differentiate among conductive, sensorineural, or mixed hearing losses. Air and bone thresholds are obtained in a similar manner.

> Automated audiometry testing is reported with Category III codes **0208T–0212T**.

- Code **92558** is reported for evoked otoacoustic emissions, screening (qualitative measurement of distortion product or transient evoked otoacoustic emissions), with automated analysis. This is used when the results are obtained automatically (ie, no interpretation and report is required). Coverage for this is typically limited to newborn screening, including follow-up newborn screening from a failed screen in the hospital and screening on younger children. Check with your payers, however.
- Code **92583** (select picture audiometry) is typically used for younger children. The patient is asked to identify different pictures with the instructions given at different intensity levels.
- Distortion product evoked otoacoustic emissions codes are reported based on the number of frequencies used. Code **92587** is used to report testing for confirmation of the presence or absence of a hearing disorder, 3 to 6 frequencies. Code **92588** is reported when a comprehensive (quantitative analysis of outer hair cell function by cochlear mapping) diagnostic evaluation with a minimum of 12 frequencies is performed. Interpretation and written report are required. Do not report these codes for automated analysis.
- Other commonly performed procedures include codes **92567** (tympanometry [impedance testing]) and **92568** (acoustic reflex testing, threshold portion). Code **92550** is reported when tympanometry and reflex threshold measurements are performed.
- Optical coherence tomography of the middle ear with interpretation and report is reported with Category III codes based on whether the service was unilateral (**0485T**) or bilateral (**0486T**). Be sure to verify payer policy prior to provision of services.
- Most audiological procedures are bundled with impacted cerumen removal services (**69209**, **69210**) and, therefore, will not be separately payable. Report only the audiology test to payers that bundle impacted cerumen removal services.

Example

➤ **Lilly is a 5-year-old whose hearing does not meet screening criteria at school and is referred to her pediatrician for additional evaluation.** She has a history of recurrent otitis media before the age of 3 years but no recent illness. Her parents report no family history of hearing loss and no concerns at home. Tympanometry reveals no evidence of effusion. Examination findings are negative for other abnormalities. Screening audiometry is performed, and its results are atypical, as indicated by the school screening. Lilly is referred to an audiologist for further evaluation. Diagnosis is abnormal auditory function with possible hearing loss in her right ear.

ICD-10-CM	**Z01.118** (encounter for examination of ears and hearing with other abnormal findings) **R94.120** (abnormal auditory function study)
CPT	**99213** (established patient office E/M, low medical decision-making) **92567** (tympanometry [impedance testing]) **92551** (screening test, pure tone, air only)

Teaching Point: *ICD-10-CM* instructs the physician to report **Z01.118** and an additional code for abnormal findings. Although the result of the screening was abnormal, the physician did not diagnose a hearing loss at this encounter. Code **R94.120** describes the abnormal screening result.

If the screening result at this visit had been negative, the physician would have been required to code **Z01.110** (encounter for hearing examination following failed hearing screening).

Emotional/Behavioral Assessment

96127   Brief emotional/behavioral assessment (eg, depression inventory, attention-deficit/hyperactivity disorder [ADHD] scale), with scoring and documentation, per standardized instrument

Code **96127**

- Represents the practice expense of administering, scoring, and documenting each standardized instrument. No physician work value is included. Physician interpretation is included in a related E/M service.
- May be used for screening but also for assessment in monitoring treatment efficacy and to support clinical decision-making.
- Not reported in conjunction with **96105**, **96125**, and **99483**.
- Two separate completions (eg, by teacher and parent) of the same form may be separately reported (ie, 2 units of service). When reporting multiple units of service, it is advisable to learn if the payer has specific guidance for reporting the total number of units as a single line item or requires splitting to multiple claim lines. Medically Unlikely Edits may apply.

Example

➤ **A 16-year-old patient receiving treatment of an initial episode of major depressive disorder returns for follow-up.** A standardized instrument is used to assess the status of the patient's depression. The physician recommends continued medication and counseling with a licensed clinical social worker. The physician's total time on the date of the encounter is 25 minutes. Diagnosis is a moderate single episode of major depressive disorder.

The established patient office E/M code **99213** is reported in addition to code **96127**. The diagnosis code **F32.1** (major depressive disorder, single episode, moderate) is reported.

Please see
- **Chapter 14 for discussion of diagnostic testing of the central nervous system**
- **Chapter 8 for discussion of developmental screening, brief emotional and/or behavioral assessment, and health risk assessment as preventive services**
- **Chapter 2 for more information on Medically Unlikely Edits**

Radiology Services

The following general guidelines are for reporting radiology services:

- Report only the service provided. See the Professional and Technical Components section earlier in this chapter for appropriate reporting when the physician does not provide the global service.
- A signed written report of the physician's or QHP's interpretation of imaging is an integral part of the professional component of a radiologic service.
- A reference to *image* in *CPT* may refer to an image on film or in digital format. Images must contain anatomical information unique to the patient for which the imaging service is provided.
- Certain health plans, including Medicaid plans, may require use of modifier **FX** (x-ray taken using film) when reporting the technical component or global radiology service (ie, combined professional and technical components). Verify health plan requirements, as payment may be reduced for radiographs taken using film.

Several categories of codes for radiology services have been revised in recent years. The following sections highlight some of these changes. Please see your coding reference for a full listing of codes and reporting instructions.

Imaging Guidance

Many procedures include imaging guidance. When a code descriptor for a procedure or *CPT* instruction indicates that the procedure includes imaging guidance, do not separately report a code for supervision and interpretation of imaging (eg, radiography, fluoroscopy, ultrasonography, magnetic resonance imaging, computed tomography, nuclear medicine).

- Do not report imaging guidance when a non–imaging-guided tracking or localizing system (eg, radar, electromagnetic signals) is used.
- If you do not own or lease the equipment but are only reporting the professional service of interpreting the image and writing the report, refer to the modifier **26** discussion in the Professional and Technical Components section earlier in the chapter.

Abdominal Radiographs

74018	Radiologic examination, abdomen; 1 view
74019	2 views
74021	3 or more views
74022	Radiologic examination, complete acute abdomen series, including 2 or more views of the abdomen (eg, supine, erect, decubitus), and a single view chest

Report code **74022** when a series of radiographs are obtained to view the abdomen and chest as workup of acute abdominal illness or pain. An acute abdomen series includes 2 abdominal views and a single chest view.

Chest Radiographs

71045	Radiologic examination, chest; single view
71046	2 views
71047	3 views
71048	4 or more views

- The types of views (eg, frontal and lateral) obtained no longer affect coding of chest radiographs.
- Do not separately report a single-view chest radiograph when obtained in conjunction with an acute abdomen series (**74022**).

Hip Radiographs

73501	Radiologic examination, hip, unilateral, with pelvis when performed; 1 view
73502	2-3 views
73503	performed minimum of 4 views
73521	Radiologic examination, hips, bilateral, with pelvis when performed; 2 views
73522	3-4 views
73523	minimum of 5 views
73525	Radiologic examination, hip, arthrography, radiological supervision and interpretation
73592	Radiologic examination lower extremity, infant, minimum of 2 views

Codes **73501–73523** include radiograph of the pelvis when performed. Do not separately report a single-view radiograph of the pelvis (**72170**) when performed in conjunction with a radiograph of the hip.

Total Spine Radiographs

72081	Radiologic examination, spine, entire thoracic and lumbar, including skull, cervical and sacral spine if performed (eg, scoliosis evaluation); one view
72082	2 or 3 views
72083	4 or 5 views
72084	minimum of 6 views

Codes **72081–72084** describe imaging of the entire thoracic and lumbar spine and, when performed, the skull, cervical, and sacral spine.

Do not separately report codes for views of the individual spinal segments or skull when performed in conjunction with radiologic examination of the spine. Rather, select the code that represents the total number of views obtained.

Chapter 11. Common Non-facility Testing and Therapeutic Services

Administrative Services and Supplies

Administrative Services

Codes in this section cover some of the administrative aspects of medical practice.

99071   Educational supplies, such as books, tapes, and pamphlets, for the patient's education at cost to physician or other qualified health care professional

99075   Medical testimony

99082   Unusual travel (eg, transportation and escort of patient)

    Codes **99071–99082** are for administrative services.

- Code **99071** may be reported when the physician incurs costs for educational supplies and provides them to the patient at cost.
- Code **99075** may be reported when a physician presents medical testimony before a court or other administrative body.
- None of these services are assigned Medicare RVUs.
- HCPCS code **S9981** (medical records copying fee, administrative) or **S9982** (medical record copying fee, per page) may be reported when it is appropriate to charge for copies of medical records. Commercial payers and some Medicaid programs may accept **S** codes.
  - State medical insurance departments or medical associations determine the amount a practice can charge for copying medical records. Be sure to know the state charge limitations and do not overcharge.
  - The Health Insurance Portability and Accountability Act (HIPAA) of 1996 regulations, where more stringent, will override state regulations. For information on charges to patients for copying health records, see www.hhs.gov/hipaa/for-professionals/privacy/guidance/access/index.html#newlyreleasedfaqs.

Physician Group Education Services

99078   Physician or other qualified health care professional qualified by education, training, licensure/regulation (when applicable), educational services rendered to patients in a group setting (eg, prenatal, obesity, or diabetic instructions)

    Code **99078** is used to report physician educational services provided to established patients in group settings (eg, obesity or diabetes classes).

- There are no time requirements.
- Modifier **25** (significant, separately identifiable E/M service) should *not* be appended to the E/M service because **99078** is an adjunct service.
- Documentation in each medical record includes the education and training provided, follow-up for ongoing education, and total time of the education.
- Services are reported on each participating child.
- Payers may require that these services be reported differently.
- For preventive medicine and risk-factor reduction counseling to patients in a group setting, see codes **99411** and **99412**.

Resources

Allergy Testing

"Allergy Skin Testing: Codes, Unit Counts, and Tips for Reporting," February 2020 *AAP Pediatric Coding Newsletter* (https://coding.solutions.aap.org/article.aspx?articleid=2759685; subscription required)

CLIA Test Categorization

Waived test systems and analytes (www.accessdata.fda.gov/scripts/cdrh/cfdocs/cfClia/analyteswaived.cfm)

US Food and Drug Administration CLIA database (www.accessdata.fda.gov/scripts/cdrh/cfdocs/cfClia/analyteswaived.cfm)

HIPAA Release of Patient Records

Individuals' Right under HIPAA to Access their Health Information: Questions and Answers About HIPAA's Access Right (45 CFR §164.524) (www.hhs.gov/hipaa/for-professionals/privacy/guidance/access/index.html#newlyreleasedfaqs)

National Drug Codes

FDA NDC Directory (www.fda.gov/drugs/drug-approvals-and-databases/national-drug-code-directory)

Chapter 11. Common Non-facility Testing and Therapeutic Services

Proprietary Laboratory Analysis

www.ama-assn.org/practice-management/cpt/cpt-pla-codes

Test Your Knowledge!

1. **Which of the following modifiers is used to indicate that a physician provided both professional and technical components of a service?**
   a. **26**
   b. **TC**
   c. **25**
   d. No modifier is required.

2. **Which phrase describes a laboratory testing platform that provides a result (ie, positive or negative) by producing a signal on the reaction chamber?**
   a. Proprietary laboratory analysis
   b. Clinical Laboratory Improvement Amendments (CLIA) waived
   c. Direct optical observation
   d. Multianalyte assays with algorithmic analyses

3. **What modifier is appended to most CLIA-waived tests?**
   a. **WT**
   b. **QW**
   c. No modifier is required.
   d. **52**

4. **What modifier is appended to the code for the audiometry service to indicate that it was performed unilaterally?**
   a. **50**
   b. Report the code without a modifier $\times$ 2 units of service.
   c. **52**
   d. No modifier is required.

5. **A physician administers 3 injections of previously prepared allergy extracts. How is the administration service reported?**
   a. **95115** $\times$ 3
   b. **95117**
   c. **95115** and **95117**
   d. **95117** $\times$ 3

Chapter 11. Common Non-facility Testing and Therapeutic Services

Management of Chronic and Complex Conditions

Contents

Outpatient Management of Chronic and Complex Conditions 287

    Tracking Time of Periodic Services 288

Coding for Management of Complex Medical Conditions 289

    Transitional Care Management Services 289

        Care Management After Transitional Care Management 292

Monthly Care Management Services 292

    Required Practice Capabilities 294

        Activities of Care Management Services 294

    Chronic Care Management (CCM) and Complex Chronic Care Management (CCCM) 295

        Reporting CCM and CCCM 297

    Principal Care Management Services 298

    Care Plan Oversight Services 298

        Home Ventilator Management 301

Medical Team Conferences 301

Advance Care Planning 303

Prolonged Services Without Direct Patient Contact 304

Related Services Discussed in Other Chapters 305

    Online Digital Evaluation and Management Services 305

    Remote Physiologic Monitoring 306

    Telephone Evaluation and Management Services 306

    Interprofessional Telephone/Internet Consultations 306

    After-hours and Special Services 306

    Reporting a Combination of Complex Medical Management Services 306

Resources 307

Test Your Knowledge! 308

Outpatient Management of Chronic and Complex Conditions

Children with chronic and complex health care needs require greater levels and amounts of multidisciplinary medical, psychosocial, rehabilitation, and habilitation services than their same-aged peers. The child with special health care needs will require extra services, such as prolonged services and care management, with an increased frequency of evaluation and management (E/M) visits.

In addition to codes for services provided on a single date of service, *Current Procedural Terminology* (*CPT*®) includes categories of codes created to recognize episodes of care for complex health care needs that go beyond the work included in preservice, intraservice, and post-service values of the traditional face-to-face visit. Several code categories include codes for reporting care management services performed by clinical staff under the supervision of a physician or other qualified health care professional (QHP).

> **New in 2022!**
> - New code +**99437** gives physicians and other qualified health care professionals the ability to report personally performed chronic care management (CCM) services of 30 minutes or more in a calendar month beyond the first 30 minutes that are reported with code 99491.
> - Principal care management codes (**99424–99427**) are added for reporting management of a single complex chronic condition (eg, severe persistent asthma with recent exacerbation). Principal care management is differentiated from CCM by the requirement for only a single complex chronic condition and no requirement that the reporting physician provide or oversee the management and/or coordination of services for all of the patient's health care needs (which is required for CCM).

Five key categories of service are discussed in this chapter.
1. Transitional care management (TCM) (**99495, 99496**) includes a combination of 1 face-to-face service and non–face-to-face services, over a 30-day period, as needed, to help patients transition from a stay in a facility to their home environment without gaps in their care management. The reporting physician or QHP provides or oversees the management and/or coordination of services, as needed, for all the patient's health care needs.
2. Chronic care management (CCM) (**99490, 99439, 99491, 99437**) and complex chronic care management (CCCM) (**99487, 99489**) are monthly services provided by a single physician to manage or coordinate services for patients with 2 or more complex chronic conditions. The reporting individual provides or oversees the management and/or coordination of services, as needed, for all the patient's health care needs.
3. Principal care management (PCM) (**99424–99427**) is monthly services provided by a physician with a focus on the medical and/or psychological needs manifested by a single complex chronic condition (eg, severe persistent asthma). Although a primary care pediatrician may provide PCM services, management and coordination of services for all of a patient's health care needs is not required.
4. Care plan oversight (CPO) (**99339, 99340; 99374, 99375; 99377, 99378; 99379, 99380**) is another monthly service provided by a single physician in supervision of health care services typically delivered by qualified nonphysician health care professionals (QNHCPs) (eg, therapists), home health, or hospice services. Care plan oversight is reported by only 1 individual who has the sole or predominant supervisory role with a particular patient.
5. Psychiatric collaborative (**99492–99494**) or general behavioral health integration (**99484**) care management services are monthly services provided by a treating physician or QHP and are focused on psychiatric and behavioral health issues. Services are provided either in collaboration with a psychiatrist (**99492–99494**) or provided by clinical staff under the supervision of a treating pediatrician or QHP (**99484**).

> **Please see Chapter 14 for information on reporting psychiatric collaborative care management services and general behavioral health integration care management services.**

Each of these categories of service are reported based on time devoted to care of the individual patient in a specified period. *CPT* includes instructions for each category of services specifying the requirements of service, eligible providers of service, required time, and whether or not other services may be separately reported within the period of each service.
- Awareness of the codes for these services and the related coding instructions may offer additional opportunities for providing and/or coordinating comprehensive care for all children.

Codes and payment policy for many of these services continue to evolve.

Chapter 12. Management of Chronic and Complex Conditions

> Care management services cannot be reported when provided during a postoperative portion of the global period of a service reported by the same physician or other physician of the same specialty and same group practice. For example, a surgeon would not report transitional care management (TCM) during a postoperative period, but a primary pediatrician may report TCM when managing all of the patient's medical conditions following hospital discharge. Care management services are not reported for postoperative care alone (eg, when reporting a surgical service code with modifier 55 for postoperative management only).

- Reporting these services and the diagnosis codes representing the patient's chronic and complex conditions can play an important role in demonstrating the higher quality, lower cost care that is a key element of emerging payment methodologies.

> See Chapter 4 for information on emerging payment methodologies such as value-based purchasing.

- Payers that have adopted value-based or enhanced payment initiatives, such as per-member, per-month payment models, may consider certain care management services bundled into the services for which the enhanced payment is made. However, practices may choose to assign codes for use in internal calculations of the cost to provide enhanced care in comparison to any enhanced payments.
- To take advantage of opportunities for providing and reporting services related to management of chronic conditions and complex health care needs, physicians must identify the services that their practice capabilities will support. For instance, provision of TCM services requires timely identification of patients who are discharged from an inpatient or observation stay so that contact may be made with the patient within 2 business days of facility discharge.
- Payers may also require specific electronic capabilities (eg, having an electronic health record [EHR] that meets specifications required by the Medicaid Promoting Interoperability Program and/or Merit-based Incentive Payment System [MIPS]).

   For more information on preparing your practice to care for patients with complex health care needs, see the American Academy of Pediatrics (AAP) policy statement, "Patient- and Family-Centered Care Coordination: A Framework for Integrating Care for Children and Youth Across Multiple Systems" (https://pediatrics.aappublications.org/content/133/5/e1451).

- This policy statement, coauthored by the AAP Council on Children With Disabilities and the Medical Home Implementation Project Advisory Committee, outlines the essential partnerships that are critical to this framework.
- To further augment and facilitate the recommendations in this policy statement, refer to the freely accessible Boston Children's Hospital Care Coordination Curriculum (www.pcpcc.org/resource/care-coordination-curriculum). This curriculum provides content that can be adapted to the needs of any entity (eg, a single practice, a network of practices, parent and family organizations, a statewide organization). By design, most of the content is universally relevant, but the curriculum is optimally used when it is adapted and customized to reflect local needs, assets, and cultures.

> Services such as chronic care management do not prevent separate reporting of preventive services when provided to children with complex health care needs. See Chapter 9 for more information on reporting preventive evaluation and management services and separately reportable services on the same date.

Tracking Time of Periodic Services

Other than TCM, care management and CPO services are reported only when a specific amount of time is spent providing the service during 1 calendar month. Services typically occur on multiple days within the month. *Each segment of time must be documented.*

> Be sure to identify the reporting period of care management services. Transitional care management services (99495, 99496) are reported for a 30-day period beginning with the date of discharge from a facility setting. Other services are reported per calendar month of service, including all chronic and principal care management, care plan oversight, psychiatric collaborative care management, and care management for behavioral health conditions.

   Documentation and tracking of time for services that are reported on a periodic basis, such as time spent in CCM activities in a calendar month, require establishment of routine processes to prevent lost revenue due to not capturing all billable services. Practice and system capabilities vary. Potential tracking mechanisms include

- Electronic health record flow sheets designed to capture each activity and the related time throughout a period of service and provide a report of time per patient within each period of service.

- Stand-alone time-tracking software may also offer a solution for documenting time of service.
- Manual systems, such as spreadsheets, that are updated at the time of each activity.
- Work-arounds in existing electronic systems, such as EHR templates for clinical staff appointments that are assigned pseudocodes to track time (see example that follows). Pseudocodes are never used on claims; instead, they provide a basis for tracking time-based services.

> Collaboration with system vendors, professional colleagues, and practice management consultants may be invaluable to successful delivery, documentation, and reporting of time-based services.

The following example illustrates one semiautomated method of using pseudocodes:

Example

➤ **A physician is providing PCM services to a child with a single high-risk disease.** The physician's clinical staff spend 35 minutes over the course of a month in PCM activities in support of the patient's plan of care. On the date of each activity, clinical staff document the nature of the activity as well as the start and stop times. They also select a pseudocode (COORD) and 1 unit of service for each minute spent providing a service. No charge is generated by entry of COORD. However, billing staff will generate a report of the patients for whom COORD was entered during a calendar month. Because the PCM service to this child was 35 minutes, the pediatrician reports code **99426** (PCM, first 30 minutes of clinical staff time directed by physician or QHP, per calendar month).

Coding for Management of Complex Medical Conditions

Management of complex medical conditions may be reported with multiple codes for individual services and/or codes that describe either a combination of face-to-face and non–face-to-face services (eg, TCM) or a period of non–face-to-face services reported with 1 or more codes based on time of service (eg, CCM, PCM).

Many inclusion and exclusion rules are applied to the services discussed in this chapter.

- Certain niche services (eg, management of end-stage renal disease) may be considered components of or an alternative to comprehensive care management.
- The same time and activity are never used to support multiple codes (eg, time used to support reporting of an online digital E/M service code is not included in time of CCM).

> More information on services that may be frequently provided as part of managing complex health conditions are found in the following chapters:
> - **Chapter 9: services provided in a patient's home, group home, or nursing facility**
> - **Chapter 13: services by qualified nonphysician health care professionals**
> - **Chapter 21: remote data collection and management services**

Transitional Care Management Services

Transitional care management (**99495, 99496**) includes services provided to a new or an established patient whose medical and/or psychosocial problems require moderate- or high-complexity medical decision-making (MDM) during the transition from the following settings to the patient's home, domiciliary, rest home, or assisted living facility:

- Inpatient hospital including partial, acute, rehabilitation, and long-term acute stays
- Observation care
- Skilled nursing or nursing facility

Transitional care management commences on the date of discharge and continues for the next 29 days. There are no specific requirements for time spent in TCM services. However, TCM activities should be documented on the dates provided.

Moderate to high MDM is a requirement for TCM. Follow-up care that includes low-intensity services such as discussion of improving or normal laboratory results, which require only straightforward or low MDM, are not reported with codes for TCM.

Transitional care management includes a combination of patient care activities by a physician or other qualified health care professional (QHP) and clinical staff working under supervision of a physician or QHP. **Table 12-1** includes code descriptors and activities that may be provided as part of a TCM service.

The 2021 Medicare Physician Fee Schedule values for TCM services were 5.96 total non-facility relative value units (RVUs) for code **99495** and 8.07 RVUs for **99496**. Total non-facility RVUs include values for physician work, practice expense, and liability. Figures for 2022 were not available at the time of publication.

- This equated to $207.96 and $281.59, respectively, for providing TCM services over a 30-day period (calculated at $34.8931 per RVU).
- 2021 physician work RVUs assigned were 2.78 for **99495** and 3.79 for **99496**. Work RVUs are often used in salary calculations for employed physicians.

> For more information on how relative value units affect payment, see Chapter 4.

Transitional care management services are not limited to the attending provider of the related facility stay (eg, hospitalist) or to physicians of any specific specialty.

- The individual reporting TCM provides or oversees the management and/or coordination of services necessary *for all* the patient's medical conditions, psychosocial needs, and activities of daily living.
- Only 1 individual may report TCM for each qualifying patient within 30 days of discharge. Another TCM service may not be reported by the same individual or group for any subsequent discharge(s) within those 30 days.
- Hospital or observation discharge services (ie, **99238**, **99239**, or **99217**) may be reported by the same individual reporting TCM services. Discharge services do not qualify as the required face-to-face visit for TCM.

The TCM services begin on the date of discharge (day 1 of 30-day period) and continue for the next 29 days.

- One face-to-face visit with the reporting physician or QHP is included in addition to non–face-to-face services performed by the physician/QHP and/or licensed clinical staff under the direction of the physician/QHP.

Table 12-1. Transitional Care Management at a Glance

Patient Population

New or established patients whose medical and/or psychosocial problems require moderate- or high-complexity MDM during a 30-day transition period beginning with date of discharge from a facility setting to the patient's home, domiciliary, rest home, or assisted living facility.

99495 Transitional care management services with the following required elements:	99496 Transitional care management services with the following required elements:
- Communication (direct contact, telephone, electronic) with the patient and/or caregiver within 2 business days of discharge - Medical decision-making of at least moderate complexity during the service period - Face-to-face visit, within 14 calendar days of discharge[a]	- Communication (direct contact, telephone, electronic) with the patient and/or caregiver within 2 business days of discharge - Medical decision-making of high complexity during the service period - Face-to-face visit, within 7 calendar days of discharge[a]

Non–face-to-face services provided by the physician or other QHP may include

- Obtaining and reviewing the discharge information - Reviewing, ordering, or following up on pending diagnostic tests and treatments - Communication or education provided to family and/or other caregivers	- Interaction with other QHPs who will assume/reassume care of the patient's system-specific problems - Scheduling assistance for necessary follow-up services - Arranging referrals and community resources as necessary

Licensed clinical staff time (under the direction of the physician or other QHP) may include face-to-face and non–face-to-face time spent

- Communicating with the patient and/or family or other caregivers about aspects of care and with other agencies and community services utilized by the patient - Patient and/or family/caregiver education to support self-management, independent living, and activities of daily living	- Assessment and support for adherence to treatment plan and medication management - Facilitating access to care and other services needed by the patient and/or family, including identification of community and health resources

Abbreviations: MDM, medical decision-making; QHP, qualified health care professional.

[a] Medication reconciliation and management must occur no later than the date of the face-to-face visit.

Codes **99495** and **99496**

- Require initial patient contact, a face-to-face visit with the reporting physician or QHP, and medication reconciliation *within specified time frames*.

> To provide direct patient contact within 2 business days of discharge and to schedule appointments within 7 or 14 days, practices must have a process for receiving notification of observation and inpatient hospital discharges. Failure to make contact within 2 business days of discharge or to provide a face-to-face visit within 14 days of discharge eliminates the possibility of reporting transitional care management services.

- Medication management must occur *no later than* the date of the face-to-face visit.
  - *Medication reconciliation* refers to the process of avoiding inadvertent inconsistencies across transitions in care by reviewing the patient's complete medication regimen at the time of admission, transfer, and discharge and comparing it with the regimen being considered for the new setting of care.
  - Clinical staff may perform and document medication reconciliation under general supervision of the physician or QHP.

> When medication management occurs in conjunction with a face-to-face visit, code **1111F** (discharge medications reconciled with the current medication list in outpatient medical record) may be reported in addition to the code for the service provided. Code **1111F** is a Category II *Current Procedural Terminology* code used for performance measurement in some quality initiatives.

- Code selection is based on the level of MDM and the date of the first face-to-face visit, as shown in **Table 12-2**. Note that all 3 components (communication within 2 business days, type of MDM, and timing of face-to-face visit) must be met to report TCM services, although only the MDM and time of the face-to-face visit differentiate code selection.
- The first face-to-face visit is included in the TCM service and is not reported separately.

  Additional face-to-face E/M services (eg, **99212–99215**) during the 30-day TCM period but provided on dates subsequent to that of the first included face-to-face visit may be separately reported.

Table 12-2. Levels of Transitional Care Management		
Type of Medical Decision-making	**Face-to-face Visit Within 7 Days**	**Face-to-face Visit Within 8 to 14 Days**
Moderate complexity	99495	99495
High complexity	99496	99495

- Documentation includes the timing of the initial post-discharge communication with the patient or caregivers, date of the face-to-face visit, and complexity of MDM over the 30-day service period. *Medical decision-making is defined by the office and other outpatient E/M service guidelines.*
- Follow payer guidelines for reporting. The Centers for Medicare & Medicaid Services (CMS) allows reporting of TCM services once the included face-to-face visit has been completed (ie, prior to the end of the service period). Other payers may not allow billing until the complete service period has elapsed.

Examples

To help illustrate the use of codes for management of complex medical conditions, examples in this chapter will focus on one patient, Isadora (Izzy) Doe, who has cystic fibrosis with failure to thrive and developmental delay.

➤ **Izzy, a child with cystic fibrosis, is discharged from the hospital after an admission for recurrent *Pseudomonas aeruginosa* infection.** Two days after discharge, the physician speaks with Izzy's mother. Clinical staff assess adherence with the treatment plan and educate the parents on management of the child. The child is seen by the physician in follow-up 10 days after discharge. The pediatrician and clinical staff monitor and coordinate the child's ongoing treatment through the 29th day following discharge. The MDM is highly complex.

Code **99495** is reported. Although the MDM is highly complex, this service did not meet the requirements for code **99496** because the face-to-face visit did not occur within 7 days of discharge. Diagnosis codes may include **E84.0** (cystic fibrosis with pulmonary manifestations), **B96.5** (*Pseudomonas* as the cause of diseases classified elsewhere), and, if pneumonia is current, **J15.1** (pneumonia due to *Pseudomonas*).

➤ **Izzy, a child with cystic fibrosis, is discharged from the hospital after an admission for recurrent *Pseudomonas aeruginosa* infection.** Two days after discharge, the physician speaks with Izzy's mother. Clinical staff assess adherence with the treatment plan and educate the parents on management of the child. The child is seen by the physician in follow-up 5 days after discharge. The pediatrician and clinical staff monitor and coordinate the child's ongoing treatment through the 29th day following discharge. The MDM is highly complex.

Code **99496** is reported. Diagnoses are as noted in the previous example.

Care Management After Transitional Care Management

A patient may require ongoing care management services after the 30-day TCM service period has ended. When a TCM service period begins or ends in the same month that other care management services are provided, each service may be reported by the same physician or QHP as long as the same period is not attributed to more than 1 service (ie, time during the TCM service period cannot be attributed to another care management service).

Example

➤ **Izzy is discharged on January 4, 2022. Transitional care management is provided through a period ending on February 2, 2022.** Izzy's pediatrician provides CCM services for the remainder of the month of February. Only the time spent in CCM services provided from February 3, 2022, through February 28, 2022, may be considered for that calendar month per *CPT*.

Transitional care management services are valued significantly higher than other care management services. If the dates and/or time for TCM and other care management services overlap, it is advantageous to report TCM, provided all required elements of service have been provided.

Monthly Care Management Services

Monthly care management services are management and support services that are not limited to the period following discharge from a facility stay. These services are provided by physicians or QHPs or by clinical staff under the direction of a physician or QHP to individuals who reside at home or in a domiciliary, rest home, or assisted living facility. The goals of care management services are to improve care coordination, reduce avoidable hospital services, improve patient engagement, and decrease care fragmentation.

CPT includes 3 types of continuous care management services. Details of patient eligibility, providers of service, and time requirements vary for these services and are discussed in detail later in this chapter.

1. *Chronic care management services*—provision or supervision of the management and/or coordination of services, as needed, *for all the patient's medical conditions, psychosocial needs, and activities of daily living*
2. *Complex chronic care management services*—CCM services that require at least 60 minutes of clinical staff time under the direction of a physician or QHP and moderate or high MDM
3. *Principal care management services*—provision or supervision of the management and/or coordination of services, as needed, for a patient's single complex chronic condition

Tables **12-3** and **12-4** list requirements for reporting care management services.

Time, activities (eg, patient education), and identification of the individual conducting each activity must be documented. Visit www.aap.org/cfp for an example of a worksheet for tracking care management activities and service times.

- Each minute of time is counted only once and only for 1 service.
- A physician or QHP may separately report a distinct time-based service (eg, an online digital E/M service) provided to the same patient during the same calendar month that clinical staff time is used to report care management services.
- Only time spent by clinical staff employed directly by or under contract and clinically integrated with the reporting professional's practice is included in the time of care management services.

The midpoint rule commonly applied for coding based on time does not apply to care management services (99424–99427, 99437, 99439, 99487, 99489, 99490, 99491).

Table 12-3. Chronic Care Management Services

A comprehensive care plan for all the patient's medical conditions, psychosocial needs, and activities of daily living must be developed, revised, or monitored and shared with the patient/caregivers for each type of CCM service.

Patient Population for All CCM Services

Patients have multiple (≥2) chronic or episodic conditions expected to last ≥12 months, or until the death of the patient, that place the patient at significant risk of death, acute exacerbation/decompensation, or functional decline.

#▲99490 Chronic care management services by clinical staff

Work Required

- ≥20 minutes of clinical staff activity directed by a physician/QHP, per calendar month
- May combine physician or QHP time of <30 minutes personally spent in CCM services with clinical staff time as long as ≥20 minutes are spent within a calendar month

#+▲99439 each additional 20 minutes of clinical staff time directed by a physician or QHP, per calendar month (List up to 2 units separately in addition to **99490**)

#▲99491 Chronic care management services by physician/QHP, first 30 minutes (≥30–59 minutes)

+●99437 each additional full 30-minute period (eg, 60–89 minutes equals 1 unit)

Work Required

- ≥30 minutes personally spent by a physician or QHP, per calendar month

---

▲99487 Complex chronic care management services by clinical staff/physician/QHP

Work Required

- Moderate- or high-complexity medical decision-making
- ≥60 minutes of clinical staff activity directed by a physician or QHP, per calendar month (may include time spent personally by a physician or QHP)

+▲99489 each additional 30 minutes per calendar month (List separately in addition to **99487**)

Abbreviations: CCM, chronic care management; QHP, qualified health care professional.

Table 12-4. Principal Care Management Services

A care plan specific to the single disease must be developed, revised, or monitored and shared with the patient/caregivers for each type of PCM service. Ongoing communication and care coordination with relevant practitioners furnishing care is also required. PCM services of <30 minutes duration in a calendar month are not reported separately.

Patient Population for All PCM Services

Patients have a single complex chronic condition expected to last ≥3 months that places the patient at significant risk of death, acute exacerbation/decompensation, or functional decline. The condition requires frequent adjustments in the medication regimen, and/or the management of the condition is unusually complex due to comorbidities.

●99424 Principal care management services by a physician/QHP

Work Required

- ≥30 minutes of physician or QHP time, per calendar month

+●99425 each additional 30 minutes of physician or QHP time, per calendar month (List separately in addition to **99424** for each full 30 minutes beyond the first 30 minutes)

●99426 Principal care management services by clinical staff/physician/QHP

Work Required

- ≥30 minutes of clinical staff activity directed by a physician or other QHP, per calendar month (may include time spent personally by a physician or other QHP)

+●99427 each additional 30 minutes per calendar month (List up to 2 units separately in addition to **99426**)

Abbreviations: PCM, principal care management; QHP, qualified health care professional.

Chapter 12. Management of Chronic and Complex Conditions

- When provided during the same calendar month as care management services, behavioral or psychiatric collaborative care management (PCCM) services (**99484**, **99492–99494**) may be separately reported. Do not count the same minutes (eg, 1:00–1:15 pm) toward care management and behavioral or PCCM services.
- Care management services are not reported by the same individual for services to the same patient in the same calendar month as end stage renal disease services (**90951–90970**), CPO (**99339**, **99340**; **99374–99380**), other care management services (eg, do not report both CCM and CCCM), or medication management services (**99605–99607**).

Required Practice Capabilities

A practice providing CCM, CCCM, or PCM services must have all of the following specific capabilities:

- Use of an EHR system that supports timely access to clinical information.
- Ability to provide access to care providers or clinical staff 24 hours a day, 7 days a week, including providing patients and caregivers with a means to contact health care professionals in the practice to address urgent needs, regardless of the time of day or day of the week.
- Ability to provide continuity of care through scheduling of the patient's successive routine appointments with a designated member of the care team.
- Provision of timely access and management for necessary follow-up when a patient is discharged from the emergency department or hospital.
- Patient and caregiver engagement and education and integration of care among all service professionals, as appropriate for each patient.
- The individual reporting care management services oversees activities of the care team.
- All care team members providing services are clinically integrated.

    CPT no longer requires use of a standardized methodology to identify patients who may qualify for care management services. However, such processes may be beneficial to identifying and offering care management services to patients. Processes may involve developing checklists or processes for identifying characteristics of patients with complex health care needs (eg, any patient with chronic or episodic conditions that are expected to last at least 12 months and increase the risk of morbidity and mortality, acute exacerbation or decompensation, or functional decline may require CCM services). Examples of such characteristics (*examples only; not a practice guideline*) include

- Number of chronic conditions
- Number of visits for nonroutine care in the past year
- Number of days the child did not attend school due to the health condition
- Emergency department visits or hospitalizations in the past 6 months
- Number of current medications or medications prescribed or revised in the last 6 months
- Number of physicians and other providers (eg, home health care provider, nutritionist)
- Lack of resources (eg, housing, health plan coverage, access to care in community)
- Assistance required for activities of daily living
- Other psychosocial considerations (eg, language barriers, multiple family members with complex care needs)

Activities of Care Management Services

Services include all clinical staff time spent in face-to-face and non–face-to-face services or a physician's time personally spent in care management activities. Time spent in other reported services (eg, time of prolonged clinical staff service [**99415**, **99416**] or time of collection and interpretation of physiologic data [**99091**]) may not be included to meet requirements for reporting care management services.

    Care management activities include

- Face-to-face and non–face-to-face time spent communicating with and engaging the patient and/or family, caregivers, other professionals, community services, and agencies
- Developing, revising, documenting, communicating, and implementing a comprehensive (CCM, CCCM) or disease-specific (PCM) care plan
- Collecting health outcomes data and registry documentation
- Teaching patient and/or family/caregiver to support patient self-management, independent living, and activities of daily living
- Identifying community and health resources
- Facilitating access to care and other services needed by the patient and/or family
- Management of care transitions not reported as part of TCM (**99495**, **99496**)
- Ongoing review of patient status, including review of laboratory and other studies not reported as part of an E/M service
- Assessment and support for adherence to the care plan

Development of a Plan of Care

A plan of care must be developed or revised *and a copy provided to each patient* receiving care management services. For CCM and CCCM services, the plan of care addresses all of the patient's health care needs. For PCM, the plan of care is focused on management of the patient's single complex chronic health condition.

- A plan of care for health problems is based on a physical, mental, cognitive, social, functional, and environmental evaluation. It is intended to provide a simple and concise overview of the patient and the patient's medical conditions and to be a useful resource for patients, caregivers, and providers. See **Figure 12-1** for an example of a plan of care.
- Creation, monitoring, or revision of a plan of care must be documented. Plans created by other entities (eg, home health agencies) cannot be substituted for a care plan established by the individual reporting CCM services.

Defining a Plan of Care

Current Procedural Terminology defines a *care plan* or *plan of care* as required for care management services (ie, chronic care management, complex chronic care management, and principal care management) as

- Based on a physical, mental, cognitive, social, functional, and environmental assessment
- Comprehensive for all health or a single complex chronic health problem, as applicable
- A typical plan of care is not limited to, but may include
  — Problem list
  — Expected outcome and prognosis
  — Measurable treatment goals
  — Cognitive assessment
  — Functional assessment
  — Symptom management
  — Planned interventions
  — Medical management
  — Environmental evaluation
  — Caregiver assessment
  — Interaction and coordination with outside resources and other health care professionals and providers
  — Summary of advance directives

These elements are intended to be a guide for creating a meaningful plan of care rather than a strict set of requirements. They should be utilized only as appropriate for the individual.

The plan should be updated periodically based on status or goals changes. The entire care plan should be reviewed at least annually.

Chronic Care Management (CCM) and Complex Chronic Care Management (CCCM)

The appropriate CCM or CCCM code(s) is reported once per calendar month by only 1 individual who has assumed the management role for all the patient's care. This may be a primary pediatrician or a subspecialist, but only the 1 individual may report CCM or CCCM services in a calendar month. Face-to-face E/M services may be separately reported by the same individual during the same calendar month.

Chronic care management and CCCM services are performed personally by a physician or QHP (**99491, 99437**) or by clinical staff under supervision by an employing (direct or contractual) physician or QHP (**99490, 99439, 99487, 99489**). Refer to **Table 12-3**, which provides requirements for CCM and CCCM services.

Chronic care management

- Is provided to patients with 2 or more chronic continuous or episodic health conditions expected to last 12 months or longer, or until the death of the patient, and that place the patient at significant risk of death, acute exacerbation/decompensation, or functional decline.
- Addresses *all* the patient's medical conditions, psychosocial needs, and activities of daily living.
- Requires creation, implementation, monitoring, and revision (as needed) of a comprehensive care plan for all the patient's health-related problems.
- Codes **99491** and **99437** are not reported for time spent by a physician or QHP on the date of a face-to-face E/M visit.

In addition to requirements for CCM, CCCM (**99487, 99489**)

- Requires moderate- or high-complexity MDM during the calendar month
- Requires at least 60 minutes of clinical staff time, under the direction of a physician or other QHP (may include time spent by the physician or QHP)

Figure 12-1. Example Plan of Care

This plan of care has been written by A Great Pediatric Practice to help us work with you to be as healthy as possible. This plan will allow you to share with us what is important to you and will let you know what to expect from us.

We will keep a copy of this plan and make changes as necessary. We will share this with other people who take care of you (for example, other doctors or therapists), as needed, to help them take care of you. You can also share this with others, such as family members, who help you take care of yourself.

Date	01/15/2022	Primary pediatrician	Dr Joe	Page 1 of 2

About Me

Name	Isadora Doe	I like to be called	Izzy	Date of birth	12/25/2014
Primary caregivers	Jenny Doe—mother; James Doe—father; Ellen Wright—mother's aunt				
Preferred contact information	Jenny Doe—MamaJ@hotmail.net, James Doe—DaddyJ@hotmail.net Ellen Wright—555/555-5555				
Secondary contact information	Jenny Doe—555/555-4444 James Doe—555/555-5554				
Preferred pharmacy	Family Drug Store	Preferred hospital		Children's Hospital-Main	

Who Do I Call When I Need Care or Have Questions?

My care coordinator	Bonnie Wood, LPN; 555/444-3333, ext 22; bwood@GreatPeds.care

Important Health Information

I am allergic to	No known allergies
I have difficulty with	Airway clearance techniques, gaining weight, infections, keeping up with schoolwork
Equipment I need (for example, wheelchair)	Percussion vest, aerosol generator
Community assistance	Mother reports no food or housing insecurity.

My Health Concerns (include concerns from patient and caregiver perspectives)

Concerns	What I can expect for each concern
Cystic fibrosis	Coordinated care with pulmonologist and respiratory therapist
Failure to thrive	Continue high calorie diet and consultation with nutritionist

My Health Goals

Goals	Plans of action
Cystic fibrosis: Maintain lung function and avoid infections.	Continue daily percussion therapy, medications, and quarterly visits to Cystic Fibrosis Clinic.
Failure to thrive: Achieve goal of >10th percentile for age.	Continue enzyme and nutrition therapy; monitor weight and height.

My Planned Care

Specialty care	Cystic Fibrosis Clinic visit quarterly or as needed
Preventive care	Next preventive visit 06/12/2022
Scheduled follow-up visit	02/25/2022 8:00 am Call for urgent appointment as needed.
Nutrition therapy	ABC Home Care biweekly appointments
Respiratory therapy	ABC Home Care weekly appointments for 1 month
School counselor	Coordinates IEP changes, available at 555/555-5555

Other: School nurse is available only 2 days a week. Alert teacher of any changes to nutrition therapy. School requires physician signature annually on chronic illness form due to potential for missed school.

Notes:	
Patient signature	
Parent signature	
Care coordinator signature	

Reporting CCM and CCCM

There are significant differences in work and practice expense required for each type of CCM and CCCM service. It is important to consider the amount and type of time (clinical staff and/or physician/QHP) and type of MDM required to determine the most appropriate code for each calendar month. A patient who requires CCM in January may require CCCM in February, or vice versa, as clinical circumstances change.

- Only 1 type of CCM or CCCM service is reported per calendar month.
  - No combination of codes **99487** and **99490** or **99491** may be reported for the same month.
  - One of these codes is reported in any calendar month when the requirements of the code descriptor are met.
- For **99491**, only count the time personally performed by the physician or other QHP. Time spent by clinical staff is not counted toward the time to support **99491**.
- More than 1 clinical staff member may spend time in CCM activities on a single date. Count all time that is not over-lapping, but do not count the same period more than once.

  If multiple clinical staff members meet about 1 patient, count the time for only 1 staff member (eg, 3 staff members spend 5 minutes discussing a patient; the total time of the CCM activity is 5 minutes).
- Do not count any time of the clinical staff spent as part of a separately reported service (eg, rooming a patient on the date of a physician or QHP visit).
- If the physician personally performs clinical staff activities, his or her time may be counted toward the required clinical staff time to meet the elements of codes **99487**, **99489**, **99490**, and **99439**. If a physician or QHP personally performs at least 30 minutes of CCM services, see codes **99491** and **99437**.

  See examples for each level of CCM in **Table 12-5**.

Table 12-5. Chronic Care Management Coding Examples

The patient in each example is Izzy, who has cystic fibrosis and failure to thrive due to exocrine pancreatic insufficiency and has just completed a 30-day period of TCM. *ICD-10-CM* diagnosis codes may include **E84.0** (cystic fibrosis with pulmonary manifestations), **B96.5** (*Pseudomonas* as the cause of diseases classified elsewhere), **E84.8** (cystic fibrosis with other manifestations), **K86** (exocrine pancreatic insufficiency), and **R62.51** (failure to thrive), in addition to codes for any other conditions addressed.

Each activity included in the CCM service must be documented in the patient record with the date and description of the activity and authenti-cated with the performing clinician's signature (electronic or written) and date signed.

Example	Code Assignment
Izzy is receiving CCM services. Time begins the day after the 30-day period of TCM was completed. Clinical staff spend 65 minutes in the remainder of the calendar month implementing the care plan and responding to questions and concerns. MDM is moderate.	Code **99487** (CCCM of at least 60 minutes with moderate to high MDM) is reported by supervising physician Dr Joe. *Tip:* No time spent during the TCM period is counted toward the time of CCM or CCCM.
Izzy is receiving continued CCM services. During the calendar month, MDM includes the decision to start tube feeding to address worsening feeding problems. A total of 95 minutes of combined physician and clinical staff time is spent in CCM activities for Izzy in the calendar month.	Dr Joe reports code **99487** for the first 60 minutes and **99489** (CCCM, each additional 30 minutes) for the additional 35 minutes. One unit of **99489** is reported for each full 30 minutes after the first 60 minutes of CCM in a calendar month.
Izzy is receiving continuing CCM services. Dr Joe spends 40 minutes revising Izzy's plan of care. Clinical staff also spend 15 minutes in CCM activities during the calendar month.	Dr Joe reports **99491** (CCM, personally performed by a physician or QHP, at least 30 minutes in the calendar month). Only Dr Joe's time is counted toward **99491**. If Dr Joe's total time in the month is at least 60 minutes, codes **99491** and **99437** are reported.
Izzy is receiving CCM services for cystic fibrosis with exocrine pancreatic insufficiency with attention to a gastrostomy and supervision of enteral nutrition. Dr Joe's clinical staff spend 20 minutes in CCM activities. Dr Joe also personally spends 10 minutes in CCM activities.	Dr Joe reports **99490** (CCM with at least 20 minutes of clinical staff time). Dr Joe and the clinical staff's combined time is counted toward **99490**. *Tip:* Dr Joe did not personally spend 30 minutes in CCM activities to support **99491**.
Izzy is receiving continued CCM services. Dr Joe personally spends 10 minutes in CCM activities in addition to 30 minutes spent by clinical staff.	**99490**, **99439** x 1 (CCM of at least 20 minutes and at least 20 minutes beyond the first 20 minutes in a calendar month) are reported for 40 minutes combined time of Dr Joe and clinical staff.

Abbreviations: CCM, chronic care management; CCCM, complex chronic care management; *ICD-10-CM, International Classification of Diseases, 10th Revision, Clinical Modification*; MDM, medical decision-making; QHP, qualified health care professional; TCM, transitional care management.

Principal Care Management Services

Principal care management services are focused on the medical and/or psychological needs manifested by a single complex chronic condition with all of the following characteristics:

- Is expected to last at least 3 months.
- Requires frequent adjustments in the medication regimen, and/or the management of the condition is unusually complex due to comorbidities.
- Places the patient at significant risk of hospitalization, acute exacerbation/decompensation, functional decline, or death.
- Requires development, monitoring, or revision of disease-specific care plan.

Refer to **Table 12-4** for codes and work descriptions for PCM services.

The patient may have multiple chronic conditions that may warrant provision of CCM or CCCM services, but the focus on the single condition differentiates PCM from these services (eg, Izzy, the patient in earlier examples, may require ongoing CCM by her pediatrician but also require a period of PCM by a pulmonologist or endocrinologist focused solely on a single condition). The same individual(s) of the same group practice *and same specialty* cannot report PCM in conjunction with CCM or CCCM.

A patient's primary care pediatrician may provide PCM services to a patient who does not have the 2 or more chronic or episodic health conditions required to report CCM services. For example, a pediatrician may provide PCM to a patient with asthma who has had severe exacerbation until the patient's condition stabilizes.

Principal care management services include

- Establishing, implementing, revising, or monitoring a care plan specific to a single disease
- 30 minutes or longer of time personally spent by a physician or QHP (**99424**, **99425**) or by clinical staff under the supervision of an employing (direct or contractual) physician or QHP (**99426**, **99427**)

  If a physician or QHP spends less than 30 minutes in a calendar month providing PCM services, codes **99426** and **99427** may be reported for 30 or more minutes of combined time of the physician and clinical staff.
- Ongoing communication and care coordination between relevant practitioners furnishing care

Unlike CCM or CCCM services, PCM services may be provided by more than 1 physician or QHP in the same calendar month for the same patient. Documentation in the patient's medical record should reflect coordination among relevant managing clinicians.

Table 12-6 includes examples of PCM services.

Table 12-6. Principal Care Management Coding Examples	
The patient in each example is Izzy, who has cystic fibrosis and failure to thrive due to exocrine pancreatic insufficiency. *ICD-10-CM* diagnosis codes may include **E84.0** (cystic fibrosis with pulmonary manifestations), **B96.5** (*Pseudomonas* as the cause of diseases classified elsewhere), **E84.8** (cystic fibrosis with other manifestations), **K86** (exocrine pancreatic insufficiency), and **R62.51** (failure to thrive), in addition to codes for any other conditions addressed.	
Example	**Code Assignment**
Izzy is receiving PCM services. An endocrinologist spends 35 minutes in the calendar month implementing a care plan focused on management of exocrine pancreatic insufficiency and responding to questions and concerns.	Code **99424** (PCM of ≥30 minutes by a physician or QHP) is reported by the endocrinologist. If time in the calendar month exceeds 59 minutes, code **99425** is reported for each additional period of ≥30 minutes in addition to code **99424**.
Izzy is also receiving PCM services focused on pulmonary manifestations of cystic fibrosis. During the calendar month, clinical staff of a pulmonologist spend 25 minutes in PCM activities. The pulmonologist also spends 20 minutes in the same calendar month in PCM activities.	The pulmonologist reports code **99426** for combined clinical staff and physician time (45 minutes). If the combined time were 60–89 minutes in a calendar month, code **99427** would also be reported with 1 unit. For any time ≥90 minutes, 2 units of service may be reported with **99427**.

Abbreviations: *ICD-10-CM, International Classification of Diseases, 10th Revision, Clinical Modification*; PCM, principal care management; QHP, qualified health care professional.

Care Plan Oversight Services

Care plan oversight is recurrent physician or QHP supervision of a complex patient or a patient who requires multidisciplinary care and ongoing physician or QHP involvement. Transitional care management or CCM/CCCM/PCM services would not be reported in conjunction with CPO services. (See the "Coding Conundrum: Chronic Care Management or Care Plan Oversight?" box later in this chapter to compare CPO with CCM services.) Care plan oversight services are not face-to-face and reflect the complexity and time required to supervise the care of the patient. The codes are reported separately from E/M office visits.

Coding Conundrum: Care Management or Care Plan Oversight?

Chronic care management (CCM) or principal care management (PCM) services personally performed by a physician or other qualified health care professional (QHP) (**99491, 99424, 99425, 99437**) is similar to care plan oversight (CPO) for patients residing at home or in a domiciliary, rest home, or assisted living facility (**99339, 99340**) or in these settings under the care of home health (**99374, 99375**) or hospice (**99377, 99378**). Which should be reported for a physician's or QHP's personally provided services?

    There are differences in code selection, as shown in this box. Additionally, practices reporting CCM/PCM must meet certain qualifications (eg, providing patients and caregivers with a means to contact health care professionals in the practice to address urgent needs, regardless of the time of day or day of the week). Specific practice qualifications are not required for CPO.

CPO	CCM/PCM
Time Requirement in Calendar Month Require ≥15 min **99339, 99374, 99377** Require ≥30 min **99340, 99375, 99378**	**Time Requirement in Calendar Month** <30 min not separately reported Require ≥30 min CCM: **99491, 99437** PCM: **99424, 99425**
Number of Chronic Conditions ≥1	**Number of Chronic Conditions** CCM: ≥2 PCM: 1 (complex)
Care Plan Work Regular development and/or revision	**Care Plan Work** Establish, implement, revise, or monitor CCM: comprehensive care plan PCM: focused on a single complex disease

Medicare requires the use of Level II Healthcare Common Procedure Coding System codes for CPO services provided to patients under the care of a home health agency (**G0181**) or hospice (**G0182**). To report these **G** codes, Medicare requires a minimum of 30 minutes of physician supervision per calendar month. Because some state Medicaid programs may follow suit, check with your payer to learn its requirements for reporting these services.

Table 12-7 provides a comparison of CPO services, including patient population, work included, and services not separately reported. (Work included and services not separately reported are the same for all CPO services).

    Care plan oversight services

- Are reported only by the individual (ie, physician/QHP) who has the predominant supervisory role in the care of the patient or is the sole provider of the services.
- A face-to-face service with the patient must have been provided by the physician prior to assuming CPO. The CMS requires a face-to-face visit within 6 months prior to CPO services.
- Include
  - Regular development and/or revision of care plans
  - Review of subsequent reports of the patient's status
  - Review of related laboratory or other diagnostic studies
  - Communication (including telephone calls) for purposes of assessment or care decisions with health care professionals, family members, surrogate decision-makers (eg, legal guardians), and/or key caregivers involved in the patient's care
  - Integration of new information into the medical treatment plan or adjustment of medical therapy
  - Team conferences
  - Prolonged E/M service before and/or after direct patient care when the same time is attributed to CPO
- Are reported once per month based on the amount of time spent by the physician during that calendar month.

Unlike care management services, time included in care plan oversight is only that of the physician or other qualified health care professional and not that of clinical staff.

Chapter 12. Management of Chronic and Complex Conditions

Table 12-7. Care Plan Oversight Service Codes at a Glance

Activity by clinical staff is not included in the time of CPO service.

Codes by Patient Population

All patients receiving CPO require complex and multidisciplinary care modalities involving regular physician development and/or revision of care plans. The patient is not present at the time of service.

Individual physician supervision of a patient *in home, domiciliary, or rest home or assisted living facility (not under the care of a home health or hospice agency)* **99339** 15–29 min **99340** ≥30 min	Supervision of patient *under care of home health agency in home, domiciliary, or equivalent environment* **99374** 15–29 min **99375** ≥30 min
Supervision of *hospice patient* **99377** 15–29 min **99378** ≥30 min	Supervision of a *nursing facility patient* **99379** 15–29 min **99380** ≥30 min

Work Included in CPO Services

- At least 15 minutes by physician in regular development and/or revision of care plans
- Review of subsequent reports of the patient's status and related laboratory or other diagnostic studies
- Communication (including telephone calls) for assessment or care decisions with individuals (eg, family, caregivers, health care professionals) involved in patient's care
- Integration of new information into the medical treatment plan or adjustment of medical therapy

May Be Separately Reported When the Time of Each Service Is Distinct and Nonoverlapping

98966–98968, 99441–99443 Telephone services
98970–98972, 99421–99423 Online digital services
99358, 99359 Prolonged E/M service before and/or after direct patient care

May Not Be Reported in the Same Calendar Month as CPO

94005 Home ventilator management care plan oversight
99091 Collection and interpretation of physiologic data
99487, 99490, 99491 Care management services
99424–99427 Principal care management services

Abbreviations: CPO, care plan oversight; E/M, evaluation and management.

- Includes all cumulative time within the same calendar month.
- Are reported based on the patient's location or status (eg, home, hospice) and the total time spent by the physician within a calendar month. Less than 15 minutes' cumulative time within a calendar month cannot be reported.
- Are reported separately from other office or other outpatient, hospital, home, nursing facility, or domiciliary E/M services.
- Do not require specific practice capabilities as are defined for CCM services.
- Require recurrent supervision of therapy.

     Time spent on the following activities may not be considered CPO:
- Travel time to or from the facility or place of domicile
- Services furnished by clinical staff (ancillary or incident-to staff)
- Very low-intensity or infrequent supervision services included in the pre- and post-encounter work for an E/M service

Example

➤ **A physician reviews a final report from a home health nurse on a patient who no longer requires home health after the first week of the calendar month.** These low-intensity services are considered part of the pre- and post-encounter work of related E/M services and are not reported as CPO services.

- Interpretation of laboratory or other diagnostic studies associated with a face-to-face E/M service
- Informal consultations with health professionals not involved in the patient's care
- Routine postoperative care provided during the global surgery period of a procedure
- Time spent on telephone calls or online digital E/M or in medical team conferences if they are separately reported with codes **99441–99443**, **99421–99423**, or **99367**

A CPO billing worksheet can be used to track time of CPO services based on documentation in the patient's medical record and used to support billing when time in a calendar month supports reporting a CPO service. A template is found online at www.aap.org/cfp. See the "Care Plan Oversight Billing Worksheet Template" box for an example of a completed CPO log. Electronic time-tracking software may be used in lieu of a worksheet.

Care Plan Oversight Billing Worksheet Template

Physician: Dr Joe   Patient Name: Izzy Doe   Month: February 2022

Supporting documentation is found in patient's medical record. Izzy is not receiving home health or hospice care and resides in her parent's home. Izzy attends a pediatric prescribed extended care facility for up to 12 hours a day and receives medical care under a plan of care approved by Dr Joe.

Date of Service	Documented Service	Start Time	End Time	Total Minutes	Monthly Subtotal
02/04/2022	Review of diet log and weights with patient's mother	12:00 pm	12:06 pm	6	6
02/04/2022	Discussion with Dr Endocrine	12:15 pm	12:21 pm	6	12
02/15/2022	Review and approval of revised care plan for extended care program[a]	5:15 pm	5:25 pm	10	22
02/16/2022	Discussion with Dr Pulmonary	5:30 pm	5:45 pm	15	37

Time Requirements per Calendar Month	Patient in Home, Domiciliary, or Rest Home (eg, assisted living facility)	Patient Under the Care of a Home Health Care Agency	Hospice Patient	Nursing Facility Patient
15–29 min	99339	99374	99377	99379
≥30 min	99340	99375	99378	99380
≥30 min Medicare code		G0181	G0182	

Code Supported: **99340**

See www.aap.org/cfp for an online version of this worksheet.

[a] Follow individual payer guidelines for reporting care plan oversight for a pediatric prescribed extended care facility. Codes **99374** and **99375** (home health care plan oversight) are required by some plans.

Home Ventilator Management

94005   Home ventilator management care plan oversight of a patient (patient not present) in home, domiciliary or rest home (eg, assisted living) requiring review of status, review of laboratories and other studies and revision of orders and respiratory care plan (as appropriate), within a calendar month, 30 minutes or more

- Services include determining ventilator settings, establishing a plan of care, and providing ongoing monitoring.
- Code **94005** is used to report home ventilator management CPO. It may only be reported when 30 or more minutes of CPO is provided within a calendar month.
- Home ventilator management CPO is distinct from CPO to patients in their home (**99339**, **99340**) or under care of a home health care agency (**99374–99378**) when provided and reported by a separate physician or QHP (eg, pulmonologist reports **94005** and primary physician reports **99374**).

Medical Team Conferences

Medical team conference codes are used to coordinate or manage care and services for established patients with chronic or multiple health conditions (eg, child who is ventilator dependent with developmental delays, seizures, and gastrostomy tube dependence for nutrition).

Chapter 12. Management of Chronic and Complex Conditions

Table 12-8 provides an overview of the patient population, code descriptors, and services not separately reported with medical team conference services.

Medical team conferences require

- *Face-to-face participation* by a minimum of 3 physicians and/or QHPs or QNHCPs from different subspecialties or disciplines (eg, speech-language pathologists, dietitians, social workers), with or without the presence of the patient, family member(s), community agencies, surrogate decision-maker(s) (eg, legal guardian), and/or caregiver(s).
  — Participation by telephone is not reported.
  — Verify payer policies for participation via interactive audiovisual communication (telemedicine). Participation in team conferences via telemedicine *has not yet been added* to the lists of services reported with modifier **95** or the Medicare list of services approved for provision via telehealth.
- Active involvement in the development, revision, coordination, and implementation of health care services needed by the patient by each participant.
- Face-to-face evaluations and/or treatments within the previous 60 days, by the participant, that are separate from any team conference.
- Only 1 individual from the same specialty may report codes **99366–99368** for the same encounter. However, physicians of different specialties may each report their participation in a team conference.

Table 12-8. Medical Team Conference Services

Patient Population

Established patients with chronic and multiple health conditions or with congenital anomalies (eg, cleft lip and palate, craniofacial abnormalities)

Physician or Qualified Health Care Professional Service

99367 Medical team conference with interdisciplinary team of health care professionals, patient and/or family not present, 30 minutes or more; participation by physician

(When patient or caregivers attend conference, report other evaluation and management codes.)

Nonphysician Service

99366 Medical team conference with interdisciplinary team of health care professionals, face-to-face with patient and/or family, 30 minutes or more; participation by nonphysician qualified health care professional

99368 Medical team conference with interdisciplinary team of health care professionals, patient and/or family not present, 30 minutes or more; participation by nonphysician qualified health care professional

Work Required

- At least 30 minutes of face-to-face services from different specialties or disciplines
- Performed face-to-face evaluations or treatments of the patient, independent of any team conference, within the previous 60 days
- Presentation of findings and recommendations
- Formulation of a care plan and subsequent review/proofing of the plan

Do not report during the service time of

99439, 99487, 99489, 99490, 99491, 99437 Chronic care management services

99424–99427 Principal care management services

- Medical record documentation supporting the reporting physician's or QHP's contributed information and subsequent treatment recommendations and the time spent from the beginning of the review of an individual patient until the conclusion of the review.
- Medical team conferences may not be reported if the facility or organization is contractually obligated to provide the service, they are informal meetings or simple conversations between physicians and other QHPs and QNHCPs, or less than 30 minutes of conference time is spent in the team conferences.

Codes differentiate provider (physician vs other health care professional) and between face-to-face and non–face-to-face (patient and/or family is not present) patient team conference services.

- *CPT* instructs that physicians *or other QHPs* who may report E/M services should report their participation in a team conference with the patient and/or family present using E/M codes for the place of service based on the instructions for the E/M service provided.

Examples

For each of the following examples, a team meets to discuss the care of Izzy, a child with cystic fibrosis with pulmonary manifestations (**E84.0**), exocrine pancreatic insufficiency (**E84.8**, **K86**), and failure to thrive (**R62.51**). Each participant in the conference has completed his or her evaluation of the patient within 60 days prior to the conference.

➤ **A primary care pediatrician, an endocrinologist, a pulmonologist, and the medical director of Izzy's pediatric prescribed extended care facility (specialized day program providing health services) participate in discussion and planning, including changes to Izzy's respiratory therapy and medications, potential side effects of treatment, and option of enteral feeding.** The conference lasts 60 minutes and neither Izzy nor her parents attend.

CPT

99367	Each participating physician (if they are different specialties and/or from different practices [ie, separate tax identification numbers])
99368	Each QNHCP (eg, medical nutrition therapist)

The medical director of the extended care facility should follow payer policy regarding separately reportable services. Physicians who provide a face-to-face visit (eg, consultation, **99241–99245**) on the same date as a *medical team conference without the patient/family present* should report codes for the individual services provided. A payer may require modifier **25** (significant, separately identifiable E/M service) on the code for the face-to-face visit.

➤ **A primary care pediatrician, endocrinologist, pulmonologist, and medical nutrition therapist participate in discussion and planning with Izzy's parents present.** The conference lasts 60 minutes. No other E/M services are provided by the physicians on this date.

CPT

99366	Each nonphysician QHP (eg, medical nutrition therapist)
99202–99499	Each participating physician (if they are different specialties and/or from different practices [ie, separate tax identification numbers]) reports an E/M service based on the place of service and applicable time-based coding instructions.

Physicians who provide a face-to-face visit on the same date as a medical team conference *with the patient/family present* should report the appropriate E/M code for the site of the visit and may also report an appropriate prolonged service code (eg, **99354**, **99355**, or, if in conjunction with an office or other outpatient code, **99417**) for time extending beyond the parameters designated by the E/M code and to the minimum time of the appropriate prolonged service code.

- If licensed QHPs (including clinical nurse specialists and clinical nurse practitioners) participated in a conference without direct physician supervision, they may report the service (**99367**) if it is within the state's scope of practice and they use their own National Provider Identifier. State Medicaid and commercial payers may follow these Medicare requirements or have their own specific rules.
- Code **99367** is the only code that may be reported by a physician, and it can only be reported when the patient and/or family is not present at the team conference.
- Time reported for medical team conferences may not be used in the determination of time for CPO (**99339**, **99340**; **99374–99380**), CCM services (**99487–99491**), prolonged services (**99354–99359**), psychotherapy (**90832–90853**), or any E/M service.

Advance Care Planning

★**99497**   Advance care planning including the explanation and discussion of advance directives such as standard forms (with completion of such forms, when performed), by the physician or other qualified health care professional; first 30 minutes, face-to-face with the patient, family member(s) and/or surrogate

★+**99498**   each additional 30 minutes (List separately in addition to code for primary procedure)

Advance care planning includes

- A face-to-face service by a physician or QHP (including telemedicine services) to a patient, family member, or surrogate spent in counseling and discussion of advance directives
- Completion of forms, when applicable (eg, Health Care Proxy, Durable Power of Attorney for Health Care, Living Will, and Medical Orders for Life-Sustaining Treatment)

Because the *CPT* prefatory language and code descriptors for advance care planning do not include other instruction on the time required for reporting, these services may be reported based on general *CPT* instruction to report when the midpoint is passed (eg, 1 unit of **99498** may be reported for services of 46–75 minutes).

- Do not report code **99497** for less than 16 minutes of physician face-to-face time. Exceptions may apply for payers with policy requiring that the time be met or exceeded.

Advance care planning services may be considered bundled to enhanced payment methodologies (eg, patient-centered medical home receiving per-member, per-month care coordination fees) and not separately paid. However, *CPT* requires reporting of the code that is specific to the service provided regardless of payment policy. Advance care planning services should not be reported as another service (eg, office visit) in an effort to avoid denial as a bundled service.

Relative value units assigned for a non-facility site of service are 2.46 for **99497** and 2.13 for **99498** ($85.84 versus $74.32, respectively, when paid at the 2021 Medicare conversion factor of $34.8931 per RVU).

CPT instructs that codes reported should accurately describe the service rendered and physicians should not report a code that merely approximates the service provided, so it would be inappropriate to report another service that may have higher RVUs and payment values.

However, when a payer does not recognize advance care planning codes or the main reason for an encounter is other than advance care planning, consultation codes **99241–99245** or other E/M service codes (eg, **99212–99215**) may be appropriately reported.

Example

➤ **A child and his parents, who have learned at a recent visit that the child's prognosis is poor, return for advance care planning.** The physician spends 50 minutes face-to-face with the patient and parents, assesses their understanding of the diagnosis, and confirms and documents the desire to limit lifesaving measures and decisions about palliative care. A plan of care is developed and documented, and an appointment with the supportive care team at the hospital is scheduled.

CPT

99497	Advance care planning, initial 30 minutes
99498 × 1	each additional 30 minutes

The physician's face-to-face time of 50 minutes spent providing the advance care planning supports reporting **99497** with 1 unit of **99498** for the final 20 minutes of service.

Prolonged Services Without Direct Patient Contact

Prolonged services without direct patient contact (**99358, 99359**) are reported when a physician or QHP provides prolonged service that does not involve face-to-face care.

Guidelines for reporting non-direct prolonged services include

- Prolonged service before and/or after direct patient care does not include time spent by clinical staff.
- Time is met when the midpoint is passed.
  - Less than 30 minutes' total duration on a given date cannot be reported.
  - Less than 15 minutes beyond the first hour or beyond the final 30 minutes is not reported separately. Use code **99359** to report the final 15 to 30 minutes of prolonged service on a given date. **Table 12-9** breaks down the time requirements.
- For time of prolonged service on the date of an office or other outpatient E/M service (**99205** or **99215**), see code **99417**.
- Service must be related to another service conducted by a face-to-face physician or other QHP.
  - Prolonged service must relate to a service or patient where direct (face-to-face) patient care has occurred or will occur and to ongoing patient management.
  - The primary service may be an E/M service (with or without an assigned time), a procedure, or other face-to-face service.

Table 12-9. Non–face-to-face Prolonged Services at a Glance	
99358	Prolonged evaluation and management service before and/or after direct patient care; first hour
+99359	each additional 30 minutes (Use in conjunction with code 99358.)

Prolonged service must be related to another service provided by the same individual.

Total Duration of Prolonged Service Without Direct Face-to-face Contact	Code(s) and Units of Service Reported
<30 min	Not separately reported
30–74 min	**99358** × 1
75–104 min	**99358** × 1 and **99359** × 1
≥105 min	**99358** × 1 and **99359** × 2

- The place of service does not affect reporting.
- May be reported on a different date than the related primary service. *CPT* does not specify a time frame (eg, within 1 week of related service) for provision of prolonged service before and/or after direct patient care.
- Cannot be reported for time spent in provision of and reported with codes for
  - Care plan oversight services (**99339, 99340; 99374–99380**)
  - Chronic care management (**99491, 99437**)
  - Principal care management (**99424, 99425**)
  - Medical team conferences (**99366–99368**)
  - Online medical evaluations (**99421–99423**)
  - Interprofessional telephone/internet/EHR consultations (**99446–99452**)
  - Anticoagulant management for a patient taking warfarin (**93792, 93793**)

Example

➤ **A physician requested and received medical records from the former physician of a child with cystic fibrosis with exocrine pancreatic insufficiency requiring enteral feeding via gastrostomy.** On a day before the date of the initial consultation service, the physician spends 35 minutes reviewing and summarizing the medical records and documents his time in the medical record. The physician reports

CPT

99358	(prolonged physician services without direct patient contact; 30–74 minutes)

International Classification of Diseases, 10th Revision, Clinical Modification

E84.8, K86	(cystic fibrosis and exocrine pancreatic insufficiency)
Z93.1	(gastrostomy status)

See Chapter 7 for prolonged service on the same date as an office or other outpatient E/M service reported with 99202–99205 or 99212–99215 and for discussion of prolonged clinical staff services.

See chapters 8 and 16 for discussion of face-to-face prolonged services.

Related Services Discussed in Other Chapters

Online Digital Evaluation and Management Services

An online digital medical evaluation (**99421–99423**) is a non–face-to-face E/M service by a physician or other QHP who may report E/M services to a patient using internet resources in response to a patient's online inquiry.

This is in contrast with telemedicine services, which represent interactive audio and video telecommunications systems that permit real-time communication between the physician, at the distant site, and the patient, at the originating site.

Codes **98970–98972** are used by a QNHCP to report an online assessment and management service. The reporting guidelines for codes **98970–98972** are the same as those required for online services provided by the physician or QHP.

Please see Chapter 20 for more information about online digital medical services.

Remote Physiologic Monitoring

#99457　　Remote physiologic monitoring treatment management services, 20 minutes or more of clinical staff/physician/other qualified health care professional time in a calendar month requiring interactive communication with the patient/caregiver during the month

#+99458　　　each additional 20 minutes

Code **99457** is reported for time spent managing care when the results from a monitoring device(s) are used for treatment management services. This code requires 20 or more minutes of time spent using the results of physiologic monitoring to manage a patient under a specific treatment plan. When the time of service extends a full 20 minutes beyond the first 20 minutes, report code **99458** in addition to **99457**.

Please see Chapter 21 for more information on remote physiologic monitoring services.

Telephone Evaluation and Management Services

Telephone services (**99441–99443**) are non–face-to-face E/M services provided at the request of a patient or caregiver by a physician or other QHP who may report E/M services provided to a patient using the telephone.

Codes **98966–98968** are used to report telephone assessment and management services by health care professionals who may not report E/M services (eg, occupational therapists, speech-language pathologists).

Please see Chapter 9 for more details on reporting telephone and consultation services.

Interprofessional Telephone/Internet Consultations

Patients with chronic conditions may often require collaboration between their primary pediatrician and a subspecialist.

A consultation request by a patient's attending or primary physician or QHP soliciting opinion and/or treatment advice *by telephone, internet, or EHR* from a physician with specialty expertise (consultant) is reported by the consultant with interprofessional consultation codes **99446–99449** or **99451**. These consultations do not require face-to-face contact with the patient by the consultant.

The physician requesting the consultation may report code **99452** when 16 to 30 minutes is spent preparing for the referral and/or communicating with the consultant in a service day. Alternatively, prolonged service codes may be reported by the requesting individual when supported by the time of service.

After-hours and Special Services

Codes **99050–99060** are used to report services that are provided after hours or on an emergency basis and are an adjunct to the basic E/M service provided.

Please see Chapter 7 for more details on after-hours and special services codes.

Reporting a Combination of Complex Medical Management Services

Services such as CCM and TCM offer a means of reporting many activities of care management with 1 or 2 codes that describe the complexity and period of care. However, when these codes do not apply (eg, patient does not meet criteria) or a payer does not provide benefits for care management services, it may be necessary to report a combination of codes for non–face-to-face services provided to a child with complex health care needs. These may include CPO, online or telephone E/M services, prolonged services, and team conference services. Some of these services may also be reported in addition to care management services when the time of each service is distinct.

- Be sure to review payer guidance on reporting of these services, as National Correct Coding Initiative edits or other payment policy may require appending modifiers to indicate distinct periods were spent in the provision of each service. For instance, prolonged E/M service is bundled to CPO, but a modifier may be appended to indicate distinct services within the same reporting period. Guidance for reporting and coverage may vary.

- Practices with the capabilities required for reporting CCM services in lieu of CPO may still report the CPO codes when the service provided and nature of the patient presentation support reporting CPO services. Physicians must determine the appropriate code selection based on the practice capabilities, services rendered, and nature of the patient presentation.

Resources

Billing Worksheets

Care Plan Oversight Billing Worksheet Template (www.aap.org/cfp)

Care Management Tracking Worksheet (www.aap.org/cfp)

Chronic Care Management

"Chronic Care Management: Coding for Services in 2022," October 2021 *AAP Pediatric Coding Newsletter˜* (https://coding.solutions.aap.org; subscription required)

Patient- and Family-Centered Care Coordination

AAP policy statement, "Patient- and Family-Centered Care Coordination: A Framework for Integrating Care for Children and Youth Across Multiple Systems" (https://pediatrics.aappublications.org/content/133/5/e1451)

Boston Children's Hospital Care Coordination Curriculum (www.pcpcc.org/resource/care-coordination-curriculum)

Principal Care Management

"Principal Care Management; Another Step Forward for Care Management Services," October 2021 *AAP Pediatric Coding Newsletter* (http://coding.aap.org; subscription required)

Transitional Care Management

"Transitional Care Management: Revisiting the Basics," July 2017 *AAP Pediatric Coding Newsletter* (https://coding.solutions.aap.org/article.aspx?articleid=2634452; subscription required)

Test Your Knowledge!

1. **Which of the following is required for principal care management (PCM)?**
   a. The patient has at least 2 chronic conditions.
   b. The patient's complex chronic condition is expected to last at least 12 months.
   c. A care plan must be established, implemented, revised, or monitored.
   d. The physician provides or oversees the management and/or coordination of services, as needed, for all medical conditions.

2. **Which is true of chronic care management (CCM) services reported with code 99491?**
   a. Clinical staff time is not included in the time of service.
   b. At least 30 minutes of clinical staff time spent in CCM activities must be documented.
   c. Physicians must provide at least 1 face-to-face service during the calendar month.
   d. The patient must have at least 1 chronic condition.

3. **Which of the following is always true of care plan oversight (CPO)?**
   a. A face-to-face visit must occur prior to provision of the CPO service.
   b. High-complexity medical decision-making is required.
   c. Physicians and clinical staff must spend at least 20 minutes in a calendar month.
   d. Services are reported for any 30-day period.

4. **Which of the following is an example of services that are never reported by the same individual in the same calendar month?**
   a. Transitional care management (TCM) and CCM
   b. Care management services and office evaluation and management services (eg, 99213)
   c. PCM and CPO
   d. Care management services and telephone services (99441–99443)

5. **Which service includes a face-to-face service that is not separately reported?**
   a. CPO
   b. PCM
   c. Complex CCM
   d. TCM

Qualified Nonphysician Health Care Professional Services

Contents

Terminology 311

Including Qualified Nonphysician Health Care Professionals in Your Practice 311

    Scope of Practice Laws 312

    National Provider Identifier 313

Incident-to Requirements: Supervision of Nonphysician Health Care Professionals 313

    Documentation Requirements and Tips When Reporting Incident-to Services 314

Nursing Evaluation and Management Visit 314

Nonphysician Assessment and Management Services 315

    Online Medical Assessment 315

    Telephone Calls 316

        Services Not Reported as Telephone Assessment and Management 316

    Medical Team Conferences 317

Patient Self-management Training Services 318

    Education and Training for Patient Self-management 318

    Payer-Specific Coding for Services Under a Disease Management Program 319

Nutritional Support Services 320

    Breastfeeding Support/Lactation Services 320

    Medical Nutrition Assessment and Intervention 321

    Payer-Specific Coding for Nutrition Assessment and Intervention 322

Other Nonphysician Qualified Health Care Professional Services 323

    Genetic Counseling Services 323

    Medication Therapy Management Services by a Pharmacist 323

    Home Health Procedures/Services 323

Resource 324

Test Your Knowledge! 325

In their quest to provide comprehensive and high-quality care to patients, pediatric physicians are including more qualified nonphysician health care professionals (QNHCPs) (eg, dieticians) in their practices and using clinical staff to their full potential.

This chapter focuses on medical services that are provided by health care professionals other than physicians and other qualified health care professionals (QHPs), such as nurse practitioners and physician assistants, who are distinguished by the ability to provide and report evaluation and management (E/M) services.

Terminology

Throughout the *Current Procedural Terminology*® code set, the use of terms such as *physician, qualified health care professional,* or *individual* is not intended to indicate that other entities may not report the service. In select instances, specific instructions may define a service as limited to professionals or other entities (eg, hospital, home health agency).

To help differentiate, the following definitions will apply in discussions and examples in this chapter:

- **Qualified health care professional:** Advanced practice providers, such as advanced practice nurses, clinical nurse specialists, and physician assistants, whose scope of practice includes E/M services beyond minimal services incident to a physician (ie, **99211**).
- **Qualified nonphysician health care professional:** A broad category of health care professionals who typically would not independently prescribe and manage, whose professional services are typically performed under the order and supervision of a physician or QHP, and whose scope of practice does not include E/M services beyond **99211**. Sometimes they are able to bill under their own National Provider Identifier (NPI). This category includes providers such as clinical psychologists, licensed counselors, dietitians/nutritionists, health educators, and lactation consultants, among others.

Please see Chapter 14 for information on reporting mental and behavioral health services provided by qualified nonphysician health care professionals.

- **Clinical staff member** (as defined by *Current Procedural Terminology* [*CPT*]): A health care team member who works under the supervision of a physician or other QHP and who is allowed by law, regulation, and facility policy to perform or assist in the performance of a specific professional service but *does not individually report that professional service.* These include, but are not limited to, registered nurses (RNs), licensed practical nurses (LPNs), and medical assistants (MAs).

  CPT references *clinical staff member* mostly in the context of staff who provide components of physician or QHP services, such as obtaining patient history, and services that are always billed by a supervising physician or QHP (eg, nurse visit, medication administration), as discussed in the Incident-to Requirements: Supervision of Nonphysician Health Care Professionals section later in this chapter.

Staff who are able to perform *administrative functions only,* such as receptionist, scheduling, billing, dictation, or scribing, are not clinical staff for coding purposes.

Including Qualified Nonphysician Health Care Professionals in Your Practice

Services by QNHCPs, provided under a physician's or QHP's order within a physician group practice, can be an integral part of providing a full scope of care in the medical home.

- Billing and coding must align not only with coding guidelines but also state scope of practice (see the Scope of Practice Laws section later in this chapter) and individual payer policies on credentialing, contracting, and billing for services of the specific QNHCP.
- *Before including QNHCPs within your group practice,* it is important to seek expert advice on related state regulations for scope of practice and supervision requirements, enrollment and payment policies of the group's most common payers, and best practices in employment and/or contractual agreements.
- The number of services that may be provided can be estimated based on current patient diagnoses or history of referral for services. Reports from electronic health records or billing software may be used in this estimation (eg, report of the number of unique patient accounts containing a diagnosis indicating mental or behavioral health conditions).

When physicians choose to arrange for services provided within their practice by QNHCPs who are not employed or contracted with their group practice, additional counsel should be obtained to avoid conflict with anti-kickback and/or self-referral regulations.

Payment for QNHCP services begins with negotiating and contracting with payers for coverage and payment of services as described by *CPT* and/or Healthcare Common Procedure Coding System (HCPCS) codes. (A list of HCPCS codes that may be used to report nonphysician education services is included in the Payer-Specific Coding for Services Under a Disease Management Program section later in this chapter.)

- Payers may pay separately for these services when your practice can demonstrate the overall cost savings (eg, decrease in physician or emergency department visits, decreased hospital care) that may be achieved through expanded care in the physician practice.

For more on quality and performance measurement, see Chapter 3.

- If payers do not agree to directly compensate for individual services, consider opportunities for shared savings and other revenue that may be realized when QNHCP services support quality improvement initiatives (eg, per-member, per-month compensation for meeting certain quality measures) and redirection of physician and QHP time to services that are restricted to or best delivered within their scope of practice.

Physicians should be especially aware of each payer's policy addressing use of E/M codes for services provided by QNHCPs or clinical staff. Medicare and payers who adopt Medicare policy do not allow reporting of E/M services other than **99211** (E/M visit not requiring physician face-to-face service) provided by QNHCPs or clinical staff. Other services that specifically indicate work of clinical staff under physician supervision (eg, transitional care management [TCM] or chronic care management [CCM]) are exceptions.

Example

➤ *CPT* **describes codes 99401–99404 as representing services provided face-to-face by a physician or other QHP for the purpose of promoting health and preventing illness or injury.** However, some payers directly instruct that codes such as **99401** may be reported for specific services by specific clinical staff or by QNHCPs such as medical nutritionists or certified lactation consultants.

Always keep a printed or electronic copy of payer guidance that conflicts with *CPT* or standard billing practices.

For more information on chronic care management and transitional care management, see Chapter 12.

Scope of Practice Laws

Scope of practice is a term used by state licensing boards for various professions to define the procedures, actions, and processes that are permitted for a licensed individual. Scope of practice may also address the delegation of health care activities to unlicensed individuals who the delegating physician or other QHP/QNHCP has ascertained has the education, training, and/or certification necessary to safely perform the activity. Additional limitations on scope of practice of QNHCPs and on delegation to clinical staff may come from Medicaid programs, health care systems, or health care professional membership organizations.

Physicians, RNs, clinical nurse practitioners, physician assistants, LPNs, physical therapists, and licensed nutritionists are among some of the professions for which scope of practice laws are defined. Some states limit the autonomous practice of advanced practice professionals and require these QHPs to have written collaboration agreements and require general or direct supervision by a physician. Prescribing authority may also be limited. Verify your state's requirements for all clinicians and appropriate inclusions in any collaboration/supervision agreements.

Every state has laws and regulations that describe the requirements of education and training for health care professionals. However, some states do not have different scope of practice laws for every level of professional (eg, LPN, lactation consultant). Health systems, government payers, and health care professional membership organizations may also define or limit the scope of practice or delegation to QNHCPs and clinical staff.

Scope of practice should be taken into consideration when delegating directly or through standing orders (eg, physician writes order that recommended screening instruments will be completed for all patients presenting for well-baby/well-child [health supervision] examinations).

While scope of practice provides guidance on what services may be performed by QNHCPs and clinical staff, certain codes also limit who can report specific services. For instance, nurses are allowed to counsel for and administer immunizations, but administration codes **90460** and **90461** are only reported when a physician or QHP has provided immunization counseling. Likewise, E/M services are reported only by a physician or QHP, although QNHCPs and clinical staff may perform tasks included in the service (eg, activities of CCM).

- Payers who follow Medicare policy on reporting of E/M services will not accept codes **99202–99205**, **99212–99215**, or **99217–99499** performed by QNHCPs. (*Note:* **99211** is typically reportable by QNHCPs and clinical staff. Payers may adopt Medicare incident-to policy requirements, as discussed in the Incident-to Requirements: Supervision of Nonphysician Health Care Professionals section later in this chapter.)

National Provider Identifier

The NPI is a unique identification number for covered health care professionals. The NPI is required on administrative and financial transactions under the Health Insurance Portability and Accountability Act (HIPAA) of 1996 administrative simplification provisions.

- Anyone who directly provides health care services (eg, physical therapist, nutritionist, audiologist) can apply for and receive an NPI.
- Usually only those who will bill for services and/or order services or prescription drugs will need an NPI.
- The NPI is included on medical claims to indicate who ordered, provided, or supervised the provision of services.

Incident-to Requirements: Supervision of Nonphysician Health Care Professionals

When physicians or other QHPs bill under their NPI for services performed by clinical staff or QNHCPs, an incident-to policy may apply. For those payers who align with Medicare policy, see detailed requirements online at www.aap.org/cfp ("Medicare Requirements for Incident-to Services by Nonphysician Professionals and Clinical Staff"). See also Chapter 12, section 30.6, of the *Medicare Claims Processing Manual*, and Chapter 15, section 60, of the *Medicare Benefit Policy Manual*, at http://cms.gov/manuals (select "Internet-Only Manuals [IOMs]").

Check with your payers and obtain a copy of their specific policies for reporting services provided by clinical staff and/or QNHCPs incident to a physician's service.

> **Incident-to provisions apply only in the office or other outpatient setting.**

- The Centers for Medicare & Medicaid Services defines *incident to* as "services incident to the service of a physician or other professional permitted by statute to bill for services incident to their services when those services meet all of the requirements applicable to the benefit."
  - Incident-to services are always provided as a continuation of a physician's services and do not address new problems (eg, a nursing visit performed at patient or caregiver request and not based on a physician's recommendation is not an incident-to service).
  - A supervising physician or QHP must be present *in the office suite* and available to assist, as needed, at the time of service.
  - A treatment plan or order must be documented by a physician or QHP prior to provision of services by a QNHCP or clinical staff provision of services billed incident to a physician or QHP.
  - The individual providing the incident-to service must be an employee (direct or leased) or working under contract with the physician practice (ie, paid as a practice expense).
- Although certain QHPs and QNHCPs otherwise may bill for their services under their own NPI when they provide medically necessary services (within their state's scope of practice), the incident-to provision allows for reporting under the name and NPI of a supervising physician when the requirements of incident-to billing are met.
  - Payment for QHPs and QNHCPs billing under the incident-to provision may be 100% of the physician payment versus 85% when reporting under the QHP's and QNHCP's individual NPI.

> **While Medicare and many other payers reduce payment to 85% of the Physician Fee Schedule amount when a qualified health care professional provides a service outside of the incident-to requirements (eg, new patient visit), this is not the case for all payers.**

— Payers may not allow reporting of a certain service as incident to a physician's service (eg, nutrition therapy) when the service is not included under the contract between the payer and physician.

- Nonphysician providers (NPPs) without their own NPIs must report services incident to a physician and must meet all incident-to requirements, including physician presence in the office suite and continuation of a physician's previously established plan of care.
- Medicare makes an exception by not requiring the physician's presence in the office suite for CCM, TCM, and behavioral health integration activities by clinical staff. Private payers may also allow inclusion of time spent by clinical staff without direct supervision when reporting these services.

Examples

➤ **A patient returns as directed by a pediatrician for evaluation of a tuberculin test result.** The physician is in the office suite at the time of service. An MA evaluates the site of the injection (48 hours earlier) and notes no reaction (0 mm). The MA instructs the patient to notify the practice if any reaction occurs within the next 24 hours.
Code **99211** (established patient E/M not requiring a physician's presence) is reported for this encounter.

➤ **An MA, as allowed under state scope of practice laws, administers an intranasal influenza vaccine that was ordered and directly supervised by the physician who documented counseling provided to the patient and/or caregivers.** Codes for the vaccine and administration (**90460**, **90672**) would be reported under the physician's NPI. If a pediatric nurse practitioner had ordered and supervised the treatment, the service would be reported under that practitioner's NPI.

Documentation Requirements and Tips When Reporting Incident-to Services

- Physicians and QHPs must document their order for a service or treatment (eg, injection) that will be performed as incident to or document their plan for a follow-up visit in the treatment plan (eg, follow-up visit in 1 week for weight check).
- To demonstrate compliant incident-to billing, QNHCPs and clinical staff providing services in continuation of a physician's plan of care *should, ideally, reference the date of the physician order for the service.* This may be documented in the chief complaint for the encounter (eg, "Patient is seen today per Dr Green's 1/2/2022 order for dressing change to left arm wound in 3 days").
- Documentation of incident-to services should fully describe the services provided, including date of service, assessment, concerns noted and addressed, details of care provided (eg, wound cleansed and new bandage applied), and education and/or instructions for home care and follow-up.
  - Inclusion of the supervising physician's name also supports that incident-to requirements were met.
  - Medical record documentation must reflect the identity, including credentials and legible or digital signature of the person providing the service.

For Medicare purposes, the physician or QHP billing the service is not required to sign documentation prepared by the clinical staff. Other payer and state regulations may require authentication by the supervising physician or QHP. Documentation might be as simple as "service performed/provided under the direct supervision of Dr X." When applicable, the signature must be legible.

Nursing Evaluation and Management Visit

99211   Office or other outpatient visit for the evaluation and management of an established patient, that may not require the presence of a physician or other qualified health care professional. Usually, the presenting problem(s) are minimal.

When clinical staff and/or QNHCPs who do not independently report E/M services provide an E/M service that is not described by another procedure code, code **99211** is reported.
Report **99211** when
- Services meet the incident-to requirements of the payer.
- Problems addressed have previously been addressed by ordering physician or QHP and services are a continuation of care.
- The service is provided based on physician orders and within scope of practice and license.
- The service is rendered face-to-face with the patient or caregiver.

Never report **99211** when

- Another procedure code describes the service provided (eg, **36415**, venipuncture).
- The physician performs a face-to-face E/M service on the same date.
- The patient is new or the problem has not been addressed by a physician.

Example

➤ **A physician orders counseling about diet and exercise by a nurse in the practice for a 16-year-old patient who has obesity with borderline hypertension (follow-up visit not on same day as physician visit).** The follow-up visit is conducted by an RN who documents the patient's weight, body mass index (BMI), and blood pressure. The nurse spends 10 minutes face-to-face with the patient going over dietary guidelines, demonstrating proper portion sizes, and encouraging him to continue an exercise routine and healthier diet.

The RN is not a registered dietitian or licensed medical nutritionist who may report medical nutrition therapy. This service was provided in continuation of the physician's plan of care and under direct (in-office) physician supervision. Code **99211** is reported. Most payers will deny code **99211** when reported on the same date as a physician's E/M service (**99202–99205**, **99212–99215**).

> Please see Chapter 7 for more information on code **99211**.

Nonphysician Assessment and Management Services

Online Medical Assessment

98970   Qualified nonphysician health care professional online digital assessment and management service, for an established patient, for up to seven days, cumulative time during the 7 days; 5-10 minutes
98971   11-20 minutes
98972   21 or more minutes

An online electronic medical assessment (**98970–98972**) is a non–face-to-face assessment and management service by a QNHCP to an established patient using internet resources in response to a patient's online inquiry.

> Online digital evaluation and management (E/M) services by a physician or other qualified health care professional (who may report E/M services) are reported with codes **99421–99423**. See Chapter 9 for information on online digital E/M services.

- *Online assessment and management* refers to use of technology such as secure email and other asynchronous digital communication.

This contrasts with *telemedicine services,* which represent interactive audio and video telecommunications systems that permit real-time communication between the QNHCP at the distant site and the patient at the originating site.

- Before providing online medical services, understand local and state laws, ensure that communications will be HIPAA compliant (eg, conducted through a secure patient portal), establish written guidelines and procedures, educate payers and negotiate for payment, and educate patients.
- Codes **98970–98972** are time-based codes used by a QNHCP to report an online assessment and management service.
- One code and 1 unit of service are reported for the sum of communications pertaining to the online encounter during a 7-day period.
- The 7-day service period begins with the initial, personal QNHCP review of the patient-generated inquiry.
- All time spent addressing the manifesting problem and any additional problems (including new unrelated problems addressed by online electronic communications) during the service period is cumulative and reported as one service.
- Online assessment and management includes
  - Review of the initial inquiry
  - Review of patient records or data pertinent to assessing the patient's problem
  - Personal QNHCP interaction with clinical staff focused on the patient's problem
  - Development of management plans
  - Timely reply to the patient's/caregiver's request for online service

— Permanent record of the service (hard copy or electronic)
— All related communications during a 7-day episode of care (eg, ordering laboratory or other testing, prescribing, conducting related phone calls)
— Cumulative time of QNHCPs in the same group that is involved in the online digital E/M service
● Online digital assessment services (**98970–98972**) are *not* reported
— For services of less than 5 minutes' cumulative time
— For new patient inquiries (although new problems may be addressed for established patients)
— For electronic communication of test results, scheduling of appointments, or other communication that does not include assessment and management
— If the online digital inquiry occurs within the postoperative period of a previously completed procedure
— If the patient generates an online digital inquiry within 7 days of a previous treatment or E/M service and both services relate to the same problem
— If a separately reported assessment service occurs within 7 days of the initial online digital inquiry
● When care plan oversight (**99339**, **99340**; **99374**, **99375**; **99377–99380**), CCM (**99487**, **99489–99491**), TCM (**99495**, **99496**), or collection of physiologic data (**99091**) are provided in the same period, do not count the time of communications related to these services toward the time of online digital medical services.

Example

➤ **Parents of a patient with moderate intermittent asthma securely email a respiratory therapist who is an asthma care coordinator, requesting advice on preparing their child for adhering to the asthma care plan on a weeklong trip with a sports team.** The asthma educator responds to the request, and emails are exchanged to further clarify concerns and provide advice. The child is to be instructed to contact the asthma educator or the treating physician by phone if questions or concerns arise during travel. The cumulative time of the communication is 15 minutes.

The social worker reports code **98971**. If the patient had been seen within the past 7 days or scheduled for an appointment within the 7-day period, this service would not be separately reported.

Telephone Calls

98966   Telephone assessment and management services provided by a qualified nonphysician health care professional to an established patient, parent, or guardian not originating from related assessment and management service provided within the previous 7 days nor leading to an assessment and management service or procedure within the next 24 hours or soonest available appointment; 5–10 minutes of medical discussion

98967   11–20 minutes of medical discussion

98968   21–30 minutes of medical discussion

Codes **98966–98968** are used to report telephone assessment and management services by QNHCPs. Those QHPs who may independently provide and report E/M services report codes **99441–99443**.

Report codes **98966–98968** when
● The patient or caregiver initiates a call that is not in follow-up to a service by the same QNHCP within the past 7 days.
● Five minutes or more is spent in assessment and management services (*time must be documented*).
● No decision to see the patient within 24 hours or at the next available appointment is made during the telephone service.

Services Not Reported as Telephone Assessment and Management

Most telephone services provided by clinical staff (eg, MA relaying physician instructions) are included in the practice expense value assigned to physician services and not separately reported.

Do not report telephone assessment and management services that
● Relate to a service provided by the QNHCP within the past 7 days, regardless of whether the service was planned or prompted by patient or caregiver concern
● Result in an appointment within the next 24 hours or in the next available appointment. When telephone assessment and management results in scheduling the patient for an appointment within 24 hours or the next available appointment, the service is considered preservice work to the face-to-face encounter
● Are within a global period of another service

Telephone services by clinical staff may contribute to time of chronic care management (CCM) or transitional care management (TCM) when the services meet the description of the clinical staff activities included in CCM or TCM.

Example

➤ **The parents of a patient with an anxiety disorder contact a licensed clinical social worker in their physician's practice to request advice on managing a transition from remote learning to classes in school.** The social worker spends 18 minutes on the phone with the parents discussing concerns and techniques for preparing the child for the transition.

The licensed clinical social worker reports code **98967** according to the time spent addressing the parents' concerns. This service would not be reported if the call were provided within 7 days of a previous service by the same provider or if the call resulted in an appointment within 24 hours or the next available face-to-face appointment.

Medical Team Conferences

99366   Medical team conference with interdisciplinary team of health care professionals, face-to-face with patient and/or family, 30 minutes or more; participation by nonphysician qualified health care professional

99368   Medical team conference with interdisciplinary team of health care professionals, patient and/or family not present, 30 minutes or more; participation by nonphysician qualified health care professional

Medical team conference codes are used to report participation by a minimum of 3 health care professionals (including physicians, QHPs, and QNHCPs) of different specialties in conferences to coordinate or manage care and services for established patients with chronic or multiple health conditions (eg, a child with ventilator dependence and developmental delays, seizures, and a gastrostomy tube for nutrition).

- Codes differentiate provider (physician or QHP vs QNHCP) and between face-to-face and non–face-to-face (patient and/or family is not present) team conference services.
- If QHPs (including clinical nurse specialists and clinical nurse practitioners) participated in the conference without direct physician supervision, they may report team conference participation *without the patient or caregiver present* as if provided by a physician (**99367**), if it is within the state's scope of practice and they use their own NPI.
- State Medicaid and commercial payers may follow these Medicare requirements or have their own specific rules.
- Medical team conferences may not be reported when
  - The facility or organization is contractually obligated to provide the service or the conferences are informal meetings or simple conversations between physicians and QNHCPs (eg, therapists).
  - Less than 30 minutes of conference time is spent in a team conference.
- One unit of service is reported for each conference of 30 minutes or more.
- Medicare assigns a bundled (B) status to team conference services in the Medicare Physician Fee Schedule and does not allow separate payment for participation in medical team conferences. Payment policies may vary among Medicaid and private health plans.

Medical team conferences require

- Face-to-face participation by a minimum of 3 health care professionals (any combination of QNHCPs, physicians, and/or QHPs) from different subspecialties or disciplines (eg, speech pathologists, dietitians, social workers), with or without the patient, family member(s), community agencies, surrogate decision-maker(s) (eg, legal guardian), and/or caregiver(s)
- Active involvement in developing, revising, coordinating, and implementing health care services needed by the patient by each participant
- That the participant has provided face-to-face evaluation(s) and/or treatment to the patient, separate from any team conference, within the previous 60 days
- Only one individual from the same specialty to report codes **99366–99368** for the same encounter
- Medical record documentation that supports the reporting individual's participation, the time spent from the beginning of review of an individual patient until the conclusion of review, and the contributed information and subsequent treatment recommendations

Examples

➤ **A care team meets to discuss the care plans for a 4-year-old girl with history of congenital heart disease, cerebrovascular injury with residual paraplegia, and developmental delays.** As the child nears entry to kindergarten, the pediatrician has requested input to the child's individualized education program and ongoing health care plan from all health care professionals. The pediatrician, cardiologist, physiatrist, occupational and physical therapists, speech pathologist, home care coordinator, and social worker attend the conference to discuss the child's current medical status, prognosis for the short and long term, and necessary accommodations for her education. The conference lasts 60 minutes. The patient and family are not present for the conference.

Qualified nonphysician health care professionals report participation by using code **99368** when the patient or caregivers are not present. Assign appropriate *International Classification of Diseases, 10th Revision, Clinical Modification* (*ICD-10-CM*) codes for the specified developmental delays (codes in categories **F80–F88**) and other health concerns addressed.

> Physicians may report code 99367 when participating in a conference without the patient or caregivers present. *Current Procedural Terminology* allows reporting of code 99368 by qualified health care professionals (eg, physician assistants). However, reporting an evaluation and management code for participation when the patient or caregivers are present may be beneficial when allowed or required by individual payer policy. See Chapter 12 for information on physician participation in team conferences.

➤ **A patient with cerebral palsy requires coordination with multiple health care professionals (eg, physical and occupational therapists, neurologist, pediatrician).** Each participant in the conference has completed their evaluation of the patient within 60 days before the conference, and a team conference of 40 minutes is held to assess the current plan of care and therapy. The patient's family is at this conference.

Code **99366** would be reported by the physical and occupational therapists. Physicians at the conference would report an E/M code that best describes their services on this date (eg, office or other outpatient E/M service based on face-to-face time with the family spent in counseling and/or coordination of care).

Patient Self-management Training Services

Education and Training for Patient Self-management

98960   Education and training for patient self-management by a qualified, nonphysician health care professional using a standardized curriculum, face-to-face with the patient (could include caregiver/family) each 30 minutes; individual patient

98961   2–4 patients

98962   5–8 patients

Report codes **98960–98962** when

- The purpose of these services is to teach the patient and caregivers how to self-manage the illness or disease or delay disease comorbidities in conjunction with the patient's professional health care team.
- A physician prescribes the services and a standardized curriculum is used. A standardized curriculum is one that is consistent with guidelines or standards established or recognized by a physician or QNHCP society, association, or other appropriate source (eg, curriculum established or endorsed by the American Academy of Pediatrics).
- Qualifications of the QNHCPs and the content of the program are consistent with guidelines or standards established or recognized by a physician or QNHCP society, association, or other appropriate source.
  - These codes apply to diabetic and asthma self-management training—important categories of patient self-management education and training. Such training can be provided by nurse educators or other clinicians who have received special education and/or certification from accreditation societies or state licensing panels.
  - These services could be reported by the supervising physician when the services are rendered by the appropriately certified professional and acknowledged by the payer via the payer contract or published guidance.
- Education and training services are provided to patients with an established illness or disease.
- When a standardized curriculum is not used in the provision of health behavior assessment and intervention, see codes **96156**, **96158**, **96159**, and **96164–96171**.

Qualifications of the qualified nonphysician health care professionals (QNHCPs) and the content of patient self-management education (98960–98962) must be consistent with guidelines or standards established or recognized by a physician or QNHCP society, association, or other appropriate source.

Code selection is based on the general *CPT* instruction for reporting services based on time. Time is met when the midpoint is passed (ie, report code **98960** for 16 or more minutes of face-to-face time and with units of service for each additional full 30 minutes and the last 16–30 minutes).

Example

➤ **A 14-year-old patient was recently diagnosed with type 1 diabetes and is referred to the diabetes educator for continued training under an approved curriculum.** The certified nurse educator assesses what the patient and caregivers have learned since diagnosis and uses a standardized curriculum to provide additional education. The total documented time of service is 30 minutes.

Code **98960** is reported for the 30 minutes of service. If the time of service extended 16 to 30 minutes beyond the first 30 minutes, an additional unit would be reported.

The content, type, duration, and patient response to the training must be documented in the medical record.

The payer contract will determine if services are reported under the name of the asthma educator, supervising physician, or QHP. If the payer credentials educators, report under the name and NPI of the educator. If the payer does not credential educators, follow payer guidance for reporting. HCPCS modifiers and/or codes may be required to indicate the service was provided by a QNHCP.

Payer-Specific Coding for Services Under a Disease Management Program

HCPCS Level II codes may be reported when the narrative differs from the *CPT* code for the service. What follows is a small sample of HCPCS codes and modifiers that may be used for services by QNHCPs when a payer accepts these codes to describe services rendered as part of a specific disease management program (eg, services specific to management of sickle cell anemia).

Note that HCPCS codes may include the term *NPP* rather than *QNHCP* or *QHP*. These codes are reported only when services are provided by NPPs unless otherwise instructed by a payer. It is advisable to retain copies of a payer's written policies and guidance for reporting HCPCS codes such as

S0315	Disease management program; initial assessment and initiation of the program
S0316	Disease management program, follow-up/reassessment
S0317	Disease management program; per diem
S0320	Telephone calls by a registered nurse to a disease management program member for monitoring purposes; per month
S9441	Asthma education, NPP; per session
S9445	Patient education, not otherwise classified, NPP, individual, per session
S9446	group, per session

Payers may also instruct certain QNHCPs to report services by appending a HCPCS modifier to the *CPT* or HCPCS code for services provided.

HA	Child/adolescent program
HN	Bachelor's degree level
HO	Master's degree level (eg, licensed master social worker)
HP	Doctoral level
HQ	Group setting
UN	Two patients served
UP	Three patients served
UQ	Four patients served
UR	Five patients served
US	Six or more patients served

See an example of how to report services as part of a disease management program for diabetes in the Payer-Specific Coding for Nutrition Assessment and Intervention section later in this chapter.

Nutritional Support Services

Breastfeeding Support/Lactation Services

Under the Patient Protection and Affordable Care Act, most health insurance plans must cover breastfeeding support, counseling, and equipment to mothers for the duration of breastfeeding. These services are not subject to a deductible, co-pay, or coinsurance. However, access to benefits for lactation counseling is not always straightforward.

In the absence of feeding problems of an infant or health problems of the mother, **Z39.1** (encounter for care and examination of lactating mother) is the diagnosis code reported for lactation counseling.

Lactation consultation services do not have a specific *CPT* code, and billing is a source of confusion for many providers. Many states do not license lactation consultants. Also, many health plans do not include lactation consultants in their networks.

Physicians and QHPs may generally use preventive medicine counseling codes **99401–99404** to report personally performed lactation counseling services. When payer policy instructs that these codes be reported for services by an RN or a QNHCP (eg, lactation consultant), a written copy of the payer policy should be kept on file.

> **Be aware, some plans bundle provision of breastfeeding support and counseling to the global obstetric service or postpartum care of the mother and do not pay separately for breastfeeding support or lactation counseling. It is important to understand contractual obligations that may limit a physician's ability to bill the patient for these covered services.**

Clinical staff services may be reported with **99211** when provided incident to a physician's plan of care for an established patient (health plan policies may or may not align with Medicare's incident-to policy).

When a pediatrician provides services related to feeding problems or maternal health issues, report E/M codes by site of service for these services (eg, office visit). Evaluation and management services provided to address maternal issues are reported to the mother's health plan. An *ICD-10-CM* code is used to identify the type of problem (eg, suppressed lactation, **O92.5**)

Other specific codes used to report these services when provided by QNHCPs may include

S9443 Lactation classes, nonphysician provider, per session

Code **S9443** is the code most specific to lactation services. This code is included in some health plan policies for preventive medicine services or breastfeeding/lactation counseling services.

S9445 Patient education, not otherwise classified, nonphysician provider, individual, per session

S9446 Patient education, not otherwise classified, nonphysician provider, group, per session

98960 Education and training for patient self-management by a qualified, nonphysician health care professional using a standardized curriculum, face-to-face with the patient (could include caregiver/family), each 30 minutes; individual patient

Key considerations for reporting lactation services include

- Unless the newborn or infant has been diagnosed with a feeding problem, the mother is typically the patient, and claims are filed to her health benefit plan.
- Payer policies may not allow separate payment for lactation counseling on the same date as an E/M service.
- Challenges might be encountered in states where licensure is not yet enacted for lactation support professionals. Hurdles include credentialing and coverage by payers who cover only services provided by licensed health care professionals, although services provided incident to a physician or QHP (eg, **99211** or **S9443**) may be allowed.
- When a medical condition (eg, feeding problem) was previously diagnosed by the physician on an earlier date, a QNHCP may see the mother and patient to identify the psychological, behavioral, emotional, cognitive, and social factors important to the prevention, treatment, or management of physical health problems. Behavioral health assessment and intervention codes **96156**, **96158** and **96159**, and **96164–96171** may be reportable for these services. Again, payer policy determines who may provide these services and what is paid for.
- Lactation counseling provided by a QNHCP in conjunction with a physician's or QHP's E/M service, although not always separately reported, may reduce the physician's time spent on history taking, counseling, and education. This may also support quality initiatives.

> **Medicaid plans often ask that physicians refer covered breastfeeding mothers to the Special Supplemental Nutrition Program for Women, Infants, and Children for lactation counseling and other support services.**

Medical Nutrition Assessment and Intervention

97802 Medical nutrition therapy, initial assessment and intervention, individual, face-to-face with the patient, each 15 minutes

97803 Reassessment and intervention, individual, face-to-face with the patient, each 15 minutes

97804   group (2 or more individuals), each 30 minutes

Medical nutrition therapy is one of the services for which *CPT* instruction excludes reporting by a physician or QHP who may report E/M services.

- Codes are reported when provided by a QNHCP who may report medical nutrition therapy services under their individual state's scope of practice.
- Many states restrict the provision of medical nutrition therapy to certain QNHCPs (eg, registered dietitians, licensed medical nutritionists). Practices providing medical nutrition therapy services should be aware of state licensing and scope of practice regulations as well as health plan credentialing policies.

  HCPCS modifiers may be required to report the type of provider for medical nutrition therapy services, such as **AE** (Registered dietitian).
- Coverage may also be limited to patients with certain conditions (eg, diabetes, kidney disease) and to a number of units of service or visits per year.
- When medical nutrition therapy is provided as a preventive service, modifier **33** may be appended to codes **97802–97804**.

> For more on modifier **33**, see chapters 2 and 8.

- Services are reported according to time. Per *CPT* instruction, a unit of time is met when the midpoint is passed.
  — Report code **97802** or **97803** with 1 unit for 8 to 22 minutes of service. An additional unit may be reported for each subsequent 15 minutes and the last 8 to 22 minutes of service.
  — Certain payers may require that the time in the code descriptor (eg, 15 minutes) be met or exceeded for each unit of service reported.
- Time must be documented.

Examples

➤ **A 14-year-old girl was seen by her physician for a health supervision visit 1 week ago.** Her BMI was at the 90th percentile, her blood pressure was at the upper limit of reference, and the results of her cholesterol screening indicated hypercholesterolemia. The patient was referred to the practice's registered dietitian for assessment and counseling on a diet to reduce the risk for cardiovascular and endocrine disorders. The dietitian meets with the child and her parents and spends 30 minutes discussing risk factors and developing a plan with goals to decrease weight, cholesterol level, and blood pressure.

ICD-10-CM	CPT
Z71.3 (dietary counseling and surveillance) **E78.00** (pure hypercholesterolemia) **Z68.53** (BMI pediatric, 85th percentile to less than 95th percentile for age)	If payer allows billing under registered dietitian's NPI **97802** × 2 (medical nutrition therapy, initial assessment and intervention, individual, face-to-face with the patient, each 15 minutes)
	If payer requires billing under the NPI of the supervising physician
	97802 AE × 2 (medical nutrition therapy as above by a registered dietitian)

Teaching Point: Some Medicaid plans and/or private payers may require that medical nutrition therapy in the physician practice be provided under a physician's order and general supervision. Services are reported as if provided by the physician, but modifier **AE** indicates that the service was provided by a registered dietitian.

Chapter 13. Qualified Nonphysician Health Care Professional Services

➤ **A group of adolescent patients with type 1 diabetes is referred to a licensed medical nutritionist for reassessment and intervention.** The patients receive both individual reassessment and group therapy services for a total time of 50 minutes.

ICD-10-CM	CPT
Z71.3 (dietary counseling and surveillance) **E10.-** (type 1 diabetes mellitus [additional characters required to indicate manifestations or lack thereof])	If payer allows billing under registered dietitian's NPI **97804** × 2 (medical nutrition therapy, reassessment and intervention, each 30 minutes) If payer requires billing under the NPI of the supervising physician **97804 AE** × 2 (medical nutrition therapy as above by a registered dietitian)

Teaching Point: The service provided to a group, even with individual reassessments in the group setting, is reported to each patient's health plan with code **97804** with 1 unit per 30 minutes. Because the time of service was 50 minutes, 2 units of service are reported (ie, the midpoint between the first and last 30-minute periods was passed).

Payer-Specific Coding for Nutrition Assessment and Intervention

HCPCS codes may be required by certain payers to provide reassessment and subsequent intervention after a change in diagnosis, medical condition, or treatment.

G0270   Medical nutrition therapy; reassessment and subsequent intervention(s) following second referral in same year for change in diagnosis, medical condition, or treatment regimen (including additional hours needed for renal disease); individual, face-to-face with the patient, each 15 minutes

G0271   group (2 or more individuals), each 30 minutes

Documentation of services should include the physician or QHP order for services, information on the medical need for services, medical nutrition therapy evaluation and plan for intervention, time, correspondence with the referring provider, date of service, and name, credentials, and signature of the provider of the medical nutrition therapy.

Payers may also offer specific benefits for nutrition assessments and counseling under specific disease management programs. HCPCS codes may be required in lieu of *CPT* codes.

G0108   Diabetes outpatient self-management training services, individual, per 30 minutes
G0109   Diabetes outpatient self-management training services, group session (2 or more), per 30 minutes
S9449   Weight management classes, NPP, per session
S9452   Nutrition class, NPP, per session
S9455   Diabetic management program, group session
S9460   nurse visit
S9465   dietitian visit
S9470   Nutritional counseling, dietitian visit

➤ **A group of adolescent patients with diabetes type 1 is referred to a licensed medical nutritionist for reassessment and intervention as part of a diabetes outpatient self-management training program.** The patients receive both individual reassessment and group therapy services for a total time of 50 minutes.

ICD-10-CM	CPT
Z71.3 (dietary counseling and surveillance) **E10.-** (type 1 diabetes mellitus [additional characters required to indicate manifestations or lack thereof])	If payer allows billing with *CPT* **97804** × 2 (medical nutrition therapy, reassessment and intervention, each 30 minutes) If payer requires billing with HCPCS **G0109** × 2 (diabetes outpatient self-management training services, group session [2 or more], per 30 minutes)

Teaching Point: The service should be reported per the individual payer's policy for the program. Note also that a payer may require that the time of service be met or exceeded (ie, a second unit of service would be reported only if time meets or exceeds 60 minutes).

Other Nonphysician Qualified Health Care Professional Services

Genetic Counseling Services

96040   Medical genetics and genetic counseling services, each 30 minutes face-to-face with patient/family

- Trained genetic counselors provide services that may include obtaining a structured family genetic history, pedigree construction, analysis for genetic risk assessment, and counseling of the patient and family.
- Only face-to-face time with the patient or caregiver is used in determining the units of service reported. Do not report genetic counseling of 15 minutes or less. Report code **96040** with units of service for the first and each additional 30 minutes and the last 16 to 30 minutes.
- Services may be provided during one or more sessions and may include review of medical data and family information, face-to-face interviews, and counseling services.
- For genetic counseling and education on genetic risks by a QNHCP to a group, see codes **98961** and **98962**.
- Genetic counseling by physicians and other QHPs who may report E/M services are reported with the appropriate E/M service code.

Medication Therapy Management Services by a Pharmacist

99605   Medication therapy management service(s) provided by a pharmacist, individual, face-to-face with patient, with assessment and intervention if provided; initial 15 minutes, new patient

99606   initial 15 minutes, established patient

+99607   each additional 15 minutes (List separately in addition to **99605** or **99606**)

    Medication therapy management services

- Are provided only by a pharmacist face-to-face with the patient or caregiver and usually in relation to complex medication regimens or medication adherence in conditions such as asthma and diabetes.
- Are provided on request of the patient or caregiver, prescribing physician, other QHPs, or prescription drug benefit plan (not reported for routine dispensing-related activities).
- Are reported with codes selected based on whether the patient is new or established and the pharmacist's face-to-face time with the patient.
- Include review of pertinent patient history (not limited to drug history).
- Include documentation of review of the pertinent patient history, medication profile (prescription and nonprescription), and recommendations for improving health outcomes and treatment compliance.
- *New patients* are those who have received no face-to-face service from the pharmacist or another pharmacist of the same clinic or pharmacy within 3 years prior to the current date of service.
- Unless otherwise specified by the payer policy, time is met when the midpoint is passed.
  - Report codes **99605** and **99606** for the first 8 to 22 minutes of face-to-face time with the patient.
  - When time exceeds 22 minutes, code **99607** may be reported for subsequent 15-minute periods and the last 8 to 22 minutes.
- Under the Medicare program, pharmacists may also provide services incident to a physician or QHP and report E/M services with code **99211** when allowed under the scope of practice as defined by state licensure.

Home Health Procedures/Services

99501   Home visit for postnatal assessment and follow-up care

99502   Home visit for newborn care and assessment

99503   Home visit for respiratory therapy care (eg, bronchodilator, oxygen therapy, respiratory assessment, apnea evaluation)

99504   Home visit for mechanical ventilation care

99505   Home visit for stoma care and maintenance including colostomy and cystostomy

99506   Home visit for intramuscular injections

99507   Home visit for care and maintenance of catheter(s) (eg, urinary, drainage, and enteral)

99509   Home visit for assistance with activities of daily living and personal care

99510   Home visit for individual, family, or marriage counseling

99511   Home visit for fecal impaction management and enema administration

99512   Home visit for hemodialysis

99600   Unlisted home visit service or procedure

Codes **99500–99600** are

- Typically reported for skilled nursing services ordered by a physician or QHP and are medically necessary services provided to a housebound patient. *Exception:* A nursing visit to a mother and newborn may be covered when provided within a specified period following hospital discharge (verify payer policy for coverage).

- Used to report services provided in a patient's residence (including assisted living apartments, group homes, nontraditional private homes, custodial care facilities, or schools).

> Physicians and other qualified health care professionals providing evaluation and management services in a patient's home report code 99341–99350.

- Not reported if another code more accurately describes the service provided (eg, report home medical nutrition therapy with **97802–97804** rather than **99509**).

Coverage of home health procedures or services by QHPs who are authorized to use E/M home visit codes (**99341–99350**) may also be reported with codes **99500–99600** if both services are performed and the patient's condition requires a significant, separately identifiable service. Modifier **25** would be appended to codes **99341–99350**.

Resource

Incident-to Billing

Medicare Claims Processing Manual Chapter 12, section 30.6, and *Medicare Benefit Policy Manual* Chapter 15, section 60 (http://cms.gov/manuals; select "Internet-Only Manuals [IOMs]")

"Medicare Requirements for Incident-to Services by Nonphysician Professionals and Clinical Staff" (www.aap.org/cfp)

Chapter 13. Qualified Nonphysician Health Care Professional Services

Test Your Knowledge!

1. **Which of the following terms describes a unique identification number for covered health care professionals?**
   a. Incident to
   b. National Provider Identifier
   c. Administrative simplification provisions
   d. Scope of practice

2. **Which of the following services may be reported for a nurse's assessment of a patient when Medicare incident-to billing requirements are met?**
   a. Any evaluation and management (E/M) service
   b. Any established patient E/M service
   c. Only **99211**
   d. Any level of E/M service addressing an established problem

3. **Which of the following is a required component of education and training for patient self-management?**
   a. A standardized curriculum is used.
   b. A physician is present when the service is provided.
   c. The service is provided to prevent an illness or injury.
   d. At least 30 minutes is spent providing the service.

4. **When is lactation counseling reported with code Z39.1 (encounter for care and examination of lactating mother)?**
   a. When the mother is experiencing a health concern related to breastfeeding
   b. Only when provided by a physician or qualified health care professional (QHP)
   c. In the absence of feeding problems of an infant or health problems of the mother
   d. When a newborn's or infant's feeding problem is evaluated

5. **Medication therapy management services (99605–99607) are reported by which type of provider?**
   a. Physician or QHP
   b. Qualified nonphysician health care professional
   c. Nurse educator
   d. Pharmacist

Chapter 13. Qualified Nonphysician Health Care Professional Services

Mental and Behavioral Health Services

Physicians and Other Mental/Behavioral Health Providers 329

    Including Nonphysician Providers in Your Practice 329

    Payment and Coverage Issues for Mental/Behavioral Health Services 329

Reporting Codes **F01–F99** 330

Current Procedural Terminology® Add-on Codes 331

Central Nervous System Assessments/Tests 331

Developmental Testing 331

Neuropsychological and Psychological Testing 332

    Neurobehavioral Status Examination 332

    Psychological and Neuropsychological Testing Services 333

        Testing Evaluation Services by a Physician or Other Qualified Health Care Professional With Interpretation and Report 333

        Testing Administration Services 334

Adaptive Behavior Assessment and Treatment Services 336

    Adaptive Behavior Assessment 336

    Adaptive Behavior Treatment 337

        Adaptive Behavior Treatment by Protocol 338

        Adaptive Behavior Treatment With Protocol Modification 338

        Family Adaptive Behavior Treatment Guidance 339

    Habilitative and Rehabilitative Modifiers 340

Health and Behavior Assessments/Interventions 340

    Health Behavior Assessment 341

    Health Behavior Intervention 341

Psychiatric Services 342

    Interactive Complexity 342

    Psychiatric Diagnostic Evaluation 343

    Psychotherapy 345

        Psychotherapy With Evaluation and Management 345

        Psychotherapy Without Evaluation and Management 346

        Psychotherapy With Biofeedback 347

        Psychotherapy for Crisis 347

        Family and Group Psychotherapy 348

        Other Psychiatric Services 348

Evaluation and Treatment of Substance Use 348

    ICD-10-CM Coding for Use, Abuse, and Dependence 349

    Management/Treatment of Alcohol and Substance Use Disorders 349

    Alcohol and/or Substance Use Screening/Testing 350

        Presumptive Drug Class Screening 350

        Definitive Drug Testing 351

Behavioral Health Integration 351

    Psychiatric Collaborative Care Management Services 351

    General Behavioral Health Integration Care Management 354

Resources 355

Test Your Knowledge! 356

Physicians and Other Mental/Behavioral Health Providers

This chapter focuses on services that are provided to diagnose, manage, or treat mental and behavioral health conditions. Mental and behavioral health services may be covered through a provider network separate from other health care services. Physicians providing these services personally and/or through nonphysician staff within their practice must be aware of the coverage and payment policies of local and regional health plans and determine how these policies affect delivery and payment of services.

Services included in this chapter may be provided by

- Physicians and other qualified health care professionals (QHPs) and qualified nonphysician health care professionals (QNHCPs), including licensed clinical psychologists and licensed clinical social workers (State regulations and payment policies are often least restrictive for these providers.)
- Allied health care professionals (AHPs), such as technicians and developmental specialists, who provide services ordered by and under the general supervision of physicians and QHPs (State regulations and payment policies are often somewhat restrictive for these providers.)
- Clinical staff working under direct physician supervision (State regulations and payment policies are typically most restrictive for these providers.)

Including Nonphysician Providers in Your Practice

Services such as behavioral health assessment by a licensed social worker or licensed psychologist may be provided within a general pediatric group practice and can be an integral part of providing a full scope of care in the medical home. However, billing and coding of these services must align not only with coding guidelines but also state scope of practice and individual payer policies on credentialing, contracting, and billing for services of the specific QNHCP.

Payment and Coverage Issues for Mental/Behavioral Health Services

Behavioral health services may be covered through a plan and provider network separate from other health care services. When arranging for or providing behavioral health services, it is very important to explore the patient's health plan policy options.

- Failure to credential and, when applicable, contract with behavioral health plans may lead to unpaid or underpaid charges.
- Payer policies may allow specific licensed professionals, such as licensed clinical psychologists and licensed clinical social workers, to directly provide and report certain services. Other QNHCPs (eg, licensed master social workers) may be limited to providing services under direct supervision and reporting in the name of the participating health care professional (eg, licensed clinical psychologist or psychiatrist).
- General pediatricians and other QHPs may be ineligible to participate in the behavioral health plan network and limited to reporting E/M services to the health plan based on time.

The American Academy of Pediatrics (AAP) Council on Early Childhood, Committee on Psychosocial Aspects of Child and Family Health, and Section on Developmental and Behavioral Pediatrics included the following information about coverage of treatment of emotional and behavioral health problems in the policy statement, "Addressing Early Childhood Emotional and Behavioral Problems" (https://pediatrics.aappublications.org/content/138/6/e20163023):

American Academy of Pediatrics Policy Statement

"Without adequate payment for screening and assessment by primary care providers and management by specialty providers with expertise in early childhood mental health, treatment of very young children with emotional and behavioral problems will likely remain inaccessible for many children. Given existing knowledge regarding the importance of early childhood brain development on lifelong health, adequate payment for early childhood preventive services will benefit not only the patients but society as well and should be supported. Mental health carve-outs should be eliminated because they provide a significant barrier to access to mental health care for children. Additional steps toward equal access to mental health and physical health care include efficient prior authorization processes; adequate panels of early childhood mental health providers; payment to all providers, including primary care providers, for mental health diagnoses; sustainable payment for co-located mental health providers and care coordination; payment for evidence-based approaches focused on parents; and payment for the necessary collection of information from children's many caregivers and for same-day services. Advocacy for true mental health parity must continue."

Chapter 14. Mental and Behavioral Health Services

Integration of psychiatric and/or developmental/behavioral health care professionals into the primary care practice may also require an understanding of health plan payment policies. Payer edits may not allow separate payment for mental and behavioral health services when E/M services are provided in the same practice on the same date. Verify coverage and billing options prior to provision of services.

> **Learn more about payer edits in Chapter 2 and about American Academy of Pediatrics payer advocacy in Chapter 4.**

- Payers often place limitations on the diagnoses that may be paid under a patient's health benefits versus a separate behavioral health benefit.
  - Pediatricians may be required to report codes for symptoms rather than diagnosed conditions (eg, sadness in lieu of depression). This conflicts with *International Classification of Diseases, 10th Revision, Clinical Modification* (*ICD-10-CM*) guidelines.
  - *ICD-10-CM* guidelines instruct, "Codes that describe symptoms and signs, as opposed to diagnoses, are acceptable for reporting purposes when a related definitive diagnosis has not been established (confirmed) by the provider."
  - Adherence to these guidelines when assigning *ICD-10-CM* diagnosis codes is required under the Health Insurance Portability and Accountability Act of 1996. Payers are required to accept codes reported in compliance with the official guidelines for code selection and reporting.
  - When payers deny claims appropriately reported with codes **F01–F99** (mental, behavioral and neurodevelopmental disorders), pediatricians may report the issue using the AAP Coding Hotline (https://form.jotform.com/ Subspecialty/aapcodinghotline) or seek the assistance of an AAP pediatric council (www.aap.org/en/practice-management/practice-financing/payer-contracting-advocacy-and-other-resources/aap-payer-advocacy/ aap-pediatric-councils).
- Healthcare Common Procedure Coding System (HCPCS) modifiers identifying the type of health care professional (eg, **AJ**, clinical social worker) may be necessary to override edits that bundle E/M services provided by a physician/ QHP and mental/behavioral health services provided by a QNHCP on the same date.
- Relevant HCPCS modifiers include

AH	Clinical psychologist
AJ	Clinical social worker
AM	Physician, team member service
HA	Child/adolescent program
HN	Bachelor's degree level
HO	Master's degree level
HP	Doctoral level
HQ	Group setting
TL	Early intervention/individualized family service plan (IFSP)
UN	Two patients served
UP	Three patients served
UQ	Four patients served
UR	Five patients served
US	Six or more patients served

Reporting Codes F01–F99

Diagnosis of behavioral and mental health conditions is typically based on the criteria set forth in the *Diagnostic and Statistical Manual of Mental Disorders,* 5th Edition (*DSM-5*) classification system.

- Often, a simple crosswalk from the *DSM-5* diagnosis to the *ICD-10-CM* code supporting the diagnosis can be made. However, the classifications are not always equivalent.

  DSM-5 does not differentiate Asperger syndrome from autism spectrum disorder (ASD). *ICD-10-CM* provides a specific code for Asperger syndrome (**F84.5**) in addition to codes for autistic disorder (**F84.0**) and other pervasive developmental disorders (eg, Rett syndrome, **F84.2**).
- It is important that documentation clearly reflects a diagnostic statement separate from the assignment of an *ICD-10-CM* code as required by official guidance for *ICD-10-CM*.
  - This statement should include the findings supporting the diagnosis (eg, observations made during the appointment, history, standardized rating scale results, pertinent physical examination findings).

International Classification of Diseases, 10th Revision, Clinical Modification codes for behavioral and emotional disorders with onset usually occurring in childhood and adolescence (F90–F98) may be reported for patients of any age. Disorders in this category typically have onset during childhood but may continue throughout life and not be diagnosed until adulthood.

— Failure to document the information supporting the diagnostic statement could affect the patient's access to care and the physician's payment for services provided.

● *ICD-10-CM* includes codes for specifying how an accident or injury happened (eg, unintentional or accidental; intentional, such as suicide or assault).

— Management of patients who have sustained injury or illness (eg, poisoning) due to intentional self-harm are reported with codes signifying the intent (eg, **T52.92XA**, toxic effect of unspecified organic solvent, intentional self-harm, initial encounter).

— If the intent of the cause of an injury or other condition is unknown or unspecified, code the intent as accidental intent. All transport accident categories assume accidental intent.

— Codes for events of undetermined intent are only for use if the documentation in the record specifies that the intent cannot be determined at the encounter (eg, suspected abuse under investigation).

Current Procedural Terminology® Add-on Codes

Many mental and behavioral health services are described by a combination of a base code with add-on codes representing extended services. Add-on codes (marked with a + before the code) are always performed in addition to a primary procedure and are never reported as a stand-alone service. Add-on codes describe additional intraservice work and are not valued to include preservice and post-service work like most other codes.

Central Nervous System Assessments/Tests

The following codes are used to report the services provided during testing of central nervous system functions. Central nervous system assessments include, but are not limited to, memory, language, visual/motor responses, and abstract reasoning/problem-solving abilities. The mode of completion can be by a person (eg, paper and pencil) or via automated means. The administration of these tests will generate material that will be interpreted and formulated into a report by a physician or other QHP or an automated result.

Standardized instruments are used in the performance of central nervous system assessment/testing services. Standardized instruments are validated tests administered and scored in the consistent or "standard" manner performed during their validation. Informal checklists created by a physician or electronic health record developer are not considered standardized instruments.

Claims for testing are typically reported after the final date of testing services, with the appropriate codes for each date of service reported on the single claim. However, payer instructions may vary, and some require reporting with only the date on which testing services are completed (see example in discussion of **96112** and **96113** in the next section).

Payers may require prior authorization of tests. Practices should adopt procedures for verifying coverage and obtaining prior authorization, when required.

Central nervous system assessments and tests are not reported in conjunction with adaptive behavior treatment (**97151–97158**, **0362T**, **0373T**).

Developmental Testing

96112   Developmental test administration (including assessment of fine and/or gross motor, language, cognitive level, social, memory and/or executive functions by standardized developmental instruments when performed), by physician or other qualified health care professional, with interpretation and report; first hour

+96113   each additional 30 minutes (List separately in addition to code for primary procedure)

Developmental screening services are described by code 96110. Developmental screening using an objective standardized instrument, including scoring and documentation, is typically done by clinical staff. Interpretation and counseling on the score are included in the related evaluation and management service.

Codes **96112** and **96113**

- Allow reporting of developmental testing in which the child is observed doing standardized tasks that are then scored, with interpretation and report.
- Include assessment of motor, language, social, and/or cognitive function by standardized developmental instruments (eg, scales of infant and toddler development) and include objective assessments as well.
- Billing time includes both face-to-face time spent in testing and time of interpretation and report.
  — Although not specifically stated in the code descriptor, interpretation and report is included as intraservice work in the assignment of work relative value units for these services.
  — Payer policies may vary on reporting of time spent in interpretation and report. Check the policies of individual health plans when reporting.
- Code selection is based on time spent per hour by the physician or QHP.

  The midpoint rule applies to developmental testing; time is met when the midpoint is passed. Thirty-one minutes are required to report 1 hour of service. Sixteen minutes are required to report the final period of service of less than 30 minutes.
- If a developmental instrument does not meet the criteria of being an objective instrument with the subjective element and does not take a minimum of 31 minutes to complete including interpretation and report, refer to code **96110** instead.

  Do not report **96110** if also reporting code **96112** or **96113** on the same day for the same patient.

Example

➤ **A 7-year-old boy presents for extended developmental testing due to long-standing social and learning difficulties at school.** Developmental tests are administered, with total testing time on this date of 75 minutes. The child returns and spends a total of 60 minutes to complete testing 1 week later. After testing is completed, the developmental pediatrician spends another 60 minutes on the same date interpreting the test results and 60 minutes formulating a report of the findings and recommendations. Code **96112** is reported for the 75 minutes of service on the first date. Because the midpoint between 60 and 90 minutes (76 minutes) was not passed, **96113** is not reported. On the second date of service, codes **96112** (first 60 minutes of testing) and **96113** with 4 units of service (2 hours interpreting the testing results and developing the report) are reported. On the final date of service (ie, the day of the feedback session), submit 1 claim for all cumulative services detailed *by separate dates of service.*

   Teaching Point: Some payers may require the entire service be reported on a single claim and single date of service. For these payers, report code **96112** (for the 60 minutes of testing on the first day) and 6 units of **96113** (for the remaining 195 minutes) on the date of the second session. It is important that staff are trained to submit the records for dates that testing services were provided, when necessary, in response to a payer's request for records.

   Remember, the midpoint must be passed for the additional units to be billed. In this case, the remaining time was only 15 minutes.

Neuropsychological and Psychological Testing

Neuropsychological and psychological testing evaluation services typically include integration of patient data with other sources of clinical data, interpretation, clinical decision-making, treatment planning, and report.

- Interactive feedback, conveying the implications of psychological or neuropsychological test findings and diagnostic formulation, is included when performed.
- Testing by a physician or QHP is separately reportable as an evaluation service on the same or a different date.
- Testing codes differentiate tests administered by a physician or other QHP, by a technician, or via an electronic platform.

Neurobehavioral Status Examination

★**96116**   Neurobehavioral status examination (clinical assessment of thinking, reasoning and judgment [eg, acquired knowledge, attention, language, memory, planning and problem solving, and visual spatial abilities]), by physician or other qualified health care professional, both face-to-face time with the patient and time interpreting test results and preparing the report; first hour

+**96121**   each additional hour

Mini-mental status examination performed by a physician is included as part of the central nervous system physical examination of an evaluation and management service and not separately reportable.

- Documentation of these services includes scoring, informal observation of behavior during the testing, and interpretation and report. It should include the date and time spent in testing, time of interpretation and report, reason for the test, and titles of all instruments used.
- Neurobehavioral status examination is reported based on the time of face-to-face testing and includes time interpreting test results and preparing a report.
- The unit of time is 60 minutes and time is met when the midpoint is passed (ie, at least 31 minutes of time is required for the first or last unit of service).
- These services may be provided via telemedicine; append modifier **95** to indicate a service provided via real-time audiovisual technology.

Example

➤ **An 8-year-old boy, previously diagnosed with attention-deficit/hyperactivity disorder (ADHD), predominantly inattentive type, is being evaluated for gradual problems with remembering directions, organizing his school materials and his room at home, and other behavior concerns.** The physician or QHP performs a neurobehavioral status examination, which involves clinical assessments and observations for impairments in acquired knowledge, attention, learning, and memory. The results indicate the need for further standardized language, memory, and intelligence testing. The total time for testing, scoring, and report writing is 3½ hours.

This service is reported with codes **96116** (neurobehavioral status examination) and **96121** with 2 units for the additional 2½ hours of testing, scoring, and report writing. The diagnosis code would be *ICD-10-CM* code **F90.0** (ADHD, predominantly inattentive type). Additional *ICD-10-CM* codes may be assigned for specific developmental disorders diagnosed following testing (eg, **F81.2**, mathematics disorder).

Psychological and Neuropsychological Testing Services

Codes for psychological and neuropsychological testing differentiate test administration by physicians and QHPs, technicians, or automated systems. A combination of testing evaluation and test administration and scoring services is typically reported on a single claim.

The tests selected, test administration, and method of testing and scoring are the same regardless of whether the testing is performed by a physician, QHP, or technician.

Testing Evaluation Services by a Physician or Other Qualified Health Care Professional With Interpretation and Report

96130   *Psychological* testing evaluation services by physician or other qualified health care professional, including integration of patient data, interpretation of standardized test results and clinical data, clinical decision making, treatment planning and report, and interactive feedback to the patient, family member(s) or caregiver(s), when performed; first hour

+96131   each additional hour (List separately in addition to code for primary procedure)

96132   *Neuropsychological* testing evaluation services by physician or other qualified health care professional, including integration of patient data, interpretation of standardized test results and clinical data, clinical decision making, treatment planning and report, and interactive feedback to the patient, family member(s) or caregiver(s), when performed; first hour

+96133   each additional hour (List separately in addition to code for primary procedure)

- These services follow standard *Current Procedural Terminology* (*CPT*) time definitions (ie, a minimum of 31 minutes must be provided to report a 1-hour unit of service). The time reported in codes **96130–96133** is the face-to-face time with the patient and the time spent integrating and interpreting data.
- *Time spent in test administration and scoring is not included in time used to support codes* **96130–96133**. Separately report psychological/neuropsychological test administration and scoring services (**96136–96139**) on the same or different days (ie, each service is separately reported on the same claim). Report the total time of evaluation and testing services at the completion of the entire episode of evaluation on a single claim with each date of service listed separately.

Time of 30 minutes or less would not be reported with codes 96132 and 96133.

- Documentation of these services includes scoring, observation of behavior, and interpretation and report. It should include the date and time spent in testing and the time spent integrating and interpreting data, reason for the testing, and titles of all instruments used.

> The time reported in codes 96130–96133 is the face-to-face time with the patient and the time spent integrating and interpreting data. Time spent in face-to-face testing and in integration and interpretation of data must be documented to support the time used in code selection. An itemization of time for each activity is preferable.

Example

➤ **An adolescent patient with history of brain surgery is referred for neuropsychological evaluation due to difficulties with memory and reading.** A physician spends 2 hours reviewing the patient's medical records, interpreting data from tests administered and scored on an earlier date by a technician, and creating a report (copied to the referring physician) of the diagnosis and recommendations for treatment. Another 40 minutes was spent providing interactive feedback to the patient and caregivers.

Code 96132 and 2 units of 96133 are reported for 2 hours and 40 minutes spent in data interpretation, interactive feedback, and report writing. If the physician also personally administered and scored tests, codes 96136 and 96137 would also be reported based on the time of testing and scoring. Test administration and scoring by a technician would be reported separately with codes 96138 and 96139 based on the time of service (see discussion of codes 96138 and 96139 in the Technician-Administered Testing section later in this chapter).

Teaching Point: Report code 96133 with 1 unit of service in addition to 96132 for time of 91 to 150 minutes. Time of 151 minutes or more supports additional units of service for code 96133 (include 1 unit for 31–59 minutes beyond the last full hour).

Testing Administration Services

Test administration and scoring services are selected based on time of service. The midpoint rule applies. Separate codes are reported based on whether testing and scoring are personally performed by a physician or QHP or are performed by a technician.

> At least 2 distinct tests must be administered and scored to report codes 96136–96139. Do not separately count subtests in a multifaceted test (eg, Wechsler Preschool and Primary Scale of Intelligence is 1 test with 14 subtests). Code 96127 (brief emotional/behavioral assessment with scoring and documentation, per standardized instrument) may be reported for administration and scoring of a single standardized test.

Physician or Qualified Health Care Professional Administration and Scoring

96136   Psychological or neuropsychological test administration and scoring by physician or other qualified health care professional, two or more tests, any method; first 30 minutes

+96137   each additional 30 minutes after first 30 minutes (List separately in addition to code for primary procedure)

- Services include administration of a series of tests, recording of behavioral observations made during testing, scoring, and transcription of scores to a data summary sheet.
- Codes are selected based on time of testing and scoring. Time is met when the midpoint is passed (ie, a minimum of 16 minutes for 30-minute codes). Refer to **Table 14-1** for more details.
- *Do not include* time spent in integration of patient data or interpretation of test results in the time reported with codes 96136 and 96137. This time is included with psychological and neuropsychological test evaluation services (96130–96133).
- Psychological or neuropsychological test administration *using a single test/instrument,* with interpretation and report by a physician or QHP, is reported with code 96127 (brief emotional/behavioral assessment [eg, depression inventory, ADHD scale], with scoring and documentation, per standardized instrument).

Table 14-1. Calculating Units of Service for Time of Test Administration and Scoring

Total Minutes of Administration and Scoring Performed by	First 30 min (16–45 min)	First Additional 30 min (46–75 min)	Second Additional 30 min (76–105 min)	Each Additional 30 min or Last 16 min Beyond Final Full 30-min Period (>106 min)
Physician/QHP	96136 (1 unit)	96136 and 96137 (1 unit each)	96136 (1 unit) and 96137 (2 units)	96136 (1 unit) and units of 96137 for each 30 min or last 16 min beyond final full 30-min period
Technician	96138 (1 unit)	96138 and 96139 (1 unit each)	96138 (1 unit) and 96139 (2 units)	96138 (1 unit) and units of 96139 for each 30 min or last 16 min beyond final full 30-min period

Abbreviation: QHP, qualified health care professional.

Examples

➤ **A physician spends 80 minutes administering tests, recording observations, scoring, and transcribing results to a data summary sheet.** Codes **96136** × 1 unit and **96137** × 2 units are reported.

  Teaching Point: Two units of code **96137** are reported in addition to **96136** because the final 20 minutes exceed the midpoint beyond the 60 minutes reported with **96136** and the first unit of **96137**.

➤ **An adolescent is referred for psychological testing evaluation.** The patient undergoes physician-administered psychological testing to evaluate emotionality, intellectual abilities, personality, and psychopathology and to make a mental health diagnosis and treatment recommendations as applicable. The total time of face-to-face testing is 45 minutes. The physician's total time of evaluation and data integration and interpretation is 75 minutes. Codes **96136** and **96130** are reported.

  Teaching Point: Test administration and scoring time of 45 minutes is reported with code **96136**. Seventy-five minutes of physician testing evaluation service is reported with code **96130**.

Technician-Administered Testing

Testing and administration services performed by a technician are reported with codes **96138** and **96139**.

96138   Psychological or neuropsychological test administration and scoring by technician, two or more tests, any method; first 30 minutes

+96139   each additional 30 minutes (List separately in addition to code for primary procedure)

● Codes **96138** and **96139** do not include the work of a physician or QHP. These codes are valued for practice expense and medical liability only.
● Evaluation services by the physician or QHP are reported with codes **96130–96133** whether provided on the same or a different date. Do not include time for evaluation services (eg, integration of patient data or interpretation of test results in the time of technician-administered testing) in time of test administration and scoring.

Example

➤ **An adolescent patient is referred for neuropsychological testing.** A technician spends 40 minutes administering and scoring tests. The technician also notes any behavioral observations. Code **96138** is reported with 1 unit of service.

  Teaching Point: When a physician or QHP provides evaluation services, including integration and interpretation of data from tests administered by a technician, on the same or different date, see codes **96132** and **96133** for those services.

Automated Testing and Result

When a single test instrument is completed by the patient via an electronic platform without physician, QHP, or technician administration and scoring, report code **96146**.

96146 Psychological or neuropsychological test administration, with single automated, standardized instrument via electronic platform, with automated result only

- Code **96146** does not include scoring by a health care professional or interpretation and report. Results are generated via the electronic platform.
- If a test is administered by a physician, QHP, or technician, do not report **96146**. For brief emotional/behavioral assessment, see code **96127**.

Example

➤ **A child who is recovering from a concussion is provided a single computerized test for post-concussion symptoms.** The patient completes the test and the automated result is included in the patient's medical record.

 Code **96146** is reported in addition to the code representing the physician's related E/M service (eg, **99213**). Append modifier **25** (significant, separately identifiable E/M service) if the payer uses National Correct Coding Initiative edits.

Adaptive Behavior Assessment and Treatment Services

Adaptive behavior services address
- Deficient adaptive behaviors, such as impaired social, communication, or self-care skills
- Maladaptive behaviors, such as repetitive and stereotype behaviors
- Behaviors that risk physical harm to the patient, others, and/or property

 Codes for adaptive behavior services are a combination of Category I and Category III (emerging technology) *CPT* codes. Adaptive behavior services may be delivered by a physician or QHP, behavioral analyst, and/or licensed psychologist working with assistant behavior analysts or technicians. Services are typically reported for conditions that present with maladaptive behaviors such as ASD.

 It is important to verify health plan policies for coverage and payment of adaptive behavior services, including any required provider qualifications (eg, certification, licensure) prior to provision of services.
- Most states mandate coverage of adaptive behavior services for patients diagnosed with ASD. Some states require that behavior analysts providing ASD-related assessment and/or treatment be certified by the Behavior Analyst Certification Board as a Board-Certified Behavior Analyst.
- In the discussion of adaptive behavior services, the QHP includes behavior analysts and licensed psychologists who can independently report these services.

 See your procedure coding reference (eg, *CPT* coding manual) for specific instructions for reporting these services.

 The general rule that time is met when the midpoint is passed applies because *CPT* doesn't include category-specific instructions on the time of service for adaptive behavior services (eg, at least 8 minutes of service is required to support a service specified as 15 minutes).

Adaptive Behavior Assessment

#97151 Behavior identification assessment, administered by a physician or other qualified health care professional, each 15 minutes of the physician's or other qualified health care professional's time face-to-face with patient and/or guardian(s)/caregiver(s) administering assessments and discussing findings and recommendations, and non-face-to-face analyzing past data, scoring/interpreting the assessment, and preparing the report/treatment plan

#97152 Behavior identification supporting assessment, administered by one technician under the direction of a physician or other qualified health care professional, face-to-face with the patient, each 15 minutes

0362T Behavior identification supporting assessment, each 15 minutes of technicians' time face-to-face with a patient, requiring the following components:
- administration by the physician or other qualified health care professional who is on site;
- with the assistance of two or more technicians;
- for a patient who exhibits destructive behavior;
- completion in an environment that is customized to the patient's behavior

 Behavior identification assessment (**97151**) is conducted by a physician or other QHP and may include
- Analysis of pertinent past data (including medical diagnosis)
- A detailed behavioral history
- Patient observation

- Administration of standardized and/or non-standardized instruments and procedures
- Functional behavior assessment
- Functional analysis
- Guardian/caregiver interview to identify and describe deficient adaptive behaviors, maladaptive behaviors, and other impaired functioning secondary to deficient adaptive or maladaptive behaviors

Documentation should include a report of the assessment and a person-centered treatment plan.

If the physician or other QHP personally performs the technician activities, his or her time engaged in these activities should be included as part of the required technician time to meet the components of the code.

- Codes **97151**, **97152**, and **0362T** may be repeated on the same or different days until the behavior identification assessment (**97151**) and, if necessary, supporting assessment(s) (**97152**, **0362T**) are complete.
- Code **97152** is reported for assessment by a technician. The reporting physician or QHP is not required to be on-site during the assessment. See code **0362T** when multiple technicians and a customized assessment environment are required due to destructive behavior(s) of the patient.
- Code **0362T** represents testing of a patient who demonstrates destructive behavior (ie, maladaptive behaviors associated with a high risk of medical consequences or property damage) and requires multiple technicians and an environment customized to the patient and behavior. The reporting physician or QHP is required to be on-site (ie, immediately available and interruptible to provide assistance and direction throughout the performance of the procedure). The reporting physician or QHP is not required to be in the room during testing.
- Only count the time of 1 technician when 2 or more technicians are present. Code **0362T** is reported based on a single technician's face-to-face time with the patient and not the combined time of multiple technicians (eg, 1 hour with 3 technicians equals 1 hour of service) despite the expectation that more than 1 technician will be needed.

Examples

➤ **A 3-year-old boy with symptoms of ASD presents for assessment.** The physician/QHP spends 1 hour face-to-face with the patient and/or guardian(s)/caregiver(s) administering assessments and discussing findings and recommendations and 38 minutes of non–face-to-face time analyzing past data, scoring/interpreting the assessment, and preparing the report/treatment plan. The total time of service is 1 hour, 38 minutes. Code **97151** is reported with 7 units (1 for each full 15 minutes of service and 1 for the last 8 minutes).

Teaching Point: If fewer than 8 minutes past the last full 15 minutes of service were provided, only the number of 15-minute periods of service would be reported (eg, 1 hour, 37 minutes equals 6 units).

➤ **An additional assessment of the 3-year-old from the previous example is required to assess behavior that interferes with acquisition of adaptive skills.** A technician, under the physician's or QHP's direction, observes and records occurrence of the patient's deficient adaptive and maladaptive behaviors and the surrounding environmental events several times in a variety of situations. The physician/QHP reviews and analyzes data from those observations. The face-to-face time of the technician is 1 hour.

Code **97152** is reported with 4 units of service.

➤ **An 11-year-old boy with ASD requires evaluation due to increased self-injury and aggression toward others.** A team of technicians conducts the assessment session in a room that is devoid of any objects that might cause injury. A physician/QHP is on-site and immediately available throughout the session. The technicians implement functional analysis as directed by the physician/QHP and record data. Graphed data are reviewed and analyzed by the physician/QHP to identify the environmental events in whose presence the level of behavior was highest and lowest. The technicians spend a total of 90 minutes face-to-face with the patient during the assessment.

Code **0362T** is reported with 6 units of service.

Adaptive Behavior Treatment

Adaptive behavior treatment services address specific treatment targets and goals based on results of previous assessments and include ongoing assessment and adjustment of treatment protocols, targets, and goals. Codes describe services to the individual patient, groups of patients, families, and an individual patient who exhibits destructive behavior.

Codes for adaptive behavior treatment specify services provided by protocol (**97153**, **97154**) or with protocol modification (**97155**, **97158**, **0373T**). Behavior treatment with protocol modification requires adjustments be made *in real time* rather than for a subsequent service.

Adaptive Behavior Treatment by Protocol

#97153   Adaptive behavior treatment by protocol, administered by technician under the direction of a physician or other qualified health care professional, face-to-face with one patient; each 15 minutes

#97154   Group adaptive behavior treatment by protocol, administered by technician under the direction of a physician or other qualified health care professional, face-to-face with two or more patients, each 15 minutes

- Adaptive behavior treatment by protocol to a single patient (**97153**) and group adaptive behavior treatment by protocol (**97154**) are administered by a technician under the direction of a physician/QHP, using a treatment protocol *designed in advance* by the physician or other QHP, who may or may not provide direction during the treatment.
  - The service described by code **97153** is face-to-face with only 1 patient.
  - Code **97154** is reported for services delivered face-to-face with 2 or more patients but not more than 8 patients.
- Codes **97153** and **97154** do not include protocol modification.
- If the physician/QHP personally performs the technician activities, his or her time spent engaged in these activities should be reported as technician time. The physician is not required to be on site during the provision of these services.

Examples

➤ **A 4-year-old girl with ASD presents with deficits in language and social skills and emotional outbursts in response to small changes in routines or when preferred items are unavailable.** A QHP directs a technician in the implementation of treatment protocols and data collection procedures. The technician conducts a treatment session in the family home with multiple planned opportunities for the patient to practice target skills. The QHP reviews the technician's recorded and graphed data to assess the child's progress and determine if any treatment protocol needs adjustment. The technician spends 1 hour at the patient's home with face-to-face time of the treatment session lasting 50 minutes. Code **97153** is reported with 3 units of service.

     Teaching Point: Only the technician's face-to-face time with the patient is used to determine the units of service. This service may also be conducted in a community setting (eg, playground, store).

➤ **Peer social skills training in a small group is recommended for a 7-year-old girl with deficits in social skills due to ASD.** A technician conducts the group session using treatment protocols and data collection procedures as previously designed by a QHP. The QHP reviews the technician's recorded and graphed data to assess the child's progress and determine if treatment protocols need adjustment. The total face-to-face time of the session is 60 minutes.

     Code **97154** is reported with 4 units.

Adaptive Behavior Treatment With Protocol Modification

#97155   Adaptive behavior treatment with protocol modification administered by physician or other qualified health care professional, which may include simultaneous direction of technician, face-to-face with one patient, each 15 minutes

#97158   Group adaptive behavior treatment with protocol modification, administered by physician or other qualified health care professional, face-to-face with multiple patients, each 15 minutes

0373T   Adaptive behavior treatment with protocol modification, each 15 minutes of technicians' time face-to-face with a patient, requiring the following components:
- administration by the physician or other qualified health care professional who is on site;
- with the assistance of two or more technicians;
- for a patient who exhibits destructive behavior;
- completion in an environment that is customized to the patient's behavior.

- Adaptive behavior treatment with protocol modification (**97155**) is administered by a physician/QHP *face-to-face with a single patient.*
  - The physician/QHP resolves 1 or more problems with the protocol and may simultaneously direct a technician in administering the modified protocol *while the patient is present.*
  - Physician/QHP direction to the technician without the patient present is not reported separately.

- Group adaptive behavior treatment with protocol modification (**97158**) is reported when a physician/QHP provides *face-to-face* protocol modification services with up to 8 patients in a group. The physician/QHP monitors the needs of individual patients and adjusts treatment techniques during the group sessions, as needed.
- Adaptive behavior treatment with protocol modification (**0373T**) is reported for services to a patient who presents with 1 or more destructive behavior(s).
  - The service time is based on a single technician's face-to-face time with the patient and not the combined time of multiple technicians.
  - The physician/QHP must be on site and immediately available during the service described by code **0373T**.

Examples

➤ **A 5-year-old boy previously showed steady improvements in language and social skills at home as a result of one-to-one intensive applied behavior analysis intervention, but skill development seems to have recently reached a plateau.** A QHP modifies the previously used written protocols to incorporate procedures designed to build the child's language and social skills into daily home routines (eg, play, dressing, mealtimes). The QHP demonstrates the procedures to the technician and directs the technician to implement the protocols with the child. The QHP then observes and provides feedback as the technician implements the procedures with the child. The technician's face-to-face time with the patient is 45 minutes. Code **97155** is reported with 3 units of service.

  Teaching Point: Time spent by the technician and QHP without the patient present is not included in the time of service.

➤ **A 13-year-old girl is reported to be isolated from peers due to poor social skills and odd behavior.** The child attends a group treatment session that focuses on peer social skills. A QHP begins the group session by asking each patient to briefly describe 2 of their recent social encounters with peers, one that went well and one that did not. The information is used to develop a group activity in which each patient has the opportunity to practice the skills she or he used in the encounters that went well and to problem-solve the interactions that did not go well. The QHP helps each patient identify social cues that were interpreted correctly and incorrectly and what she or he could have done differently. The QHP also provides prompts and feedback individualized to each patient's skills. The QHP ends the session by summarizing the discussion. The total time of the session was 70 minutes, including a 10-minute break (ie, 60 minutes of group session). Code **97158** is reported with 4 units of service.

  Teaching Point: Only the QHP's face-to-face time spent providing the service is reported.

➤ **A 16-year-old boy has had 2 surgeries to relieve esophageal blockages due to pica involving repeated ingestion of small metal objects (eg, paper clips, pushpins).** The patient's pica behavior has not responded to previous treatment. The QHP supervising the patient's treatment plan has previously developed written protocols for reducing the patient's pica. A technician carefully inspects the room before the session to make sure there are no potential pica items on the floor. Two technicians are present, with one presenting the patient with a series of trials in which the patient is presented with a food item and a nonhazardous item that resembles a pica item. The second technician prompts the patient to choose the food item and blocks attempts to choose the pica item. The patient's response to each trial is recorded. The QHP is on site and available to assist as needed. The total session lasts 40 minutes. Code **0373T** is reported with 3 units.

  Teaching Point: Although 2 technicians were present, time is counted only once. The midpoint rule allows reporting a unit of service for the final 10 minutes of service.

Family Adaptive Behavior Treatment Guidance

Family adaptive behavior treatment guidance (**97156**) and multiple-family group adaptive behavior treatment guidance (**97157**) are administered by a physician or QHP face-to-face with guardian(s)/caregiver(s) and involve identifying potential treatment targets and training guardian(s)/caregiver(s) to implement treatment protocols designed to address deficient adaptive or maladaptive behaviors.

#**97156** Family adaptive behavior treatment guidance, administered by physician or other qualified health care professional (with or without the patient present), face-to-face with guardian(s)/caregiver(s), each 15 minutes

Chapter 14. Mental and Behavioral Health Services

#97157 Multiple-family group adaptive behavior treatment guidance, administered by physician or other qualified health care professional (without the patient present), face-to-face with multiple sets of guardians/caregivers, each 15 minutes

● Family adaptive behavior treatment guidance (**97156**) provided to the caregiver(s) of one patient may be performed with or without the patient present.

   Adaptive behavior treatment where the parent(s) or guardian(s) are present but not part of the therapy would not qualify as family adaptive behavior treatment.

● Family adaptive behavior treatment guidance provided to the caregiver(s) of multiple patients (**97157**) is performed without the patients present. The group must be no larger than the caregiver(s) of 8 patients. *CPT* does not include a code for reporting services to a group of 9 or more patients.

Examples

➤ **The parents of a 6-year-old boy seek training on procedures for helping the child communicate using picture cards during typical family routines (a skill he previously developed in adaptive behavior treatment therapy sessions with technicians).** A physician/QHP trains the parents. The service includes reviewing the written treatment and data collection protocols with the parents, demonstrating how to implement the cards in role-plays and with the child, and having the parents implement the protocols with the child while the provider observes and provides feedback. The time of service is 1 hour.

   Code **97156** is reported with 4 units of service.

➤ **The parents of a 3-year-old boy who has pervasive hyperactivity and no functional play, social, or communication skills seek training on how to manage his hyperactive and disruptive behavior and help him develop appropriate play, social, and communication skills.** The parents attend a group session (without the patient) led by a physician who asks each set of parents to identify 1 skill to be increased or 1 problem behavior to be decreased in their own child. The physician describes how behavior analytic principles and procedures could be applied to the behavior identified by the parents of this 3-year-old patient. The physician demonstrates a procedure (eg, prompting the child to speak instead of whining when he wants something; not giving him preferred items when he whines). The parents then role-play, implementing that procedure. Other group participants and the physician provide feedback and make constructive suggestions. That process is repeated for skills/behaviors identified by other sets of parents. The group session ends with the physician summarizing the main points, answering questions, and giving each set of parents a homework assignment to practice the skills they worked on during the session. The session lasts 110 minutes. Code **97157** is reported with 7 units.

   Teaching Point: The last 5 minutes are not reported because the midpoint of 8 minutes beyond the last full 15-minute period (105 minutes) was not passed.

Habilitative and Rehabilitative Modifiers

Adaptive behavior services may be either habilitative or rehabilitative. *Habilitative* services are those provided to help an individual learn skills not yet developed and to keep and/or improve those skills. *Rehabilitative* services help a patient keep, get back, or improve skills that have been lost or limited due to illness, injury, and/or disability. Because the Patient Protection and Affordable Care Act provides that certain health plans must provide equal coverage for habilitative and rehabilitative services and count each type of service separately, it may be necessary to indicate that a service is habilitative or rehabilitative. Modifiers **96** (habilitative services) and **97** (rehabilitative services) are appended to procedure codes to designate the nature of a service. Modifiers **96** and **97** may not be adopted for use by all payers or may have limited utility. Verify payer policies for these modifiers when providing habilitative and rehabilitative services.

Health and Behavior Assessments/Interventions

Health and behavior assessment and intervention procedures (**96156, 96158, 96159,** and **96164–96171**) are used to identify and address psychosocial, behavioral, emotional, cognitive, and interpersonal factors important to the assessment, treatment, or management of physical health problems.

Chapter 14. Mental and Behavioral Health Services

The patient's primary diagnosis must be a medical (physical) issue, and the focus of the assessment and interventions is on factors complicating medical conditions and treatments. These codes describe assessments and interventions to improve the patient's health and well-being using psychological and/or psychosocial interventions designed to ameliorate specific disease-related problems.

These services do not represent preventive medicine counseling and risk factor reduction interventions.

- Physicians and QHPs who can provide and report E/M services do not report **96156, 96158, 96159,** or **96164–96171.** Evaluation and management codes including preventive medicine services are reported instead depending on the type of service provided.
- When an E/M service is provided by a physician or QHP on the same date that an AHP provides health and behavior assessment/intervention, each service is separately reported by the individual providing the service. The same provider cannot report both services.
- May be reported by psychologists, clinical social workers, licensed therapists, and other AHPs within their scope of practice who have specialty or subspecialty training in health and behavior assessment or intervention procedures.
- Are not reported with psychiatric codes (**90785–90899**) when provided on the same day. Only the primary service is reported (ie, **96156, 96158, 96159,** and **96164–96171** or **90785–90899**).
- Are not reported with adaptive behavior assessment or treatment (**97151–97158, 0362T, 0373T**).
- Are not used in conjunction with a primary diagnosis of mental disorder. (Payers may deny claims when a diagnosis code indicating mental disorder is included for these services.)

Health Behavior Assessment

96156   Health behavior assessment, or re-assessment (ie, health-focused clinical interview, behavioral observations, clinical decision making)

Health behavior assessment includes evaluation of the patient's responses to disease, illness or injury, outlook, coping strategies, motivation, and adherence to medical treatment. Assessment is conducted through health-focused clinical interviews, observation, and clinical decision-making.

Code **96156** is not reported based on time. Report only 1 unit of service.

Example

➤ **A 13-year-old girl with multiple food allergies and newly increased anxiety is assessed for response to management of food allergies.** The patient notes feelings of social isolation at home and school due to restricted diet. She is fearful of having an allergic reaction in front of her peers. The patient is assessed using standardized questionnaires. The child's parents are also interviewed.

Code **96156** would be reported with, for example, *ICD-10-CM* code **Z91.010**, allergy to peanuts. If the patient has been diagnosed with an anxiety disorder, report also a code for the anxiety disorder (eg, **F41.9**, anxiety disorder, unspecified). However, codes for mental and behavioral health conditions should not be reported as the first-listed or primary reason for health behavior assessment.

When neuropsychological and/or psychological testing is performed at the same session as health behavior assessment or reassessment, payer edits may require modifier **59** to be appended to the code for the testing to indicate a distinct service.

Health Behavior Intervention

Codes **96158, 96159,** and **96164–96171**

- Are time-based services requiring documentation of the time spent face-to-face with the patient(s) and/or family.
- Do not report **96158, 96164, 96167,** or **96170** for less than 16 minutes of service.
- Include promotion of functional improvement, minimizing psychological and/or psychosocial barriers to recovery, and management of and improved coping with medical conditions.
- Emphasize active patient/family engagement and involvement. These interventions may be provided individually, to a group (≥2 patients), and/or to the family, with or without the patient present.

Refer to **Table 14-2** for a breakdown of the health behavior intervention codes.

Table 14-2. Health Behavior Intervention Codes

Health Behavior Intervention Provided to	Initial Code	Add-on Code
Individual, face-to-face;	96158 initial 16–30 min	+96159 each additional 15 min (List separately in addition to code 96158)
Group (2 or more patients), face-to-face;	#96164 initial 16–30 min	#+96165 each additional 15 min (List separately in addition to code 96164)
Family (with the patient present), face-to-face;	#96167 initial 16–30 min	#+96168 each additional 15 min (List separately in addition to code 96167)
Family (without the patient present), face-to-face;	#96170 initial 16–30 min	#+96171 each additional 15 min (List separately in addition to code 96170)

Examples

➤ **Health behavior intervention is provided to a 13-year-old girl with multiple food allergies and newly increased anxiety.** Results from a health behavior assessment are used to develop a plan for coping and gaining confidence and self-reliance in social settings. Thirty minutes is spent with the patient discussing the behavior and suggested coping skills.

Code 96158 with 1 unit of service would be reported with diagnosis codes for the food allergies and any diagnosed anxiety disorder.

➤ **Three patients with type 1 diabetes and identified needs for better treatment adherence take part in a group intervention.** Based on assessments conducted at previous encounters, the clinical psychologist works with the patients to gain understanding and acceptance of their physician's care plan, addresses barriers to compliance, and helps each patient develop goals for better compliance. A total of 55 minutes is spent face-to-face with the group of patients.

Code 96164 (1 unit for first 30 minutes) and 96165 with 2 units of service (1 full 15-minute period and 1 unit for the last 10 minutes because the midpoint of 8 minutes beyond the last full period was passed). *ICD-10-CM* codes appropriate to each patient's condition (eg, appropriate codes from category E10, type 1 diabetes, and codes for any manifestations) are reported.

Psychiatric Services

Psychiatric services include diagnostic services, psychotherapy, and other services to an individual, a family, or a group. Comprehensive services may be provided by a multidisciplinary team (eg, a psychiatrist, developmental-behavioral pediatrician, nurse practitioner, psychologist, clinical social worker, and/or clinical counselor).

However, in many parts of the country, children's mental and behavioral health professionals are not available. General pediatricians must often take on management of minor mental health problems and, when possible, consult with a mental/behavioral health professional at a distant location or arrange for services via telemedicine services. (See the Payment and Coverage Issues for Mental/Behavioral Health Services section earlier in this chapter for important considerations for general pediatricians providing psychiatric services.)

An emerging method of delivering mental health services is *psychiatric collaborative care management* (PCCM), in which care is directed by a primary care pediatrician or QHP and provided in collaboration with a psychiatric consultant. See the Psychiatric Collaborative Care Management Services section later in this chapter for more information.

Interactive Complexity

★+90785　Interactive complexity

Psychiatric services to children may include interactive complexity. According to *CPT*, psychiatric procedures may be reported "with interactive complexity" when at least one of the following is present:

Chapter 14. Mental and Behavioral Health Services

- The need to manage maladaptive communication (related to, eg, high anxiety, high reactivity, repeated questions, disagreement) among participants that complicates delivery of care
- Caregiver emotions or behavior interfering with the caregiver's understanding and ability to assist in the implementation of the treatment plan
- Evidence or disclosure of a sentinel event and mandated report to third party (eg, abuse or neglect with report to state agency) with initiation of discussion of the sentinel event and/or report with the patient and other visit participants
- Use of play equipment or other physical devices to communicate with the patient to overcome barriers to therapeutic or diagnostic interaction between the physician or other QHP and a patient who has not developed or has lost either the expressive language communication skills to explain his or her symptoms and response to treatment or the receptive communication skills to understand the physician or other QHP if he or she were to use typical language for communication

Add-on code **90785** is reported when interactive complexity complicates delivery of psychiatric services, including diagnostic psychiatric evaluation (**90791, 90792**), psychotherapy (**90832–90834, 90836–90838**), and group psychotherapy (**90853**). Report code **90785** in conjunction with code **90853** for the specified patient when group psychotherapy includes interactive complexity.

- Interactive complexity indicates an *increased complexity of work* as opposed to an extended duration of services. The increased complexity of the psychiatric service is due to specific communication factors that can result in barriers to diagnostic or therapeutic interaction with the patient.
- Interactive complexity is not billed in conjunction with psychotherapy for crisis (**90839, 90840**) or with psychiatric or neuropsychiatric testing (**96130–96134, 96136–96139, 96146**).
- Interactive complexity applies only to the psychiatric portion of a service including both psychiatric and E/M components. Code **90785** is never reported alone and is not reported in conjunction with E/M services alone.

    When provided in conjunction with time-based psychotherapy services, the time spent providing interactive complexity services is reflected in the time of the psychotherapy service and must relate to the psychotherapy service only.
- Do not report code **90785** in conjunction with adaptive behavior assessment or treatment services (**97151–97158, 0362T, 0373T**).

Examples

➤ **A 10-year-old patient undergoes psychiatric evaluation.** The child is accompanied by separated parents, reporting the child has recently demonstrated significant anxiety when leaving either or both parents. The child's teachers report that the child appears to feign illness and seek reasons to contact a parent during the school day. The parents are extremely anxious and repeatedly ask questions about the treatment process. Each parent continually challenges the other's observations of the patient.

    Codes **90791** (psychiatric diagnostic evaluation) and **90785** (interactive complexity) are reported.

➤ **A 6-year-old girl is seen for psychotherapy.** The child was placed in foster care following hospitalization for injuries sustained due to physical abuse and neglect by her mother 3 years before this evaluation. The service includes the psychologist's review of the child's medical record and telephone interviews with the child's social worker and teacher. The mother refuses a request for interview. The psychologist interviews current and former foster parents, who express concerns that the child is easily offended and retaliates against perceived offenses with violent outbursts. The psychologist uses play to gain trust and evaluate the child. The psychologist and foster mother agree on a treatment plan and then discuss the plan with the child in terms she can understand. Following the service, the psychologist provides a report to the patient's social worker.

    Codes **90791** (psychiatric diagnostic evaluation) and **90785** (interactive complexity) are reported.

Psychiatric Diagnostic Evaluation

★**90791**   Psychiatric diagnostic evaluation
★**90792**   Psychiatric diagnostic evaluation with medical services

Psychiatric diagnostic evaluation (**90791**) and psychiatric diagnostic evaluation with medical services (**90792**) include an integrated biopsychosocial assessment, including history, mental status, and recommendations. When medical services (ie, medical assessments and physical examination other than mental status, when indicated) are included, code **90792** is reported.

- Psychiatric diagnostic evaluation or reevaluation (**90791**, **90792**) is reported once per day. Do not report psychotherapy codes (**90832–90839**) on the same date of service as **90791** or **90792**.
- The same individual may not separately report E/M services on the same date as psychiatric diagnostic evaluation.
- Report code **90785** for interactive complexity in addition to code **90791** or **90792**, when applicable.

Health plans may not cover mental health consultation, testing, or evaluation that is performed to assess custody, visitation, or parental rights.

- **Verify health plan contractual obligations prior to providing services that may lack medical necessity and determine if a waiver of liability must be signed by the patient(s) prior to beginning the service.**
- **A waiver of liability (similar to Medicare's advance beneficiary notice) is the patient's agreement to pay out of pocket for services not covered by his or her health plan.**
- **Modifier GA (waiver of liability statement issued as required by payer policy, individual case) may be appended to the code reported to indicate the waiver is on file.**

When services are requested for purposes that a health plan may not consider medically necessary, failure to obtain the responsible party's signature on a waiver of liability *prior to the service* may release the patient from the obligation to pay based on contractual agreement between the provider and health plan.

Examples

➤ **A 14-year-old girl is referred by her primary care pediatrician for evaluation and treatment of depression with suicidal ideation.** The psychologist obtains information on the presenting problem and situation. A statement of need and expectations is documented. Current symptoms and behaviors are documented. The patient has no history of previous psychiatric treatment. The patient denies previous substance use treatment and current use of alcohol or drugs. Her current medication regimen of fluoxetine 10 mg once a day is documented. She has no current medical problems and is not allergic to any medications. The patient's family and social status (current and historical), school status/functioning, and resources are obtained and documented. A diagnosis of moderate major depressive disorder, single episode, and parent-child relationship problem is documented.

Code **90791** is reported in conjunction with *ICD-10-CM* codes **F32.1** (major depressive disorder, single episode, moderate) and **Z63.8** (other specified problems related to primary support group).

➤ **A 15-year-old girl was admitted through the emergency department (ED) following a suicide attempt.** The girl is evaluated by a psychiatrist for admission to inpatient psychiatric care. The psychiatrist performs a psychiatric diagnostic evaluation of this patient, who previously attempted suicide at age 13 years and has a history of recurrent major depressive disorder. The patient also expresses fear that she may be pregnant and has been exposed to a sexually transmitted infection. Medical history includes nausea with vomiting for the last week and last menstrual period 6 weeks ago. Laboratory tests are ordered to rule out pregnancy and/or infection, and consultation with a gynecologist is ordered. Diagnoses are severe major depressive disorder without psychosis (**F33.2**), nausea with vomiting (**R11**), and pregnancy test, unconfirmed (**Z72.40**).

Code **90792** is reported for combined psychiatric and medical evaluations.

➤ **A 17-year-old girl wishes to be evaluated for purposes of determining her ability to accept responsibility for herself.** The girl is seeking emancipation from her mother, who is currently living with an abusive boyfriend and will not allow her to move in with her aunt while finishing high school. An attorney has advised obtaining a psychological evaluation to support the girl's claims that she is psychologically prepared to take this action. The girl's health plan considers this service not medically necessary but allows for patient payment when a waiver of liability is obtained prior to the service. She agrees to sign the waiver and pay for the service. An evaluation is completed, and a report of the evaluation is provided to the girl and her attorney.

The service is reported to the health plan with modifier **GA** (waiver of liability statement issued as required by payer policy, individual case) appended to code **90791**.

● =New code   ▲ =Revised code   # =Re-sequenced code   + =Add-on code   ★ =Telemedicine

Psychotherapy

CPT defines *psychotherapy* as the treatment of mental illness and behavioral disturbances in which the physician or QHP, through definitive therapeutic communications, attempts to alleviate the emotional disturbances, reverse or change maladaptive patterns of behavior, and encourage personality growth and development.

Progress notes for psychotherapy services should include
- **Start and stop times of psychotherapy**
- **Service type**
- **Diagnosis**
- **Interval history (eg, increase/decrease in symptoms, current risk factors)**
- **Names and scores of standardized rating scales used in monitoring progress**
- **Therapeutic interventions (eg, type of therapy, medications)**
- **Summary of goals and progress**
- **An updated treatment plan**
- **Date and signature of performing provider**

These elements should be documented in the progress note in the patient record rather than the protected psychotherapy notes. Protected psychotherapy notes *are not disclosed* for purposes of receiving or supporting accurate payment.

- Services include ongoing assessment and adjustment of psychotherapeutic interventions and may include involvement of informants in the treatment process.
- Codes differentiate psychotherapy services to individuals (with and without E/M services), an individual family or groups of families, and groups of patients. Codes for each are provided in the following discussions.
- Separate codes (**90839**, **90840**) are reported for psychotherapy for crisis (see the Psychotherapy for Crisis section later in this chapter).

  Pertinent instructions for coding for all psychotherapy services are
- Psychotherapy times are for face-to-face services with a patient and/or family member. The patient must be present for all or some of the service except when reporting family psychotherapy without the patient present (**90846**). This allows for the participation of others in the psychotherapy session for the patient as long as the patient remains the focus of the intervention. Documentation must support that the patient was present for a significant portion of the session.
- For psychotherapy with biofeedback (**90875**, **90876**), see Psychotherapy With Biofeedback section later in this chapter.
- Psychotherapy differs from family psychotherapy (**90846**, **90847**). Family psychotherapy uses techniques to benefit the patient (eg, attempting to improve family communication or alter family interactions that negatively affect the patient; encouraging interactions to improve family functioning). Family psychotherapy includes sessions with the entire family as well as sessions that may not include the patient.
- In reporting, choose the code closest to the actual time (**Table 14-3**). Do not report psychotherapy of less than 16 minutes' duration.
- Do not report psychotherapy codes in conjunction with codes for adaptive behavior assessment or treatment services (**97153–97158, 0362T, 0373T**).
- Psychotherapy of more than 45 minutes is often considered unusual and may require health plan precertification.

Psychotherapy With Evaluation and Management

★+**90833**   Psychotherapy, 30 minutes with patient when performed with an evaluation and management service
★+**90836**   45 minutes with patient when performed with an evaluation and management service
★+**90838**   60 minutes with patient when performed with an evaluation and management service

  Psychiatrists and other physicians who provide a combination of psychotherapy and E/M services (eg, **99213**) on the same date may report an E/M code and an add-on code for psychotherapy (**90833**, **90836**, **90838**).
- To report both E/M and psychotherapy, the 2 services must be significant and separately identifiable.
- Time may not be used as the basis of E/M code selection. Evaluation and management code selection must be based on the level of key components of history, examination, and medical decision-making (MDM), *or MDM alone in the case of office and other outpatient E/M services*, when reported in conjunction with psychotherapy.
- Prolonged services *may not* be reported when psychotherapy with E/M (**90833**, **90836**, **90838**) is reported.

Table 14-3. Reporting Psychotherapy Services	
Duration of Psychotherapy	***CPT* Codes**
<16 min	Do not report.
16–37 min	**90832, 90833**
38–52 min	**90834, 90836**
53–89 min	**90837, 90838**
≥26 min	**90846, 90847** (family psychotherapy)

Abbreviation: *CPT*, Current Procedural Terminology.

Example

➤ **An 8-year-old boy presents for psychotherapy.** The psychiatrist provides psychotherapy services with face-to-face time of 40 minutes and also provides an E/M service to reevaluate the effectiveness and patient reaction to current medications. The office E/M service includes low-complexity MDM based on the low number and complexity of problems (1 stable chronic illness) with moderate risk of morbidity of prescription drug management. Codes reported are **99213** and **90836**.

The 40 minutes of time is only the face-to-face time of psychotherapy services and does not include the time of the E/M service. Because the midpoint between 30 and 45 minutes was passed, code **90836** (45 minutes) is reported in lieu of **90833** (30 minutes). No modifier is required (eg, modifier **25**) because the add-on codes were assigned values that took into account the overlapping practice expense of the 2 services (eg, same clinical staff and examination room).

Psychotherapy Without Evaluation and Management

★**90832** Psychotherapy, 30 minutes with patient and/or family member
★**90834** 45 minutes with patient and/or family member
★**90837** 60 minutes with patient and/or family member
★+**90863** Pharmacologic management, including prescription and review of medication, when performed with psychotherapy services

When psychotherapy is provided without an E/M service on the same date, codes **90832**, **90834**, and **90837** are reported based on the face-to-face time of service.

● To accommodate reporting of pharmacologic management by psychologists who have prescribing privileges but who cannot provide E/M services, add-on code **90863** is reported in addition to the appropriate code for psychotherapy without E/M.

Only a psychologist with prescribing authority may provide pharmacologic management. Other QHPs may provide psychotherapy but must collaborate with a physician or advance practice professional who provides pharmacologic management.

● Physicians and QHPs providing pharmacologic management report the service with an E/M code.

● Prolonged services in the outpatient setting (**99354**, **99355**) or inpatient or observation setting (**99356**, **99357**) may be reported in addition to the psychotherapy service code **90837** when 90 minutes or longer of face-to-face time with the patient and/or family member is spent performing psychotherapy services, *which are not performed with an E/M service.*

● Code **90863** is an add-on code and may only be reported in addition to one of the stand-alone psychotherapy codes (ie, **90832, 90834, 90837**). Time spent providing medication management is not included in the time spent in psychotherapy.

Example

➤ **An 8-year-old boy presents for psychotherapy.** The physician or licensed clinical psychologist (whose state scope of practice includes prescribing authority) provides psychotherapy services with face-to-face time of 40 minutes and also provides a pharmacologic management service to reevaluate the effectiveness and patient reaction to current medications. Codes reported are **90834** and **90863**.

Psychotherapy With Biofeedback

90875   Individual psychophysiological therapy incorporating biofeedback training by any modality (face-to-face with the patient), with psychotherapy (eg, insight oriented, behavior modifying or supportive psychotherapy); 30 minutes

90876   45 minutes

When psychotherapy incorporates biofeedback training, code **90875** or **90876** is reported based on the face-to-face time of the combined services. Do not separately report codes for psychotherapy (**90832–90838**) or biofeedback training (**90901**).

Example

➤ **A child with frequent tension headaches is provided psychotherapy and biofeedback training to help her cope with and control her pain.** The face-to-face time of service is 45 minutes.

Code **90876** is reported for the combined services. Were biofeedback training provided on a date when no psychotherapy was provided, code **90901** would be reported. Time of service is not a factor in reporting code **90901**.

Psychotherapy for Crisis

★**90839**   Psychotherapy for crisis; first 60 minutes

★+**90840**   each additional 30 minutes (List separately in addition to code **90839**)

Psychotherapy for crisis is provided on an urgent basis to a patient requiring mobilization of resources to defuse a crisis and restore safety. It also incorporates implementation of psychotherapeutic interventions to minimize the potential for psychological trauma.

- This includes assessment and history of a crisis state, a mental status examination, and a disposition.
- The presenting problem is typically life-threatening or complex and requires immediate attention to a patient in high distress.
- Codes **90839** and **90840** are reported based on the total face-to-face time the physician or QHP spends with the patient and/or family providing psychotherapy for crisis on a single date of service. Time is cumulative for all psychotherapy for crisis on the same date even if time is not continuous.
  - Code **90839** is reported for the first 30 to 74 minutes of psychotherapy for crisis on a single date of service. For psychotherapy for crisis with face-to-face time of less than 30 minutes' duration, report individual psychotherapy codes (**90832** or **90833**).
  - Add code **90840** for each additional block of time (each 30 minutes beyond the first 74 minutes and once for up to 30 minutes beyond the last full 30-minute period).
- Do not report psychotherapy for crisis (**90839**, **90840**) for service of less than 30 minutes or on the same date as other psychiatry services (**90785–90899**).

Example

➤ **A psychologist or psychiatrist is consulted in the ED for a patient who was brought to the hospital after trying to injure his parents due to paranoia.** The psychologist speaks to the parents to determine the nature of the crisis. The parents agree to evaluation and possible inpatient admission. The psychologist examines the patient, obtains agreement for inpatient treatment, and makes arrangements for admission. The total face-to-face time of the encounter is 45 minutes.

Code **90839** is reported. Although the code descriptor states, "first hour," the instructions for reporting psychotherapy for crisis instruct that code **90839** is reported for the first 30 to 74 minutes of face-to-face service.

Chapter 14. Mental and Behavioral Health Services

    ●=New code   ▲=Revised code   #=Re-sequenced code   +=Add-on code   ★=Telemedicine

Family and Group Psychotherapy

★90846   Family psychotherapy (without the patient present), 50 minutes

★90847   Family psychotherapy (conjoint psychotherapy) (with patient present), 50 minutes

90849   Multiple-family group psychotherapy

　　While family members may act as informants during individual psychotherapy, psychotherapy using family psychotherapy techniques is reported with codes 90846 and 90847 based on whether the patient is present for the service.

● Psychotherapy to a group of individual patients includes discussion of individual and/or group dynamics. Processes may include interpersonal interactions, support, emotional catharsis, and reminiscing.

● The focus of family psychotherapy is on family dynamics and/or subsystems within the family (eg, parents, siblings) and on improving the patient's functioning by working with the patient in the context of the family.

● Do not report family psychotherapy for services of fewer than 26 minutes.

● Prolonged service may also be reported in conjunction with code 90847 (family psychotherapy, 50 minutes) when 80 minutes or longer of face-to-face time with the patient and family are spent performing psychotherapy.

● Codes for individual psychotherapy (90832–90838) may be reported on the same day as family psychotherapy codes 90846 and 90847 when the services are separate and distinct. Append modifier 59 (distinct procedural service) to the group psychotherapy code when both services are reported on the same date.

● When multiple families participate in family psychotherapy at the same session, code 90849 is reported once for each family.

90853   Group psychotherapy (other than of a multiple-family group)

● Report code 90853 with 1 unit of service for each group member. Documentation should support the individual patient's involvement in the group session, the duration of the session, and issues that were presented.

● No time is assigned to code 90853. This service is reported with 1 unit of service regardless of the time of service.

Other Psychiatric Services

The following services are often bundled under payer contracts (ie, considered components of other services) or non-covered. However, check plan benefits, especially for Medicaid patients, as there may be circumstances in which these services are separate benefits. Plan-specific modifiers are often required when coverage of the following services is a health plan benefit:

90882   Environmental intervention for medical management purposes on a psychiatric patient's behalf with agencies, employers, or institutions

90885   Psychiatric evaluation of hospital records, other psychiatric reports, psychometric and/or projective tests, and other accumulated data for medical diagnostic purposes

> Code 90885 may be reported in addition to psychotherapy services (90832–90838) when both services are provided by the same individual on the same date of service.

90887   Interpretation or explanation of results of psychiatric, other medical examinations and procedures, or other accumulated data to family or other responsible persons, or advising them how to assist patient

　　Do not report code 90887 in conjunction with adaptive behavior services (97151–97158, 0362T, 0373T).

90889   Preparation of report of patient's psychiatric status, history, treatment, or progress (other than for legal or consultative purposes) for other individuals, agencies, or insurance carriers

　　Code 90889 should not be reported in conjunction with psychological or developmental testing, as the codes for these services include time for report writing.

Evaluation and Treatment of Substance Use

The initial evaluation of a child for alcohol and/or substance use is often in the context of an E/M service. When more than 50% of the physician/QHP time with the patient is spent in counseling and/or coordinating care, E/M codes are selected based on the total face-to-face time of the service in a non-facility setting or total unit/floor time in a facility setting (eg, ED, hospital unit). Office E/M services (99202–99205, 99212–99215) may be reported for the physician or other QHP's total time on the date of service, as described in **Chapter 7**.

● =New code   ▲ =Revised code   # =Re-sequenced code   + =Add-on code   ★ =Telemedicine

Chapter 14. Mental and Behavioral Health Services

ICD-10-CM Coding for Use, Abuse, and Dependence

The guidelines for *ICD-10-CM* offer specific guidance for reporting diagnoses of mental and behavioral disorders due to psychoactive substance use.

- Code **Z71.41** is reported as the first-listed code when an encounter is primarily focused on alcohol abuse counseling and surveillance. An additional code for alcohol abuse or dependence (**F10.-**) is additionally reported.
- Code **Z71.51** is reported as the first-listed code when an encounter is primarily for drug abuse counseling and surveillance of drug abuser. Codes for drug abuse or dependence (**F11–F16**, **F18**, or **F19**) are reported in addition to code **Z71.51**.
- When substance use is addressed and/or affects patient management during an encounter that is primarily for management or treatment of other conditions, report first a code for management of the other condition(s) followed by a code for substance use.
- The codes for psychoactive substance *use* disorders (**F10.9-**, **F11.9-**, **F12.9-**, **F13.9-**, **F14.9-**, **F15.9-**, **F16.9-**) are to be used only when the psychoactive substance use is associated with a physical, mental, or behavioral disorder and such a relationship is documented by the provider. Note that codes for inhalant use (**F18.9-**) and polysubstance or indiscriminate drug use (**F19.9-**) are not included in this instruction.

> For a diagnosis of nicotine vaping, assign code **F17.29-**, nicotine dependence, other tobacco products. Electronic nicotine delivery systems are noncombustible tobacco products.

- Subcategories of codes for mental and behavioral disorders due to psychoactive substance use indicate *use* and *abuse* of and *dependence* on various psychoactive substances. These categories do not include abuse of nonpsychoactive substances such as antacids, laxatives, or steroids that are reported with category **F55**. Each subcategory offers a spectrum of use, abuse, and dependence with extended information such as *with intoxication, with withdrawal,* and *with delusions.*
- When documentation refers to use of, abuse of, and dependence on the same substance (eg, alcohol, opioid, cannabis), only 1 code should be assigned to identify the pattern of use based on the hierarchy shown in **Figure 14-1**. Report a code for the condition farthest to the right in the figure.

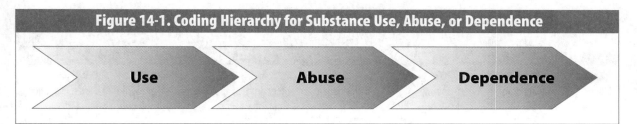

Figure 14-1. Coding Hierarchy for Substance Use, Abuse, or Dependence

Use → Abuse → Dependence

- Selection of codes for mental and behavioral disorders due to psychoactive substance use for substance abuse or dependence in remission (categories **F10–F19** with **-.11**, **-.21**) requires the provider's clinical judgment. The appropriate codes for in remission are assigned only on the basis of provider documentation unless otherwise instructed by the classification.
- Mild substance use disorders in early or sustained remission are classified to the appropriate codes for substance abuse in remission, and moderate or severe substance use disorders in early or sustained remission are classified to the appropriate codes for substance dependence in remission.

Management/Treatment of Alcohol and Substance Use Disorders

Coding for management/treatment of alcohol and substance use disorders is largely payer driven. Psychotherapy codes may be applicable, or E/M codes may be selected based on time of counseling and/or coordination for ongoing counseling on alcohol and/or substance use disorders. However, many health plans and Medicaid programs require use of HCPCS codes and/or modifiers for reporting assessments and management/treatment of alcohol and/or substance use disorders.

Examples of HCPCS codes include

H0016   Alcohol and/or drug services; medical/somatic (medical intervention in ambulatory setting)

T1007   Alcohol and/or substance abuse services, treatment plan development and/or modification

Modifiers **HF–HI** provide details such as integrated mental health/substance abuse program. See payer guidelines for use of these modifiers.

Individual health and Medicaid plans may have different definitions for the services reported with HCPCS codes. Prior authorization of services is often required.

General behavioral health integration (GBHI) care management services (99484) may also be provided for substance use disorders; see the General Behavioral Health Integration Care Management section later in this chapter for a discussion.

Alcohol and/or Substance Use Screening/Testing

> Codes for findings of drugs and other substances not normally found in blood (R78.-) are not reported in conjunction with codes for substance use (F10–F19).

Presumptive Drug Class Screening

Presumptive drug class screening is typically used to identify possible use or nonuse of a drug or drug class. These tests are often used to verify compliance with treatment, identify undisclosed drug use, and monitor for relapse in patients with known use or dependence.

Urine is often the specimen used for testing in outpatient settings. *ICD-10-CM* codes for use or dependence (F10–F19) or counseling (eg, Z71.51) are often sufficient to support the need for testing. However, payer policies may vary, so it is advisable to verify each plan's policy and any coding requirements.

When the specimen used for alcohol/drug testing is blood, report *ICD-10-CM* code Z02.83 (encounter for blood-alcohol and blood-drug test). When blood test findings are positive in a patient not diagnosed with substance use (F10–F19), report codes from category R78.- (findings of drugs and other substances, not normally found in blood) in addition to code Z02.83.

When findings of blood alcohol testing are positive, codes in category Y90.- are used to report the alcohol level. Codes in category Y90 are reported secondary to codes for associated alcohol-related disorders. See **Table 14-4** for a listing of related codes in categories R78 and Y90.

Presumptive drug class screening includes all drugs and drug classes performed by the respective methodology (eg, dipstick kit with direct optical observation) on a single date of service. Sample validation is included in presumptive drug screening service. Venipuncture to obtain samples for drug testing may be separately reportable with code 36415 (collection of venous blood by venipuncture).

Table 14-4. *International Classification of Diseases, 10th Revision, Clinical Modification* Abnormal Finding Drug Blood Test

R78.0 blood[a]	R78.1 opiate drug	R78.2 cocaine	R78.3 hallucinogen	R78.4 other drugs of addictive potential	R78.5 other psycho-tropic drug	R78.6 steroid agent

Finding of
R78.89 other specified substances, not normally found in blood
R78.9 unspecified substance, not normally found in blood

ICD-10-CM Evidence of Alcohol Involvement Determined by Blood Alcohol Level[b]
Blood alcohol level (mg/100 mL)

Y90.0 <20	Y90.1 20–39	Y90.2 40–59	Y90.3 60–79	Y90.4 80–99	Y90.5 100–119	Y90.6 120–199	Y90.7 200–239	Y90.8 ≥240

Y90.9 Presence of alcohol in blood, level not specified

Abbreviation: ICD-10-CM, International Classification of Diseases, 10th Revision, Clinical Modification.

[a] Use additional external cause code (Y90.-) for detail regarding alcohol level.
[b] Code first any associated alcohol-related disorders (F10).

When testing is performed with a method using direct optical observation to determine the result, code 80305 is reported. Tests that have a waived status under the Clinical Laboratory Improvement Amendments may be reported with modifier QW (waived test).

80305   Drug test(s), presumptive, any number of drug classes, any number of devices or procedures; capable of being read by direct optical observation only (eg, utilizing immunoassay [eg, dipsticks, cups, cards, or cartridges]), includes sample validation when performed, per date of service

When a reader is used to determine the result of testing (eg, a dipstick is inserted into a machine that determines the final reading), code 80306 is reported.

80306   read by instrument assisted direct optical observation (eg, utilizing immunoassay [eg, dipsticks, cups, cards, or cartridges]), includes sample validation when performed, per date of service

Testing that uses a chemistry analyzer or more effort than tests represented by codes 80305 and 80306 is reported with code 80307.

> *International Classification of Diseases, 10th Revision, Clinical Modification* code F40.231 (fear of injections and transfusions) may be used for patients who have a phobia of needles.

80307   by instrument chemistry analyzers (eg, utilizing immunoassay [eg, EIA, ELISA, EMIT, FPIA, IA, KIMS, RIA]), chromatography (eg, GC, HPLC), and mass spectrometry either with or without chromatography, (eg, DART, DESI, GC-MS, GC-MS/MS, LC-MS, LC-MS/MS, LDTD, MALDI, TOF); includes sample validation when performed, per date of service

Some plans require use of HCPCS codes for reporting alcohol/drug screening or testing. Code H0048 is reported for the collection and handling of specimens other than blood for alcohol and/or drug testing. Code H0003 is used to report the analysis of a screening test for alcohol and/or drugs.

H0003   Alcohol and/or drug screening; laboratory analysis of specimens for presence of alcohol and/or drugs
H0048   Alcohol and/or other drug testing: collection and handling only, specimens other than blood

Examples

➤ **A psychologist is consulted by an ED physician to evaluate and recommend treatment options for a 17-year-old patient who presented with symptoms of abdominal pain and vomiting for several days.** The patient admits to smoking and consuming cannabis products on a daily basis for at least 2 years. The psychologist recommends treatment for cannabis abuse through a local community health center. The documented diagnosis is cannabis abuse with cannabis hyperemesis syndrome.

ICD-10-CM codes reported are Z71.51 (drug abuse counseling and surveillance of drug abuser), F12.188 (cannabis abuse with other cannabis-induced disorder), and R11.2 (nausea with vomiting, unspecified).

➤ **A patient who is dependent on cannabis is seen in follow-up.** A urine sample is tested for the presence of drugs and the result is negative. The patient's diagnosis is cannabis dependence, in remission.

Codes Z02.83 (encounter for blood-alcohol and blood-drug test) and F12.21 (cannabis dependence, in remission) are reported.

Definitive Drug Testing

When necessary to identify specific drugs or metabolites, a definitive drug test may be ordered. Definitive drug identification methods identify individual drugs and distinguish between structural isomers but not necessarily stereoisomers. Definitive drug tests are reported with codes 80320–80373 based on drug classes (eg, alcohol[s] or non-opioid analgesics) as identified in the Definitive Drug Classes Listing in the Pathology and Laboratory section of *CPT* references.

Behavioral Health Integration

Behavioral health integration services are differentiated by the required elements of service. Psychiatric collaborative care management services (99492–99494) include a defined team of health care professionals providing care using a specific care method. General behavioral health integration (99484) services do not include specific types of providers or a specified method of delivery.

Psychiatric Collaborative Care Management Services

▲99492   Initial psychiatric collaborative care management, first 70 minutes in the first calendar month of behavioral health care manager activities, in consultation with a psychiatric consultant, and directed by the treating physician or other qualified health care professional, with the following required elements:

- ● outreach to and engagement in treatment of a patient directed by the treating physician or other qualified health care professional,
- ● initial assessment of the patient, including administration of validated rating scales, with the development of an individualized treatment plan,
- ● review by the psychiatric consultant with modifications of the plan if recommended,
- ● entering patient in a registry and tracking patient follow-up and progress using the registry, with appropriate documentation, and participation in weekly caseload consultation with the psychiatric consultant, and
- ● provision of brief interventions using evidence-based techniques such as behavioral activation, motivational interviewing, and other focused treatment strategies.

▲99493   Subsequent psychiatric collaborative care management, first 60 minutes in a subsequent month of behavioral health care manager activities, in consultation with a psychiatric consultant, and directed by the treating physician or other qualified health care professional, with the following required elements:

- ● tracking patient follow-up and progress using the registry, with appropriate documentation,
- ● participation in weekly caseload consultation with the psychiatric consultant,
- ● ongoing collaboration with and coordination of the patient's mental health care with the treating physician or other qualified health care professional and any other treating mental health providers,
- ● additional review of progress and recommendations for changes in treatment, as indicated, including medications, based on recommendations provided by the psychiatric consultant,
- ● provision of brief interventions using evidence-based techniques such as behavioral activation, motivational interviewing, and other focused treatment strategies,
- ● monitoring of patient outcomes using validated rating scales, and
- ● relapse prevention planning with patients as they achieve remission of symptoms and/or other treatment goals and are prepared for discharge from active treatment.

+99494   Initial or subsequent psychiatric collaborative care management, each additional 30 minutes in a calendar month of behavioral health care manager activities, in consultation with a psychiatric consultant, and directed by the treating physician or other qualified health care professional (List separately in addition to code for primary procedure)

(Use **99494** in conjunction with **99492, 99493**)

Psychiatric collaborative care management includes use of validated rating scales in monitoring patient outcomes. Do not separately report use of standardized rating scales (eg, **96127**).

Psychiatric collaborative care management services are reported by a physician or QHP who supervises a behavioral health care manager (BHM) who delivers the services. Psychiatric collaborative care management services are provided to patients who have a new or existing psychiatric disorder that requires a behavioral health assessment; care plan implementation, revision, or monitoring; and provision of brief interventions. The treating physician or QHP reports codes **99492–99494** when all requirements for reporting are met. Evaluation and management and other services may be reported separately by the same physician or QHP during the same calendar month.

Each team member's role is defined in *CPT* as follows:

- ● The treating physician or QHP
  - — Directs the BHM and continues to oversee the patient's care, including prescribing medications, providing treatments for medical conditions, and making referrals to specialty care when needed.
  - — Engages the services of the psychiatric consultant who does not directly bill for PCCM services (ie, the treating physician's or QHP's practice contracts with the psychiatric consultant for this component of the PCCM service).
  - — Acts in a supervisory role to the BHM (may be a direct employee or contractual employee but should represent a practice expense like other clinical staff and QNHCPs).
  - — May personally perform behavioral health care management activities. When those activities are not used to meet criteria for a separately reported service (eg, office E/M), his or her time may be counted toward the required time for PCCM.
  - — Is ultimately responsible for delivery, documentation, and billing of PCCM services in compliance with *CPT* and payer policies.
- ● The BHM is a QNHCP or clinical staff member with master- or doctoral-level education *or* specialized training in behavioral health who provides behavioral health care management services under the treating physician's or QHP's supervision and in consultation with a psychiatric consultant. The BHM provides the following services, as needed:
  - — Assessment of needs including the administration of validated rating scales.
  - — Development of a care plan.

— Provision of brief face-to-face and non–face-to-face interventions.
— Ongoing collaboration with the treating physician or QHP.
— Consultation with the psychiatric consultant at least weekly (typically non–face-to-face).
— Maintenance of a registry.
— May also provide and report other services (within BHM's scope of practice) in the same calendar month as PCCM. These may include psychiatric diagnosis, psychotherapy, smoking and tobacco use cessation counseling (**99406**, **99407**), and alcohol and/or substance use structured screening and brief intervention services (**99408**, **99409**).

- The psychiatric consultant is a medical professional trained in psychiatry or behavioral health *and qualified to prescribe a full range of medications*. The psychiatric consultant typically does not see the patient or prescribe medications, except in rare circumstances. The psychiatric consultant advises and makes recommendations to the treating physician or QHP (typically via consultation with the BHM). The psychiatric consultant's services include recommending the following services, as needed:
  — Psychiatric and other medical differential diagnosis.
  — Treatment strategies addressing appropriate therapies.
  — Medication management.
  — Medical management of complications associated with treatment of psychiatric disorders.
  — Referral for specialty services.
  — The psychiatric consultant may directly provide and separately report E/M or psychiatric services, such as psychiatric evaluation (**90791**, **90792**), to a patient within a calendar month when the same patient receives PCCM services.

  Reporting requirements for PCCM services include

- Time of service is met when the midpoint is passed. Documentation must support provision of PCCM services for the required time.

  When service time does not meet the midpoint (ie, 36 minutes for **99492**, 31 minutes for **99493**, 16 minutes beyond last full period for **99494**), do no report PCCM.

- Services are provided for an episode of care defined as beginning when the treating physician or QHP directs the patient to the BHM and ending with
  — The attainment of targeted treatment goals, which typically results in the discontinuation of care management services and continuation of usual follow-up with the treating physician or other QHP
  — Failure to attain targeted treatment goals culminating in referral to a psychiatric care provider for ongoing treatment
  — Lack of continued engagement with no PCCM services provided over a consecutive 6-month calendar period (break in episode)

- A new episode of care starts after a break in episode of 6 calendar months or more.
- Medical necessity of PCCM services may be supported by documentation such as
  — A newly diagnosed condition
  — A patient's need for help engaging in treatment
  — A patient who has not responded to standard care delivered in a nonpsychiatric setting or who requires further assessment and engagement prior to consideration of referral to a psychiatric care setting

  These are typical patient scenarios. Other reasons for services may support medical necessity.

- Documentation of the patient's behavioral health conditions, psychosocial needs, and other factors influencing patient care may help support the necessity of services when health plans implement specific coverage criteria and/or prior authorization for PCCM services.

  Psychiatric collaborative care management services do not require establishment of a care plan for *all* the patient's health care needs. The services are directed to behavioral health needs. Patients may or may not have comorbid conditions that affect treatment and management.

- Psychiatric collaborative care management services may be reported in the same month as chronic or principal care management services (**99439**, **99487**, **99489**–**99491**, **99424**–**99427**, **99437**) when the requirements for each service are met without overlap.
- Provision of PCCM services may support quality initiatives such as use of an electronic clinical data system to track care and administration of a validated rating scale (eg, depression screening instrument) during a 4-month period for patients diagnosed with major depression or dysthymia.

● =New code   ▲ =Revised code   # =Re-sequenced code   + =Add-on code   ★ =Telemedicine

Chapter 14. Mental and Behavioral Health Services

Example

➤ **A pediatrician orders PCCM services for a 15-year-old patient diagnosed with moderate depression, single episode.** A licensed clinical psychologist acting as the BHM discusses PCCM services with the patient and performs an initial assessment. Standardized assessment instruments are used in the assessment and a treatment plan including psychotherapy is agreed on. Later, the BHM enters the patient information into a registry that will be used to track medication compliance and progress. At a regularly scheduled conference call between the BHM and a consulting psychiatrist the patient's assessment is reviewed and the treatment plan approved. The supervising pediatrician is also consulted and approves the treatment plan. The BHM, whose scope of practice includes psychotherapy, provides 3 separately reportable individual psychotherapy sessions within the calendar month in addition to PCCM services. During the calendar month, the BHM documents 60 minutes of time spent in PCCM services.

ICD-10-CM	*CPT*
F32.1 (major depressive disorder, single episode, moderate)	**99492** (initial month PCCM service, first 70 minutes)
	90832, **90834**, or **90837** (psychotherapy without E/M based on time of service; 30, 45, or 60 minutes)

Teaching Point: Time of service for PCCM services is met when the midpoint is passed. In this example, the 60 minutes spent by the BHM supports reporting of code **99492**, which includes the first 70 minutes of PCCM services in the initial month of service.

Psychotherapy services may be reported on a separate claim prior to fulfilling the time requirement for PCCM. No time spent in provision of psychotherapy may be attributed to the time of PCCM services. If psychotherapy services were not within the scope of practice for the BHM, the patient might be referred to another provider (eg, the consulting psychiatrist), who would report the services rendered.

General Behavioral Health Integration Care Management

#▲99484 Care management services for behavioral health conditions, at least 20 minutes of clinical staff time, directed by a physician or other qualified health care professional, per calendar month, with the following required elements:

- Initial assessment or follow-up monitoring, including the use of applicable validated rating scales,
- Behavioral health care planning in relation to behavioral/psychiatric health problems, including revision for patients who are not progressing or whose status changes,
- Facilitating and coordinating treatment such as psychotherapy, pharmacotherapy, counseling and/or psychiatric consultation, and
- Continuity of care with a designated member of the care team

General behavioral health integration care management (**99484**) is reported by a physician or QHP for supervision of clinical staff who provide at least 20 minutes of GBHI services within a calendar month to a patient with a behavioral health condition (includes substance use). A treatment plan must be documented and address the patient's behavioral health condition(s), but a comprehensive health care plan is not required. General behavioral health integration is an outpatient service.

Clinical staff providing GBHI services are not required to have qualifications that would permit them to separately report services (eg, psychotherapy), but, if qualified and they perform such services, they may report such services separately. The time of the separately reported service is not used to support reporting **99484**.

Services must be provided under general physician supervision and in accordance with the licensing and scope of practice requirements of the state where services are provided. The individual supervising and reporting GBHI care management services must be able to report E/M services.

All the required elements of service listed in the code descriptor must be provided and documented.

Example

➤ **A 17-year-old presents to the primary care pediatrician with complaint of anxiety and stress about planning for college.** The primary care physician diagnoses the patient with a behavioral health disorder and recommends that the patient receive behavioral health care management as part of the treatment plan. Clinical staff provide behavioral health care planning and coordination of care with a psychologist in another practice as directed by the pediatrician. At least 20 minutes of clinical staff time is documented for contact with the patient and psychologist throughout the calendar month to assess progress using standardized rating scales and coordinating care, including facilitating access to community resources, as needed.

  If clinical staff time of fewer than 20 minutes is documented in a calendar month, code **99484** is not reported. Code **99484** does not include requirements for a BHM or collaboration with a psychiatrist.

- *Use of validated rating scales is required and is not separately reported* (ie, do not report code **96127** for rating scales administered during the period of behavioral health care management services).
- Time may be face-to-face but more typically may be non–face-to-face. Clinical staff must be available to provide face-to-face services to the patient when requested.
- Evaluation and management and/or psychiatric services may be reported on the same date or in the same calendar month as GBHI services when performed, but these services cannot be used to support reporting of GBHI (ie, time of separately reported services is not counted toward the time of GBHI services).
- General behavioral health integration (**99484**) may be reported in the same month as chronic or principal care management services (**99439**, **99487**, **99489–99491**, **99424–99427**, **99437**) when the requirements for each service are met without overlap.
- The reporting individual may personally provide GBHI services and combine the time of service with that of clinical staff to support reporting code **99484**. However, the time of services that are separately reported (eg, 20 minutes' total time spent providing an E/M service reported with code **99213**) cannot be included in the time supporting **99484**.
- General behavioral health integration (**99484**) and PCCM (**99492–99494**) may not be reported by the same provider in the same month.
- Clinical staff time spent coordinating care with the ED may be reported using **99484**, but time spent while the patient is an inpatient or is admitted to observation status may not be reported using **99484**.

Resources

AAP Policy Statement

"Addressing Early Childhood Emotional and Behavioral Problems" (https://pediatrics.aappublications.org/content/138/6/e20163023)

Payment/Denial Advocacy

AAP Coding Hotline (Hassle Factor Form) (https://form.jotform.com/Subspecialty/aapcodinghotline)

AAP Pediatric Councils (www.aap.org/en/practice-management/practice-financing/payer-contracting-advocacy-and-other-resources/aap-payer-advocacy/aap-pediatric-councils/)

Chapter 14. Mental and Behavioral Health Services

Test Your Knowledge!

1. **Which code or codes are appropriate to use to report developmental screening using a standardized instrument during a well-child visit?**
   a. The screening is included in the preventive medicine service (eg, **99391**).
   b. **96110** and the preventive medicine service (eg, **99391**)
   c. **96112** and the preventive medicine service (eg, **99391**)
   d. **96146** and the preventive medicine service (eg, **99391**)

2. **What *Current Procedural Terminology* codes are reported for 2 hours and 40 minutes spent in neuropsychological testing data interpretation, interactive feedback, and report creation?**
   a. **96132** × 2
   b. **96132, 96133** × 1
   c. **96132, 96133** × 2
   d. **96138, 96139** × 3

3. **True or false? When family members act as informants during individual psychotherapy, codes 90846 and 90847 are always reported.**
   a. True
   b. False

4. **A diagnosis of abusive alcohol use with dependence is documented. Which type of code is reported?**
   a. Use
   b. Abuse
   c. Dependence
   d. All of the above

5. **Which of the following is not separately reported when reporting general behavioral health integration care management (99484)?**
   a. Evaluation and management services provided by a physician or other qualified health care professional
   b. Psychotherapy provided by a psychologist or licensed clinical social worker
   c. Care management for chronic conditions
   d. Brief emotional/behavioral assessment using a standardized instrument

Part 3
Primarily for Hospital Settings

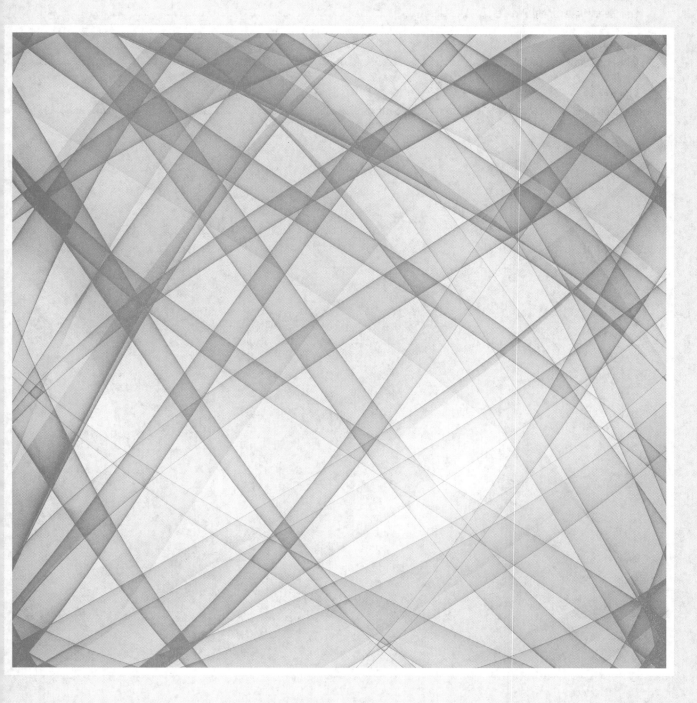

Part 3. Primarily for Hospital Settings

Chapter 15
Hospital Care of the Newborn 359

Chapter 16
Noncritical Hospital Evaluation and Management Services 377

Chapter 17
Emergency Department Services 401

Chapter 18
Critical and Intensive Care 423

Chapter 19
Common Surgical Procedures and Sedation in Facility Settings 447

Hospital Care of the Newborn

Contents

Perinatal Care...361
    Definitions of the Perinatal and Neonatal Periods...361
    Expectant Parent Visits...361

Normal Newborn Care 361
    ICD-10-CM Codes for Newborn Services..363

Hospital Care of the Ill Newborn 364
    Attendance at Delivery...364
    Diagnosis Codes for Perinatal Conditions...366
    Hospital Evaluation and Management Services to the Newborn...367
    Normal Newborn Care or Hospital Care?...367
        Initial Hospital Care...367
        Subsequent Hospital Care 369
        Discharge Day Management 369
        Prolonged Services 370
        Consultations 371
    Coding for Transitions to Different Levels of Neonatal Care 372

Other Newborn Hospital Care 373
    Circumcision 373
    Frenotomy..374
    Car Safety Seat Testing...374

Resources...374

Test Your Knowledge! 375

Perinatal Care

This chapter focuses on coding for care of the typical newborn and those with conditions not requiring intensive monitoring or critical care.

The American Academy of Pediatrics (AAP) Section on Neonatal-Perinatal Medicine, in conjunction with state chapters and councils of the AAP, has developed strategies that have been successful in addressing payment concerns for neonatal care. Contact your state chapter, its pediatric council, your section district AAP Executive Committee representative, a neonatal trainer, or the AAP Committee on Coding and Nomenclature for assistance in addressing any payment inequities for neonatal services in your state.

Definitions of the Perinatal and Neonatal Periods

For coding purposes, the *perinatal period* commences at 32 completed weeks of gestation through the 28th day following birth (the World Health Organization definition). Based on this definition, the *neonatal period* begins at birth and continues through *the completed 28th day after birth*, ending on the 29th calendar day after birth. The day of birth is considered day 0 (zero). Therefore, the day after birth is considered day 1. This definition is important for selecting the correct diagnosis code for conditions that originate in the perinatal period. (It is also important for selection of codes for neonatal critical care and initial intensive care.)

Expectant Parent Visits

When expectant parents request a visit to meet the pediatrician and learn about the practice, these meet and greet visits are typically not considered a medically necessary service. However, many pediatric practices establish policies for managing this type of visit (often at times when the practice is least busy) as a non-billable service used for marketing the practice.

> See Chapter 9 for consultations provided to expectant parents at the request of another physician or other appropriate source (eg, to address risk reduction and plan newborn care in the presence of identified or suspected abnormalities).

Normal Newborn Care

99460	Initial hospital or birthing center care, per day, for evaluation and management of normal newborn infant
99461	Initial care, per day, for evaluation and management of normal newborn infant seen in other than hospital or birthing center
99462	Subsequent hospital care, per day, for evaluation and management of normal newborn
99463	Initial hospital or birthing center care, per day, for evaluation and management of normal newborn infant admitted and discharged on the same date
99238	Hospital discharge day management; 30 minutes or less
99239	more than 30 minutes

Current Procedural Terminology (*CPT*®) codes for care of a normal newborn typically follow a pathway of daily care from initial care to subsequent care and/or discharge day management depending on the length of the newborn's hospital stay. See **Figure 15-1** for notable exceptions.

A *normal newborn* may be defined as a newborn who

- Transitions to life in the usual manner
- May require delivery room intervention (discussed later in this chapter) but is normal after transition
- May require some testing or monitoring (eg, bilirubin, complete blood cell count [CBC], culture)
- Does not require significant intervention
- May be observed for illness but is not sick
- May be late preterm but requires no special care
- May be in house with sick mother/twin

> Normal newborn codes can be reported for care provided to neonates who are acting normally but recovering from fetal stress or a low Apgar score or who are being observed for a potential problem but are asymptomatic.

Figure 15-1. Normal Newborn Care Coding Pathways

99460 Initial day hospital or birthing center care → **99462** Subsequent hospital care, per day → **99238** or **99239** Discharge day management

99463 Initial hospital or birthing center care, per day, normal newborn *admitted and discharged on the same date*

99461 Initial care, per day, *seen in other than hospital or birthing center* (eg, care in the office following home birth)

Codes **99460**, **99462**, **99463**, **99238**, and **99239** are used to report evaluation and management (E/M) services provided to the healthy newborn in a health care facility such as a hospital (including birthing room deliveries) or birthing center. They are reported when the neonate is cared for in the mother's room (rooming-in), a labor and delivery room, a postpartum floor, or a traditional newborn nursery and when a normal neonate is cared for after the mother is discharged (eg, awaiting foster care).

Code **99461** may be appropriate for E/M of a neonate born at home and evaluated in the physician practice soon after birth (ie, same day or next day).

Guidelines for reporting include

- The neonate is considered admitted at the time of leaving the delivery room. There is no code for observation of a newborn.
- Code **99463** (history and examination of the normal newborn, including discharge) should be reported when an initial history and physical examination and the discharge management are performed *on the same calendar date* for a normal newborn.
- *Do not report* **99463** when discharge occurs on the next calendar date even if less than 24 hours have passed since the initial newborn care.
- Code **99460** (history and examination of the normal newborn, initial service) is reported only once on the first day that the physician provides a face-to-face service in the facility. This date may not necessarily correlate with the date the patient is born or the hospital admission date.
- Code **99462** (subsequent hospital care, normal newborn) is reported once per calendar date on the date(s) subsequent to the initial normal newborn care service but *not* on the discharge date.
- Discharge management services performed on a day subsequent to initial newborn care are reported with code **99238** (hospital discharge day management; 30 minutes or less) or **99239** (hospital discharge day management; more than 30 minutes) when discharging a normal newborn.

Include time spent in final examination of the patient, discussion of the hospital stay, instructions for continuing care, and preparation of discharge records, prescriptions, and referral forms. Time must be documented when reporting **99239**.

> **Discharge day management codes 99238 and 99239 are valued (2.07 and 3.05 total facility relative value units [RVUs]) to include the physician's time and work such as counseling parents about care of the neonate that is not captured by 99462, subsequent newborn hospital care (1.19 total facility RVUs).**

- Any additional procedures (eg, circumcision) should be reported in addition to normal newborn care codes. Modifier **25** (significant, separately identifiable E/M service) should be appended to the E/M code when a procedure is performed on the same day of service.

When reporting an E/M service based on time (eg, discharge day management), do not include the time spent providing a separately reported service (eg, circumcision) in the time of the E/M service (eg, obtaining consent, postprocedural care instruction).

ICD-10-CM Codes for Newborn Services

International Classification of Diseases, 10th Revision, Clinical Modification (ICD-10-CM) codes from category **Z38** are used to report live-born neonates according to type of birth and are the first-listed codes for care by the attending or admitting physician during the entire birth admission. Other physicians providing care during the birth admission do not report **Z38** codes but instead report codes for the conditions managed at each encounter. Category **Z38** codes for a single and twin live-born neonates are shown in **Table 15-1**.

Table 15-1. *International Classification of Diseases, 10th Revision, Clinical Modification* Codes for Single and Twin Live-born Neonates	
Z38.00 (single liveborn infant, delivered vaginally)	**Z38.30** (twin liveborn infant, delivered vaginally)
Z38.01 (single liveborn infant, delivered by cesarean)	**Z38.31** (twin liveborn infant, delivered by cesarean)
Z38.1 (single liveborn infant, born outside hospital)	**Z38.4** (twin liveborn infant, born outside hospital)
Z38.2 (single liveborn infant, unspecified as to place of birth)	**Z38.5** (twin liveborn infant, unspecified as to place of birth)

See the *ICD-10-CM* manual for **Z38** codes for other multiple-birth neonates.

Report *ICD-10-CM* code **Z76.2** (encounter for health supervision and care of other healthy infant and child) when a healthy newborn continues to receive daily visits pending discharge of the mother or foster care placement, or for other reasons. Code **Z76.2** is useful for indicating the reason for an extended stay of a healthy newborn. Report code **Z76.2** secondary to the appropriate **Z38** code for services by the attending physician during the birth admission.

Examples

➤ **The physician receives a late-night call about the vaginal delivery of a healthy term boy.** A nurse relates that the newborn has been admitted and seems fine. The physician's standing admission orders are followed, and the physician examines the newborn the following morning. The physician reviews the record, examines the neonate, and speaks with the mother. The newborn and mother remain in the hospital until the next day, when both are then discharged home. Discharge management takes 25 minutes.

ICD-10-CM	Diagnosis code for all days **Z38.00** (single liveborn delivered vaginally)
CPT	**Day 1:** No charge (no face-to-face services provided) **Day 2:** **99460** (initial normal newborn care) **Day 3:** **99238** (hospital discharge day management; 30 minutes or less)

➤ **A baby is born vaginally in the hospital on March 3 at 4:00 pm.** The physician first sees the baby on March 4 at 7:00 am and, later the same date, determines that the newborn is ready for discharge. A history and examination of the newborn, discussion of the hospital stay with the parents, instructions for continuing care, family counseling, and preparation of the final discharge records are performed.

ICD-10-CM	**Z38.00** (single liveborn, delivered vaginally)
CPT	**99463** (initial normal newborn care and discharge on the same date)

➤ **A baby is born by cesarean delivery in the hospital on March 3 at 10:00 am.** The pediatrician provides initial newborn care on that date. On March 4, the pediatrician provides subsequent normal newborn care. On March 5, the physician determines that the newborn is ready for discharge and spends 25 minutes in discharge day management. Each service is appropriately documented.

Chapter 15. Hospital Care of the Newborn

ICD-10-CM	Diagnosis code for each day **Z38.01** (single liveborn, delivered by cesarean section)	
CPT	**Day 1: 99460** (initial normal newborn care) **Day 2: 99462** (subsequent normal newborn care) **Day 3: 99238** (discharge day management)	

➤ **A subsequent hospital visit is performed in the well-baby nursery on a vaginally delivered 2-day-old who is being observed due to risk of jaundice; however, no interventions are noted, and baby is doing well. Diagnosis is neonatal hyperbilirubinemia.**

Code **99462** (subsequent normal newborn care) is reported. The first-listed diagnosis code is **Z38.00**. For neonatal hyperbilirubinemia, report *ICD-10-CM* code **P59.9** (neonatal jaundice, unspecified).

➤ **During a subsequent newborn care visit, the physician notes that the newborn failed the routine hearing screen.** The attending physician spends 15 minutes discussing the results with the parents and refers to an audiologist for testing to confirm or rule out hearing abnormality.

ICD-10-CM	**Z38.00** (single liveborn, delivered vaginally) **R94.120** (abnormal auditory function study)
CPT	**99462** (subsequent normal newborn care)

Teaching Point: The time spent providing the subsequent newborn care does not affect code selection, as normal newborn care services are reported per day, not per hour. Only code **Z38.00** would be reported when the result of an auditory screening is normal.

An audiologist performing confirmatory testing would report code **Z01.110** (encounter for hearing examination following failed hearing screening) and codes for any identified conditions.

Hospital Care of the Ill Newborn

Attendance at Delivery

99464 Attendance at delivery (when requested by the delivering physician or other qualified health care professional) and initial stabilization of newborn

Attendance at delivery (**99464**) is not reported when hospital-mandated attendance is the only underlying basis for providing the service. When physician on-call services are mandated by the hospital (eg, attending all repeat cesarean deliveries) and not physician requested, report code **99026** (hospital-mandated on-call service; in hospital, each hour) or **99027** (hospital-mandated on-call service; out of hospital, each hour).

Attendance at delivery (**99464**)

● Service is only reported when requested by the delivering physician and indicated for a newborn who may require immediate intervention (ie, stabilization, resuscitation, or evaluation for potential problems).

● Medical record documentation must include the request for attendance at the delivery and substantiate the medical necessity of the services performed. If there is no documentation by the delivering physician for attendance at delivery, the verbal request and the reason for the request should be documented in the attendance note.

● Includes initial drying, stimulation, suctioning, blow-by oxygen, or continuous positive airway pressure or high-flow air/oxygen without positive-pressure ventilation (PPV); a cursory visual inspection of the neonate; assignment of Apgar scores; and discussion of the care of the newborn with the delivering physician and parents. A quick look into the delivery room or examination after stabilization is not sufficient to report **99464**. See the "Coding Conundrum: What Service Can Be Reported When a Physician Arrives After Delivery?" box later in this chapter for more information on reporting less than full attendance at delivery services.

● May be reported in addition to initial normal newborn (**99460**), initial sick newborn (**99221–99223**), initial intensive care of the neonate (**99477**), or critical care (**99468; 99291, 99292**) codes.

● Is not reported in conjunction with standby service codes **99026** and **99027**.

See Chapter 16 for guidelines for standby service codes 99026 and 99027. Standby services *may be* reported with the newborn resuscitation services (99465) per *Current Procedural Terminology* guidelines.

Examples

➤ **A physician is called at the request of an obstetrician to attend a cesarean delivery.** The physician stands by until the neonate is delivered and provides stabilization of the neonate, who initially requires blow-by oxygen but steadily becomes more vigorous (99464). The same physician then provides initial normal newborn care (99460) later that same day.

➤ **A delivering physician asks a neonatologist to be present at delivery of a neonate whose mother has active infection.** The neonatologist documents stabilization, including use of continuous positive airway pressure without PPV and a comprehensive examination of the neonate, in addition to the maternal and fetal history. Although a history and examination were performed, this does not equate to initial hospital care of the newborn. The neonatologist reports code 99464.

The newborn is admitted to the newborn nursery under the orders of another physician. This attending physician provides a comprehensive history and examination, orders screening tests and prophylactic interventions, and counsels the family that the neonate will be monitored closely for signs of illness. The physician also counsels about topics such as feeding, sleep, and safety. The attending physician reports code 99460 or initial hospital care (99221–99223) if the newborn required any significant intervention on that date.

When qualifying resuscitative efforts including PPV are provided to a neonate with respiratory or cardiac instability, code 99465 (delivery/birthing room resuscitation, provision of PPV and/or chest compressions in the presence of acute inadequate ventilation and/or cardiac output) is reported instead of 99464. Do no report both 99464 and 99465 (ie, report only 99465, when provided).

See the "Stillborn Deliveries and Unsuccessful Resuscitation" box later in this chapter for discussion of billing for services provided to a mother and/or neonate when the outcome is a stillborn neonate or unsuccessful resuscitation of an ill neonate.

See Chapter 18 for more information on delivery/birthing room neonatal resuscitation and guidelines for coding intensive or critical care services.

Coding Conundrum: What Service Can Be Reported When a Physician Arrives After Delivery?

There are no specific time requirements for reporting attendance at delivery. Remember, this service requires a request for attendance at delivery by the delivering physician and includes physician work to perform the initial drying, stimulation, suctioning, blow-by oxygen, or continuous positive airway pressure without positive-pressure ventilation; a cursory visual inspection of the neonate; assignment of Apgar scores; and discussion of the care of the newborn with the delivering physician and parents. When a physician arrives in the delivery room after the delivery and some or all this work has been performed, should attendance at delivery be reported? Physicians might want to consider

- When the newborn continues to require intervention or stabilization in the delivery room, code 99464 (attendance at delivery) may be reported if the physician work and medical necessity are related to the delivery and are not a component of a sick, intensive, or critical admission and the nature of the intervention is documented in the medical record.
- When the work provided in the delivery room is related more to the initial hospital care (eg, neonate is examined and the physician sends the neonate to the well-baby nursery), only the initial normal newborn care code (99460) is reported.

For example, attendance at delivery was requested by the delivering physician and the physician arrives after the delivery.

- The 1-minute Apgar score has been assigned; the neonate has been dried, stimulated, and suctioned by the nurses; and the neonate is ready to be sent to the newborn nursery by the time the pediatrician appears in the delivery room. The delivering physician acknowledges that assistance is no longer needed. The attending pediatrician will report initial normal newborn care (99460) after completing the initial examination of the newborn. However, if the pediatrician is not the attending pediatrician, no service can be reported.
- In the previous example, the delivering physician wants continued assistance. The pediatrician assigns the 5-minute Apgar score, performs a cursory examination, and discusses the care of the newborn with the delivering physician and parents. Code 99464 can be reported because most of the basic elements of the attendance at delivery were performed and documented in the medical record.

●=New code ▲=Revised code #=Re-sequenced code +=Add-on code ★=Telemedicine

Stillborn Deliveries and Unsuccessful Resuscitation

Questions arise on documentation, coding, and billing for services provided to a baby who is stillborn or thought to be viable (eg, showing fetal distress prior to delivery) but who, shortly after birth, despite resuscitative efforts, never shows active signs of a heartbeat.

If a baby is delivered but is known to have expired in utero, a separate chart will not be created. Therefore, any services performed by a pediatrician or neonatologist would be documented in the maternal record. The physician could be called on to perform an examination and/or discuss any known or discovered fetal anomalies. In this circumstance, the physician could charge a new patient hospital visit (with the mother as the patient) with counseling only, using time to determine to code level (99221–99223), which includes floor/unit time. In practice, many physicians may not charge for this service.

Similar to a known intrauterine fetal demise, a neonate who was felt to be viable may be born without evidence of a heart rate or respiratory effort. Resuscitative efforts may be started and then stopped after a determined amount of time. While neonatal resuscitation (99465) could be coded and billed for, a separate medical record may not be created for the neonate. The service may be billed using the mother as the patient; however, medical records would likely have to accompany the claim. Most payers will deny this claim, so an appeal would be required. It would be best to create a record for the baby so the services could be documented for both the physician and nursing staff. Again, in practice, many physicians do not charge for this service.

For a live-born neonate who is in distress and dies in the delivery room, an individual medical record should be created to document the care. This service will be reported as neonatal resuscitation services (99465) with the deceased as the recipient of care. Remember to also document and report any other separately billable services (eg, surfactant administration), when performed.

While all services and procedures performed must be clearly documented in the maternal or neonate's medical record (if one is created), billing for the services will be up to the individual physician.

Diagnosis Codes for Perinatal Conditions

There are some important guidelines for reporting conditions that originate in the perinatal period. In *ICD-10-CM*, these conditions are classified to Chapter 16 and codes **P00–P96**. Codes in this chapter are used only on the neonate's record and not that of the mother.

The ordering of codes for neonates at the birth hospital are as follows:

1. Birth outcome (Z38-, reported only by the attending/admitting physician)
2. Codes from the perinatal chapter (P00–P96)
3. Codes from the congenital anomalies chapter (Q00–Q99)
4. All other chapters

Other important guidelines include

- Perinatal condition codes are assigned for any condition that is clinically significant. In addition to clinical indications for reporting codes from other chapters, perinatal conditions are considered clinically significant if the condition has implications for future health care needs. Other clinical indications that apply to all conditions are those requiring
  - Clinical evaluation
  - Therapeutic treatment
  - Diagnostic procedures
  - Extended hospital stay
  - Increased nursing care and/or monitoring
- Should a condition originate in the perinatal period and continue past the 28th day after birth, the perinatal code should continue to be used regardless of the patient's age.

  Typical scenarios that may require exclusive use of perinatal or neonatal codes beyond the perinatal period are those related to care of a critically ill or recovering neonate, such as necrotizing enterocolitis in newborn (**P77.-**), chronic respiratory disease arising in the perinatal period (**P27.-**), and preterm birth (**P07.-**).
- Note that these codes are not reported for conditions with *onset after the patient is 28 days old*. For example, necrotizing enterocolitis with onset after the neonatal period is reported with codes **K55.30–K55.33**.
- If a newborn has a condition that could be due to the birth process or community acquired and documentation does not indicate which it is, the condition is reported as due to the birth process. Community-acquired conditions are reported with codes other than those in *ICD-10-CM* Chapter 16.
- Codes in categories **P00–P04**, newborn affected by maternal factors and by complications of pregnancy, labor, and delivery, may be reported when the conditions are suspected but have not yet been ruled out.

Chapter 15. Hospital Care of the Newborn

> If a neonate is suspected of having an abnormal condition that, after examination and observation, is ruled out, assign codes for signs and symptoms or, in the absence of signs or symptoms, a code from category **Z05** (encounter for observation and evaluation of newborn for suspected diseases and conditions ruled out).

Examples

➤ **A neonate was born at 36 weeks' gestation to a mother whose group B β-hemolytic streptococcal culture result was still pending at the time of delivery.** The newborn appeared typical in the delivery room and was admitted to the newborn nursery. The newborn was managed per current guidelines, with no indication of illness. On day 2, the mother's group B β-hemolytic streptococcal culture result was negative. The patient was found to be a normal newborn.

ICD-10-CM	**Day 1: Z38.00** (single liveborn, delivered vaginally), **P00.89** (newborn affected by other maternal conditions) **Day 2: Z38.00** (single liveborn, delivered vaginally), **Z05.1** (observation and evaluation of newborn for suspected infectious condition ruled out)
CPT	**Day 1: 99460** **Day 2: 99462**

Teaching Point: On day 1, the patient was suspected of being affected by a localized maternal infection (**P00.89**), but by day 2, the condition was ruled out (**Z05.1**). Normal newborn care codes are reported rather than hospital care because the neonate, while at risk for infection in this case, was not treated but observed and did not develop infection.

Hospital Evaluation and Management Services to the Newborn

Levels of hospital E/M services are based on all hospital care services on the same date by the same physician or physicians of the same group practice (billing under the same tax identification number) and same exact specialty.

When multiple physicians of the same specialty and same group practice provide separate initial or subsequent hospital care to a newborn on the same date, report with a single code representing the combined work (eg, comprehensive history and examination with high-complexity medical decision-making [MDM]).

Normal Newborn Care or Hospital Care?

The choice between coding for normal newborn care and coding for hospital care is based on a physician's judgment. Services to newborns that require an increased level of physician care, nursing observation, or physiologic monitoring (but not intensive care as described by codes **99477–99480**) are typically reported with codes for initial or subsequent hospital care. **Table 15-2** shows the differences in relative value units and potential monetary values for normal and sick newborn care services.

- A sick visit will have a presenting problem that supports the need for diagnostic investigation or therapy. *Therapeutic intervention is typically necessary for the sick newborn.*
- The nature of the presenting problem and extent of work required to diagnose and manage the problem should be considered when determining the appropriate procedure code to describe the service.

Initial Hospital Care

Codes **99221–99223** are used to report the initial hospital care of a sick neonate who does not require intensive observation and monitoring or critical care services.

> Refer to Chapter 16 and Table 16-2 for the specific coding and documentation requirements for reporting initial hospital care.

Chapter 15. Hospital Care of the Newborn

Table 15-2. Comparison Values of Newborn and Hospital Care		
Code	**Total Facility RVUs**[a]	**Monetary Value Example (Based on $40 per RVU)**
99460	2.74	$109.60
99221	2.90	$116.00
99222	3.90	$156.00
99223	5.74	$229.60
99462	1.19	$47.60
99231	1.10	$44.00
99232	2.06	$82.40
99233	2.96	$118.40

Abbreviation: RVU, relative value unit.

[a] Not geographically adjusted.

Examples

➤ **The pediatrician sees a newborn boy admitted to the well-baby nursery.** The baby is O+ DAT+. He was born to a mother with blood type O- who has a history of 2 previous newborns with jaundice secondary to Rh incompatibility. At 8 hours of age, the neonate appears jaundiced. A bilirubin and CBC with a reticulocyte count are ordered, results are evaluated, the newborn's risks for kernicterus are discussed with the family, and phototherapy is started. The pediatrician performs a comprehensive history (maternal history of pregnancy and delivery, significant family history) and physical examination. Medical decision-making is of moderate complexity for this new problem with moderate risk.

ICD-10-CM	**Z38.00** (single liveborn, delivered vaginally) P55.0 (Rh isoimmunization of newborn)
CPT	**99222** *MDM:* Moderate *History:* Comprehensive *Physical examination:* Comprehensive

Teaching Point: When reporting initial hospital care, all 3 key components (ie, history, physical examination, MDM), or average total floor/unit time if more than 50% of time spent is in counseling and/or coordination of care, must be met. The level of service is based on all hospital care services on the same date by the same physician or physicians of the same group practice and same specialty. If the minimum key components are not sufficiently met (eg, an expanded history is performed rather than detailed or comprehensive), the initial care must be reported using subsequent hospital care codes (**99231–99233**).

While code **P55.0** does not specifically mention "jaundice," the *ICD-10-CM* Index entry for newborn jaundice due to maternal/fetal Rh incompatibility directs only to code **P55.0**.

➤ **The pediatrician admits a term neonate, born vaginally, with Rh incompatibility (mom AB– and baby B+/ Coombs test result positive).** The otherwise normal neonate is monitored for elevated bilirubin.

ICD-10-CM	**Z38.00** (single liveborn, delivered vaginally) **P55.0** (Rh isoimmunization of newborn)
CPT	**99460** (initial newborn care)

Teaching Point: The neonate is being observed but not treated, supporting **99460**.

Subsequent Hospital Care

Subsequent hospital care codes (99231–99233) are reported for each day of service subsequent to initial care for the newborn who continues to be sick (ie, not a typical neonate but not in critical condition and not requiring intensive observation and interventions).

Refer to Chapter 16 and Table 16-3 for detailed coding and documentation requirements for codes 99231–99233.

- When a neonate is not treated but only observed for the potential development of illness, normal newborn codes would be reported.
- Report the appropriate code for the highest acuity on each date of service. On subsequent dates when a previously sick neonate is improved and requires no more care than a normal newborn, the subsequent normal newborn care code (99462) should be reported.

It is useful to consider the typical patient when reporting subsequent hospital care. These are

- **99231**: Usually, the patient is stable, recovering, or improving.
- **99232**: Usually, the patient is responding inadequately to therapy or has developed a minor complication.
- **99233**: Usually, the patient is unstable or has developed a significant complication or a significant new problem.

Example

➤ **On day 2 of the birth admission, the attending pediatrician provides subsequent hospital care to a term neonate, born vaginally, with ABO incompatibility (mom O+/antibody negative and baby B+/Coombs test result negative).** The total serum bilirubin is elevated. The pediatrician orders phototherapy and follow-up laboratory tests. An expanded problem-focused interval history and examination are documented.

ICD-10-CM	Z38.00 (single liveborn, delivered vaginally) P55.1 (ABO incompatibility)
CPT	99232 (subsequent hospital care)

Teaching Point: On day 2, the neonate requires MDM of moderate complexity (new diagnosis with prescription of phototherapy). This, along with the expanded problem-focused history or examination, supports code 99232.

Discharge Day Management

Either code 99238 or 99239 (hospital day discharge management) is reported on the day the newborn is discharged (when on a separate day from the initial hospital care).

- A newborn who dies on the date of birth is not discharged from the hospital. The attending physician should report a code for the level of hospital care provided (ie, initial hospital care, intensive care, or critical care) as appropriate. Codes for discharge services are not reported.
- When a neonate is transferred to another facility, the physician providing care prior to transfer reports the appropriate code for the type of care provided on that date (eg, 99291, 99292; hourly critical care) prior to the transfer, not discharge day management.
- Time must be documented to support code 99239 (ie, time of >30 minutes).

Chapter 16 includes more information on discharge day management codes 99238 and 99239.

Chapter 15. Hospital Care of the Newborn

Example

➤ **The physician performs a follow-up visit for a neonate who will be discharged with a home apnea monitor.** The parents are counseled on their neonate's condition and given instructions for home care and follow-up. Forty-five minutes was spent on the floor reviewing the hospital course and expected follow-up and in counseling the parents.

CPT	**99239** (more than 30 minutes)
	Time (45 minutes unit/floor time dedicated to the patient) is the key controlling factor.

Teaching Point: If time spent in discharge day management is not documented, code **99238** must be reported.

Find more information and examples of coding for an ill neonate in the June 2020 *AAP Pediatric Coding Newsletter* article, "General Pediatrics: Care of Newborn Who Becomes Ill" (https://coding.solutions.aap.org/article.aspx?articleid= 2765188; subscription required), or challenge your newborn hospital care coding skills with the January 2020 *AAP Pediatric Coding Newsletter* article, "You Code It! Assigning Appropriate Codes for Hospital Care of Newborns" (https:// coding.solutions.aap.org/article.aspx?articleid=2758028; subscription required).

Prolonged Services

+**99356**   Prolonged service in the inpatient or observation setting, requiring unit/floor time beyond the usual service; first hour (30–74 min)

+**99357**   each additional 30 minutes (minimum 15 min)

99358   Prolonged evaluation and management service before and/or after direct patient care; first hour

+**99359**   each additional 30 minutes (minimum 15 min)

● Codes for direct (face-to-face) prolonged services in the inpatient or observation setting (**99356**, **99357**) are add-on codes and include direct care as well as unit/floor care for that patient. When time requirements are met, codes **99356** and **99357** are reported in addition to the code for the basic service—consultation (**99241–99245**, **99251–99255**), an initial hospital service (**99221–99223**), or a subsequent hospital service (**99231–99233**).

● Direct prolonged services are not reported with normal newborn codes, intensive care codes, or neonatal/pediatric critical care codes because these services do not include an assigned typical time by *CPT*.

● *Time must be documented.*

Prolonged clinical staff services (**99415** and **99416**) are not reported for inpatient care.

> The specific coding guidelines for reporting face-to-face (**99354–99357**) and non–face-to-face (**99358**, **99359**) prolonged service codes are detailed in Chapter 16.

Examples

➤ **The physician performs an expanded problem-focused history and physical examination on a term neonate born via cesarean delivery who is experiencing mild tachypnea on a subsequent day.** The physician obtains and reviews a chest radiograph and CBC and requests that an oxygen saturation (SpO_2) monitor be placed on the neonate for 5 minutes. The chest radiograph and CBC are normal and the SpO_2 is persistently greater than 95%. The physician spends 65 minutes of total time on the floor with the patient, speaking with the mother and reviewing the chart.

CPT	**99232** (typical time is 25 minutes)
	MDM: Low complexity
	History: Expanded problem focused
	Physical examination: Expanded problem focused
	99356 (direct prolonged services, first 30–74 minutes)

Teaching Point: In addition to code **99232**, code **99356** will be reported based on total documented time spent on the floor or unit dedicated to the 1 patient. Time is not the controlling factor in selection of the subsequent hospital care code because there is no documentation of time spent counseling and coordinating care.

➤ **An infant is transferred from a Level III neonatal intensive care unit (NICU), following a 30-day hospital stay, to a community Level II unit to complete recovery before home discharge.** A large volume of records accompanies the infant. A comprehensive history and physical examination are performed on admission; MDM is moderately complex. The physician spends another 1 hour and 20 minutes reviewing the extensive transfer records while off the unit.

CPT	**99222** (typical time is 50 minutes)
	MDM: Moderate complexity
	History: Comprehensive
	Physical examination: Comprehensive
	99358 (prolonged non–face-to-face services, first hour)
	99359 (each additional 30 minutes)

Teaching Point: This service included 80 minutes of prolonged service time spent off the unit/floor (ie, the time is not combined with the unit/floor time of the patient encounter). Code **99358** represents the first 60 minutes. Code **99359** is reported for the final 20 minutes of prolonged service. If fewer than 75 minutes of prolonged services were provided, code **99359** would not be reported because this code is reported for time that goes at least 15 minutes beyond the first hour or final 30 minutes.

Consultations

A consultation is reported when a physician or other appropriate source requests an opinion and/or advice from another physician or appropriate source. This request must be in writing or given verbally by the requestor and documented in the consultation record. The consulting physician renders advice, records it, and returns a report to the requesting physician or appropriate source.

A requested service to determine whether to accept responsibility for ongoing management of the patient's entire care or for the care of a specific condition or problem is also a consultation per *CPT*. However, when an agreement for transfer of care from one physician to another occurs prior to an initial encounter with the receiving physician, this is not a consultation. Documentation should be clear that the transferring physician requested a determination regarding transfer of care.

Chapter 16 details the specific reporting, documentation, and coding requirements for inpatient consultations. See Table 16-5 for inpatient consultation codes.

Example

➤ **At the request of a primary care physician, a neonatologist evaluates a full-term gestation neonate with moderate tachypnea after birth.** A detailed history is obtained from the mother noting she has a history of a positive group B streptococcal screening result. Review of labor and delivery records reveals that she received 1 dose of intravenous ampicillin 2 hours prior to delivery. Due to fetal tachycardia, a cesarean delivery was performed. After birth, the newborn had Apgar scores of 7 and 9 but was noted to be tachypneic with mild substernal retractions. A detailed physical examination was performed. Physical examination and growth parameters are consistent with term gestation. The neonatologist recommends obtaining blood cultures and beginning antibiotics pending the results of the cultures, as well as follow-up CBC at 12 hours. The neonatologist spends 10 minutes explaining the evaluation and plan and counseling the baby's parents. The neonatologist writes a detailed chart note and discusses her recommendations with the attending physician by phone. The attending physician does not want the neonatologist to assume care but requests follow-up consultation. At follow-up, the 12-hour CBC is reassuring, the blood culture results have remained negative, and the tachypnea has resolved. The neonatologist recommends continuing the antibiotics until culture results are negative at 48 hours but otherwise signs off on the case, remaining available for further questions.

ICD-10-CM	**P70.4** (hypoglycemia, newborn) **P07.38** (preterm newborn, gestational age 35 completed weeks)
CPT	**99253** *MDM:* Low complexity *History:* Detailed *Physical examination:* Detailed Or, if payer does not recognize consultations, **99221** (initial hospital care)

Coding for Transitions to Different Levels of Neonatal Care

During a hospital stay, a newborn or readmitted neonate may require multiple levels of care. A normal newborn may end up becoming sick, intensively ill, or critical during the same hospital stay. Neonates who were initially sick may also improve to require lower levels of care (eg, normal neonatal care).

It is important to remember

- When a patient qualifies for normal newborn care and, at a subsequent encounter on the same day, becomes ill and requires an additional encounter at a higher service level, normal newborn care (**99460** or **99462**) may be reported in addition to the following on the same day:
  — Hospital care (**99221–99223**)
  — Initial intensive care (**99477**)
  — Initial critical care (**99468**)
  — Time-based critical care (**99291**, **99292**)
- *CPT* instructs to report the appropriate E/M code with modifier **25** for these services in addition to the normal newborn code.

Examples

➤ **A neonate who was initially normal becomes ill 5 hours after birth.** A pediatrician, who provided initial newborn care earlier the same day, provides a second E/M service to evaluate the neonate's condition and determines that a transfer to a NICU is necessary. Following transfer, a neonatologist provides initial intensive care to the newborn.

The pediatrician reports **99460** and **99221–99223 25**	The neonatologist reports **99477**

Teaching Point: The second E/M service on the same date as the initial newborn care is reported with modifier **25** appended.

➤ **A neonate who was initially normal becomes ill several hours after Physician A provided normal newborn care.** Physician B of another group practice assumes management of the newborn's care and provides an initial hospital care service with a comprehensive history and examination and moderate MDM.

Physician A reports **99460**	Physician B reports **99222**

Teaching Point: No modifier is required because the physicians are not of the same group practice, although they may each be general pediatricians (eg, community physician provides normal newborn care but hospitalist assumes care of ill newborn).

- Once an initial-day care code for a higher service level has been reported, an *initial* code for a lower service level within the same hospital stay will not be reported.
  — If an ill neonate has required intensive care (**99477–99480**) but no longer qualifies for intensive care and is transferred to the care of a physician of a different specialty or different group practice, the receiving physician will report subsequent hospital care (**99231–99233**) based on the level of service provided.
  — The receiving physician *will not report* initial hospital care (**99221–99223**) for the first encounter after the transfer. If the neonate is no longer ill, the receiving physician will report subsequent normal newborn care (**99462**).

— The transferring physician may report initial neonatal intensive care (**99477**) if provided earlier on the date of transfer. However, when the ill neonate improves and is transferred on a date after the date of initial intensive care, a transferring physician will report subsequent hospital care (**99231–99233**), and not subsequent neonatal intensive care (**99478–99480**). The level of care determines the code, not the location of the newborn. Care provided in the NICU does not automatically support intensive care.

Example

➤ **A neonate (2,600 g) is transferred from neonatal intensive care by Dr A to Dr B, who is of a different specialty, to complete recovery before home discharge.** On the day of transfer, Dr A determines the ill but recovering neonate no longer requires intensive care and documents 25 minutes spent on the unit/floor arranging the transfer. Dr B provides a face-to-face visit to the neonate, documenting a detailed interval history, comprehensive examination, moderate-complexity MDM, and 75 minutes of time on the unit reviewing the patient's record and consulting with the family.

Dr A reports	Dr B reports
99232 (subsequent intensive care, 25 minutes)	**99233** (subsequent hospital care, typical time 35 minutes)
	99356 (direct prolonged services, first 30–74 minutes)

Teaching Point: Dr B may not report initial hospital care for services to the patient who has received prior initial hospital services (eg, initial neonatal intensive care). The typical time of code **99233** was exceeded by more than 30 minutes, supporting code **99356**.

Payers that use the Medicare or Medicaid National Correct Coding Initiative (NCCI) will not allow separate payment of

- **Normal newborn hospital care (99460, 99462, 99463)** by the same physician or a physician of the same specialty and same group practice on the same date as initial hospital care (**99221–99223**)
- **Initial hospital care (99221–99223)** by the same physician or a physician of the same specialty and same group practice on the same date as initial inpatient neonatal critical care (**99468**)
- **Subsequent hospital care (99231–99233)** by the same physician or a physician of the same specialty and same group practice on the same date as subsequent normal newborn care (**99462**)

When reporting to these payers, report only the most extensive level of care provided; the code in column 1 of the NCCI edit table is considered the more comprehensive code. See Chapter 2 for more information on NCCI edits and where to find them.

Other Newborn Hospital Care

Circumcision

54150   Circumcision, using clamp or other device with regional dorsal penile or ring block

- If the circumcision using a clamp or other device is performed without dorsal penile or ring block, append modifier **52** (reduced services) to **54150**.
- Medicare has a global period of 0 (zero) assigned to code **54150**.
- When performing a circumcision and a separately identifiable E/M service on the same day (eg, **99462**, subsequent normal newborn care; **99238**, discharge services <30 minutes), append modifier **25** to the E/M code. Link the appropriate *ICD-10-CM* code (eg, **Z38.00**) to the E/M service and to the circumcision code.
- The American Hospital Association *Coding Clinic* instructs that code **Z41.2** (encounter for routine and ritual male circumcision) *is not assigned* during the birth admission, as circumcision is a routine part of the newborn's hospital care.

54160   Circumcision, surgical excision other than clamp, device, or dorsal slit; neonate (28 days of age or less)
54161   older than 28 days

Unlike code **54150**, Medicare has a global period of 10 days assigned to codes **54160** and **54161**. A physician who performs a procedure with a 10-day global period must append modifier **24** (unrelated E/M service by the same physician or other qualified health care professional during a postoperative period) to the E/M code for subsequent newborn or hospital care or discharge management (eg, **99238 24**) provided in the 10-day period following the procedure for general care of the newborn unrelated to the procedure.

See Chapter 10 for information on coding for circumcisions performed in the office.

Frenotomy

40806   Incision of labial frenum (frenotomy)

41010   Incision of lingual frenum (frenotomy)

Often, a newborn will experience issues with latching or feeding due to a tight frenulum. If the issues are severe enough to warrant intervention by means of incising the frenulum, report code **41010** for lingual frenotomy or **40806** for labial frenotomy. This may be completed in the hospital before discharge. Link *ICD-10-CM* codes **P92.5** (neonatal difficulty in feeding at the breast) and **Q38.1** (ankyloglossia) to the procedure code on the claim.

- If the physician performing the incision is also performing newborn care on the same date, be sure to append modifier **25** to the hospital care service also being reported. Link this service to the appropriate **Z38** code followed by **P92.5** and **Q38.1**.
- Do not report *CPT* code **41115** (excision of lingual frenum [frenectomy]) when the frenulum is only incised or clipped.

Car Safety Seat Testing

Codes **94780** and **94781** (car seat testing) are reported for monitoring to determine if *an infant through 12 months of age* may be safely transported in a car seat or must be transported in a car bed.

- Car seat testing codes may be reported in addition to the subsequent hospital or discharge day management codes when performed and documented. *Note:* These codes cannot be reported in addition to critical or intensive care services.
- Time spent in car seat testing is not counted as time spent in discharge day management.
- Car seat testing may also be provided to an infant in an outpatient setting to determine if the infant can safely move from car bed to car seat transportation.

See Chapter 18 for more information on car seat testing.

Resources

Discharge Day Management

"Hospital Discharge Day Management: Are You Coding Correctly?" February 2019 *AAP Pediatric Coding Newsletter* (https://coding. solutions.aap.org/article.aspx?articleid=2720944; subscription required)

Hospital Care of the Newborn

"You Code It! Assigning Appropriate Codes for Hospital Care of Newborns," January 2020 *AAP Pediatric Coding Newsletter* (https:// coding.solutions.aap.org/article.aspx?articleid=2758028; subscription required)

"General Pediatrics: Care of Newborn Who Becomes Ill," June 2020 *AAP Pediatric Coding Newsletter* (https://coding.solutions.aap.org/ article.aspx?articleid=2765188; subscription required)

Newborn Coding Decision Tool

American Academy of Pediatrics *Newborn Coding Decision Tool* (available for purchase online at https://shop.aap.org/ newborn-coding-decision-tool-2022)

Test Your Knowledge!

1. **A neonate is born on January 1. How old is the neonate on January 29?**
   a. 30 days old
   b. 29 days old
   c. 28 days old
   d. 31 days old

2. **When a normal newborn (born late on February 15, 2022) receives initial normal newborn hospital care on February 16, 2022, what code does the attending physician report?**
   a. **99460**
   b. **99461**
   c. **99462**
   d. **99463**

3. **What code is the first-listed *International Classification of Diseases, 10th Revision, Clinical Modification* code by a pediatrician providing subsequent care to a neonate who is being observed for jaundice during the birth admission?**
   a. **P59.9** (neonatal jaundice unspecified)
   b. A category **Z38** code (liveborn infant)
   c. Either **P59.9** or a category **Z38** code
   d. **Z05.42** (observation and evaluation of newborn for suspected metabolic condition ruled out)

4. **What code(s) are reported when the same physician provides subsequent normal newborn care and circumcision on the same date?**
   a. Subsequent hospital care (**99231–99233**)
   b. Normal newborn care (**99460**)
   c. Only the appropriate code for the circumcision (eg, **54150**)
   d. **99462 25** and the appropriate code for the circumcision (eg, **54150**)

5. **What codes does a pediatrician report for assuming management of a neonate who no longer requires critical or intensive care but is not a normal newborn?**
   a. **99231–99233** (subsequent hospital care)
   b. **99251–99255** (inpatient consultation)
   c. **99221–99223** (initial hospital care)
   d. Any of the above if supported by documentation

Noncritical Hospital Evaluation and Management Services

Chapter 16. Noncritical Hospital Evaluation and Management Services

Contents

Coding for Noncritical Hospital Evaluation and Management Services...379

    Progression of Care 379

    Key Components 380

    Time-Based Code Selection...380

    Split/Shared Billing 381

Observation Care 382

    Initial Observation Care..382

    Subsequent Observation Care 385

    Observation Care Discharge Day Management 386

Same Date Admission and Discharge Services..386

    When Payers Use Medicare Observation Policy 386

Inpatient Hospital Care 388

    Initial Inpatient Hospital Care..388

    Subsequent Hospital Care...390

    Hospital Discharge Day Management 391

    Discharge Versus Subsequent Hospital Services 392

Hospital Services by Other Physicians 392

    Concurrent Care...392

    Consultations..393

    Medicare Consultation Guidelines..393

        Consultations for Patients in Observation 394

        Inpatient Consultations 395

    Interprofessional Telephone/Internet/Electronic Health Record Consultation...........................396

Prolonged Evaluation and Management Services Provided in the Inpatient Setting 397

    Direct Prolonged Service 397

    Prolonged Service Before or After Direct Patient Care...398

Medical Team Conferences 398

Advance Care Planning 399

Continuing Care After Hospitalization...399

Hospital-Mandated On-Call Services 399

Resources..400

Test Your Knowledge! 400

Coding for Noncritical Hospital Evaluation and Management Services

This chapter includes tables with descriptions of the required key components (ie, history, physical examination, medical decision-making [MDM], and time) for all evaluation and management (E/M) services that are described in the observation and inpatient hospital setting.

Codes and selection requirements for observation and inpatient hospital care are based on key components (ie, history, examination, and MDM) or floor/unit time.

> **See Chapter 6 for specific documentation requirements. See also the American Academy of Pediatrics Pediatric Evaluation and Management: Coding Quick Reference Card 2022 (available for purchase at https://shop.aap.org).**

The following are basic guidelines for reporting noncritical/non-intensive observation and inpatient hospital E/M services. There are no distinctions between new and established patients.

- Codes are reported based on the cumulative services (performance of the required key components and/or time when appropriate) provided by an individual physician or any combination of physicians or other qualified health care professionals (QHPs)
  - Of the same specialty within a group
  - With the same tax identification number (or group National Provider Identifier [NPI])
  - During a single calendar day

> **When additional separately reported procedures are performed on the date of the evaluation and management (E/M) service, do not include the time spent performing those procedures in the time of the E/M service.**

- Services may be performed and reported by any physician of any specialty (eg, hospitalist, primary care physician, specialist) or other QHPs.
- Any procedure or other service with a *Current Procedural Terminology* (*CPT*®) code may be reported separately when performed by the reporting provider or group and documented.

Progression of Care

Selecting the appropriate level of service from the appropriate family of codes depends on the documentation of the child's condition, admission order(s) (observation vs inpatient), and intensity of the service provided on a particular day of service. **Figure 16-1** indicates the category of codes that should be reported based on the progression of care provided. Remember that the level of service reported is based on cumulative work (ie, key components or time applicable to the code category) performed during the calendar day by the same physician or physicians of the same specialty and same group practice.

Report only the applicable service that is farthest to the right (applies to encounters for the same or related problem by the same individual or physicians and/or other QHPs of the same group practice and specialty).

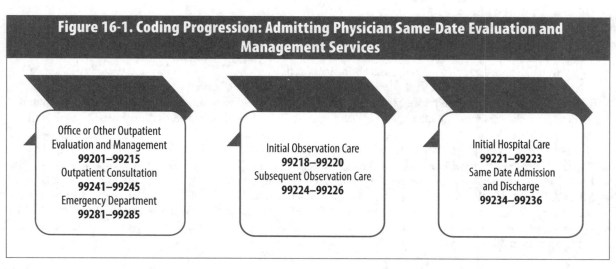

Figure 16-1. Coding Progression: Admitting Physician Same-Date Evaluation and Management Services

Office or Other Outpatient Evaluation and Management
99201–99215
Outpatient Consultation
99241–99245
Emergency Department
99281–99285

Initial Observation Care
99218–99220
Subsequent Observation Care
99224–99226

Initial Hospital Care
99221–99223
Same Date Admission and Discharge
99234–99236

Chapter 16. Noncritical Hospital Evaluation and Management Services

Key Components

Table 16-1 provides specific detail of required elements within each level of history and physical examination (eg, problem focused, detailed) and MDM (eg, straightforward, moderate) of an E/M code. Services may be reported using either the 1995 or 1997 documentation guidelines. The nature of the presenting problem (ie, reason for the encounter) is included as a contributory factor for levels of MDM but is not 1 of the 3 required elements. Evaluation and management coding guidelines are more fully discussed in **Chapter 6**.

Table 16-1. Evaluation and Management Key Components[a]

History (must meet or exceed HPI, ROS, and PFSH)	Problem focused	Expanded	Detailed	Comprehensive
	HPI: 1–3 elements ROS: 0 PFSH: 0	HPI: 1–3 elements ROS: 1 PFSH: 0	HPI: 4+ elements or status of 3 chronic or inactive conditions ROS: 2–9 PFSH: 1	HPI: 4+ elements or status of 3 chronic or inactive conditions ROS: 10+ PFSH: 3
Physical Examination (choose either the 1995 [based on the specified number of body areas/systems] or 1997 guidelines [requires certain bulleted elements])	**Problem focused** 1995: 1 body area/organ system 1997: 1–5 bulleted elements (●) in ≥1 areas or systems	**Expanded** 1995: Limited examination—total 2–7[b] 1997: at least 6 bulleted elements (●) in ≥1 areas or systems	**Detailed** 1995: Extended examination—total 2–7[b] 1997: at least 2 bulleted elements (●) in ≥6 areas or systems or ≥12 bulleted elements (●) in ≥12 areas or systems	**Comprehensive** 1995: 8+ organ systems or complete examination of a single organ system 1997: <u>Multisystem examination</u>—9 systems or areas[c] <u>Single organ system examination</u>[d]—all bulleted elements
MDM Complexity (must meet 2 of 3—DMO, data, and risk) Usual PP severity	**Straightforward** DMO: Minimal Data: Minimal Risk: Minimal PP: Self-limited or minor	**Low** DMO: Limited Data: Limited Risk: Low PP: Moderate	**Moderate** DMO: Multiple Data: Moderate Risk: Moderate PP: Moderate to high	**High** DMO: Extensive Data: Extensive Risk: High PP: Moderate to high

Abbreviations: DMO, number of diagnoses and management options; HPI, history of present illness; MDM, medical decision-making; PFSH, past, family, and social history; PP, presenting problem; ROS, review of systems.

[a] See **Chapter 6** for a detailed description of the guidelines and components of evaluation and management services with documentation requirements and tips.

[b] Includes affected body area/organ system and other related areas/systems (total 2–7).

[c] A comprehensive multisystem examination includes 9 systems or areas with performance of all elements identified by a bullet (●) in each area/system examined and documentation of at least 2 elements identified by a bullet (●) of each area(s) or system(s).

[d] A comprehensive single system examination includes performance of all elements identified by a bullet (●) and documentation of every element in box with shaded border and at least 1 element in box with unshaded border.

Time-Based Code Selection

- Time in the observation and inpatient setting is defined as *floor or unit time* (dedicated to the 1 patient) and includes time spent
  - At the patient's bedside—counseling family or patient (or those who may have assumed responsibility for the care of the patient [eg, foster parents, legal guardians, persons acting in place of a parent])
  - On the floor, performing and documenting the history and examination, and reviewing diagnostic tests or communicating with physicians and other clinicians participating in the patient's care and/or communication with family/caregivers
  - Coordinating care with care team members
- Time is the basis for code selection in lieu of key components only when more than 50% of the unit/floor time is spent in counseling and/or coordination of care. Time includes counseling provided to the patient and/or caregiver(s).
- When time is used as the controlling factor in the selection of the code, the cumulative time spent and the notation that *more than half* the time was spent in counseling and/or coordination of care *must be documented* in the medical record.
- When time is spent off the unit/floor (eg, reviewing and/or discussing medical imaging studies in the radiology department rather than digitally on the unit), do not include that time in the unit/floor time.

See also the Prolonged Evaluation and Management Services Provided in the Inpatient Setting section later in this chapter for discussion of prolonged services.

> The American Academy of Pediatrics *Pediatric Evaluation and Management: Coding Quick Reference Card 2022* is an easy-to-use card that will help you to navigate the steps to ensuring proper code-level reporting for many of your evaluation and management services (eg, provides tables showing key component and time requirements for each type of code). This card is available for purchase at https://shop.aap.org/pediatric-evaluation-and-management-coding-quick-reference-card-2022.

Split/Shared Billing

A split/shared E/M service is one in which a physician and a QHP, such as a nurse practitioner or physician assistant, from the *same group practice* each personally perform a medically necessary and substantive portion of 1 or more face-to-face E/M encounters on the same date. Split/shared billing may allow a physician to report the combined work and receive payment at a higher fee schedule rate than would be paid if reported by the QHP. (Some health plans pay for QHP services at 85% of the plan's physician fee schedule.)

The following requirements apply to all split/shared services:

- A portion of the key components of the service must be provided face-to-face by the physician to report under the physician's NPI.
- Split/shared services were defined and implemented for services to Medicare beneficiaries. Private payers may adopt the same or a similar policy.
- The physician and QHP must each document and sign their portion of the service.
- A physician cannot merely sign off on the documentation of the work by the QHP.
- If the E/M service is reported based on counseling and/or coordination of care, the physician and the QHP must each document their time supporting the level of service reported.
- Documentation must support the total time, the portion of time (ie, >50%) spent in counseling and/or coordination of care, and a summary of the issues discussed and/or coordination of care provided.
- Shared services are not permitted if the QHP is a hospital employee.
- Services may be reported by the QHP or physician (if QHP may bill).
- Shared services are allowed when sick hospital care services are reported (combined physician and QHP time) and with discharge services. (*Critical care is never a split/shared service* because critical care services reflect the work of only 1 individual.)

> Split/shared billing differs from incident-to billing, which is only allowed in a non-facility setting. See Chapter 13 for more information on incident-to rules.

> Notice: At the time of publication, CMS has proposed, but not finalized, significant changes to the Medicare policy for split/shared visits. Please visit the American Academy of Pediatrics website (www.aap.org/cfp or www.aap.org/errata) to check for updates.

Example

▶ **A physician and QHP from the same group practice see a patient on the same date.** The QHP provides and documents initial hospital care, including a comprehensive history, detailed examination, and MDM of moderate complexity. Later that day, the physician is called to see the patient, who is exhibiting new symptoms, and to review new laboratory test results. Taking into account both services, which have been individually documented and signed, the examination and history are comprehensive and MDM is of high complexity.

   Teaching Point: Because both health care professionals are from the same group practice and have signed off on their individually provided services, the services may be shared and billed under the physician as code **99223**. The combined time spent by the physician and QHP may also be used in code selection when more than 50% of that time was spent in counseling and/or coordination of care.

Observation Care

- Hospital observation services are provided to patients who require monitoring and treatment to determine if inpatient admission will be required. For example, a patient with asthma who is not responding adequately to treatment but is not quite sick enough for immediate inpatient care and may be able to later be discharged home would be admitted to observation.
- Hospitals do not need to designate a separate area for these patients; rather, designation of observation versus inpatient status is dependent on the physician's order and the likelihood that the patient's treatment may avoid inpatient admission.
- Initial observation care is reported by the admitting physician or QHP using codes **99218–99220**. Subsequent-day observation care is reported with codes **99224–99226** and observation care discharge management with code **99217**.
- Admission (ie, initial care) and discharge services (observation or inpatient status) provided on the same day are reported with codes **99234–99236**.
- See the Hospital Services by Other Physicians section later in this chapter for guidance on reporting observation or inpatient care by a physician or QHP of a different group practice and/or different specialty from the admitting physician or QHP.
- When the patient's status changes from observation to inpatient status or vice versa (eg, utilization review staff request that the physician change status from inpatient to observation), the physician should write an order to reflect the change and report only the code that reflects care consistent with the patient's final status on that date.

Initial Observation Care

99218–99220 Initial observation care, per day, for the evaluation and management of a patient

See the full code requirements in **Table 16-2**. The examples included here and throughout the chapter are coded based on the 1995 E/M documentation guidelines.

When reporting based on key components
- The history and physical examination to support code **99218** may be detailed or comprehensive. The MDM is of straightforward to low complexity.
- Codes **99219** and **99220** require comprehensive history and examination and are differentiated by the complexity of MDM (moderate [**99219**] or high [**99220**]).

Initial observation care codes are reported
- On the first day that the admitting physician provides face-to-face services to the patient in the observation setting.
- Using the code that reflects the overall care provided by the admitting physician to the patient on that calendar date. When "observation status" is initiated in the course of an encounter in another site of service (eg, emergency department [ED], physician's office), all E/M services performed by the same physician (or physicians of the same specialty in the same group practice) are considered part of the initial observation care when performed on the same calendar date.

Important guidelines to remember include
- If the patient is admitted for observation and subsequently is formally admitted to the hospital on the same day, only the initial inpatient hospital code (**99221–99223**) is reported.
- Observation services are reported with place of service code **22** (on campus—outpatient hospital).

> Chapter 9 addresses the guidelines for selection of codes **99241–99245** and Chapter 7 for **99202–99215**; see Chapter 4 for more information on place of service codes.

- Code selection is dependent on the performance and documentation of all 3 key components. Time may be used as the key or controlling factor in the selection of the code if more than 50% of the total face-to-face encounter and/or floor/unit time is spent in counseling and/or coordination of care.
- Observation care codes are not reported for initial transitional care of hospital-born neonates. (See code **99463** for initial E/M of a normal newborn admitted and discharged on the same date.)

Use **Table 16-2** to help you in the selection of the appropriate codes in the following clinical examples:

Chapter 16. Noncritical Hospital Evaluation and Management Services

Table 16-2. Observation Care

Key Components (For a description of key components, see Table 16-1.)

Initial Day (99218–99220) or Admission and Discharge on the Same Date (99234–99236): 3 of 3 key components must be performed to at least the degree specified for the codes in each row. A chief complaint is required for each level of history.

CPT Code/Time[a]	Medical Decision-making[b]	History	1995 Examination[c]
99218 30 min 99234 40 min	Straightforward to low complexity PP: Usually low severity	HPI: ≥4 or 3 CC; ROS: 2–9; PFSH: 1/3	2–7 detailed
99219 50 min 99235 50 min	Moderate complexity PP: Usually responding inadequately to therapy or minor complication	HPI: ≥4 or 3 CC; ROS: ≥10; PFSH: 3/3	≥8 body areas/ systems
99220 70 min 99236 55 min	High complexity PP: Usually patient is unstable or develops significant complication or new problem.	HPI: ≥4 or 3 CC; ROS: ≥10; PFSH: 3/3	≥8 body areas/ systems

Subsequent Observation Care: 2 of 3 key components must be performed to at least the degree specified for the codes in each row. A chief complaint is required for each level of service.

99224 15 min	Straightforward to low complexity PP: Usually stable, recovering, or improving	HPI: 1–3; ROS: 0; PFSH: 0	1 body area/system
99225 25 min	Moderate complexity PP: Usually responding inadequately to therapy or minor complication	HPI: 1–3; ROS: 1; PFSH: 0	2–7 limited
99226 35 min	High complexity PP: Usually patient is unstable or develops significant complication or new problem.	HPI: ≥4 or 3 CC; ROS: 2–9; PFSH: 0	2–7 detailed

Abbreviations: CC, chronic condition; *CPT, Current Procedural Terminology;* HPI, history of present illness; PFSH, past, family, and social history; PP, presenting problem; ROS; review of systems.

[a] Typical time is an average and represents a range of times that may be higher or lower depending on clinical circumstances.

[b] The presenting problem is considered to be a contributory factor and does not need to be present to the degree specified.

[c] Number of body areas or organ systems examined; see **Table 16-1** for details.

Examples

➤ **A 5-month-old boy is admitted to observation due to suspected viral bronchiolitis.**

History: Patient presented to the ED with low-grade fever, rapid respiratory rate, cough, and wheezing. History of present illness: duration, several days; quality, coughing and now wheezing today; severity, trouble breathing with retractions; timing, especially while feeding; associated signs and symptoms, runny nose and fever; irritability; and feeding intolerance. Review of systems: all systems reviewed and notable for temperature as high as 38.8°C (101.8°F) today, alternately sleepy and fussy, a productive and deep-sounding cough, clear runny nose, taking longer to feed because of cough and nasal drainage but able to finish some bottles, and no vomiting or diarrhea; urinary, fewer wet diapers but still urinating every 4 to 6 hours. Past history: immunizations are up to date, normal obstetric and perinatal course, early milestones met, no known allergies. Family history: asthma in mother and sister and seasonal allergies in father; no genetic or immunologic disease. Social history: no tobacco exposure; goes to child care 3 days a week; lives with mother and father.

Physical examination: Comprehensive examination of constitutional (temperature, 38.6°C [101.5°F]; pink with mild cyanosis during coughing spasm; respiratory rate, 60 breaths per minute; oxygen saturation, 88%), eyes, ears, mouth, nose, throat, cardiovascular, respiratory, gastrointestinal, genitourinary, musculoskeletal, skin, neurologic, and lymphatic systems performed. Tachypnea with retractions, heart rate at the high end of reference range, and mild dehydration are noted.

Laboratory tests: Respiratory viral panel, basic metabolic panel, complete blood cell count (CBC), and chest radiograph are ordered.

Assessment/plan: Assessment is respiratory distress, probable viral bronchiolitis without pneumonia. The plan is chest radiograph, continuous oxygen saturation monitoring, intravenous (IV) fluids if feeding attempts fail, albuterol every 3 hours, admit to observation status, and continue to suction secretions and supply supplemental oxygen.

International Classification of Diseases, 10th Revision, Clinical Modification (ICD-10-CM)	*CPT*
R06.03 (respiratory distress) **R09.02** (hypoxemia) **E86.0** (dehydration)	**99219** (requires comprehensive history and examination and moderate MDM) *MDM:* Moderate complexity (new problem with additional workup and acute illness with systemic symptoms) *History:* Comprehensive *Physical examination:* Comprehensive

Teaching Point: Remember, all 3 key components must be met for the level of initial observation care reported. The level of history and examination are comprehensive. Medical decision-making is moderate. This supports code **99219**. If MDM were of high complexity, code **99220** would be reported.

➤ **An established patient presents to her physician's office on Monday.** During the evaluation of the patient, the physician decides to admit to observation care for further treatment and monitoring for fever, abdominal pain, abnormal urinalysis, and presumed acute pyelonephritis, with mild dehydration. The physician does not see the patient in the observation setting until the next morning (Tuesday) but phones in orders for IV fluids and antibiotics and coordinates care with the nursing staff on Monday. On Tuesday, the physician performs a face-to-face initial observation care service (detailed history and examination, moderate-complexity MDM) on the patient and determines the patient is not improving enough to be discharged.

ICD-10-CM	*CPT*
N10 (acute pyelonephritis) **E86.0** (dehydration)	Monday's visit **99212–99215** (office E/M, established patient) Tuesday's visit **99218** (initial observation care) or, if admitted as an inpatient on Tuesday, **99221** (initial hospital care)

Teaching Point: Initial observation care and initial inpatient care (**99218–99220**, **99221–99223**) require a face-to-face service with the patient by the reporting physician in the facility. Entry of the history, physical examination, and orders directly into a facility electronic health record (EHR) by online connection without a face-to-face visit in the facility does not support reporting (and, because this information will be date stamped, could be interpreted as fraudulent). Also, an outpatient office building connected physically to the hospital does not count as the patient being seen in the hospital.

➤ **Same patient; however, the physician sees the patient in the office and in the hospital on the same day.** The combined E/M service in the office and hospital results in a comprehensive history and physical examination with moderately complex MDM.

Teaching Point: Only the initial observation care (**99219**) is reported because that code represents all of the physician's E/M services to the patient on the date of admission.

Subsequent Observation Care

99224–99226 Subsequent observation care, per day, for the evaluation and management of a patient

- Codes include all E/M services by a physician, QHP, or physicians in the same group and same specialty provided on a given day.
- Level of service reported will be dependent on the total services provided on that calendar date and documented.
- Codes require that 2 of the 3 key components be performed and documented.

> **Some payers may require medical decision-making as 1 of the 2 key components performed and documented.**

- Time may be used as the key or controlling factor in code selection if more than 50% of the total encounter (ie, floor/unit time) is spent in counseling and/or coordination of care.
- An interval history is required for subsequent observation visits (ie, additional or updated history obtained since the last physician assessment, including history of present illness and problem-pertinent system review). A past, family, and social history is not required.

> **Documentation of an updated history of present illness (eg, "patient's oral intake is improved from yesterday") and assessment and plan based on the patient's present status and plan for discharge or continued hospital care may be important for future utilization review and payer approval of continued observation or inpatient care.**

- Individual documentation for each encounter should contain all information necessary to determine the level of service provided. It is important to document the chief complaint and other factors of the patient presentation that affect management at each encounter.

> **Be careful to avoid the temptation to simply cut and paste your previous day's note even if little has changed overnight.**

The complexity of the presenting problems is often an indicator of the medically necessary level of subsequent observation services required. *CPT* indicates the patient presentation for each level of subsequent observation care. See the MDM row of **Table 16-2** for presenting problems for each code.

Use **Table 16-2** to help you select the appropriate codes in the following clinical example:

Example

➤ **A patient is seen by her attending physician for subsequent observation care following an observation admission the previous evening for head injury.** She was admitted to observation due to recurrent vomiting and confusion and a working diagnosis of concussion syndrome. She is now also experiencing a severe headache with nausea. The attending physician discusses the case with a consultant and orders computed tomography (CT) and additional nonnarcotic pain medications in addition to obtaining an expanded problem-focused history and examination.

ICD-10-CM	CPT
S06.0X1A (concussion with loss of consciousness [LOC] of 30 minutes or less, initial encounter) **G44.309** (posttraumatic headache, unspecified, not intractable) **R11.10** (vomiting)	**99225** *MDM:* Moderate complexity *History:* Expanded problem focused *Physical examination:* Expanded problem focused

Teaching Point: The condition of the patient in this example is worsening. Medical decision-making is moderate based on discussion of the case with another physician and an order for a CT scan in conjunction with the risk of an internal cerebral injury and/or bleed (an acute complicated injury). Additional diagnosis codes for the external cause of injury (**W21.07XA**, struck by softball, initial encounter; **Y93.64**, activity, baseball [includes softball]) may be required by state or facility policy. Seventh character **A** is appropriate for active management of the injury.

Chapter 16. Noncritical Hospital Evaluation and Management Services

Observation Care Discharge Day Management

99217   Observation care discharge day management

Code **99217** is to be used to report all services provided to a patient on discharge from observation status (ie, final examination of the patient, discussion of the hospital stay, counseling, instructions for continuing care, and preparation of discharge records) if the discharge *is on a day other than the initial date of observation status.*

- Performance of the key components is not required.
- Typical time has not been established for code **99217**, so time spent in discharge management is not a factor in the selection of this code.
- A face-to-face encounter is required on the date that code **99217** is reported. Even if some of the discharge work was performed on the day prior to discharge, code **99217** would be reported on the discharge date if a face-to-face encounter occurred on that date.

Example

➤ **A 13-year-old girl is seen by her hospitalist for subsequent observation care (third day of admission) for a concussion with LOC of less than 5 minutes after being hit by a softball.** She experienced no vomiting overnight, headache has resolved, and she successfully passed a concussion protocol. The CT scan result was negative, and neurology found no evidence of complications from her injury. The patient ate a light breakfast without nausea or vomiting. She is discharged with home care instructions and precautions. Code **99217** (observation care discharge day management) is reported and linked to diagnosis code **S06.0X1A**. Additional codes (**W21.07XA**, struck by softball, initial encounter; **Y93.64**, activity, baseball [includes softball]) may be reported to indicate the cause of the condition.

Same Date Admission and Discharge Services

When a patient is admitted and discharged from observation or inpatient services on the *same date of service,* report codes **99234–99236**.

- Code selection is based on the performance and documentation of all 3 key components.
  - Include the combined services provided by the same physician or physicians of the same specialty within a group during a calendar day.
  - At times, an attending physician may see the patient only once (eg, when admitted by phone and not seen face-to-face until the discharge on the next date). However, the documentation should support that initial observation care and discharge day management services were both provided (eg, describe physician's involvement over course of the stay).
- Time may be used as the key or controlling factor in the selection of the code if more than 50% of the total face-to-face encounter (eg, floor/unit time) is spent in counseling and/or coordination of care.
- Except where payer guidance specifies otherwise, reporting of initial observation or inpatient care is based on the date of the face-to-face assessment and not the date of admission or designation of a status by a facility (eg, when changed on physician order).

When Payers Use Medicare Observation Policy

Medicaid and private payers may adopt a Medicare policy that limits reporting of codes **99234–99236** to services provided to a patient who was admitted to observation or inpatient status for *at least 8 hours and not more than 24 hours.* Under this policy, when a patient is admitted to observation or inpatient care for fewer than 8 hours on the same calendar date, only the initial observation (**99218–99220**) or inpatient care (**99221–99223**) shall be reported by the physician. A separate code for discharge services is not reported.

Medicare also requires that there must be a medical observation record for the patient that contains dated and timed physician's orders for the observation services the patient is to receive, nursing notes, and progress notes prepared by the physician indicating physical presence and personal performance of services. This record must be in addition to (and not a copy and paste of) any record prepared as a result of an ED or outpatient clinic encounter.

Use **Table 16-2** to review the required components used to select level of service in the following examples:

Examples

➤ **6:00 am: An 8-year-old girl is admitted to observation for generalized abdominal pain.** Encounter includes comprehensive history and examination and MDM of moderate complexity. The physician orders monitoring of regular vital signs and small amounts of clear fluids pending test results. Nursing staff monitors the patient periodically. The physician adds an order for a stool softener and suppository, which produce stooling, and symptoms are slowly resolved. Decision for discharge to home is made at 11:00 am. Diagnosis is abdominal pain due to fecal impaction.

ICD-10-CM	CPT
K56.41 (fecal impaction)	99235
	MDM: Moderate complexity
	History: Comprehensive
	Physical examination: Comprehensive

Teaching Point: Face-to-face services performed include initial care and discharge management. A code from the **99234–99236** series would be reported because observation admission and discharge services were provided on the same date. Alternatively, if the payer requires an observation stay of 8 hours to report **99234–99236**, code **99222** (initial observation care) would be reported for this 5-hour stay.

➤ **An established 14-year-old patient is seen in the physician's office with acute exacerbation of asthma that was not responsive to treatment. The patient was admitted for observation at 6:00 pm on Tuesday.** The attending physician telephones the observation admission orders and does not see the child again until the next morning (Wednesday). On Wednesday, the physician completes a history and physical examination and, later that afternoon, discharges the child.

ICD-10-CM	CPT
J45.41 (moderate persistent asthma with exacerbation)	Tuesday's visit
	99212–99215 (office E/M, established patient)
(same for both dates of service)	Wednesday's visit
	99234–99236 (observation care, same-day admission and discharge)

Teaching Point: Because the physician first saw the patient in observation on Wednesday, the office visit on Tuesday and the admission and discharge on Wednesday are separately reported. The call to admit the patient is counted as part of the office E/M code reported.

➤ **A 14-year-old patient with an acute exacerbation of asthma is admitted from the ED at 6:00 am on Monday.** An attending physician, from a different group than the ED physician who reports an ED service (**99281–99285**), orders the observation stay and performs the initial history and physical examination. Another physician from the attending physician's same specialty and group practice returns to the hospital at 5:00 pm and, after evaluation of the child, discharges the patient home. The combined service is a comprehensive history and physical examination with moderate-level MDM.

ICD-10-CM	CPT
J45.41 (moderate persistent asthma with exacerbation)	**99235** (observation care, same-day admission and discharge)
	MDM: Moderate complexity
	History: Comprehensive
	Physical examination: Comprehensive

Teaching Point: Because the 2 physicians who provided care in the observation setting are of the same specialty and same group practice, the code representing the combined work of the 2 visits is reported. If more than 50% of the total unit/floor time of the 2 physicians who provided observation care were spent in counseling and/or coordination of care, the level of service would be selected based on time (eg, 50 minutes for **99235**).

➤ **A 14-year-old patient with an acute exacerbation of asthma presents to the ED.** The patient has presented to the ED twice in the last year and has not scheduled follow-up appointments with the primary care physician between ED visits. The patient's mother notes transportation difficulties, and it is noted that the adolescent's emergency-use inhaler is beyond its expiration date. An allergy and asthma specialist is consulted in the ED and admits the patient to observation. The patient improves over the course of the day, and a new asthma action plan is agreed to by the patient's mother, who is also assisted with scheduling follow-up care and community transportation services. Assessment is poorly controlled moderate persistent asthma with exacerbation. The adolescent is discharged to home that afternoon after 9 hours in observation status. The specialist's total face-to-face time with the patient was 60 minutes, with more than 50% spent in counseling and/or coordination of care.

ICD-10-CM	CPT
J45.41 (moderate persistent asthma with exacerbation)	**99236** (observation care, same-day admission and discharge, typical time 55 minutes)

Teaching Point: The specialist reports only the observation admission and discharge because the consultation in the ED is included in the work of the observation services. The total face-to-face time of 60 minutes supports code **99236**.

Inpatient Hospital Care

Initial Inpatient Hospital Care

99221–99223 Initial hospital care, per day, for the evaluation and management of a patient
- Initial inpatient hospital service codes are used to report initial face-to-face services provided to a hospital inpatient.
- Initial inpatient encounters by more than 1 physician must be reported based on payer guidelines. (See the Hospital Services by Other Physicians section later in this chapter.)
- Selection of the code is based on performance and documentation of the 3 required key components or on time if more than 50% of the encounter is spent in counseling and/or coordination of care (**Table 16-3**).
- The lowest level of initial hospital care (**99221**) requires at least a detailed history and detailed physical examination. If the level of history and/or physical examination performed and documented is expanded or problem focused, initial inpatient hospital care must be reported using subsequent hospital visit codes (**99231–99233**) because the required key components for code **99221** have not been met.
- The code is reported on the first day that a face-to-face (physician–patient) service is provided.
- The date of initial hospital care that the physician reports does not need to correlate with the facility's date of admission.
- Report only an initial hospital care code when a patient is admitted to inpatient status from observation status.

Use **Table 16-3** to review the required components used to select level of service in the following examples:

Examples

➤ **An 8-week-old is seen in the ED and admitted by Physician A.** Over the past 2 days, the mother reported that the infant seemed warm to the touch, seemed irritable, fed much less than normal, and was harder to arouse. The mother had noticed only 2 wet diapers and 1 stool in the past 24 hours.

Review of systems: Fever; no history of heart murmur; no vomiting or diarrhea; no apnea or cyanosis; no wheeze or respiratory distress.

Past, family, and social history: Full-term male; no reported problems with pregnancy or delivery; delivered by repeat cesarean. No maternal complications with delivery; rupture of membranes at the time of cesarean delivery, no fever prior to cesarean delivery. Discharged on day 4 with mother breastfeeding well. No prior ED visits or hospitalizations since birth hospitalization, no febrile or sick contacts at home, and lives with parents and 2 older female siblings. Two-month well-child vaccinations were received last week.

Physical examination: Comprehensive examination includes vital signs with temperature 38.0°C (100.4°F), mildly irritable, decreased tearing, and somewhat sleepy, with examination of head, mucous membranes, clavicles, heart, lungs, abdomen, hips, genitalia, skin, and general neurologic assessment demonstrating no significant findings.

Table 16-3. Inpatient Hospital Care

Initial Day (**99221–99223**) or Admission and Discharge on the Same Date (**99234–99236**): 3 of 3 key components (see **Table 16-1**) must be performed to at least the degree specified for the codes in each row. A chief complaint is required for each level of history.

CPT Code/Time[a]	Medical Decision-making[b]	History	1995 Examination[c]
99221 30 min **99234** (A&D) 40 min	Straightforward to low complexity PP: Usually low severity	HPI: ≥4 or 3 CC; ROS: 2–9; PFSH: 1/3	2–7 detailed
99222 50 min **99235** (A&D) 50 min	Moderate complexity PP: Usually responding inadequately to therapy or minor complication	HPI: ≥4 or 3 CC; ROS: ≥10; PFSH: 3/3	≥8 body areas/systems
99223 70 min **99236** (A&D) 55 min	High complexity PP: Usually patient is unstable or develops significant complication or new problem.	HPI: ≥4 or 3 CC; ROS: ≥10; PFSH: 3/3	≥8 body areas/systems

Subsequent hospital care: 2 of 3 key components (see **Table 16-1**) must be performed to at least the degree specified for the codes in each row.

99231 15 min	Straightforward to low complexity PP: Usually stable, recovering, or improving	HPI: 1–3; ROS: 0; PFSH[d]: 0	1 body area/system
99232 25 min	Moderate complexity PP: Usually responding inadequately to therapy or minor complication	HPI: 1–3; ROS: 1; PFSH[d]: 0	2–7 limited
99233 35 min	High complexity PP: Usually patient is unstable or develops significant complication or new problem.	HPI: ≥4 or 3 CC; ROS: 2–9; PFSH[d]: 0	2–7 detailed

Abbreviations: A&D, admission and discharge on same day; CC, chronic conditions; *CPT, Current Procedural Terminology*; HPI, history of present illness; PFSH, past, family, and social history; PP, presenting problem; ROS, review of systems.

[a] Typical time is an average and represents a range of times that may be higher or lower depending on clinical circumstances.
[b] The presenting problem is considered to be a contributory factor and does not need to be present to the degree specified.
[c] Number of body areas or organ systems examined; see **Table 16-1** for details.
[d] Past, family, and social history is not required for interval history.

Assessment: 8-week-old with fever, mild dehydration, and lethargy. Laboratory evaluation: CBC with white blood cells 12,000, no left shift on differential; urinalysis normal or negative with pH 7.0, specific gravity 1.020; fever. Due to patient's age and continued symptoms, concern for sepsis or undetected bacterial infection; doubt pyelonephritis given normal urinalysis; less likely meningitis given mild clinical findings; doubt bronchiolitis given lack of viral symptoms. Urine and blood culture results pending.

Plan: Admit for IV antibiotics and IV fluids, pending culture results. Continue breastfeeding ad lib. Discussed current diagnostic and treatment plans with parents and advised that the physician's partner, Physician B, will visit later today to discuss further.

Unit/floor time is 35 minutes with 15 minutes spent in counseling and/or coordination of care. Moderate-complexity MDM, detailed history, and comprehensive examination support the reporting of code **99221**.

➤ **Later that same calendar day, Physician B from the same group practice sees the infant.** She adds to the history (particularly under review of systems), examines the infant, and spends 25 minutes of a 40-minute visit talking with the parents.

ICD-10-CM	CPT
R50.9 (fever, unspecified) **E86.0** (dehydration) **R53.83** (lethargy)	**99223** *Combined unit/floor time:* 75 minutes with 40 minutes spent in counseling and/or coordination of care *MDM:* Moderate complexity *History:* Comprehensive *Physical examination:* Comprehensive

Teaching Point: The total E/M services provided on this date now include key components supporting code **99222**. However, Physician A and Physician B provided hospital care on the admission date with a combined time of 75 minutes with documentation that more than 50% of the unit/floor time was spent in counseling and/or coordination of care. This supports code **99223**. Physician A submits no bill, and Physician B submits the bill for the calendar day's service.

See Chapter 1 for more information on code selection based on time.

Subsequent Hospital Care

99231–99233 Subsequent hospital care, per day, for the evaluation and management of a patient
- Codes include all E/M services by a physician or QHP of the same specialty and same group practice provided on a subsequent day. The level of service reported will be dependent on the total services provided and documented.
- Selection of the code is based on performance and documentation of *2 of 3 key components* or time if more than 50% of the encounter is spent in counseling and/or coordination of care (see **Table 16-3**).
- An interval history is required for subsequent hospital visits (ie, additional or updated information obtained since the last physician assessment, including chief complaint, history of present illness, and problem-pertinent system review [documentation of review of systems can state "reviewed and unchanged from yesterday"]).

Past, family, and social history is not required as part of an interval history.

See additional discussion of subsequent hospital care in the February 2021 *AAP Pediatric Coding Newsletter* article, "Subsequent Hospital Care: Patient Status Can Guide Code Selection" (https://coding.solutions.aap.org/article.aspx?articleid=2765279; subscription required).

Use **Table 16-3** to help you in the selection of the appropriate codes in the following examples:

Example

➤ **Same patient as previous example (ie, 8-week-old with fever, dehydration, and lethargy).** No new reported problems overnight; breastfeeding has improved; however, patient continues to have low-grade fever (38.2°C [100.8°F] maximum temperature) overnight; no reported apnea or cyanosis; no respiratory distress. Drinking better, more wet diapers, more alert.

Physical examination: Expanded problem-focused examination, including vital signs and general appearance, heart, lungs, genitourinary, neurologic, and skin.

Laboratory: No growth in blood or urine cultures at less than 24 hours.

Assessment/plan: Continued fever. Continued concern for sepsis; suspect viral etiology given negative workup so far for common serious bacterial infections, such as pyelonephritis, pneumonia, meningitis, and bacteremia. Continue IV antibiotics until culture results are negative for 48 hours; continue breastfeeding ad lib. Spoke with mother and reviewed overnight events, morning laboratory results, current plan, and possible discharge home tomorrow.

ICD-10-CM	CPT
R50.9 (fever)	**99232** *MDM:* Straightforward *History:* Expanded interval history *Physical examination:* Limited (2–7 systems or body areas)

Teaching Point: In this example, the MDM is straightforward based on 2 of 3 MDM elements being limited: a limited number and complexity of problems and management options (stable established problem); limited amount and complexity of data reviewed (laboratory results); and moderate risk of an undiagnosed problem requiring IV antibiotics. A payer may require MDM as 1 of 2 key components supporting subsequent hospital care. This example would be limited to code **99231** if MDM were a required component.

Time cannot be used as the controlling factor in selection of the code because the documentation does not indicate the total floor/unit time or time spent in counseling and/or coordination of care.

➤ **Same progress note as in previous vignette but with the following additional documentation: Spoke with mother, who is still quite concerned, for 30 minutes and reviewed overnight events, morning laboratory results, and current plan; anticipate discharge home tomorrow.** Total visit time: 40 minutes.

Time would be used as the controlling factor in selection of the code because a total of 40 minutes was spent on the unit/floor with the patient and more than 50% of the time was spent in counseling. The appropriate code would be **99233**.

Hospital Discharge Day Management

99238   Hospital discharge day management; 30 minutes or less
99239   more than 30 minutes

Codes **99238** (≤30 minutes) and **99239** (>30 minutes) are reported by the attending physician providing discharge services on a day subsequent to the date of the admission service. Discharge codes are not reported when a patient is transferred to another physician or another unit in the same facility.

> If the total time spent in performing discharge management is not documented in the medical record, code **99239** cannot be supported.

- Subsequent hospital care is reported in lieu of discharge day management (and initial hospital care) when a patient is transferred to another hospital and receives care from the same physician or a physician of the same group and specialty.
- When a patient is transferred to another facility and into the services of a physician who is not in the same group practice and same specialty as the transferring physician, each physician reports the appropriate E/M code for the service provided.
- A face-to-face physician-patient encounter in the hospital is required, although time is unit/floor time.
- Reporting is based on the total time (does not have to be continuous) spent performing all final discharge services, including, as appropriate, examination of the patient, discussion of the hospital stay, patient and/or family counseling, instructions for continuing care to all relevant caregivers, and preparation of referral forms, prescriptions, and medical records.

> Only unit or floor time spent on the date of the discharge management is reported with codes **99238** and **99239**. Do not include time spent documenting discharge on a date after the service was rendered.

- May be used to report discharge services provided to patients who die during their hospital stay. An exception is a neonate who dies on the date of birth; report only the appropriate level of hospital care (ie, initial hospital care, intensive care, or critical care) in this instance.
- Services are reported on the day the physician sees the patient and performs discharge services, even if the patient leaves the hospital on a different day.
- Only the attending physician or physician providing services on behalf of the attending physician (eg, covering physician, physician of same group and same specialty) may report discharge management services. If another physician is providing concurrent care, that physician's services would be reported using subsequent hospital visit codes (**99231–99233**).
- Time spent in discharge services must be documented in the medical record to report code **99239**. If the total time spent performing the discharge management is not documented in the medical record, report code **99238** instead of **99239**. Only time spent on the day of discharge may be counted.
- Time spent on the day of discharge performing separately reported services (eg, interpretation and report of electroencephalography results) is not included in the discharge day management time.

●=New code   ▲=Revised code   #=Re-sequenced code   +=Add-on code   ★=Telemedicine

Examples

➤ **A physician provides an updated history and examination and a decision is made to discharge a patient.** Examination is performed as relevant to determine if discharge is appropriate. New test results and/or reports from other clinicians since the last visit are reviewed. Therapeutic treatments are discontinued. Patient is discharged home with detailed instructions for home care and follow-up provided to both parents. The physician spends 35 minutes on the floor reviewing the hospital course, expected follow-up, and signs and symptoms of possible complications with the mother.

This visit would be reported with code **99239** because 35 minutes were spent in the provision of discharge management services and the time was documented in the medical record.

➤ **An attending physician is notified by phone of the death of a patient who was an inpatient.** The physician comes into the facility the next morning and completes documentation. Discharge day management services (**99238**, **99239**) are not reported when no face-to-face encounter (eg, pronouncement of death or hospital discussion with family) is provided by the attending physician.

Discharge Versus Subsequent Hospital Services

Codes **99238** and **99239** are underused and often reported incorrectly. Subsequent hospital visit codes should not be reported on the day of discharge alone or in addition to the discharge code. Code **99239** is one of the most underreported *CPT* codes, even though it often more accurately reflects the service performed than codes for subsequent hospital care. Physicians often spend longer than 30 minutes in discharge management, especially when the patient is seen several times that day. Time spent in charting *on the day of discharge* is counted in the total unit/floor time. *Note:* The 2022 relative value units (RVUs) were not available at time of publication.

CPT Code	2021 Medicare RVUs and Payment at $40 per RVU	
99231	1.10	$44.00
99232	2.06	$82.40
99233	2.96	$118.40
99238	2.07	$82.80
99239	3.05	$122.00

Teaching Point: The RVUs for discharge service codes reflect the additional services provided on the day of discharge. Each final day of hospital care reported with code **99231** instead of code **99238** would result in loss of approximately $38.80 (at $40 per RVU). If time is not documented when more than 30 minutes is spent in discharge day management, reporting code **99238** instead of **99239** could result in loss of approximately $39.20 (at $40 per RVU).

Hospital Services by Other Physicians

Observation or hospital care is often provided by a physician or QHP who is not the admitting physician and not of the same group practice and same exact specialty as the admitting physician. These services may be consultations (ie, requests for advice/opinions) and/or concurrent care of problems (ie, following patients for a specific component of their illness) other than those managed by the admitting physician. For example, a patient with cerebral palsy admitted with pneumonia also has a seizure disorder and requires medication adjustment by a neurologist.

If a consulting physician accepts a transfer of care after the initial consultation and assumes the role of attending physician, continuing care is reported as subsequent observation or hospital care until the day of discharge, when discharge day management is reported. If the consultant continues to provide care in addition to an attending physician's care, daily subsequent observation or hospital care is reported for each date including any service provided on the date of discharge.

Concurrent Care

Concurrent care is defined by *CPT* as the provision of similar services to the same patient by more than 1 physician on the same day. Concurrent care may be provided by physicians from different practices or physicians from the same practice but different specialties. When concurrent care is provided, the diagnosis code(s) reported by each physician should reflect the medical necessity for the provision of services by more than 1 physician on the same *date* of service. Although it is easier to justify concurrent care when each treating physician reports different diagnoses, if the *diagnosis* code is reported for the same condition, it does not prevent billing for the services.

Example

➤ **The attending physician wants the consultant to provide ongoing management of 1 problem (eg, heart failure) while the attending physician provides ongoing management for other active problems (eg, pneumonia, inadequate weight gain).**

Both physicians would report subsequent hospital care codes and link the *CPT* codes to the appropriate *diagnosis* codes.

See **Figure 1-1** for an example of linking diagnoses to procedure codes on a claim.

Consultations

CPT defines *consultations* as services provided by a physician at the request of another physician or "other appropriate source" to provide advice or opinion about the management or evaluation of a specific problem. Medicare does not recognize consultation codes but pays for the services using codes for other E/M services (discussed later in this chapter). Detailed information on the *CPT* and Centers for Medicare & Medicaid Services Medicare guidelines for reporting consultations for office and outpatient consultations appears in **Chapter 7**. Please review those guidelines carefully as general guidelines that apply for all consultations.

Consultation codes should not be reported by the physician who has agreed to accept transfer of care before an initial evaluation. Consultation codes are appropriate to report if the decision to accept transfer of care is not made until after the consultant's initial evaluation, regardless of site of service.

Medicare Consultation Guidelines

Payers that adopt Medicare guidelines require that consultations provided to patients in observation status will be reported with office or outpatient E/M codes **99202–99215**. If the patient is new to the physician (ie, has not received any face-to-face professional services from the physician or another physician of the same specialty who belongs to the same group practice *within the past 3 years*), codes **99202–99205** are reported based on the performance and documentation of the required key components. If the patient does not meet the requirements of a new patient, an established patient office or outpatient E/M code **99202–99215** is reported.

Prolonged service in addition to office or outpatient E/M codes **99202–99215** is also subject to payer policy. *CPT* instructs to report code **99417** when the physician's total time on the date of the encounter exceeds the *minimum* time in the code descriptor for **99205** (includes 60–74 minutes) or **99215** (includes 40–54 minutes) by 15 minutes. However, Medicare policy instructs that prolonged service time begins when the *maximum* time in the code descriptor has been exceeded by 15 minutes and requires reporting of **G2212** instead of **99417**. **Table 16-4** includes the required times per *CPT* and Medicare guidelines.

Table 16-4. Prolonged Office Evaluation and Management Service Time Requirements		
E/M Service Code	**CPT Guidelines**	**Medicare Guidelines**
New patient **99205**	**99417** 75 minutes or more	**G2212** 89 minutes or more
Established patient **99215**	**99417** 55 minutes or more	**G2212** 69 minutes or more
Abbreviations: *CPT, Current Procedural Terminology*; E/M, evaluation and management.		

Learn more about reporting prolonged office or other outpatient evaluation and management services in Chapter 7.

Consultations provided to inpatient hospital patients are reported using initial inpatient hospital care codes (**99221–99223**). The admitting physician must report the initial hospital care services with modifier **AI** (principal physician of record) appended to the appropriate code to distinguish the services from the consulting physician. Subsequent face-to-face services, including new consultations within the same admission, are reported with subsequent hospital care codes **99231–99233** (**Table 16-5**).

Table 16-5. Consultation Codes Using *Current Procedural Terminology* and Medicare Guidelines

Codes Used by Payers That Follow *CPT* Consultation Guidelines		Codes Used by Payers That Follow Medicare Consultation Guidelines	
Observation[a]	**Inpatient**	**Observation**	**Inpatient**
99241–99245, 99224–99226	99251–99255, 99231–99233	99202–99205, 99212–99215	99221–99223, 99231–99233

Abbreviation: CPT, Current Procedural Terminology.

[a] A second consultation, with new request from the attending, during the same observation stay may be reported with codes 99241–99245.

Check with your commercial payers to learn if they follow Medicare consultation guidelines or have otherwise adopted consultation guidelines that differ from *CPT*.

Consultations for Patients in Observation

99241–99245 Office or other outpatient consultation for a new or established patient (See key components and time in **Table 16-6.**)

Table 16-6. Observation Consultation Codes

Key Components (For a description of key components, see Table 16-1.)
3 of 3 key components must be performed to at least the degree specified under the code.

CPT Code/Time[a]	Medical Decision-making	History[b]	1995 Examination[c]
99241 15 min	Straightforward	HPI: 1–3; ROS: 0; PFSH: 0	1 body area/system
99242 30 min	Straightforward	HPI: 1–3; ROS: 1; PFSH: 0	2–7 limited
99243 40 min	Low complexity	HPI: ≥4 or 3 CC; ROS: 2–9; PFSH: 1/3	2–7 detailed
99244 60 min	Moderate complexity	HPI: ≥4 or 3 CC; ROS: ≥10; PFSH: 3/3	≥8 body areas/systems
99245 80 min	High complexity	HPI: ≥4 or 3 CC; ROS: ≥10; PFSH: 3/3	≥8 body areas/systems

Abbreviations: CC, chronic conditions; CPT, Current Procedural Terminology; HPI, history of present illness; PFSH, past, family, and social history; ROS; review of systems.

[a] Typical time is an average and represents a range of times that may be higher or lower depending on clinical circumstances.

[b] A chief complaint is required for all levels of history.

[c] Number of body areas or organ systems examined; see **Table 16-1** for details.

- Level of care is determined by performing and documenting the required 3 key components (ie, history, physical examination, and MDM) or time as described for other E/M services that are assigned a typical time. Follow-up visits that are initiated by the physician consultant are reported using codes for subsequent observation care services (**99224–99226**).
- If an additional request for an opinion or advice on the same or a new problem is received from the attending physician and documented in the medical record, office or outpatient consultation codes, unlike inpatient consultation codes, may be used again.
- In the observation care setting, report prolonged service in the outpatient setting with a direct patient contact code (**99354, 99355**) in addition to the appropriate outpatient consultation code (**99241–99245**) when the typical time of the consultation is exceeded by 30 minutes or more.

Use **Table 16-6** to help you in the selection of the appropriate codes in the following example:

Example

➤ **Dr A requests that Dr B, a pediatric surgeon, evaluate a patient with complaint of generalized abdominal pain and recommend options for diagnosis and management.** Dr B reviews Dr A's documentation of initial observation care and also 3 unique test results before obtaining a comprehensive history from the patient and mother and performing a comprehensive examination. Dr B recommends additional testing in a report to Dr A. Dr B reports an outpatient consultation.

ICD-10-CM	*CPT*
R10.84 (generalized abdominal pain)	**99244** *MDM:* Moderate *History:* Comprehensive *Physical examination:* Comprehensive Or, if payer does not recognize consultations, office or other outpatient E/M service with moderate-complexity MDM **99204** (new patient) **99214** (established patient)

Teaching Point: If the payer does not allow payment for consultation codes, the appropriate office or other outpatient E/M code is reported. Level 4 (**99204, 99214**) codes are supported based on the moderate complexity of MDM (supported by evaluation of an undiagnosed new problem with uncertain prognosis and a moderate amount and complexity of data to review and analyze). See **Chapter 7** for more information on office and other outpatient E/M code selection.

Inpatient Consultations

99251–99255 Inpatient consultation for a new or established patient

- Codes **99251–99255** are to be used only once by the reporting physician for an individual hospital patient for a particular admission. There are no specific guidelines for the length of stay.
- Follow-up visits provided in the hospital by the same physician must be reported using subsequent care codes (**99231–99233**). Examples of a follow-up visit might be to complete the initial consultation when test results become available or in response to a change in the patient's status.

Table 16-7. Inpatient (99251–99255) Consultation Codes

Key Components (For a description of key components, see Table 16-1.)

3 of 3 key components must be performed to at least the degree specified under the code. A chief complaint is required for all levels of history.

CPT Code/Time[a]	Medical Decision-making[b]	History	1995 Examination[c]
99251 20 min	Straightforward	HPI: 1–3; ROS: 0; PFSH: 0	1 body area/system
99252 40 min	Straightforward	HPI: 1–3; ROS: 1; PFSH: 0	2–7 limited
99253 55 min	Low complexity	HPI: ≥4 or 3 CC; ROS: 2–9; PFSH: 1/3	2–7 detailed
99254 80 min	Moderate complexity	HPI: ≥4 or 3 CC; ROS: ≥10; PFSH: 3/3	≥8 body areas/systems
99255 110 min	High complexity	HPI: ≥4 or 3 CC; ROS: ≥10; PFSH: 3/3	≥8 body areas/systems

Abbreviations: CC, chronic conditions; *CPT, Current Procedural Terminology;* HPI, history of present illness; PFSH, past, family, and social history; ROS, review of systems.

[a] Typical time is an average and represents a range of times that may be higher or lower depending on clinical circumstances.

[b] The presenting problem is considered to be a contributory factor and does not need to be present to the degree specified.

[c] Number of body areas or organ systems examined; see **Table 16-1** for details.

- If a second consultation by a physician or physicians of the same specialty and same group practice is requested by the attending physician to address a completely different problem during the same hospital stay, subsequent hospital care codes (99231–99233) must be reported. The subsequent role of a consultant in the ongoing care of the patient must be clearly stated in the medical record by the attending physician. If the attending physician turns over the care of the patient to the consultant, the consultant, now the new attending physician, should use subsequent hospital care codes (99231–99233) to indicate the level of service provided until the day of discharge management (99238, 99239).
- The attending physician and consultant may continue to provide care to the patient. Each would code for subsequent hospital care as long as the problems they manage are different. (The attending and consulting physicians should use different *diagnosis* codes to indicate they are managing different problems.) When 2 physicians provide care for the same diagnosis on 1 date, the medical necessity for each service must be clearly documented.
- If a patient is readmitted for the same or a different problem (ie, a new hospital stay), an initial inpatient consultation code may be reported if it meets the definition and requirements for reporting a consultation.
- When an inpatient consultation is performed on a date a patient is admitted to the hospital, all E/M services provided by the consultant (including any outpatient encounters) related to the admission are reported with the inpatient consultation service code. If a patient is admitted after an outpatient consultation (eg, office, ED) and the patient is not seen on the unit on the date of admission, only the outpatient consultation code is reported.
- Procedures performed by the consultant will be separately reported, although the time spent performing the procedure is not added to the time of the E/M service.

Use **Table 16-7** to help you in the selection of the appropriate codes in the following example:

Example

➤ **A 13-year-old patient is seen by Dr A in the ED and is subsequently admitted to observation status for vomiting and general abdominal pain.** Dr A consults Dr B, a pediatric surgeon, and, following further workup, Dr B diagnoses acute appendicitis without rupture and recommends to Dr A that the patient transfer to inpatient status with plan for surgery the next morning. Dr A asks Dr B to assume management and order the admission. Dr B documents his written report in the medical record, speaks to the parents, and arranges for the surgery. Dr B reports initial hospital care with the code selected based on the cumulative work of the consultation and initial hospital care. Dr A reports initial observation care for the cumulative work of the services provided while the patient was an ED patient and in observation status.

ICD-10-CM	CPT
K35.80 (unspecified acute appendicitis)	**99223 57** (initial hospital visit) *MDM:* High complexity *History:* Comprehensive *Physical examination:* Comprehensive

Teaching Point: Dr B's combined services on this day are reported as initial inpatient hospital care (99223) rather than consultation to a patient in observation (99241–99245). Modifier 57 indicates a decision for surgery was made at the encounter and may prevent bundling of the initial hospital care with the preservice work of the procedure.

Test your inpatient consultation coding skills further with the March 2020 *AAP Pediatric Coding Newsletter* challenge, "You Code It! Two Consultations in One Admission" (https://coding.solutions.aap.org/article.aspx?articleid=2761970; subscription required).

Interprofessional Telephone/Internet/Electronic Health Record Consultation

A consultation request by a patient's attending or primary physician or other QHP soliciting opinion and/or treatment advice by telephone, internet, or EHR from a physician with specialty expertise (consultant) is reported by the consultant with interprofessional consultation codes 99446–99451. Codes are selected based on the minutes of medical consultative discussion and review. Code 99452 may be reported by a requesting physician who spends 16 to 30 minutes on the date of service preparing for the referral and/or communicating with the consultant.

- When reporting codes 99446–99449 (consultation with verbal and written report), the consultant must spend at least 5 minutes, with more than 50% of the time reported as interprofessional consultation spent in medical consultative verbal or internet discussion rather than review of data (eg, medical records, test results).

- The service time for code 99451 (consultation with written report only) is based on total review and interprofessional communication time. No face-to-face contact between the patient and consultant is required. The patient may be in the inpatient or outpatient setting.

For information on reporting interprofessional consultation or other digital medicine services, see Chapter 20.

Prolonged Evaluation and Management Services Provided in the Inpatient Setting

Prolonged service codes are reported when a physician provides services that *are 30 minutes or more beyond the usual service duration* described in an E/M code or other codes with a published maximum time. The code categories for prolonged service are subdivided into service with direct (ie, face-to-face) patient contact and service without direct patient contact.

Direct Prolonged Service

+99356   Prolonged service in the inpatient or observation setting, requiring unit/floor time beyond the usual service; first hour (30–74 min)

+99357   each additional 30 minutes (List separately in addition to the code for prolonged physician service.) (Report code 99357 in conjunction with code 99356.)

According to *CPT,* the prolonged services inpatient add-on codes 99356 and 99357 may be reported in addition to observation codes (99218–99220, 99224–99226, 99234–99236) because, although observation care services are performed in an outpatient setting, the intraservice times for the codes are defined as unit or floor time.

- Direct inpatient/observation setting prolonged services (99356 and 99357) may only be reported in conjunction with the following codes:
  — 99218–99220 (initial observation care)
  — 99221–99223 (initial hospital care)
  — 99234–99236 (admission/discharge same day)
  — 99224–99226 (subsequent observation care)
  — 99231–99233 (subsequent hospital care)
  — 99251–99255 (inpatient consultations)
  — 99304–99310 (nursing facility services)
  — And when provided in an observation or inpatient setting,
    - 90837 (psychotherapy without E/M, 60 minutes)
    - 90847 (family psychotherapy [conjoint psychotherapy] [with patient present], 50 minutes)
- If a code does not have a typical time listed (eg, hospital discharge [99238, 99239]), direct prolonged services may not be reported in conjunction with it.
- Time in the inpatient facility is defined as unit/floor time dedicated to the patient. (*Note:* It is Medicare's policy that time spent reviewing charts or discussion of a patient with house medical staff and not with direct face-to-face contact with the patient cannot be billed as prolonged service. It is important to be aware of Medicaid and private payers that adopt Medicare policy [ie, allow only face-to-face time].)
- When an E/M service is reported using time as the key or controlling factor, prolonged services can be reported only when the prolonged service exceeds 30 minutes beyond the highest level of E/M service (eg, 99220, 99223).
- The medical record must reflect the total time of the service and medical need for the service. **Table 16-8** shows the time requirements for codes 99356 and 99357.

Table 16-8. Coding Direct Prolonged Services for Inpatient and Observation Care	
Total Duration of Prolonged Services, min	**Code(s)**
<30	Not reported separately
30–74	99356 × 1
75–104	99356 × 1 and 99357 × 1
≥105 (≥1 h 45 min)	99356 × 1 and 99357 × 2 (or more for each additional 30 min)

Example

➤ **Dr A admits a 3-year-old patient for workup of daily fever for several weeks and new complaint of neck stiffness during periods of fever.** Dr A obtains a comprehensive history from the child's parents about the child's recurring fever. Dr A reviews laboratory and radiology results from tests ordered in the ED. Dr A writes an order for infectious disease consultation. Later that same day, after the infectious disease consultant visits the patient, Dr A spends 15 minutes in discussion with the consultant, followed by 45 minutes spent counseling the patient's parents about test results and the need for an additional consultation with a rheumatologist. Dr A documents the total unit/floor time of 120 minutes, with more than 50% spent in counseling and/or coordination of care, in the medical record.

Dr A reports her services with codes **99223** and **99356**.

Teaching Point: Dr A reports initial inpatient hospital code **99223** based on unit/floor time. The typical time assigned to code **99223** is 70 minutes. This leaves an additional 50 minutes of unit/floor time that Dr A may report with prolonged services code **99356**.

Prolonged Service Before or After Direct Patient Care

99358   Prolonged evaluation and management service before and/or after direct patient care; first hour
99359   each additional 30 minutes (Use code **99359** in conjunction with code **99358**.)

● Non-direct (non–face-to-face) prolonged physician services (**99358** and **99359**) may be reported on a different date than the related primary service. The related primary service may be an E/M service (with or without an assigned typical time), a procedure, or other service.
● Non-direct prolonged E/M services must relate to a face-to-face service that has occurred or will occur and must be relevant to ongoing care.

Example

➤ **Dr A spends 40 minutes reviewing extensive medical records that are received the day after a patient is admitted.**

Code **99358** would be reported. Prolonged service of less than 30 minutes' total duration would not be separately reported.

> Refer to Chapter 7 for details of the specific requirements for reporting physician prolonged services in conjunction with office or outpatient evaluation and management services (**99202–99205**, **99212–99215**).

Medical Team Conferences

99366   Medical team conference with interdisciplinary team of health care professionals, face-to-face with patient and/or family, 30 minutes or more, participation by nonphysician qualified health care professional
99367   Medical team conference with interdisciplinary team of health care professionals, patient and/or family not present, 30 minutes or more; participation by physician
99368   Medical team conference with interdisciplinary team of health care professionals, patient and/or family not present, 30 minutes or more; participation by nonphysician qualified health care professional

Codes **99366–99368** are used to report participation by physicians or other health care professionals in conferences to coordinate or manage care and services for established patients with chronic or multiple health conditions (eg, cerebral palsy) or with congenital anomalies (eg, craniofacial abnormalities).

> See Chapter 12 for a complete summary of the reporting requirements for medical team conferences.

Code **99367** is the only code that may be reported by a physician, and it can only be reported *when the patient and/or family is not present* at the team conference. When the physician or QHP who may report E/M services (eg, advanced practice nurse) participates in a medical team conference with the patient and/or family present, the appropriate-level E/M code (eg, **99231–99233**) will be reported based on the place of service and total face-to-face time spent in counseling and/or coordination of care.

Advance Care Planning

99497   Advance care planning, including the explanation and discussion of advance directives such as standard forms (with completion of such forms, when performed), by the physician or other qualified health care professional; first 30 minutes, face-to-face with the patient, family member(s) and/or surrogate

+99498   each additional 30 minutes (List separately in addition to code for primary procedure)

Codes **99497** and **99498** include

- Face-to-face service by a physician or QHP to a patient, family member, or surrogate spent in counseling and discussion of advance directives
- Completion of forms, when applicable (eg, Health Care Proxy, Durable Power of Attorney for Health Care, Living Will, Medical Orders for Life-Sustaining Treatment)

Face-to-face time spent by the physician or QHP is required and the total time must be documented.

Active management of problems is not included in advance care planning. Other E/M services (eg, subsequent hospital care) provided on the same date as advance care planning may be separately reported. However, *do not report* codes **99497** and **99498** in conjunction with hourly critical care services (**99291** and **99292**), inpatient neonatal and pediatric critical care (**99468** and **99469**; **99471–99476**), and initial and continuing intensive care services (**99477–99480**).

Example

➤ **An adolescent with cystic fibrosis wishes to discuss and be involved in planning her care after learning she will require a lung transplantation.** Her pulmonologist spends 50 minutes face-to-face with the patient and her parent assessing their understanding of the diagnosis and prognosis, the continued hope that treatment is successful, and the patient's wishes to be included in decisions about her care. A plan of care is developed and documented and an appointment with the supportive care team at the hospital is scheduled to provide additional counseling and support services to the patient and family.

The physician may report codes **99497** and **99498** for the 50 minutes of face-to-face time spent providing the advance care planning. Because the *CPT* prefatory language and code descriptors for advance care planning do not include other instruction on the time required for reporting, these services may be reported based on general *CPT* instruction to report when the midpoint is passed (eg, 1 unit of **99498** may be reported for 46–75 minutes). Exceptions may apply for payers with policy requiring that the time be met or exceeded.

Continuing Care After Hospitalization

A key goal of many quality improvement programs is avoidance of readmittance and/or ED visits following hospitalization. In recent years, *CPT* and payers have recognized a need for codes to capture services related to care coordination and management of chronic and episodic conditions that may lead to emergency and inpatient care. For physicians continuing patient care after hospital discharge, services such as transitional care management, principal (ie, single serious disease) care management, or chronic (ie, multiple chronic illnesses) care management offer opportunities to provide and be compensated for care aimed at reducing the risk of decline, exacerbation, and/or functional decline.

> **See Chapter 12 for more information on care management services.**

Hospital-Mandated On-Call Services

99026   Hospital mandated on-call service; in-hospital, each hour

99027   out of hospital, each hour

- Codes **99026** and **99027** describe services provided by a physician who is on call per hospital mandate as a condition of medical staff privileges.
- Used to report on-call time spent by the physician when he or she is not providing other services.
- Time spent performing separately reportable services should not be included in time reported as mandated on-call services.
- Most payers do not cover these services because they consider this a contract issue between the hospital and physician. However, these codes may be used for tracking purposes.

Resources

Evaluation and Management Code Selection

American Academy of Pediatrics *Pediatric Evaluation and Management: Coding Quick Reference Card 2022* (available for purchase at https://shop.aap.org/pediatric-evaluation-and-management-coding-quick-reference-card-2021)

Hospital Discharge Day Management

"Hospital Discharge Day Management: Are You Coding Correctly?" February 2019 *AAP Pediatric Coding Newsletter* (https://coding.solutions.aap.org/article.aspx?articleid=2720944; subscription required)

Inpatient Consultation

"You Code It! Two Consultations in One Admission," March 2020 *AAP Pediatric Coding Newsletter* (https://coding.solutions.aap.org/article.aspx?articleid=2761970; subscription required)

Observation Services

"Observation Services: Reporting Care by Multiple Physicians," May 2019 *AAP Pediatric Coding Newsletter* (https://coding.solutions.aap.org/article.aspx?articleid=2731589; subscription required)

Subsequent Hospital Care

"Subsequent Hospital Care: Patient Status Can Guide Code Selection," February 2021 *AAP Pediatric Coding Newsletter* (https://coding.solutions.aap.org/article.aspx?articleid=2765279; subscription required)

Test Your Knowledge!

1. **When can a physician select an initial hospital care service based on time?**
   a. Inpatient hospital care codes are always selected based on time.
   b. Physicians should select a code based on medical decision-making or time.
   c. When more than 50% of the total unit/floor time was spent in counseling and/or coordinating care
   d. Only when the unit/floor of the highest level of initial hospital care has been met

2. **Which term describes an evaluation and management (E/M) service in which a physician and a qualified health care professional from the same group practice each personally perform a medically necessary and substantive portion of 1 or more face-to-face E/M encounters on the same date?**
   a. Incident to
   b. Split/shared
   c. Consultation
   d. Interprofessional consultation

3. **Which of the following would prevent a physician from reporting an initial observation care service (99218–99220)?**
   a. The physician provides initial hospital care and discharge day management on the same date.
   b. The history or examination is less than detailed or comprehensive.
   c. The physician provides inpatient care on the same date.
   d. All of the above

4. **Which of the following describes observation discharge management code 99217?**
   a. All services provided to a patient on discharge from observation status if the discharge is on other than the initial date of observation status
   b. Observation discharge management services of more than 30 minutes
   c. Completion of documentation with or without a face-to-face service
   d. Discharge services reported when a patient is transferred from observation to initial hospital care (99221–99223)

5. **Which codes are reported when a physician provides a second consultation to a patient within the same inpatient admission?**
   a. A second consultation service cannot be reported.
   b. 99251–99255
   c. 99241–99245
   d. 99231–99233

CHAPTER 17

Emergency Department Services

Contents

Reporting the Diagnosis Code for Emergency Department (ED) Visits 403

    Reporting External Cause of Injury 403

    Reporting Suspected or Confirmed Abuse 404

ED Evaluation and Management Codes 404

    Comanagement of ED Patients 409

Modifiers Used With ED Codes 410

Reporting Procedures in the ED 411

    Fracture Care 412

        Nasal Fractures 413

    Point-of-Care Ultrasound 413

Sedation 415

    Moderate Sedation 415

    Deep Sedation 416

Directing Emergency Medical Technicians 416

Critical Care in the ED 416

Special Service Codes 418

Continuum Model for Fever 419

Resources 421

Test Your Knowledge! 421

Reporting the Diagnosis Code for Emergency Department (ED) Visits

Emergency department (ED) physicians play critical roles in care and documentation. While multiple symptoms may be listed as the chief complaint during the ED triage process, the physician must designate only 1 sign, symptom, disease, or injury as the chief complaint. Hospitals depend on the physician's designation of the chief complaint because only 1 diagnosis code may be reported for this category on the hospital claim form. This diagnosis is used to help support the urgency of the ED visit under prudent layperson guidelines. This may be different from conditions that are "present on admission" that must now be tracked by hospitals.

The diagnoses on the physician's claim for professional services are equally important to support the level of ED service reported (**99281–99285**). Some health plans now compare diagnosis codes submitted on physician claims that include codes **99284** and **99285** to a predetermined list of diagnosis codes indicating conditions that typically require these levels of service. When a claim for **99284** or **99285** is submitted with diagnosis codes not included on the list, the claim may be down-coded (eg, **99283**) and paid at the rate of the lesser code. **Figure 17-1** illustrates the corresponding decrease in relative value units (RVUs) (2021 RVUs, not geographically adjusted) when a payer down-codes **99284** or **99285** to **99283**. Relative value units for 2022 were not available at the time of publication. Learn more about payment based on RVUs in **Chapter 4**.

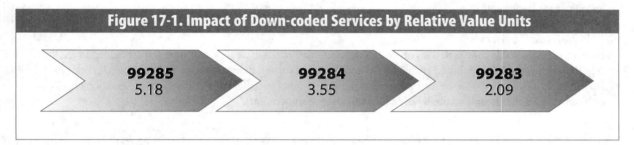

Figure 17-1. Impact of Down-coded Services by Relative Value Units

99285	99284	99283
5.18	3.55	2.09

Medicaid plans also significantly limit the amount paid for any condition not included on a diagnosis list, regardless of the level of service reported. To receive the payment most appropriate under the health plan contract

- List first the diagnosis that is most responsible for the level of service provided and report the code for that diagnosis first on your claim. Some plans consider only the first 2 diagnoses listed on the claim.
- Document and report codes for all current conditions that require or affect patient care treatment or management.

Some plans take into account all diagnoses on the claim, including

- Complicating factors (eg, **F84.0**, autism spectrum disorder)
- Social determinants of health (eg, **Z59.0**, homelessness)
- External cause of injury (eg, **W13.0XXA**, fall [on] [from] balcony)

Physicians should document all diagnoses including factors that increased the complexity of medical decision-making (MDM) of an encounter. To appeal the down-coded claim, medical records supporting the higher level of service typically must be submitted to the health plan.

Reporting External Cause of Injury

States may require EDs to report codes describing the circumstances of an injury. These codes are referred to as *external cause* codes in *International Classification of Diseases, 10th Revision, Clinical Modification* (ICD-10-CM). These codes capture the cause, intent, place of occurrence, activity of the patient at the time of the event, and patient status (eg, employee, military, volunteer, student).

> External cause of injury codes are found in the *International Classification of Diseases, 10th Revision, Clinical Modification* External Cause of Injuries Index. For example, under the term *struck*, sub-terms allow reporting of external causes such as a struck by baseball (**W21.03-**) or baseball bat (by accident [**T75.0-**] or assault [**Y08.02-**]). Combination codes allow for reporting multiple details, such as striking against an object with subsequent fall (**W18.0-**).

External cause codes provide information that is valuable for research on the cause and occurrence of injuries as well as evaluation of injury prevention strategies (eg, reduced reporting of injuries due to automobile crashes following prohibition of cell phone use while driving). This is particularly important in pediatrics, as injuries remain the leading cause for death and disability. While the physician may not be required to add the specific external cause code with the discharge diagnosis, there should be sufficient documentation in the record to allow a coder to extract the proper diagnosis code.

Examples of assignment of external cause codes are provided later in this chapter.

Key points for reporting external cause codes include

- External cause codes may be reported in conjunction with any health condition that is related to an external cause (eg, adverse effect of medical treatment).
- External cause codes are never the principal or first-listed diagnosis code.
- In *ICD-10-CM,* only external cause codes for the cause and intent of an injury or illness are reported for the duration of treatment, with the seventh character of the code indicating whether an encounter is for initial care, subsequent care, or care for sequela (late effect) of the injury or illness.

> Seventh character A is often reported for management of injuries other than fracture in the emergency department. It may be helpful to remember that seventh character A (initial encounter) is reported for active treatment and not for care during the healing phase of an injury. For example, S61.411A (laceration without foreign body of right hand, initial encounter) is reported for active management of the wound versus care during the healing phase or to address a late effect.

- External cause codes indicating place of occurrence, activity, and patient status are reported only at the initial encounter for treatment.
- If the intent (eg, accident, self-harm, assault) of the cause of an injury or other condition is unknown or unspecified, code the intent as *accidental.*
- No external cause code should be assigned when the cause and intent of an illness or injury are included in another reported code (eg, T58.11XA, initial encounter for toxic effect of carbon monoxide from utility gas, accidental).
- No external cause code should be assigned when an injury is ruled out after examination and observation (eg, Z04.1, encounter for examination and observation following transport accident).

> Read more about assigning *International Classification of Diseases, 10th Revision, Clinical Modification* codes for injuries in the May 2020 *AAP Pediatric Coding Newsletter*™ article, "Don't Get Bitten When Coding Injuries!" (https://coding.solutions.aap.org/article.aspx?articleid=2765180; subscription required).

Reporting Suspected or Confirmed Abuse

Suspected (T76.-) or confirmed abuse (T74.-) is reported as the first-listed diagnosis when this is the reason for the encounter. Codes for associated mental health or injury are reported secondary to the code for suspected or confirmed abuse. See **Table 17-1** for *ICD-10-CM* codes for abuse that may be reported by ED physicians caring for children.

- Codes are selected based on documentation. The record should clearly state whether abuse is suspected, ruled out, or confirmed.
- If a suspected case of child abuse, neglect, or mistreatment is ruled out during an encounter, code Z04.72 (encounter for examination and observation following alleged child physical abuse, ruled out) should be used, not a code from T76.
- If a suspected case of forced sexual exploitation or forced labor exploitation is ruled out during an encounter, code Z04.81 (encounter for examination and observation of victim following forced sexual exploitation) or Z04.82 (encounter for examination and observation of victim following forced labor exploitation) should be used, not a code from T76.
- When reporting confirmed abuse, report also codes for assault (X92–Y04; Y08, Y09) and perpetrator (Y07.-).

ED Evaluation and Management Codes

- Evaluation and management (E/M) codes 99281–99285 are only reported when care is provided in an ED. An ED is defined as an organized hospital-based facility for the provision of unscheduled episodic services to patients who present for immediate medical attention. The facility must be available 24 hours a day, 7 days a week.
  - Some states allow for freestanding EDs that are not hospital affiliated. Payers may or may not allow the use of ED codes in these circumstances.
  - Physician services provided in a freestanding hospital-affiliated ED may be subject to specific billing rules. Check payer contracts for payment and billing policies.
- Services performed in an urgent care center, a nonhospital facility, or a facility that is not open 24 hours a day should be reported with the appropriate *Current Procedural Terminology* (CPT®) office or outpatient visit codes (99202–99215) and with the appropriate place of service code (eg, 20 for urgent care facility). These facilities are not considered freestanding EDs.
- Selection of the appropriate E/M code is primarily driven by the risk involved in the presenting problem, evaluation measures, and/or treatment options.

Table 17-1. Abuse or Neglect: *ICD-10-CM* Codes for Suspected, Confirmed, or Ruled Out

The appropriate seventh character is to be added to each code from categories **T74** and **T76**. **A**, initial encounter; **D**, subsequent encounter; **S**, sequela

Suspected Abuse/Neglect	Confirmed	Ruled Out
T76.02X- Child neglect or abandonment, suspected	**T74.02X**- Child neglect or abandonment, confirmed	Encounter for examination and observation **Z04.42** following alleged child rape (ruled out)
T76.12X- Child sexual abuse, suspected	**T74.12X**- Child physical abuse, confirmed	**Z04.72** following alleged child physical abuse (ruled out)
T76.32X- Child psychological abuse, suspected	**T74.22X**- Child sexual abuse, confirmed	**Z04.81** of victim following forced sexual exploitation
T76.52X- Child sexual exploitation, suspected	**T74.32X**- Child psychological abuse, confirmed	**Z04.82** of victim following forced labor exploitation
T76.62X- Child forced labor exploitation, suspected	**T74.4XX**- Shaken infant syndrome	
	T74.52X- Child sexual exploitation, confirmed	
	T74.62X- Child forced labor exploitation, confirmed	

- Performance and documentation of all 3 key components (ie, history, physical examination, and MDM) are used to select the level of an ED E/M code.

Emergency Department Caveat: Code 99285

The emergency department evaluation and management code 99285 allows an exception to the "3 key components" rule (Level 5 caveat) for patients whose clinical condition, mental status, or lack of available history may not permit obtaining a comprehensive history and/or physical examination. Therefore, code 99285 may be reported for patients presenting with a high-severity condition that requires a high level of medical decision-making when circumstances prevent the physician from obtaining a comprehensive history and/or completing a comprehensive physical examination. When such urgency exists, the physician must document the condition or reason why a comprehensive history and/or comprehensive physical examination could not be obtained.

- Time spent in counseling and/or coordination of care *cannot* be used as a key or controlling factor in the selection of the E/M code; nor can prolonged services be reported with ED codes. Because of the unpredictability and inconsistency in the intensity of these services, there are presently no time values assigned to this family of codes.
- There is no differentiation between new or established patients for ED encounters. All problems for encounters in the ED are considered new to the attending physician for purposes of determining MDM.
- The ED codes are not reported if the treating ED physician admits the patient to their service for observation or inpatient status on the same date of service as the ED encounter. Only the appropriate initial observation (99218–99220), initial hospital care (99221–99223), or initial observation or inpatient hospital admission and discharge, same day (99234–99236), codes are reported instead of ED codes. All the E/M work performed in the ED should be combined with any additional work performed for admission (and, when appropriate, discharge) when selecting the correct code and level of care.

Table 17-2 summarizes the key components required for each ED E/M code based on the 1995 and 1997 Centers for Medicare & Medicaid Services *Documentation Guidelines for Evaluation and Management Services.* Also refer to **Chapter 6**, Evaluation and Management Documentation Guidelines, for more details on E/M coding guidelines. Medical necessity is an overarching criterion for selecting the level of E/M service. Physicians should always consider whether the nature of the presenting problem supports the medical necessity of services rendered when selecting the level of E/M service.

Use **Table 17-2** to help you in the selection of the appropriate level of ED E/M service in the examples for each level of service that follow.

For more information on coding evaluation and management services in the emergency department, see "Evaluation and Management Coding in the Emergency Department" in the May 2018 *AAP Pediatric Coding Newsletter* (https://coding.solutions.aap.org/article. aspx?articleid=2679117; subscription required).

Table 17-2. Emergency Department Services

Key Components

3 of 3 key components must be performed to at least the degree specified for each code. All patients in the emergency department are considered new patients.

Code	MDM	History	Physical Examination
99281	**Straightforward** # Diagnoses/options: Minimal Data: Minimal Risk: Minimal	**Problem focused** HPI: 1–3 elements ROS: 0 PFSH: 0	**Problem focused** **1995:** One body area/organ system **1997:** 1–5 elements identified by a bullet (●) in ≥1 areas or systems
99282	**Low complexity** # Diagnoses/options: Limited Data: Limited Risk: Low	**Expanded problem focused** HPI: 1–3 elements ROS: 1 PFSH: 0	**Expanded problem focused** **1995:** Limited examination—affected body area/organ system and 1–6 other related areas/systems **1997:** ≥6 elements identified by a bullet (●) in ≥1 areas or systems
99283	**Moderate complexity** # Diagnoses/options: Multiple Data: Moderate Risk: Moderate	**Expanded problem focused** HPI: 1–3 elements ROS: 1 PFSH: 0	**Expanded problem focused** **1995:** Limited examination—affected body area/organ system and 1–6 other related areas/systems **1997:** ≥6 elements identified by a bullet (●) in ≥1 areas or systems
99284	**Moderate complexity** # Diagnoses/options: Multiple Data: Moderate Risk: Moderate	**Detailed** HPI: 4+ elements or status of 3 chronic or inactive conditions ROS: 2–9 PFSH: 1	**Detailed** **1995:** Extended examination—affected body area(s) and 1–6 other symptomatic or related organ system(s) **1997:** ≥2 elements identified by a bullet (●) in ≥6 areas or systems or ≥12 elements identified by a bullet (●) in ≥2 areas or systems
99285	**High complexity** # Diagnoses/options: Extensive Data: Extensive Risk: High	**Comprehensive** HPI: 4+ elements or status of 3 chronic or inactive conditions ROS: 10+ PFSH: 2 Or clinical condition or mental status did not permit performance of history (must document reason that comprehensive history could not be performed).	**Comprehensive** **1995:** 8+ organ systems or complete examination of a single organ system **1997:** Multisystem examination—≥9 organ systems or body areas with performance of all elements identified by a bullet (●) in each area/system examined Documentation is expected for ≥2 elements identified by a bullet (●) of each area(s) or system(s). Single organ system examination—Performance of all elements identified by a bullet (●) and documentation of every element in each box with a shaded border and at least 1 element in a box with an unshaded border Or clinical condition or mental status did not permit performance of examination.

Abbreviations: HPI, history of present illness; MDM, medical decision-making; PFSH, past, family, and social history; ROS, review of systems.

Examples

➤ **A 3-year-old presents with a splinter in his right forefoot.** History of present illness (HPI): Patient was playing on a wooden deck with bare feet about an hour ago and complained of a splinter. Immunizations are up to date. Mother reports trying to remove the splinter with tweezers, but child refused to be still and wants a doctor to remove the splinter. The child appears well and is in no discomfort. Examination reveals a visible wood splinter that is readily grasped with tweezers and removed. Antibiotic ointment and a bandage are applied.

> *ICD-10-CM*
> **S90.851A** (superficial foreign body, right foot, initial encounter)

> *CPT*
> **99281**
> *Documentation must support all 3 elements (ie, MDM, history, and examination).*
>
> MDM: Straightforward (number of diagnoses/options: minimal [self-limiting condition]; data: limited; risk: minimal)
>
> History: Problem focused (HPI: 1–3 elements [location of splinter]; review of systems [ROS]: 1 system [musculo-skeletal]; past, family, and social history [PFSH]: past history [immunization history])
>
> Examination: Problem focused (1995) (limited examination of affected body area)

    Teaching Point: The key components support code **99281**. If the splinter removal had required an incision, a code for incision and removal of a foreign body from subcutaneous tissue is reported with code **10120** when simple or **10121** when complicated.

➤ **An 11-year-old patient presents with an injury to his left ankle.** The patient reports hurting his ankle by tripping during a basketball game approximately an hour earlier. The ankle is mildly painful, but patient is able to bear his full weight. The patient reports no prior ankle injury. Review of systems: constitutional—no complaints; musculoskele-tal—positive for left ankle pain, otherwise negative. After an expanded problem-focused examination, the need for a radiograph is ruled out and a compression wrap is applied. The patient and parents are instructed on home care and follow-up with primary care physician. Diagnosis is sprain of the anterior talofibular ligament of the left ankle.

> *ICD-10-CM*
> **S93.492A** (sprain of other ligament of left ankle, initial encounter)
> **W01.0XXA** (fall on same level from slipping, tripping and stumbling without subsequent striking against object, initial encounter)
> **Y93.67** (activity, basketball)
> **Y92.310** (basketball court as the place of occurrence of the external cause)
> **Y99.8** (other external cause status [leisure activity])

> *CPT*
> **99282**
> *Documentation must support all 3 elements (ie, MDM, history, and examination).*
>
> MDM: Low complexity (number of diagnoses/options: moderate [new problem without additional workup planned]; data: minimal [decision to not order a radiograph]; risk: low)
>
> History: Expanded problem focused (HPI: 3 elements; ROS: 2; PFSH: past history [no prior injury])
>
> Examination: Expanded problem focused (1995) (extended examination of affected body area/organ system plus 1–6 other related body areas/organ systems)

    Teaching Point: The expanded problem-focused history and examination with low-complexity MDM supports code **99282**.

> For purposes of medical decision-making, a new problem without additional workup is indicative that the diagnosis is known at the end of the encounter, although treatment will follow. In contrast, a new problem requiring additional workup indicates further workup is necessary to fully diagnose the patient's problem(s).

Chapter 17. Emergency Department Services

➤ **An 11-year-old patient presents with an injury to his left ankle.** The patient reports hurting his ankle by tripping during a basketball game approximately an hour earlier and is not able to bear full weight on the ankle. The patient gives history of a prior broken ankle. Review of systems: constitutional—no complaints; musculoskeletal—positive for left ankle pain, otherwise negative. After an expanded problem-focused examination, a radiograph is ordered and reviewed. The ED physician chooses to speak with the radiologist about the interpretation of the radiograph. Current fracture is ruled out, and the patient and parents are provided with a walking boot and instructed on home care and follow-up with primary care physician. Diagnosis is sprain of the anterior talofibular and calcaneofibular ligaments of the left ankle.

ICD-10-CM

S93.412A (sprain of calcaneofibular ligament of left ankle, initial encounter)
S93.492A (sprain of other ligament of left ankle, initial encounter)
W01.0XXA (fall on same level from slipping, tripping and stumbling without subsequent striking against object, initial encounter)
Y93.67 (activity, basketball)
Y92.310 (basketball court as the place of occurrence of the external cause)
Y99.8 (other external cause status [leisure activity])

CPT

99283

Documentation must support all 3 elements (ie, MDM, history, and examination).

MDM: Moderate complexity (number of diagnoses/options: moderate [new problem without additional workup planned]; data: moderate [order of radiograph, independent visualization of images, discussion with performing physician]; risk: low to moderate)

History: Expanded problem focused (HPI: 3 elements; ROS: 2; PFSH: past history [prior broken ankle])

Examination: Expanded problem focused (1995) (extended examination of affected body area/organ system plus 1–6 other related body areas/organ systems)

Teaching Point: The expanded problem-focused history and examination with moderate-complexity MDM support code **99283**. In the future, ED codes may be revised to align with office E/M code selection guidelines (ie, moderate-complexity MDM would support **99284**). However, this is not an option for ED code selection in 2022.

➤ **An adolescent is brought to the ED by his parents for evaluation after an all-terrain vehicle (ATV) accident.** History of present illness is headache. The patient reports his ATV rolled over on an incline in his family's cow pasture about 2 hours ago. He believes he hit his head on something and "blacked out" for a minute, but a fellow rider did not witness this and reported the patient was alert within a minute of the accident. The patient's helmet is lightly scarred. All systems reviewed are normal other than a headache and minor body aches. Parents report immunizations are up to date, and patient has no known health problems. The patient denies alcohol or substance use. A comprehensive examination is performed with normal findings other than contusions on the left forearm and left outer thigh. The patient is discharged with instructions for follow-up.

ICD-10-CM

R51.9 (headache, unspecified)
S50.12XA (contusion of left forearm, initial encounter)
S70.12XA (contusion of left thigh, initial encounter)
V86.55XA (driver of 3- or 4-wheeled ATV injured in nontraffic accident, initial encounter)
Y92.73XA (farm field as the place of occurrence of the external cause)

> **CPT**
>
> **99284**
>
> *Documentation must support all 3 elements (ie, MDM, history, and examination).*
>
> MDM: Moderate complexity (number of diagnoses/options: multiple [new problems without additional workup planned]; data: minimal; risk: moderate due to acute complicated injury)
>
> History: Detailed (HPI: 4+ elements or status of 3 chronic or inactive conditions; ROS: complete; PFSH: 1 [past medical])
>
> Examination: Comprehensive (1997) (≥2 elements identified by a bullet [●] in ≥6 areas or systems or ≥12 elements identified by a bullet [●] in ≥2 areas or systems)

Teaching Point: The patient's presentation with possible traumatic brain injury as well as other injuries supports the clinical indication for moderate-complexity MDM.

➤ **An adolescent boy is brought to the ED by ambulance after a rollover automobile accident. Attempts to contact the patient's parents were unsuccessful.** Emergency medical technicians relay that the patient was driving and wearing a seat belt but the older model vehicle did not have airbags. Witnesses to the accident reported the patient lost consciousness for several minutes prior to arrival of the ambulance. The ED physician performs a comprehensive examination on the patient, whose Glasgow Coma Scale score is 13 due to confusion. Radiographs of the chest and left shoulder and a computed tomography scan of the head are ordered. The patient is found to have a closed frontal skull fracture and fractured left clavicle. Neurology and orthopedic consultations are obtained and the patient is admitted for observation by the neurologist.

> **ICD-10-CM**
>
> **S02.0XXA** (fracture of vault of skull, initial encounter for closed fracture)
> **S42.021A** (displaced fracture of shaft of right clavicle, initial encounter for closed fracture)
> **R40.2412** (Glasgow coma scale score 13-15, at arrival to emergency department)
> **V48.5XXA** (car driver injured in noncollision transport accident in traffic accident, initial encounter)
> **Y92.413** (state road as the place of occurrence of the external cause)

> **CPT**
>
> **99285** (ED visit code)
>
> *Documentation must support all 3 elements (ie, MDM, history, and examination).*
>
> MDM: High complexity (number of diagnoses/options: extensive; data: moderate; risk: high)
>
> History: Comprehensive (Level 5 caveat with information obtained from emergency medical services [EMS])
>
> Examination: Comprehensive (1995) (8+ organ systems)

Teaching Point: The Level 5 caveat regarding unobtainable history would apply because this patient's condition prohibited a reliable history, other than that from EMS. Evaluation and management services by the orthopedist would be reported with office or other outpatient consultation codes (likely **99244** or **99245**). The neurologist will report initial observation care (**99218–99220**). Each physician will report the diagnoses for the conditions confirmed at the conclusion of the encounter (eg, the ED physician reports what was known at the time the patient is transferred to the neurologist's care).

Comanagement of ED Patients

Only 1 physician should report an ED E/M service for a patient who receives care in the ED. In general, this will be the emergency physician or pediatric emergency medicine specialist who is staffing the ED. At times, other physicians (eg, generalists, specialists) may provide care for a patient in the ED.

The type of service reported will depend on whether the other physician is providing consultative services, a specific intervention (eg, diagnostic or therapeutic procedure), or primary management of the patient. The ED physician will typically report the ED E/M code or time-based critical care (when provided) and the other physician will report services as follows:

Chapter 17. Emergency Department Services

- *Consultation:* An outpatient consultation (**99241–99245**) may be reported with place of service **23** (ED) when the ED physician requests the opinion of and/or advice from the other physician. See **Chapter 9** for full requirements for codes **99241–99245**.
- If a payer follows Medicare guidelines and does not cover consultations or the second physician is called in to assume management of the patient's care, services should be reported using the office or outpatient E/M codes (**99202–99215**) with place of service **23**. See **Chapter 7**, Office and Other Outpatient Evaluation and Management Services, for detailed requirements for reporting consultations.
- *Observation or inpatient admission:* See **Chapter 16** for discussion of codes reported when a consulting physician admits the child to the hospital for observation or inpatient services after stabilization and/or provision of care in the ED. For inpatient intensive or critical care services, see codes discussed in **Chapter 18**.
- *Critical care:* If the patient is critically ill or injured, the physicians providing critical care services may report the services using time-based critical care codes **99291** and **99292** (see **Table 18-2**).

Modifiers Used With ED Codes

Physicians need to understand when it is appropriate to report modifiers in addition to E/M or procedural service codes. Modifiers **25** (significant, separately identifiable E/M service) and **57** (decision for surgery) may be appended to ED E/M codes to indicate E/M beyond the preservice work of a procedure. Procedures performed in the ED may require reporting of modifiers such as **26** (professional component), **54** (surgical care only), or **59** (distinct procedural service) or, when accepted by the payer in lieu of modifier **59**, modifier **XE** (separate encounter), **XP** (separate practitioner), **XS** (separate structure), or **XU** (unusual nonoverlapping service). **Table 17-3** lists modifiers commonly used in the ED. (See **Chapter 2**, Modifiers and Coding Edits, for more detail on the use of modifiers.)

Table 17-3. Common Modifiers Used in the Emergency Department	
Modifier	**When to Use**
24	An unrelated E/M service is provided during the global period of a previously performed procedure by the same physician or group.
25	A significant, separately identifiable E/M service is performed by the same physician on the same day of the procedure or other service.
26	Reporting professional component only of a service for which payment includes equipment (or technical services) cost (eg, radiograph)
32	A service is mandated by third-party payer, regulation, or governmental entity.
51	Multiple procedures are performed on the same day other than E/M, physical medicine and rehabilitation services, or provision of supplies (eg, vaccines).
54	Only the surgical care component of a procedure was provided. Another physician will provide postoperative care.
57	Decision for surgery was made. Some payers may require this modifier be appended to the E/M code only with procedures with 90-day global periods.
59	Distinct procedural service (non-E/M) was performed on the same day as another procedural service and was at a different encounter or a different surgery or procedure or was performed on a different body site or organ system.
63	Procedures (**20000–69999**) and certain procedures in the Medicine section of *CPT* performed on an infant weighing <4 kg if the code descriptor does not include a descriptor of "young infant or neonate"
76	The same physician repeats a procedure or service on the same date of service.
77	Another physician repeats a procedure or service already performed by another physician on the same day of service.
79	An unrelated procedure is performed during the global period of a previously provided procedure by the same physician or group.
CR	Catastrophe/disaster related
XE	The service was provided at a separate encounter on the same date.
XP	The non-E/M service or procedure was performed by a separate practitioner of the same group on the same date.
XS	The procedure or service was performed on a separate structure.
XU	Unusual nonoverlapping service

Abbreviations: *CPT, Current Procedural Terminology;* E/M, evaluation and management.

Example

➤ **The ED physician is caring for a 9-year-old who has a 4-cm–long, deep laceration of the right calf and a separate 1-cm–long laceration of the right ankle from broken glass in his backyard.** The physician performs a detailed history and physical examination. A radiograph of the extremity shows no retained radiopaque foreign bodies. The child's immunizations are current, with the last tetanus booster less than 5 years ago. The physician irrigates, carefully explores both wounds, and performs a 2-layer repair on the calf. The ankle laceration requires only single-layer closure. The child is discharged with appropriate follow-up plans.

ICD-10-CM	*CPT*
S81.811A (laceration without foreign body, right lower leg, initial encounter)	**99283 25**
	12032 (intermediate repair of the extremities, 2.6–7.5 cm)
S91.011A (laceration without foreign body, right ankle, initial encounter)	**12001 59** or **XS** (simple repair of the extremity, ≤2.5 cm)
W25.XXXA (contact with sharp glass, initial encounter)	
Y92.007 (garden or yard of noninstitutional residence)	

Teaching Point: Modifiers are used to indicate the laceration repairs were distinct procedures (**59**) or of a separate structure (**XS**). Append modifier **25** only when providing an E/M and other service with an E/M component (pre- and post-service work) on the same date to indicate the E/M was significantly beyond the preservice work of the other service and distinctly documented.

Verify payer policy on reporting of modifier **59** (distinct procedural service) versus **XS** (separate structure). (See **Chapter 2**, Modifiers and Coding Edits, for more information on these modifiers and appropriate modifier placement.)

See Chapter 10, Surgery, Infusion, and Sedation in the Outpatient Setting, for more examples of coding for laceration repairs.

See also "You Code It! Integumentary Repair," in the April 2020 *AAP Pediatric Coding Newsletter* (https://coding.solutions.aap.org/article. aspx?articleid=2763375; subscription required).

Reporting Procedures in the ED

Many procedures performed in the ED have an associated global period assigned by Medicare and other payers and/or are subject to the *CPT* surgical package. The global period affects reporting of pre- and post-procedural care. The *CPT* surgical package defines the work included in each surgical procedure. (See **Chapter 19**, Common Surgical Procedures and Sedation in Facility Settings, for the definition of the *CPT* surgical package and Medicare global period and examples of reporting procedures when follow-up care is provided by another physician.)

To report an E/M service in addition to a procedure, there must be documentation of performance of a significant and separately identifiable E/M service beyond the pre- and post-procedural work typical for the procedure (eg, evaluation for a concussion and repair of wounds at 1 encounter). Post-procedural prescriptions for pain control or prophylactic antibiotics may be included in the procedure performed.

Table 17-4 contains a list of procedures (with assigned Medicare global periods) commonly performed in the ED.

Any separately identifiable procedure that is personally performed by the physician may be reported, with the exception of

- Procedures that are bundled in time-based critical care codes (See **Table 18-1** for a list of services and procedures that are included in hourly critical care codes.)
- Services performed by hospital personnel because they are billed by the hospital facility (If a nurse or other clinical staff assist in part of a procedure, the ED physician may bill for the professional services if the ED physician provides the primary or key component of the procedure.)
- Hydration, infusion, and/or injection procedures (**96360–96379**) because the physician work associated with the procedures involves only confirmation of the treatment plan and not direct supervision of staff
- Procedures involving use of hospital-owned equipment (eg, pulse oximetry), unless the procedure includes a technical and professional component (If performed and documented, the professional component, such as interpretation and report of x-ray findings, may be reported with modifier **26** [professional component] appended to the procedure code.)

Table 17-4. Common Emergency Department Procedures
Procedures Not Assigned a Global Period
These procedures have an **X** *or* **M** *status in the Medicare Physician Fee Schedule.*
Arterial puncture (**36600**)
Venipuncture, >3 y requiring physician skill (**36410**)
Venipuncture, <3 y requiring physician skill, femoral/jugular (**36400**)
Procedures With 0-Day Global Period
Bladder aspiration (**51100**)
Burn care, <5% TBSA (**16020**); 5%–10% TBSA (**16025**); >10% TBSA (**16030**)
Cardiopulmonary resuscitation (**92950**)
Cardioversion (**92960**)
Chest tube insertion (**32551**)
Endotracheal intubation, emergency (**31500**)
Foreign body removal, conjunctiva (**65205**), ear (**69200**)
Gastric intubation and aspiration(s), therapeutic, including lavage (if performed) (**43753**)
Intraosseous needle placement (**36680**)
Laceration repair, simple, ≤2.5 cm, face/ears/lips (**12011**)
Repair, simple, scalp/trunk/extremities ≤2.5 cm (**12001**), 2.6–7.5 cm (**12002**)
Repair, simple 2.6–5.0 cm, face/ears/lips (**12013**)
Lumbar puncture (**62270**), with fluoroscopic or CT guidance (**62328**)
Pleural drainage, percutaneous, with insertion of indwelling catheter; without imaging guidance (**32556**); with imaging guidance (**32557**)
Splint, finger (**29130**); short arm (**29125**); short leg (**29515**); ankle (**29540**)
Strap, knee (**29530**); shoulder (**29240**)
Subungual hematoma evacuation (**11740**)
Thoracentesis, needle or catheter, without imaging (**32554**); with imaging (**32555**)
Procedures With 10-Day Global Period
Foreign body removal, nose (**30300**)
Foreign body removal with incision, subcutaneous, simple (**10120**)
Incision and drainage, abscess, simple (**10060**)
Incision and drainage, finger, complicated (eg, felon) (**26011**)
Incision and drainage, perianal abscess (**46050**)
Laceration repair, intermediate, face/ears/lips ≤2.5 cm (**12051**); 2.6–5.0 cm (**12052**)
Repair, intermediate, hands/feet/neck ≤2.5 cm (**12041**); 2.6–7.5 cm (**12042**)
Repair, intermediate, scalp/trunk/arms/legs ≤2.5 cm (**12031**); 2.6–7.5 cm (**12032**)
Nursemaid elbow reduction (**24640**)
Puncture aspiration of abscess, hematoma, bulla, or cyst (**10160**)
Repair, nail bed (**11760**)
Procedures With 90-Day Global Period
Dislocation, shoulder, reduction (**23650**)
Fracture, clavicle (**23500**)
Fracture, finger distal, each (**26750**)
Fracture, finger shaft, each (**26720**)
Abbreviations: CT, computed tomography; TBSA, total body surface area.

- Modifier **54** is appropriately appended to procedure codes with 10- or 90-day global periods when the patient will not return to the ED for follow-up care (eg, removal of sutures or fracture care follow-up visits). Some payers require modifier **54** only on codes assigned a 90-day global period.

Fracture Care

New in 2022: Changes to coding for treatment of fractures of the nasal bone (See discussion on next page.)

Fracture care in the ED is typically limited to initial care. Most codes for fracture care include a 10- or 90-day period of care related to the fracture. Correct coding requires appending modifier **54** (surgical care only) to codes for fracture care when follow-up care will be provided by another physician. The physician who assumes management during the follow-up period reports the same fracture care code with modifier **55** (postoperative management only) and the same date of service. Some payers require that both physicians document the transfer of care.

> Casting, splinting, or strapping used solely to temporarily stabilize the fracture for patient comfort is not considered closed fracture treatment and is included in the related evaluation and management service.

Example

➤ **A 16-year-old patient is seen in the ED for right shoulder pain that occurred following a fall while playing soccer at a community sports field.** The patient is examined for additional injuries (expanded problem-focused history, detailed examination). Diagnosis is anterior glenohumeral dislocation of the right shoulder. The patient agrees to an attempt at reduction without analgesia, which is successful. A sling is applied. The physician refers the patient to another physician for follow-up care and documents the transfer of care.

ICD-10-CM	CPT
S43.014A (anterior dislocation of right humerus, initial encounter)	**99283 57**
W18.30XA (unspecified fall on same level, initial encounter)	**23650 54** (closed treatment of shoulder dislocation, with manipulation; without anesthesia)
Y93.66 (activity, soccer)	
Y92.322 (soccer field as place of occurrence)	

Teaching Point: The use of modifier **54** (surgical care only) alerts payers that another physician will report follow-up care for this procedure, which typically includes 90 days of postprocedural care. Medical decision-making for the ED visit is moderate based on a new problem without additional workup and moderate risk related to the decision for closed treatment of the dislocation. Modifier **57** indicates the decision for surgery during the E/M service. If a detailed history were indicated and performed, code **99284** would be supported.

> See the February 2021 *AAP Pediatric Coding Newsletter* article, "Initial Fracture Care: Musculoskeletal or Evaluation and Management," for more examples of initial fracture care (https://coding.solutions.aap.org/article.aspx?articleid=2765276; subscription required).

Nasal Fractures

Code **21310** (closed treatment of nasal bone fracture without manipulation) is deleted in 2022. This service must now be reported with an E/M code based on the key components performed and documented (ie, **99283** or **99284**). As shown codes **21315** and **21320** are revised to include "with manipulation" in the code descriptor.

▲**21315**   Closed treatment of nasal bone fracture with manipulation; without stabilization
▲**21320**   with stabilization

Point-of-Care Ultrasound

Point-of-care ultrasound services performed by the ED physician (**Table 17-5**) are separately reportable in addition to the ED E/M service when *all 3 of the following conditions apply:*
- Thorough evaluation of organ(s) or anatomical region is performed.
- There is permanent image documentation (with measurements, when clinically indicated).
- A written report equivalent to that typically produced by a radiologist is documented.

> Use of handheld or portable ultrasound that does not include all 3 of the listed elements is not separately reported.

Without all these elements, the examination is not separately reported and would be considered part of any E/M service provided. (*Exception:* Permanent image documentation is not required for ophthalmic ultrasound for biometric measurement.)

Chapter 17. Emergency Department Services

Table 17-5. Codes for Common Point-of-Care Ultrasound Procedures

76536	Soft tissues of head and neck (eg, thyroid, parathyroid, parotid)
76604	Chest (includes mediastinum when performed)
76700	Abdominal; complete
76705	Abdominal; limited (eg, single organ, quadrant, follow-up)
76770	Retroperitoneal (eg, renal, aorta, nodes), complete
76775	Retroperitoneal (eg, renal, aorta, nodes), limited
76857	Pelvis (nonobstetric); limited or follow-up
76870	Scrotum and contents[a]
76881	Complete joint (eg, joint space and periarticular soft tissue structures)[b]
76882	Joint or other nonvascular extremity structure(s), limited[b]
76885	Infant hips; dynamic (requiring physician or other QHP manipulation)
76886	Infant hips; limited, static (not requiring physician or other QHP manipulation)
+76937	Ultrasound guidance for vascular access requiring ultrasound evaluation of potential access sites, documentation of selected vessel patency, concurrent real-time ultrasound visualization of vascular needle entry, with permanent recording and reporting (List separately in addition to code for primary procedure.)
93976	Duplex scan of arterial inflow and venous outflow of abdominal, pelvic, scrotal contents and/or retroperitoneal organs; limited study[a]

Abbreviation: QHP, qualified health care professional.

[a] Evaluation of vascular structures using color and spectral Doppler is separately reportable. However, color Doppler alone, when performed for anatomical structure identification in conjunction with a real-time ultrasound examination, is not reported separately.

[b] Code **76881** requires ultrasound examination of all the following joint elements: joint space (eg, effusion), periarticular soft-tissue structures that surround the joint (eg, muscles, tendons, other soft tissue structures), and any identifiable abnormality. When fewer than all the required elements for a "complete" examination (**76881**) are performed, report the "limited" code (**76882**).

Point-of-care ultrasound services in the ED are reported by the physician with the professional service only modifier (**26**). (See **Table 17-3** and the Modifiers Used With ED Codes section in this chapter for more information.) The technical component (eg, equipment cost, facility overhead costs) is typically reported by the facility. (Payers may limit physicians to reporting the professional component only for all facility-based services even if the physician performs the ultrasound and/or owns the equipment used for the service. The technical component includes all associated overhead costs. Check individual payer policies for reporting.)

One use of point-of-care ultrasound in the ED is the focused assessment with sonography for trauma (FAST) examination. This may consist of 2 distinct components: limited transthoracic echocardiogram and limited abdominal ultrasound. When 2 distinct procedures are performed, 2 codes are reported.

76705	Ultrasound, abdominal, real-time with image documentation; limited
93308	Echocardiography, transthoracic, real-time with image documentation (2D), includes M-mode recording, when performed, follow-up or limited study

When a limited ultrasound examination of the chest is included (eg, for pneumothorax), report code **76604** (ultrasound, chest [includes mediastinum when performed], real-time with image documentation). Limited studies are defined in *CPT* as those that include examination of less than the required elements for a "complete" examination (eg, limited number of organs, limited portion of region evaluated). See your *CPT* reference for required components of complete examinations.

Please see the discussion of central venous access in **Chapter 19** for appropriate reporting of ultrasound guidance for vascular access (**76937**). This code is reported separately in addition to a code for primary vascular access procedure (eg, **36555**).

When ultrasound guidance is used for needle placement for procedures such as aspiration of an abscess, code **76942** is reported. Do not report code **76942** in conjunction with a service for which the code descriptor includes ultrasound guidance (eg, joint aspiration). Code **76937** (ultrasound guidance for vascular access) is not reported in conjunction with code **76942**.

Example

➤ **A child is seen in the ED for injuries sustained in a traffic accident.** The physician performs a trauma assessment, including a FAST examination. This examination may consist of 2 distinct components: limited transthoracic echocardiogram and limited abdominal ultrasound. When 2 distinct procedures are performed, 2 codes are reported.

In addition to the appropriate E/M service code, the physician reports **76705 26** (ultrasound, abdominal, real-time with image documentation; limited) and **93308 26** (echocardiography, transthoracic, real-time with image documentation [2D], includes M-mode recording, when performed, follow-up or limited study). Modifier **26** signifies the physician is reporting the professional component of each service. The facility will report the same codes with modifier **TC** to indicate reporting of the technical component of each service. When applicable and all requirements for reporting are met, an ultrasound performed with physician-owned equipment is reported without a modifier (ie, modifiers **26** and **TC** are not applicable).

Sedation

Moderate Sedation

Moderate sedation (**99151–99157**) is a drug-induced depression of consciousness during which patients may respond purposefully to verbal commands, either alone or accompanied by light tactile stimulation. Moderate sedation may be necessary for the performance of certain procedures in the ED.

99151	Moderate sedation services provided by the same physician or other qualified health care professional performing the diagnostic or therapeutic service that the sedation supports, requiring the presence of an independent trained observer to assist in the monitoring of the patient's level of consciousness and physiological status; initial 15 minutes of intraservice time, patient younger than 5 years of age
99152	initial 15 minutes of intraservice time, patient age 5 years or older
+99153	each additional 15 minutes intraservice time (report with **99151** or **99152**)
99155	Moderate sedation services provided by a physician or other qualified health care professional other than the physician or other qualified health care professional performing the diagnostic or therapeutic service that the sedation supports; initial 15 minutes of intraservice time, patient younger than 5 years of age
99156	initial 15 minutes of intraservice time, patient age 5 years or older
+99157	each additional 15 minutes intraservice time (report with **99155** or **99156**)

> See Chapter 10 and Table 10-5 for a full discussion of coding for moderate sedation.

- Codes are selected based on intraservice time. Intraservice time
  - Begins with the administration of the sedating agent(s)
  - Ends when the procedure is completed, the patient is stable for recovery status, and the physician or other qualified health care professional (QHP) providing the sedation ends personal continuous face-to-face time with the patient
  - Includes ordering and/or administering the initial and subsequent doses of sedating agents
  - Requires continuous face-to-face attendance of the physician or other QHP
  - Requires monitoring patient response to the sedating agents, including
    - Periodic assessment of the patient
    - Further administration of agent(s) as needed to maintain sedation
    - Monitoring of oxygen saturation, heart rate, and blood pressure
- Moderate sedation services of less than 10 minutes' intraservice time are not separately reported.

Example

➤ **A 5-year-old requires a procedure in the ED.** A physician other than the ED physician performs the procedure. The ED physician provides the moderate sedation and documents 25 minutes of service, beginning with administration of the sedating agent and ending when the patient is sufficiently recovered so that the physician's continuous face-to-face monitoring is no longer necessary.

> *CPT*
> **99281–99285 25**
> **99156** (moderate sedation by other than physician performing procedure, first 15 minutes)
> **99157** (moderate sedation, each additional 15 minutes)

Teaching Point: The ED physician reports an E/M code as appropriate for care prior to the pre-sedation evaluation (eg, initial evaluation of illness or injury) and appends modifier **25** to indicate the service was significant and is separately identifiable in the documentation. Code **99157** is reported for the final 10 minutes because the midpoint between the first and second 15-minute period was passed.

Deep Sedation

Deep sedation or analgesia is a drug-induced depression of consciousness during which patients cannot be easily aroused but respond purposefully after repeated verbal or painful stimulation (eg, purposefully pushing away the noxious stimuli). The ability to independently maintain ventilatory function may be impaired. Patients may require assistance in maintaining a patent airway, and spontaneous ventilation may be inadequate. Cardiovascular function is usually maintained. A state of deep sedation may be accompanied by partial or complete loss of protective airway reflexes.

Although ED physicians may provide deep sedation, payment for these services is limited.

Deep sedation provided by a physician also performing the services for which the sedation is being provided is reported by appending modifier **47** (anesthesia by surgeon) to the procedure code for the service for which sedation is required. Many health plans do not pay separately for anesthesia by the physician or surgeon performing the procedure.

National Correct Coding Initiative (NCCI) edits do not allow payment of an ED visit (**99281–99285**) and deep sedation when provided by the same ED physician or 2 ED physicians of the same group practice. No modifier will override the NCCI edits. Payers that have adopted Medicare or Medicaid NCCI edits will deny the ED visit when reported on the same date as deep sedation.

Please see **Chapter 19**, Common Surgical Procedures and Sedation in Facility Settings, for more information on deep sedation.

Directing Emergency Medical Technicians

99288   Physician or other qualified health care professional direction of emergency medical systems (EMS) emergency care, advanced life support

- Report code **99288** (physician direction of EMS) when
  - The physician directing the services is in the hospital and in 2-way communication with EMS personnel who are in the prehospital setting providing advanced life support that requires direct or online medical control.
  - The documentation includes the times of all contacts, any orders provided, and/or directions provided to the EMS team.
- Code **99288** may be reported on the same day as ED E/M or hourly critical care services. Modifier **25** would be appended to code **99288** to alert payers that this was a significant and separately identifiable service from ED E/M (**99281–99285**) or the critical care (**99291**, **99292**) service provided.
- The supervising physician cannot report the actual procedures and interventions performed by the EMS team because he or she is not physically present during the transport.
- Code **99288** is designated as a bundled procedure (included in the work value of other services) by Medicare. There are no relative values assigned under the Medicare Resource-Based Relative Value Scale. Check with your major payers and negotiate for coverage of this service.
- See codes **99485** and **99486** in **Chapter 18**, Critical and Intensive Care, for information on supervision of inter-facility transport of a critically ill or injured patient, 24 months or younger, via direct 2-way communication with a transport team.
- When a QHP (eg, nurse practitioner) provides critical care services during transport, and those services will be reported under the QHP's National Provider Identifier or by the employing hospital, the ED physician does not report **99288**.

Critical Care in the ED

99291   Critical care, E/M of the critically ill or critically injured patient; first 30 to 74 minutes
+99292   each additional 30 minutes (Use in conjunction with **99291**.)

To report **99291** and **99292**, the patient's condition must meet the specific *CPT* definition of a critically ill or injured patient.

> A *critical illness* or *injury* is defined in *CPT* as one that acutely impairs 1 or more vital organs such that there is a high probability of imminent or life-threatening deterioration of the patient's condition.

Guidelines for reporting critical care codes **99291** (critical care, E/M of the critically ill or injured patient; first 30–74 minutes) and **99292** (each additional 30 minutes) are described in detail in **Chapter 18**, Critical and Intensive Care.

- Time-based critical care codes (**99291**, **99292**) should be used to report the provision of critical care when performed in the ED. The global codes for pediatric or neonatal critical care should not be reported by a physician providing critical care in the ED unless that physician (eg, an intensivist) will continue to provide critical care services in the inpatient setting.
- Time spent providing critical care does not need to be continuous and includes time at the bedside as well as time in the ED reviewing data specific to the patient, discussing the patient with other physicians, and discussing the patient's management or condition with the patient's family.

> Time of any learner (eg, student, resident) involved in the patient's care may not be reported by the attending physician. Only the time specifically spent by the attending physician may be reported.

- Time reported for critical care must be devoted to the critically ill or injured patient. Therefore, the "critical care clock" stops when attention is turned to the care of another patient or the physician is not readily available in the ED.
- See **Table 18-1** for a list of services and procedures that are included in hourly critical care codes.
- Those procedures *not bundled* with codes **99291** and **99292** and personally performed by the reporting provider may be reported separately (eg, starting an intravenous line on a child younger than 3 years, placing an intraosseous or central venous line, endotracheal intubation, cardiopulmonary resuscitation [CPR], cardioversion). Time spent performing these separately reported services must be subtracted from the critical care time calculated and reported.

Example

➤ **A 13-month-old with apparent sepsis and hypotension is brought to the ED.** The child requires placement of an intraosseous needle to achieve vascular access and subsequently receives parenteral fluids, antibiotics, and vasopressors. The child experiences cardiopulmonary arrest, prompting the ED physician to intubate the child. Cardiopulmonary resuscitation is performed for 20 minutes. The child is in the ED for a total of 45 minutes before transfer to the intensive care unit.

> **ICD-10-CM**
> **I46.9** (cardiac arrest)
> If the physician included sepsis in the diagnosis, codes **A41.9** (sepsis, unspecified organism), **R65.21** (severe sepsis with septic shock), and **I46.8** (cardiac arrest due to other underlying condition) would be appropriate.

> **CPT**
> **99285 25**
> **92950** (CPR)
> **36680** (placement of intraosseous needle)
> **31500** (endotracheal intubation, emergency)

Teaching Point: Critical care time does not accrue during the performance of non-bundled, separately billable procedures. Because CPR is a separately billable, non-bundled procedure, the ED physician did not spend a minimum of 30 minutes providing critical care. Because the E/M service is reported rather than critical care, coding is based on documented key components of history, examination, and MDM. However, the caveat for code **99285** allows reporting based on the extent of history and examination possible within the constraints imposed by the urgency of the patient's clinical condition and mental status.

Chapter 17. Emergency Department Services

> *International Classification of Diseases, 10th Revision, Clinical Modification* codes for severe sepsis (R65.20) and septic shock (R65.21) are reported secondary to the underlying infection (eg, A41.9, sepsis, unspecified organism) and followed by codes for related organ failure (eg, J96.01, acute respiratory failure with hypoxia).

● Critical care may be reported on the same day as an ED E/M code when provided by the same physician as long as 2 independent services are provided. Modifier 25 should be appended to the ED E/M code when this occurs.

Examples

➤ **The ED physician performs a comprehensive history and physical examination on a 13-month-old patient with severe stridor and respiratory distress believed to be secondary to croup.** Medical decision-making is highly complex. The patient's condition does not improve with nebulized epinephrine and then worsens, evidenced by progressive lethargy. The patient goes into respiratory failure and 75 minutes of critical care is provided. Ten minutes of the critical care time is spent performing endotracheal intubation.

ICD-10-CM
J96.00 (acute respiratory failure)
J05.0 (croup)

CPT
99285 25 (ED visit code)
99291 25 (critical care, first 30–74 minutes)
31500 (endotracheal intubation, emergency)

Teaching Point: Endotracheal intubation is not bundled with critical care; therefore, time spent in the provision of the service (10 minutes for this patient) is not considered in the total critical care time, so only the base code, 99291, can be used. Modifier 25 is appended to codes 99285 and 99291 to indicate they were significant and separately identifiable services from each other and the endotracheal intubation.

➤ **The ED physician saw a 10-year-old for moderate asthma exacerbation in the morning.** The child responded well to an aerosolized bronchodilator treatment and was discharged home. The child returns to the ED a few hours later with a more severe exacerbation and is seen by the same physician. The child now has respiratory failure with hypoxia. The child receives oxygen, a continuous bronchodilator nebulizer treatment, and, subsequently, a parenteral bronchodilation drug. The child improves enough to be admitted to a monitored medical ward bed with diagnosis of respiratory failure due to status asthmaticus. The ED physician spends a total of 60 minutes in patient-directed critical care.

ICD-10-CM
J96.01 (acute respiratory failure with hypoxia)
J45.42 (moderate persistent asthma with status asthmaticus)

CPT
99284 25
99291

Teaching Point: The patient received oxygen, continuous inhalation treatment, and parenteral bronchodilator in the ED. However, these services include no professional component. The facility will report the services because the cost of supplies and clinical staff time are an expense to the facility.

Special Service Codes

99053	Service(s) provided between 10:00 pm and 8:00 am at 24-hour facility, in addition to basic service
99056	Service(s) typically provided in office, provided out of office at request of patient, in addition to basic service
99060	Service(s) provided on an emergency basis, out of office, which disrupts other scheduled office services, in addition to basic service

Special service codes may be used to report services that are an adjunct to the basic service provided. *CPT* guidelines do not restrict the reporting of adjunct special service codes in the ED. However, third-party payers will have specific policies for coverage and payment. Communicate with individual payers to understand their definition or interpretation of the service and coverage and payment policies.

These codes are intended to describe services that are provided outside the normal time frame and location.

Code **99053** would be reported when services are provided between the designated time limits in an ED.

CPT does not restrict reporting of any procedure or service to any specific specialty. However, it would be inappropriate for an ED physician to report code **99056** or **99060** for services provided in the ED.

If appropriate, a non-ED physician could report *CPT* code **99056** or **99060** when he or she provides services in the ED in addition to an outpatient office or clinic visit, ED visit, or consultation E/M code.

Continuum Model for Fever

The continuum model is a teaching tool that gives examples of how common conditions in the ED might be reported based on the severity and/or complexity of the presenting problem(s). The following table presents fever as the presenting complaint across the continuum of codes **99281–99285** plus critical care.

Although the actual assignment of a code for an individual patient may vary from the examples, members of the American Academy of Pediatrics Committee on Coding and Nomenclature generally agree that these examples provide an accurate representation of how 1 condition typically flows across the family of codes.

Additional continuums for 3 common conditions—asthma, head injury, and laceration—are provided online at www.aap.org/cfp.

It is important to remember that all 3 key components (ie, history, examination, and MDM) must be met to support the code selected. Past, family, and social history elements are required only for codes **99284** (1 of 3) and **99285** (2 of 3).

Continuum Model for Fever in the Emergency Department			
CPT Code Vignette	History	Physical Examination (systems)	Medical Decision-making (1. diagnoses; 2. data; 3. risk)
99281 5-month-old with temperature of 99.8°F (37.7°C)	***Problem focused*** CC: fever, fussy HPI: fussy all day, feels warm (not measured at home) ROS: constitutional, respiratory, GI, GU	***Problem focused (Detailed provided in this example.)*** Constitutional, eyes, ENMT, neck, respiratory, cardiovascular, GI, lymphatic, musculoskeletal, neurologic, skin	***Straightforward*** 1. Self-limited problem 2. History from someone other than patient 3. Advice for home care
99282 5-year-old with temperature of 101.0°F (38.3°C) last night and URI symptoms	***Expanded problem focused*** CC: fever, upper respiratory symptoms HPI: started 1 day ago, runny nose, sore throat, nighttime cough, ibuprofen last night (none today) ROS: constitutional, eyes, ENMT, respiratory, cardiovascular, GI, GU, skin PFSH: current medications reviewed, no hospitalizations	***Expanded problem focused*** Constitutional (height, weight, temperature), respiratory system (effort and auscultation), eyes, and ENMT (nasal and oral mucosa)	***Low complexity*** 1. Self-limited problem 2. History from someone other than patient 3. Ibuprofen/acetaminophen as needed
99283 5-year-old with temperature of 101.0°F (38.3°C) and URI symptoms	***Expanded problem focused*** CC: fever, respiratory symptoms HPI: fever for 2 days, runny nose, cough, less active than usual, alternating ibuprofen and acetaminophen (last dose 5 hours ago) ROS: fever; runny nose with dry cough; denies shortness of breath or wheezing; no GI or GU symptoms, musculoskeletal pain PFSH: current medications and allergies updated; no known ill contacts	***Expanded problem focused*** Constitutional (temperature, weight, height, pulse oxygen), eyes, ENMT, respiratory (effort and auscultation), and other pertinent organ systems	***Moderate complexity*** 1. New problem with no additional workup 2. Influenza and SARS-CoV-2 tests, pulse oxygen 3. Antiviral medication prescribed

●=New code   ▲=Revised code   #=Re-sequenced code   +=Add-on code   ★=Telemedicine

	Continuum Model for Fever in the Emergency Department (*continued*)		
CPT Code Vignette	History	**Physical Examination** (systems)	**Medical Decision-making** (1. diagnoses; 2. data; 3. risk)
99284 2-month-old with temperature of 102.2°F (39.0°C)	*Detailed* CC: fever HPI: timing of symptom onset, severity, feeding, elimination, disposition ROS: constitutional, eyes, ENMT, respiratory, cardiovascular, gastrointestinal, urinary, neurologic PFSH: birth history, ill contacts	*Detailed* Constitutional, eyes, ENMT, neck, respiratory, cardiovascular, GI, lymphatic, musculoskeletal, neurologic, skin	*Moderate complexity* 1. New problem to examiner with or without additional workup planned 2. Urinalysis and urine culture, history from someone other than patient 3. Antibiotic prescribed
99285 Neonate presenting with fever	*Comprehensive* CC: fever HPI: duration and severity of symptoms, disposition, feeding, elimination ROS: constitutional, eyes, ENMT, respiratory, cardiovascular, GI, urinary, and at least 3 more (all others reviewed and negative) PFSH: maternal/fetal and birth history, no ill family members or social contacts, no tobacco use or exposure	*Comprehensive* Constitutional, eyes, ENMT, neck, respiratory, cardiovascular, GI, lymphatic, musculoskeletal, neurologic, skin	*High complexity* 1. New problem, additional workup planned (Transfer to inpatient care.) 2. CBC, CMP, blood culture, urine culture, lumbar puncture 3. Empiric antibiotics, acyclovir, admission
99291, 99292 **Critical Care** Febrile neonate with gray appearance	CC: fever seizure, cardiovascular distress		*High complexity* 1. High probability of imminent or life-threatening deterioration requires >30 min of directed patient care. 2. Assess, manipulate, and support vital system function(s) to treat organ/system failure and/or to prevent further life-threatening deterioration of the patient's condition.

Abbreviations: CBC, complete blood cell count; CC, chief complaint; CMP, comprehensive metabolic panel; *CPT, Current Procedural Terminology*; ENMT, ear, nose, mouth, throat; GI, gastrointestinal; GU, genitourinary; HPI, history of present illness; PFSH, past, family, and social history; ROS, review of systems; SARS-CoV-2, severe acute respiratory syndrome coronavirus 2; URI, upper respiratory infection.

Resources

Evaluation and Management

Coding continuums for asthma, head injury, and laceration (www.aap.org/cfp)

"Evaluation and Management Coding in the Emergency Department," May 2018 *AAP Pediatric Coding Newsletter* (https://coding. solutions.aap.org/article.aspx?articleid=2679117; subscription required)

Fracture Care

"Initial Fracture Care: Musculoskeletal or Evaluation and Management," February 2021 *AAP Pediatric Coding Newsletter* (https://coding. solutions.aap.org/article.aspx?articleid=2765276; subscription required)

ICD-10-CM Coding

"Don't Get Bitten When Coding Injuries!" May 2020 *AAP Pediatric Coding Newsletter* (https://coding.solutions.aap.org/article. aspx?articleid=2765180; subscription required)

Repair of Integumentary Lacerations

"You Code It! Integumentary Repair," April 2020 *AAP Pediatric Coding Newsletter* (https://coding.solutions.aap.org/article. aspx?articleid=2763375; subscription required)

Test Your Knowledge!

1. **Which of the following are described by codes for reporting abuse or neglect?**
   a. Suspected, ruled out, or confirmed abuse
   b. Signs, symptoms, or injuries
   c. External cause, activity, and place of occurrence
   d. Initial encounter, subsequent encounter, or encounter for sequela

2. **Which of the following is true for emergency department (ED) service codes (99281–99285)?**
   a. These codes are reported for evaluation and management (E/M) services in any 24-hour care setting.
   b. These codes are reported for care at an urgent care facility.
   c. These codes are reported only by an ED physician.
   d. These codes are only reported for care in an ED as defined by *Current Procedural Terminology* or state regulation.

3. **Which level(s) of ED E/M service includes moderate-complexity medical decision-making?**
   a. **99282**
   b. **99283**
   c. **99284**
   d. Both **99283** and **99284**

4. **Which is true of fracture care in the ED?**
   a. Fracture care without manipulation is reported with an E/M code.
   b. Initial fracture care is reported with modifier **54** if another physician will provide follow-up care.
   c. Initial fracture care is reported with modifier **55** if another physician will provide follow-up care.
   d. Fracture care includes all E/M services by the same physician on the same date.

5. **How much time is included in the service reported with code 99291?**
   a. 60 minutes
   b. Up to 30 minutes
   c. 30–74 minutes
   d. 15 minutes or more

Critical and Intensive Care

Contents

Critical Care Services..425
    Critical Illness or Injury..425
    Hourly Critical Care...425
        Time Units of Hourly Critical Care...427
    Procedures *Not* Bundled With Critical/Intensive Care Services 428

Definition of Neonatal/Perinatal Periods...430
    ICD-10-CM Guidelines and Neonatal Critical Care 430

Attendance at Delivery and Newborn Resuscitation...431
    Attendance at Delivery...431
    Neonatal Resuscitation 431

Neonatal and Pediatric Daily Critical Care Codes..432
    Neonatal Critical and Intensive Care Supervision Requirements...432
        Guidelines for Reporting Neonatal or Pediatric Inpatient Critical Care 433
    Neonatal Critical Care..433
    Pediatric Critical Care..435
    Patients Critically Ill After Surgery 436
    Remote Critical Care Services..436

Initial and Continuing Intensive Care 437
    Coding for Transitions to Different Levels of Neonatal Care 438

Emergency Medical Services Supervision and Patient Transport...439
    Pediatric Critical Care Patient Transport...439
        Face-to-face Critical Care Patient Transport...439
        Non–face-to-face Pediatric Critical Care Patient Transport..440
    Direction of Emergency Medical Services..441

Total Body Systemic and Selective Head Hypothermia 442

Extracorporeal Membrane Oxygenation (ECMO) or Extracorporeal Life Support (ECLS) Services 442
    ECMO/ECLS Cannula Insertion, Repositioning, and Removal 443
    ECMO/ECLS Initiation and Daily Management 444

Sedation...444

Car Seat/Bed Testing...444

Values and Payment...445
    Payment Advocacy..445

Resources...446

Test Your Knowledge!..446

    ●=New code   ▲=Revised code   #=Re-sequenced code   +=Add-on code   ★=Telemedicine

This chapter focuses on correctly coding critical and intensive care, including attendance at delivery; neonatal resuscitation; hourly critical care; critical care of the neonate, infant, and child younger than 6 years; and intensive care of the recovering or low birth weight neonate and infant. Services commonly reported before and after intensive or critical care services, such as consultations and care during emergency transport, are included.

Evaluation and management (E/M) of the child who no longer requires intensive or critical care is discussed in **Chapter 16**, Noncritical Hospital Evaluation and Management Services.

Critical Care Services

Critical Illness or Injury

- A *critical illness or injury* is defined by *Current Procedural Terminology* (*CPT®*) as one that acutely impairs 1 or more vital organs such that there is a high probability of imminent or life-threatening deterioration of the patient's condition.
- Services qualify as critical care *only if both* the injury or illness *and* the treatment being delivered meet the following criteria:
  — The illness or injury acutely impairs 1 or more vital organs as defined previously.
  — The treatment delivered involves high-complexity medical decision-making (MDM) to prevent life-threatening deterioration of the patient's condition.
- Critical care involves high-complexity MDM to assess, manipulate, and support vital organ system function(s); treat single or multiple organ system failure; and/or prevent further life-threatening deterioration of the patient's condition.
- Immaturity alone, or any of the specific procedures, equipment, or therapies associated with care of the immature neonate, does not define critical care.
- Coding critical care is not determined by the location in which the care is delivered but by the nature of the care being delivered and the condition of the patient requiring care.
- Critical care is not limited to an inpatient setting or a critical care area, and a physician of any specialty can provide these services. Services must be provided directly by the physician or other qualified health care professional (QHP).
- Many typically performed procedures are included (bundled) in the work valuation of each critical care code and cannot be reported separately (**Table 18-1**). (See also the Procedures *Not* Bundled With Critical/Intensive Care Services section later in this chapter for commonly provided services not bundled with hourly and/or neonatal and pediatric critical care service.)

Hourly Critical Care

99291   Critical care, E/M of the critically ill or critically injured patient; first 30 to 74 minutes
+99292   each additional 30 minutes (Use in conjunction with **99291**.)

  Guidelines for reporting codes **99291** and **99292**
- Reported when critical care is provided for 30 minutes or more
  — In the outpatient setting (eg, emergency department [ED], office, clinic) *regardless of age*
  — To an inpatient 6 years or older (Daily critical care of a child younger than 6 years is discussed later in this chapter.)
  — Concurrently by a second physician from a different specialty to a critically ill or injured patient, regardless of age
  — To an inpatient aged 5 years or younger when the patient is being transferred to another facility where a receiving physician of the same specialty but different medical group will be reporting the daily inpatient critical care service codes (**99468** and **99469**; **99471** and **99472**; **99475** and **99476**)
  — By the physician physically transporting a critically ill child older than 2 years or when payer policy does not recognize codes **99466** and **99467** (face-to-face transport care of the critically ill or injured patient 24 months or younger [discussed later in this chapter])
- Many procedures typically performed are included (*bundled*) in the work valuation of the code and cannot be reported separately (see **Table 18-1**). (See also the Procedures *Not* Bundled With Critical/Intensive Care Services section later in this chapter for commonly provided services not bundled with hourly and/or neonatal and pediatric critical care services.)
- Procedures not included as bundled may be reported separately (eg, lumbar puncture, endotracheal intubation, thoracentesis).

The reported time of critical care cannot include any time spent performing procedures or services that are reported separately.

Table 18-1. Critical Care Bundled Services			
CPT Code and Procedure	Hourly Critical Care 99291, 99292	Pediatric Transport 99466, 99467	Neonatal/Pediatric Critical and Intensive Care 99468–99476, 99477–99480
Interpretation and Monitoring			
71045 X-ray, chest; single view 71046 X-ray, chest; 2 views	X	X	X
●+93598 Cardiac output measurement(s), thermodilution or other indicator dilution method, performed during cardiac catheterization for the evaluation of congenital heart defects	X	X	X
94760 Pulse oximetry; single determination 94761 multiple determinations (eg, during exercise) 94762 by continuous overnight monitoring	X	X	X
Vascular Access Procedures			
36000 Introduction of needle or intracatheter, vein	X	X	X
36140 Catheterization extremity artery			X
36400 Venipuncture, <3 years, requiring physician or QHP skill; femoral or jugular vein 36405 scalp vein 36406 other vein		X	X
36410 Venipuncture, ≥3 years, requiring physician or QHP skill	X		X
36415 Collection of venous blood by venipuncture	X	X	X
36420 Venipuncture, cutdown; younger than age 1 year			X
36430 Transfusion, blood or blood components 36440 Push transfusion, blood, 2 years or younger			X
36510 Catheterization of umbilical vein, newborn			X
36555 Insertion of non-tunneled CICC; <5 years of age			X
36591 Collection blood from venous access device	X	X	X
36600 Arterial puncture, withdrawal of blood for diagnosis	X	X	X
36620 Arterial catheterization, percutaneous 36660 Catheterization, umbilical artery, newborn			X
Other Procedures			
31500 Endotracheal intubation, emergency			X
43752 Nasogastric/orogastric intubation, fluoroscopic guidance	X	X	X
43753 Gastric intubation including lavage if performed	X	X	X
51100 Aspiration of bladder; by needle			X
51701 Insertion of non-indwelling bladder catheter 51702 Temporary indwelling bladder catheter; simple			X
62270 Spinal puncture, lumbar, diagnostic			X
92953 Temporary transcutaneous pacing	X	X	X

	Hourly Critical Care 99291, 99292	Pediatric Transport 99466, 99467	Neonatal/Pediatric Critical and Intensive Care 99468–99476, 99477–99480
Table 18-1 (*continued*)			
***CPT* Code and Procedure**			
Other Procedures (*continued*)			
94002 Ventilation initiation; inpatient/observation, initial day **94003** each subsequent day	x	x	x
94004 Ventilation initiation; nursing facility, per day	x		x
94375 Respiratory flow volume loop			x
94610 Intrapulmonary surfactant administration			x
94660 CPAP initiation and management **94662** CNP, initiation and management	x	x	x
94780 Car seat/bed testing, infants through 12 months; 60 minutes **94781** each additional full 30 minutes			x

Abbreviations: CICC, centrally inserted central venous catheter; CNP, continuous negative pressure ventilation; CPAP, continuous positive airway pressure; *CPT, Current Procedural Terminology*; QHP, qualified health care professional.

- Critical care is not permitted to be reported as a split/shared service (ie, the times of a physician and QHP cannot be combined and reported as a single service). When the physician and neonatal nurse practitioner (NNP) provide critical care services to a patient, only one may report the code.

Notice: At the time of publication, CMS has proposed, but not finalized, significant changes to the Medicare policy for split/shared visits. Please visit the American Academy of Pediatrics website (www.aap.org/cfp or www.aap.org/errata) to check for updates.

- Codes **99291** and **99292** may be reported by an individual of a *different specialty* from either the same or a different group on the same day that neonatal or pediatric critical care services are reported by another individual (**99468–99476**).
- A teaching physician may report time-based critical care services only when he or she was present for the entire period for which the claim is submitted and that time is supported in documentation of the service.
- When inpatient and outpatient critical care services are provided to a neonate, infant, or child younger than 6 years on the same date by the same physician (or physician of the same group and specialty), only the *inpatient* critical care codes are reported (**99468–99476**). See exceptions included in the Neonatal and Pediatric Daily Critical Care Codes and Emergency Medical Services Supervision and Patient Transport sections later in this chapter.
- Other significant, separately identifiable E/M services (eg, **99212–99215, 99281–99285**) can be reported in addition to time-based critical care services as appropriate. Do not count time spent in separately reported E/M services in critical care time.

  National Correct Coding Initiative (NCCI) edits bundle ED E/M codes **99281–99285** with codes **99291** and **99292**. Appending a modifier will not override the edits. Payers who use these edits will not pay for both services on the same date by the same physician or physicians of the same group practice and same specialty.

Time Units of Hourly Critical Care

- Reporting is time based. **Table 18-2** lists times and billing units. The total floor or unit time devoted to the patient in the provision of critical care is used in code selection. Critical care time includes physician–patient face-to-face time or time spent on the patient's *unit or floor* directly related to the patient's care (eg, hands-on care at the bedside, reviewing test results, discussing care with other medical staff or family, documenting services in the medical record).
- Time spent in the provision of critical care does not need to be continuous. The cumulative time of critical care provided on a single date of service is used to calculate the units of service provided.

Chapter 18. Critical and Intensive Care

When a *continuous period* of critical care occurs before and after midnight, report the total time on the date that the period of care was initiated. Do not report a second initial hour of critical care for the period beginning at midnight.

Table 18-2. Reporting Hourly Critical Care Services

Do not report services of <30 minutes as critical care; report the appropriate E/M service for the site where service is provided.

Duration of Face-to-face Critical Care	30–74 min	75–104 min	105–134 min	135–164 min	165–194 min
CPT Codes and Units of Service	99291	99291 × 1, 99292 × 1	99291 × 1, 99292 × 2	99291 × 1, 99292 × 3	99291 × 1, 99292 × 4

Abbreviations: *CPT, Current Procedural Terminology;* E/M, evaluation and management.

- The physician must be immediately available to the patient during time reported as critical care. No time spent in activities that take place out of the unit, off the patient's floor, or consulting with other caregivers from home is included in critical care time.
- The time required to report code **99291** must be met by a single physician. If multiple physicians and other QHPs from the same group practice and same specialty care for a patient after a single physician has provided the initial 30 minutes of critical care, combine the total time and report with code **99292** as appropriate. Do not report **99291** more than once per day. All services must be reported under the name and National Provider Identifier of a single physician.
- Code **99291** is reported once on a given date of service when 30 to 74 minutes of critical care is performed. If less than 30 minutes of critical care is provided, an appropriate E/M service (eg, **99202–99215** for office services, **99221–99233** for inpatient hospital care) is reported.
- Code **99292** is reported with 1 unit for each additional period up to 30 minutes beyond the previous period. Time spent providing critical care services must be documented in the medical record.

Examples

➤ **A 4-year-old with asthma arrives to the ED with acute respiratory distress.** The ED physician provides an hour of critical care before the child is admitted to the intensive care unit by an intensivist.

Code **99291** with 1 unit of service (30–74 minutes) is reported by the ED physician. The intensivist will report the appropriate level of daily hospital and/or hourly critical care.

➤ **A pediatrician is called to see a 1-day-old neonate in the newborn nursery who received subsequent hospital care earlier in the day by the same physician or a physician or QHP of the same specialty and same group practice.** The neonate is pale and hypotensive; perioral cyanosis is noted with oxygen saturation of 80%. Despite the pediatrician starting the patient on 100% oxygen, the patient continues to deteriorate, requiring intubation, umbilical vein catheter placement, and referral for a transport to a higher-level neonatal intensive care unit (NICU). The physician spends 2 hours stabilizing the neonate, including antibiotics, intravenous (IV) fluids, and prostaglandin drip. The physician explains to the family the need to transfer and assisted the transport team.

Codes **99291** × 1 (first 30–74 minutes) and **99292** × 2 (75–134 minutes) are reported in addition to the E/M code reported for the visit earlier in the day. Codes **31500** (endotracheal intubation, emergency) and **36510** (catheterization of umbilical vein for diagnosis or therapy, newborn) are separately reported.

Some payers may require modifier **25** to be appended to the code for the subsequent hospital care (eg, **99231 25**). However, NCCI edits do not bundle subsequent hospital care and critical care services. (For more on edits, see **Chapter 2**, Modifiers and Coding Edits.)

Procedures *Not* Bundled With Critical/Intensive Care Services

When reporting hourly critical or neonatal and pediatric critical and intensive care services, many services commonly performed in the provision of critical care are not bundled into the intensive or critical care services. However, claim edits may require appending a modifier to indicate the services were distinct. Examples of procedures that are not bundled with critical care services include (not all-inclusive)

- Thoracentesis (**32554**, **32555**) (via needle or pigtail catheter)
- Percutaneous pleural drainage with insertion of indwelling catheter (**32556**, **32557**)

- Complete (double volume) exchange transfusion (**36450**, newborn; **36455**, other)
- Partial exchange transfusion (**36456**)
- Abdominal paracentesis (**49082**, **49083**)
- Bone marrow aspiration (**38220**)
- Circumcision (**54150**)
- Cardioversion (**92960**)
- Cardiopulmonary resuscitation (**92950**)
- Extracorporeal membrane oxygenation (ECMO) (**33946–33949**)
- Peripherally inserted central catheter (**36568–36573**)
- Insertion of non-tunneled centrally inserted central venous catheter, older than 5 years (**36556**)
- Replacement (rewire) of non-tunneled centrally inserted central venous catheter (**36580**)
- Therapeutic apheresis (**36511–36514**)
- Insertion of cannula for hemodialysis, other purpose (separate procedure); vein to vein (**36800**)
- Placement of needle for intraosseous infusion (**36680**)
- Initiation of selective head or total body hypothermia in the critically ill neonate (**99184**)

Payer edits may vary, and certain services are bundled unless performed for diagnostic purposes rather than monitoring. The following instructions from the Medicaid NCCI manual demonstrate reporting of diagnostic services:

Lumbar puncture (**62270**, **62328**) and suprapubic bladder aspiration (**51100**) are separately reportable with hourly critical care (**99291**, **99292**) but are *not separately reportable* with the pediatric and neonatal critical care service codes (**99468–99472**, **99475**, **99476**) and the intensive care services codes (**99477–99480**).

> **Emergency cardiac defibrillation is included in cardiopulmonary resuscitation (92950). Per the Medicaid National Correct Coding Initiative manual, if emergency cardiac defibrillation without cardiopulmonary resuscitation is performed in the emergency department or critical/intensive care unit, the cardiac defibrillation service is not separately reportable. Report code 92960 only for elective cardioversion.**

Example

➤ **During an encounter with a child who was found unconscious in a swimming pool, a physician spends 10 minutes performing cardiopulmonary resuscitation (CPR) and then another 45 minutes providing critical care before the patient is transferred to another facility.** Critical care service (**99291**) time is documented and distinctly identifiable in the patient record from the time spent performing the separately reportable CPR (**92950**), for which start and stop times were documented.

Diagnostic rhythm electrocardiogram (ECG) codes **93040–93042** are reported only when there is a sudden change in a patient status associated with a change in cardiac rhythm that requires a diagnostic rhythm ECG and return to the critical care unit. When separately reporting a diagnostic ECG, do not include the time for this service in the time spent providing critical care. Modifier **59** is appended to the ECG code when indicated by patient status and performed on the same date as critical care services.

Transesophageal echocardiography (TEE) monitoring (**93318**) without probe placement is not separately reportable by a physician performing critical care E/M services. However, if a physician places a transesophageal probe to be used for TEE monitoring on the same date of service that the physician performs critical care E/M services, code **93318** may be reported with modifier **59** or **XU** (unusual nonoverlapping service). The time necessary for probe placement *shall not be included* in the critical care time reported with *CPT* codes **99291** and **99292**. This is true for all separately reportable procedures performed on a patient receiving critical care E/M services. Diagnostic TEE services may be separately reportable by a physician performing critical care E/M services.

> **American Academy of Pediatrics Tip: Payers may require modifier 25 to be appended to the codes for critical care services rather than appending modifier 59 to the procedure code. Modifier 59 is intended to distinguish 2 distinct non–evaluation and management services.**

Many practice management and billing systems include claim scrubbers that provide an alert that claim edits apply and a modifier may be appropriate based on clinical circumstances. Payers may also offer online tools for determining when code pair edits apply.

Definition of Neonatal/Perinatal Periods

For coding purposes, the neonatal period begins at birth and continues through the completed 28th day after birth, ending on the 29th calendar day after birth. The day of birth is considered day 0 (zero). Therefore, the day after birth is considered day 1.

This definition is important in selecting the initial- and subsequent-day neonatal critical care codes **99468** and **99469** as well as code **99477** for the initial hospital care of the neonate, 28 days or younger, who requires intensive observation, frequent interventions, and other intensive care services.

ICD-10-CM Guidelines and Neonatal Critical Care

It is important to correctly assign *International Classification of Diseases, 10th Revision, Clinical Modification* (*ICD-10-CM*) codes that reflect the diagnoses for which critical care services were required. Assign codes for neonatal conditions that require treatment or further investigation, prolong the length of stay, or require resource utilization as well as codes for conditions that have implications for future health care needs.

> When care is provided by the attending physician during the birth admission, report first a code from category **Z38** (liveborn infants according to place of birth and type of delivery). Codes for abnormal conditions are reported secondary to the code for live birth. When a neonate is transferred to another facility after birth, the admission to the receiving facility is not a birth admission and **Z38** codes are not reported.

- *ICD-10-CM* contains codes (**P00–P96**) for conditions originating in the perinatal period described as having their origin in the fetal or perinatal period (before birth through the first 28 days after birth) even if morbidity occurs later. Again, this period includes the completed 28th day after birth with the day of birth being counted as day 0 (zero).
  - These codes are only to be reported when the condition originates in this time, but they can be reported beyond the perinatal period if the condition(s) causes morbidity or is the primary reason for or contributing to the reason the patient is receiving health care.
  - The perinatal code should continue to be used regardless of the patient's age if a condition originates in the perinatal period and continues throughout the patient's life.

Example

> ➤ **A 30-day-old who was a 26-weeks' gestation preterm neonate continues to require critical or intensive care due to a condition originating in the perinatal period.** The *ICD-10-CM* code that is linked to the critical or intensive care service is the appropriate perinatal code (**P00–P96**) for the condition(s) managed or treated.

- Any condition *originating* after the perinatal period (29th calendar day after birth and beyond) is not reported with codes for perinatal conditions.
- A diagnosis of prematurity must be documented to support reporting of a code for prematurity. Coders cannot assign codes for prematurity based solely on documented gestational age.
- Codes in category **P05** are reported for the newborn affected by fetal growth restriction or slow intrauterine growth.
  - Codes in subcategory **P05.0** are used to report that the neonate is light for gestational age but not small (weight below but length above the 10th percentile). These neonates have often been said to exhibit *asymmetrical growth restriction*.
  - Codes in subcategory **P05.1** are used to report the neonate is small and light (both weight and length below the 10th percentile) for gestational age. These newborns have often been said to exhibit *symmetrical growth restriction* or *intrauterine growth restriction*.
- Code **P05.2** is provided for reporting fetal (intrauterine) malnutrition affecting a newborn whose weight is not below the 10th percentile and has a significant disparity between weight and length percentiles.

> Learn more about reporting codes in category **P05** in the December 2020 *AAP Pediatric Coding Newsletter™* article, "Coding for Abnormalities in Fetal Growth" (https://coding.solutions.aap.org/article.aspx?articleid=2765246; subscription required).

- Codes from category **P07** (disorders of newborn related to short gestation and low birth weight [not due to fetal malnutrition]) are reported based on the recorded birth weight (*not less than the 10th percentile*) and estimated gestational age to indicate these conditions are the cause of morbidity or reason for additional care of the newborn.

— When both are documented, weight is sequenced before age.

— These codes may be reported for a child as well as for an adult who was preterm or had a low birth weight as a newborn and this is affecting the patient's current health status.

Codes in subcategory **P07.3-** (preterm newborn) should be reported for neonates born at 36 weeks' gestation who stay in the newborn nursery or who are cared for in the NICU.

> Codes in subcategory **P07.0-** (extremely low birth weight newborn) and **P07.1-** (other low birth weight newborn) are not reported in conjunction with codes in category **P05** (disorders of the newborn due to slow fetal growth and fetal malnutrition). However, subcategory **P07.2-** (extreme immaturity of newborn) and **P07.3-** (preterm newborn) may be reported in addition to category **P05**.

Attendance at Delivery and Newborn Resuscitation

Attendance at Delivery

99464   Attendance at delivery (when requested by the delivering physician or other qualified health care professional) and initial stabilization of newborn

Attendance at delivery (**99464**) is only reported when the physical presence of the provider is requested by the delivering physician and indicated for a newborn who may require immediate intervention (ie, stabilization, resuscitation, or evaluation for potential problems).

● Includes initial drying, stimulation, suctioning, blow-by oxygen, or continuous positive airway pressure (CPAP) without positive-pressure ventilation (PPV); a cursory visual inspection of the neonate; assignment of Apgar scores; and discussion of the care of the newborn with the delivering physician and parents. A quick look in the delivery room or examination after stabilization is not sufficient to support reporting of **99464**.

— When qualifying resuscitative efforts are provided, code **99465** (delivery/birthing room resuscitation) is reported instead. Codes **99464** and **99465** cannot be reported on the same day of service.

See **Chapter 15**, Hospital Care of the Newborn, for further discussion and coding examples.

Neonatal Resuscitation

99465   Delivery/birthing room resuscitation, provision of positive pressure ventilation and/or chest compressions in the presence of acute inadequate ventilation and/or cardiac output

Attendance at delivery with neonatal resuscitation (**99465**)

● Requires PPV delivered by any means (resuscitation bag or T-piece resuscitator) and/or cardiac compressions.

● Do *not* report when T-piece resuscitator is used to provide CPAP only. If the neonate responds to provision of CPAP with an adequate respiratory effort, code **99464** should be reported.

● May be reported in addition to any initial care service, including initial critical care (**99468**), hourly critical care (**99291**, **99292**), initial neonatal intensive care (**99477**), or normal newborn care (**99460**) if the resuscitation results in a stable term neonate.

> Payers may require modifier **25** (significant, separately identifiable evaluation and management [E/M] service) appended to the code for E/M services reported in addition to code **99464** or **99465**. However, National Correct Coding Initiative edits do not bundle these services.

● Medically necessary procedures (eg, **31500**, intubation, endotracheal, emergency procedure; **31515**, laryngoscopy, direct, for aspiration; **36510**, catheterization of umbilical vein for diagnosis or therapy, newborn; **94610**, surfactant administration) essential to successful resuscitation that are performed in the delivery room prior to admission may also be reported in addition to codes **99465** and **99468** or **99477** (initial neonatal critical or intensive care).

— Do not separately report services performed as a convenience before admission to the NICU.

— Medical record documentation must clearly support that the services are provided as a required measure for emergency resuscitation and not as part of an admission protocol.

> Documentation of neonatal resuscitation should explicitly state that the neonate demonstrated respiratory and/or cardiac instability requiring intervention, including apnea or inadequate respiratory effort to support gas exchange; that the provider instituted positive-pressure ventilation (PPV); and the neonate's response to the PPV.

Example

➤ **A neonatologist attends an emergency cesarean delivery of a 34-weeks' gestation neonate whose mother has known, poorly controlled diabetes mellitus and a history of drug misuse. The neonate is born limp and cyanotic with no spontaneous respiratory activity.** The resuscitation includes PPV, intubation, and placement of an umbilical vein catheter with physiologic (normal) saline bolus (solution). The newborn, who is continuously bradycardic and pale, is admitted to the NICU where the neonatologist administers surfactant and initiates red blood cell transfusion.

The intubation and umbilical vein catheterization are separately reported procedures provided as part of the resuscitation and not as a convenience to the physician prior to admission.	**CPT** **99465** (delivery/birthing room resuscitation) **31500** (endotracheal intubation, emergency) **36510** (catheterization of umbilical vein for diagnosis or therapy, newborn) **99468 25** (initial neonatal critical care) **36450** (exchange transfusion, blood; newborn)

Teaching Point: Modifier **25** is appended to code **99468** to signify a significant, separately identifiable E/M service provided in addition to codes **31500** and **36510** because these services are bundled by NCCI edits. Codes **99465** and **99468** are not bundled by NCCI edits, but individual payers may require modifier **25** to designate separately identifiable critical care services on the same date. The surfactant administration is not separately reported when performed in conjunction with neonatal critical care. However, the red blood cell transfusion is separately reported.

Neonatal and Pediatric Daily Critical Care Codes

Codes are
- Reported for critical care of children younger than 6 years in the inpatient setting.
- Global—they encompass all E/M services by a single provider (or provider of the exact same specialty in the same group) on 1 calendar date. Other physicians and QHPs providing critical care must report hourly critical care code **99291** or **99292**. (See exceptions under the Guidelines for Reporting Neonatal or Pediatric Inpatient Critical Care section later in this chapter.)
- Bundled—they have commonly performed procedures included in the E/M codes. See **Table 18-1** for services and procedures that are included with neonatal critical care codes.
- Not time based. Prolonged services *may not* be reported in conjunction with neonatal or pediatric critical care services.
- Not based on typical E/M rules and the performance and documentation of key components (ie, history, physical examination, MDM, and/or time).
- Reported based on postnatal age (see the Definition of Neonatal/Perinatal Periods section earlier in this chapter) and initial or subsequent care (**Table 18-3**).

Table 18-3. Neonatal and Pediatric Global Critical Care			
Inpatient Neonatal Critical Care	**28 Days or Younger**	**29 Days Through 24 Months of Age**	**2 Through 5 Years of Age**
Initial inpatient neonatal critical care	99468	99471	99475
Subsequent inpatient neonatal critical care	99469	99472	99476

Neonatal Critical and Intensive Care Supervision Requirements

Under the heading Inpatient Neonatal and Pediatric Critical Care Service, *CPT* states that codes **99468**, **99469**, and **99471–99476** are used to report services provided by a physician "directing the inpatient care" of a critically ill neonate, infant, or child through 5 years of age. Constant in-house attendance by the supervising physician is not a requirement of neonatal critical and intensive care. However, the codes' values were established assuming the physician is physically present and participating directly in the patient's care for a significant portion of the reported service.
- Documentation in the patient's chart should reflect this active participation, including documentation of hands-on care, such as a personal physical examination.

- Supervision of all the care from a distance without face-to-face care is not reported as critical or intensive care.
- Care must be provided by the reporting physician, but it also includes the services provided by the health care team functioning under the direct supervision of the physician *or an advanced nurse practitioner who is employed by the physician or physician group* and when allowed under state licensure requirements.
- Typically, a neonate or infant is evaluated during numerous intervals throughout a calendar day, depending on the clinical needs of the patient. While the critical care team is continuously present with the neonate or infant, overnight in-house care by the reporting physician is determined by the complexity of the total population of neonates cared for in a nursery or the changes in a specific neonate's or infant's condition that cannot be adequately assessed or managed over the telephone.
- Medical record documentation must support the need for and meet the definition of critical care (eg, complex MDM, high probability of imminent or life-threatening deterioration, organ system failure).

> **For more information, refer to "Global Per Diem Critical Care Codes: Direct Supervision and Reporting Guidelines," available online at www.aap.org/cfp.**

Documentation must support the physician's presence and supervision of the team as well as the critical nature of the child's disease. As noted previously, the directing physician is not required to be present or in the facility for the entire day. Rather, because neonatal and pediatric critical and intensive care may require numerous encounters to reevaluate and manage the patient each day, neonatal and pediatric critical and intensive care codes encompass all the sick care provided within a calendar day.

Coding Conundrum: Selecting the Appropriate Code

Many diagnoses or conditions, such as respiratory distress, infection, seizures, mild to moderate hypoxic-ischemic encephalopathy, and metabolic disorders, can be reported with codes **99468**, **99477**, or **99221–99223**. The patient's clinical status, required level of monitoring and observation, and present body weight will determine which of these code sets is chosen. Selection of the service must be justified by medical record documentation.

Guidelines for Reporting Neonatal or Pediatric Inpatient Critical Care

- The physician or NNP (subject to state regulations, scope of practice, and hospital privilege credentials) primarily responsible for the patient on the date of service should report the neonatal or pediatric critical care codes. When both the physician and NNP provide critical care services to a patient, only one may report the code.
- If critical care is provided in both the outpatient and inpatient settings by the same physician or a physician of the same specialty and group, only the inpatient code is reported.
- Codes are reported only once per day, per patient.
- When the same physician or physicians of the same specialty and group practice provide pediatric critical care during transport of a child 24 months or younger (**99466**, **99467**, **99485**, **99486**) and critical care after admission to the receiving facility, both services are reported and modifier **25** is appended to the transport code.
- Initial critical care codes (**99468**, **99471**, **99475**) are only reported once per calendar day and *once per hospital stay* for a given patient. For a second episode of critical care during the same hospital stay, report a subsequent critical care code (**99469**, **99472**, **99476**).
- Subsequent critical care may be reported on multiple days even if there is no change in the patient's condition if the patient continues to meet the critical care definition and documentation supports this level of service.
- Care may be provided on any unit of a hospital facility.

Subsequent-day neonatal and pediatric intensive care codes (**99478–99480**) are reported when critical care is no longer required and the neonate who weighs 5,000 g or less on the day of service requires more intensive care than what is typically provided under routine subsequent hospital care (**99231–99233**). Once a neonate weighing at least 5,001 g no longer requires critical care services, report an appropriate level of subsequent-day inpatient hospital care codes (**99231–99233**).

Neonatal Critical Care

99468	Initial inpatient neonatal critical care, per day, for the evaluation and management of a critically ill neonate, 28 days of age or younger
99469	Subsequent inpatient neonatal critical care, per day, for the evaluation and management of a critically ill neonate, 28 days of age or younger

Chapter 18. Critical and Intensive Care

Selection of the appropriate code will depend on the newborn's or infant's condition and the intensity of the service provided and documented on a particular day of service.

- Codes may be reported in addition to normal newborn care (**99460** or **99462**) or neonatal consultation (**99251–99255**) when the patient receives normal newborn care or consultation and then, at a subsequent separate encounter on the same day, requires critical care. Each service should be reported with the appropriate diagnosis code to support the service (eg, diagnosis codes for well newborn and the defined illness). However, the neonatologist would report only critical or intensive care services if a transfer of care occurs at the initial consultation.

> National Correct Coding Initiative edits bundle normal newborn care to neonatal critical care, but you may use modifier 25 (significant, separately identifiable evaluation and management service) to override the edit under appropriate circumstances (eg, separate encounters).

- Only a single code representing the highest level of service performed and documented is reported if all the care was provided by a single physician or physicians of the same specialty and group practice. However, if the intensity of care progresses over the day and services are provided by physicians from different groups or specialties, or the patient is transferred to another facility, each physician reports a different level of service.

Coding Conundrum: Applying the Critical Care Definition

While immaturity commonly leads to many levels of organ dysfunction that will increase the risk of a critical illness in a newborn, neither immaturity alone nor any of the specific procedures or therapies associated with care of the immature neonate or infant qualifies alone for reporting critical care. The physician must use his or her experience and judgment in assigning the *Current Procedural Terminology* definition of critical care. In summary, these are patients presently at clear risk of death or serious morbidity, requiring close observation and frequent interventions and assessments, and high-complexity medical decision-making (MDM) is apparent in the medical record documentation. No single criterion places or excludes a patient from this category, and the patient is not required to demonstrate all the characteristics listed in this chapter. The most convincing way to demonstrate the appropriate application of a critical care code is to clearly document the neonate's condition in the medical record, noting the risks to the patient, frequency of needed assessments and interventions, degree and type of organ failure(s) the patient is presently experiencing, and complexity of the MDM.

Examples

➤ **A term 3,500-g neonate is born cyanotic following a vaginal delivery.** He has minimal respiratory distress and appears otherwise vigorous. He is brought to the NICU, where a chest radiograph shows dramatic cardiomegaly and a marked increase in pulmonary markings. An umbilical artery catheter and umbilical vein catheter are inserted to determine blood gases. An ECG is performed, and a pediatric cardiologist is consulted to obtain an emergency echocardiogram.

It is important to remember that respiratory support (ie, mechanical ventilation) is not required to report critical care services. In this case, serious cyanosis and clear evidence of cardiac decompensation qualify as critical care. Code **99468** would be reported for initial date of neonatal critical care services. The umbilical vessel catheterizations are bundled with **99468**. Depending on the findings on the echocardiogram and a need for cardiac intensive care, the cardiologist may report hourly critical care for any additional time beyond the echocardiogram. If critical care is not provided, the cardiologist would report consultative services (**99251–99255**) or subsequent hospital care (if requirements for reporting a consultation are not met). (See **Chapter 16**, Noncritical Hospital Evaluation and Management Services, for more information on reporting consultations and reporting to payers who do not recognize consultation codes.) If the neonate were transferred to a cardiac center by the neonatologist, the neonatologist would report time-based critical care codes (**99291**, **99292**) for the care provided prior to the transfer rather than **99468**. The receiving physician in the cardiac center would report code **99468** for the initial date of critical care.

> Only 1 individual reports daily critical care services for each patient per date of service. Initial critical care is reported only once per admission.

➤ **A 6-day-old born at 31 weeks' gestation with unstable apnea is weaned off the ventilator to CPAP.** She is continued on caffeine, partial parenteral nutrition by central vein, and IV antibiotics.

Code **99469** is reported because the medical record continues to document the neonate's instability and the continued need for critical care services.

Coding Conundrum: Apnea in Neonates

Apnea in neonates may be an expected component of preterm birth and may be effectively managed by manual stimulation, pharmacological stimulation, high-flow nasal oxygen, or continuous positive airway pressure. At other times, this symptom is associated with a serious underlying problem(s) and reflects the instability of a critically ill neonate. When this is the case, one or more of the same interventions will be required. The physician must employ his or her best clinical judgment and clearly document the factors that make the patient's present condition critical (or require intensive care). The same requirements for organ failure, risk of imminent deterioration, and complex medical decision-making apply. With apnea and many other conditions, the following drive correct code selection: the total picture of the neonate with the diagnosis, clinical presentation, and immediate threat to life; amount of hands-on and supervisory care provided by the physician; and the level of intervention needed to manage that neonate's conditions on a given day. When critical care codes are reported, the documentation must support the physician's judgment that the patient is critically ill and services provided are commensurate with the condition on that day of service on which critical care codes are reported.

Pediatric Critical Care

99471   Initial inpatient pediatric critical care, per day, for the evaluation and management of a critically ill infant or young child, 29 days through 24 months of age

99472   Subsequent inpatient pediatric critical care, per day, for the evaluation and management of a critically ill infant or young child, 29 days through 24 months of age

99475   Initial inpatient pediatric critical care, per day, for the evaluation and management of a critically ill infant or young child, 2 through 5 years of age

99476   Subsequent inpatient pediatric critical care, per day, for the evaluation and management of a critically ill infant or young child, 2 through 5 years of age

Codes **99471–99476** are used to report direction of the inpatient care of a critically ill infant or young child outside of the neonatal period. Only 1 physician reports the daily critical care codes for each calendar day of care. Services are provided to patients who are at least 29 days of age (postnatal age with day of birth being 0 [zero]) until the child reaches 6 years of age. Initial pediatric critical care for children of these ages is reported with code **99471** (29 days through 24 months of age—up to, but not including, the second birthday) or **99475** (2 through 5 years of age—up to, but not including, the sixth birthday).

Initial pediatric critical care codes (**99471**, **99475**) are only reported by a single physician once per calendar day, *per hospital stay,* for a given patient. If the patient is stepped down from critical care to continued hospital care and then requires a subsequent episode of critical care during the same hospital stay, report a subsequent critical care code (**99472**, **99476**) on the initial and each subsequent date the child remains critical.

Examples

➤ **A 22-month-old girl with status epilepticus is initially treated by the ED physician (1 hour of critical care).** Although seizures were initially controlled, pharmacologic management led to irregular respiratory activity, lethargy, and hypotension. The patient was admitted to the pediatric intensive care unit at 11:00 pm that evening by the critical care attending physician, who intubated her, placed her on a ventilator, began fluid expansion, used dobutamine to control her blood pressure, and made arrangements for a bedside electroencephalogram (EEG).

The ED physician would report 1 hour of critical care (**99291**). The pediatrician or intensivist would report their services with the initial inpatient pediatric critical care code (**99471**) for that calendar day, even though only 1 hour of care was provided. One hour later, after midnight, a new date of service would begin. The intubation is bundled with **99471** and cannot be separately billed.

➤ **A hospitalist admits a 5-year-old to observation for exacerbation of asthma that initially improved with treatment.** Later the same day, the patient is found to be in respiratory failure and the hospitalist provides 35 minutes of critical care services before transferring the patient's care to a pediatric intensivist. The pediatric intensivist assumes management of the critically ill patient at 10:00 pm.

The hospitalist reports initial observation care (**99218–99220**) based the level of service provided and appends modifier **25** to indicate that this service is significant and separately identifiable from critical care services reported with code **99291**. The intensivist reports code **99475** (initial inpatient pediatric critical care, per day, for the E/M of a critically ill infant or young child, 2 through 5 years of age). The intensivist will report code **99476** for each subsequent calendar day on which critical care services are provided.

➤ **A 1-month-old is admitted by a surgeon following consultation in the ED.** The patient presented with 2-day history of vomiting, initial inconsolable crying and now lethargy, and decreased urine output. The patient is diagnosed with malrotation and is taken to the operating room where volvulus is found, necessitating bowel resection. Eight days later, the patient is recovering well and is in preparation for discharge. On day 9, the patient's temperature is 38.4°C (101.1°F). The incision area is swollen and erythematous. Sepsis evaluation is initiated and antibiotics are started. Within hours the patient becomes hypotensive, requiring vasopressors. The surgeon requests a transfer of care to an intensivist, who accepts the transfer and provides critical care to the critically ill patient. The intensivist reports code **99471** (initial inpatient pediatric critical care, per day, for the E/M of a critically ill infant or young child, 29 days through 24 months of age). The intensivist will report **99472** for each subsequent calendar day on which critical care services are provided. The surgeon's postoperative care, other than a return to the operating room, is included in the global period of the surgery.

Patients Critically Ill After Surgery

Postoperative care of a surgical patient is included in the surgeon's global surgical package. For some neonatal surgical care, critical care days are included in the work values assigned to surgical procedures (eg, **39503** [repair of diaphragmatic hernia], **43314** [esophagoplasty, thoracic approach; with repair of tracheoesophageal fistula], **49605** [repair of large omphalocele or gastroschisis; with or without prosthesis]).

However

- If a second physician (eg, intensivist, hospitalist) provides care for the routine postoperative patient, the surgeon must append modifier **54** (surgical care only) to the surgical code. (A formal transfer of care should be documented.)
- If the surgeon provides and reports the complete surgical care package, a request for consultation from another specialist may be made.
- If the patient's course is not typical and an unexpected complication occurs that requires concurrent care from another specialist, both may report their service.

Example

➤ **If a surgeon first requests a consultation, an initial consultation code (or other appropriate E/M code based on the payer's payment policy for consultations) would be reported by the consultant.** If the surgeon requests concurrent care for a specific medical problem, time-based critical care (**99291**, **99292**) or subsequent hospital care (**99231–99233**) codes would be reported dependent on the child's condition and care provided. The diagnosis code representing the condition or symptom being treated should be reported with the concurrent *CPT* code. The rationale for the need for concurrent care must be documented in the surgeon's notes.

Remote Critical Care Services

G0508 Telehealth consultation, critical care, physicians typically spend 60 minutes communicating with the patient via telehealth (initial)

G0509 Telehealth consultation, critical care, physicians typically spend 50 minutes communicating with the patient via telehealth (subsequent)

Remote critical care is the direct delivery of medical care by a physician(s) for a critically ill or critically injured patient from an off-site location (ie, when a critically ill or injured patient requires additional critical care resources that are not available on-site). *CPT* instructs to report code **99499** (unlisted E/M service) appended with modifier **95** (synchronous telemedicine service rendered via a real-time interactive audio and video telecommunications system) for neonatal and pediatric critical care via telemedicine. Other payers may allow reporting with codes **G0508** or **G0509** with place of service **02**. It is recommended that practices verify health plan policies for provision of critical care services via telemedicine before initiating these services.

See **Chapter 20**, Digital Medicine Services: Technology-Enhanced Care Delivery, for more information on reporting telemedicine services, including remote critical care.

Initial and Continuing Intensive Care

99477   Initial hospital care, per day, for the evaluation and management of the neonate, 28 days of age or younger, who requires intensive observation, frequent interventions, and other intensive care services

99478   Subsequent intensive care, per day, for the evaluation and management of the recovering very low birth weight infant (present body weight less than 1500 grams)

99479   Subsequent intensive care, per day, for the evaluation and management of the recovering low birth weight infant (present body weight of 1500–2500 grams)

99480   Subsequent intensive care, per day, for the evaluation and management of the recovering infant (present body weight of 2501–5000 grams)

> Continuing intensive care services provided to an infant weighing more than 5,000 g (approximately 11.02 lb) are reported with subsequent hospital care codes (99231–99233). Documentation of these services must support 2 of 3 key components or the total unit or floor time and time spent counseling and/or coordinating care.

Neonatal and pediatric intensive care codes (**99477–99480**) may be used to report care for neonates or infants who are not critically ill but have a need for intensive monitoring, observation, and frequent assessments by the health care team and supervision by the physician. This includes

- Neonates who require intensive but not critical care services from birth
- Neonates who are no longer critically ill but require intensive physician and health care team observation and interventions
- Recovering low birth weight infants who require a higher level of care than that defined by other hospital care services

These neonates or infants often have a continued need for oxygen, parenteral or gavage enteral nutrition, treatment for apnea of prematurity, and thermoregulation from an Isolette or radiant warmer, and may be recovering from cardiac or surgical care. The intensive services described by these codes include intensive cardiac and respiratory monitoring, continuous and/or frequent vital sign monitoring, heat maintenance, enteral and/or parenteral nutritional adjustments, and laboratory and oxygen saturation monitoring when provided. Patients are under constant observation by the health care team, which is under direct physician supervision.

- **Table 18-4** illustrates codes for initial- and subsequent-day neonatal and pediatric intensive care services (**99477–99480**) by age and present body weight.
- These are bundled services and include the same procedures that are bundled with neonatal and pediatric critical care services (**99468–99476**). See **Table 18-1** for a list of all the services and procedures that are included.

Code **99477** is used to report the more intensive services that an ill but not critically ill neonate (28 days or younger) requires on the day of admission to inpatient care. Code **99477** includes all E/M services on that date, excluding

- Attendance at delivery (**99464**) or newborn resuscitation (**99465**), which may be reported in addition to code **99477**, when performed.
- Normal newborn care (**99460–99462**), when performed.
- Append modifier **25** to code **99477** when reporting on the same date as **99460–99462**, **99464**, or **99465**.

> Payers that have adopted the Medicare National Correct Coding Initiative (NCCI) edits will not allow payment of codes 99460–99462 and 99477 for services by the same physician or physicians of the same specialty and group practice on the same date. Only code 99477 is reported under these circumstances. See more about NCCI edits in Chapter 2, Modifiers and Coding Edits.

- If the infant is older than 28 days at admission but weighs less than 5,000 g, codes **99221–99223** should be used for intensive care on the date of hospital admission (typically **99223**, assuming documentation of comprehensive history and physical examination and high-level MDM).
- Services are typically (but not required to be) provided in a NICU or special care unit and require a higher intensity of care than would be reported with codes **99221–99223** (initial hospital care of sick patient).
- Do not report code **99477** twice in the same hospital admission. If a patient requires a new episode of intensive care during the same hospital stay, report subsequent intensive care services (**99478–99480**) for the first and each successive day that the patient requires intensive care services.

●=New code   ▲=Revised code   #=Re-sequenced code   +=Add-on code   ★=Telemedicine

Table 18-4. Neonatal and Pediatric Intensive Care				
Description	Present Weight <1,500 g	Present Weight 1,500–2,500 g	Present Weight 2,501–5,000 g	Present Weight ≥5,001 g
Initial intensive care of a neonate (28 days or less)	99477			99221–99223
Initial intensive care of an infant (29 days or older)	99221–99223			
Subsequent intensive care	99478	99479	99480	99231–99233

- Codes 99478–99480 are reported by only 1 individual and once per calendar day of subsequent intensive (but not critical) care for the E/M of the recovering infant weighing 5,000 g or less. Selection of the code will be dependent on the present body weight of the infant, not the infant's age, on the date of service. Therefore, code selection may change from one day to the next depending on the infant's present body weight and condition.
- Codes 99478–99480 are typically used for subsequent days, as long as the neonate or infant continues to require intensive care, and include all the E/M services (and bundled procedures) provided to the patient on the date of service.
- Once the baby's weight exceeds 5,000 g, subsequent hospital care codes (99231–99233) are reported until the date of discharge (99238, 99239).

Examples

➤ **A 1,500-g neonate has mild respiratory distress.** She is on 30% oxygen by nasal cannula, a cardiorespiratory monitor, and continuous pulse oximetry. Laboratory tests and radiographs are ordered, and IV fluids and antibiotics are started. Frequent monitoring and observation are required and ordered.

Code 99477 (initial hospital care for the ill neonate, 28 days of age or less, who requires intensive observation and monitoring) would be reported by the admitting physician.

➤ **A 1,250-g infant, now 40 days old, is stable on 1.5 L oxygen by nasal cannula with fraction of inspired oxygen of 30%. The patient is on caffeine for apnea of prematurity, tolerates orogastric feeds, and requires use of an Isolette for temperature stability.**

Code 99478 would be reported.

➤ **A 15-day-old, 1,600-g neonate remains in an Isolette for thermoregulation and is on methylxanthines for intermittent apnea and bradycardia, for which the neonate requires continuous cardiorespiratory and pulse oximetry monitoring.** The physician adjusts the neonate's continuous gavage feeds based on tolerance and weight.

Code 99479 would be reported.

➤ **A baby requires intensive care and weighs 2,500 g on Monday.** The following day, she continues to require intensive care and her weight is 2,504 g.

Code 99479 would be reported for the care provided on Monday. Code 99480 would be reported for the continuing intensive care provided the following day.

In these examples, the neonate is not critically ill but continues to require intensive monitoring and constant observation by the health care team under direct physician supervision.

Coding for Transitions to Different Levels of Neonatal Care

During a hospital stay, a newborn or readmitted neonate may require different levels of care. A normal newborn may end up becoming sick, intensively ill, or critical during the same hospital stay. Neonates who were initially sick may also improve to require lower levels of care (eg, normal neonatal care).

An initial-day critical or intensive care code (eg, 99468, 99477) is reported only once per hospital stay. If the patient recovers and is later stepped up again to that higher level of care, only the subsequent-level codes (99469, 99478–99480) are reported.

Figure 18-1 provides an illustration of coding for a newborn who transitions from critical care to intensive care and hospital care before discharge. Note that all services take place during the same admission and the physicians are of 2 different specialties. Dr A is a pediatric hospitalist and Dr B is a neonatologist. Each physician individually reports the services provided, and each may only report 1 initial hospital or intensive or critical care service. You can also refer to the American Academy of Pediatrics (AAP) *Newborn Coding Decision Tool* (available for purchase at https://shop.aap.org) for numerous scenarios of coding for newborn care throughout admissions and transfers of care.

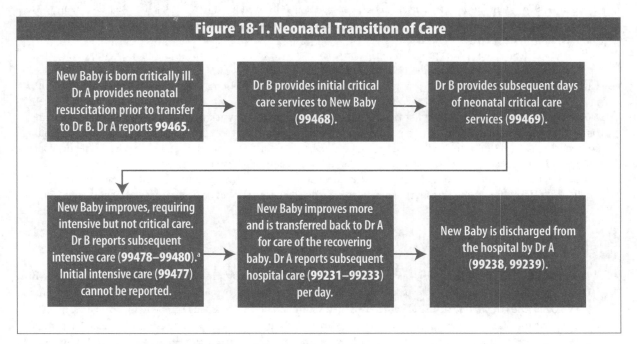

Figure 18-1. Neonatal Transition of Care

New Baby is born critically ill. Dr A provides neonatal resuscitation prior to transfer to Dr B. Dr A reports **99465**. → Dr B provides initial critical care services to New Baby (**99468**). → Dr B provides subsequent days of neonatal critical care services (**99469**).

New Baby improves, requiring intensive but not critical care. Dr B reports subsequent intensive care (**99478–99480**).ª Initial intensive care (**99477**) cannot be reported. → New Baby improves more and is transferred back to Dr A for care of the recovering baby. Dr A reports subsequent hospital care (**99231–99233**) per day. → New Baby is discharged from the hospital by Dr A (**99238, 99239**).

ª Assumes patient's current weight supports code assignment.

Emergency Medical Services Supervision and Patient Transport

Pediatric Critical Care Patient Transport

Face-to-face Critical Care Patient Transport

99466 Critical care face-to-face services, during an interfacility transport of critically ill or critically injured pediatric patient, 24 months of age or younger; first 30–74 minutes of hands-on care during transport

99467 each additional 30 minutes (List separately in addition to code **99466**)

Codes **99466** and **99467** are used to report the physical attendance and direct face-to-face care provided by a physician or QHP during the inter-facility transport of a critically ill or injured patient aged 24 months or younger.

- The patient's condition must meet the *CPT* definition for critical care.
- Face-to-face time begins when the physician or other QHP assumes primary responsibility for the patient at the referring hospital or facility and ends when the receiving hospital or facility accepts responsibility for the patient's care. Only the time the physician spends in direct face-to-face contact with the patient during transport should be reported.
  — Less than 30 minutes of face-to-face time cannot be reported.
  — Time must be documented.
  — Code **99467** is used to report each additional 30 minutes of physician face-to-face time of critical care provided on the same day of service beyond the first 74 minutes.
- Codes include the bundled services listed in **Table 18-1**. Codes **99466** and **99467** may be reported separately from any other procedures or services that are not bundled and performed on the date of transfer. The time involved in performing any procedures that are not bundled and are reported separately should not be included in the face-to-face transport time.

- Procedures or services that are performed by other members of the transport team with the physical presence, participation, and supervision of the accompanying physician may be reported by the physician. Documentation must support the physician's participation.
- Medical record documentation must include the total face-to-face time spent with the patient, the critical nature of the patient's condition, and any performed procedures that are not bundled.
- The pediatric critical care transport codes are preadmission codes and may be reported in addition to neonatal (**99468**) or pediatric (**99471**) initial-day critical care codes. For payers that have adopted NCCI edits, modifier **25** is required to indicate the significant and separately identifiable E/M services. Append modifier **25** to code **99466** when reporting in conjunction with daily critical care codes.
- Face-to-face critical care services provided during an inter-facility transport of a child older than 24 months are reported with hourly critical care codes (**99291** and **99292**).
- If an NNP employed by the neonatal group is on the transport team, the NNP may report codes **99466** and **99467** if independent billing by an NNP is allowed by the state and the activities are covered in the scope of practice. The neonatologist from that same group would not report codes **99485** and **99486** (physician direction of pediatric critical care transport) or **99288** (physician direction of emergency medical systems emergency care). The facility (hospital) could also report these services if the NNPs are employed by the hospital. In this case, the neonatologist would report codes **99485** and **99486** for supervision of interfacility transport because the NNP is not of the same group practice.
- *CPT* does not include specific codes for face-to-face transport of a patient when criteria for critical care are not met. When face-to-face care during transport of a patient is medically necessary but critical care is not, report code **99499** (unlisted E/M service).

Example

➤ **A 4-week-old with tetralogy of Fallot is brought to the local ED with complaints of feeding intolerance, blue lips, labored breathing, and crying.** Transport is dispatched form the regional neonatal center. On arrival, the transport neonatologist finds a cyanotic neonate, with low oxygen saturation despite receiving supplemental oxygen. The ED nurse reports that baby was irritable on arrival but now seems sleepy and not very responsive. The neonatologist intubates the patient and administers morphine, which, over time, improves oxygen saturation. A peripheral IV line is placed and fluids are initiated. The neonatologist spends 50 minutes face-to-face evaluating and stabilizing the newborn. The newborn is then transferred to the helicopter and back to the receiving nursery. Total time from bedside back to the receiving nursery is 45 minutes. Frequent assessments of vital signs and ventilator settings are performed on the transport back. The neonatologist spent a total of 95 minutes of face-to-face critical care time with the neonate; 10 minutes are subtracted for the performance of non-bundled procedures. The time spent in critical care during the transport is 85 minutes. The neonatologist continues care of the newborn in the NICU.

99466 25	(first 74 minutes)
99467 25 × 1 unit	(final 11 minutes)
31500	(endotracheal intubation, emergency)
99468 25	(initial neonatal critical care)

Modifier **25** is appended to each of the services to designate a significant and separately identifiable E/M service provided by the same physician on the same date of service. Endotracheal intubation is bundled with daily neonatal critical care but is separately reported when provided during transport of the critically ill or injured neonate.

Non–face-to-face Pediatric Critical Care Patient Transport

#99485   Supervision by a control physician of interfacility transport care of the critically ill or critically injured pediatric patient, 24 months of age or younger, includes two-way communication with transport team before transport, at the referring facility and during the transport, including data interpretation and report; first 30 minutes

#99486   each additional 30 minutes (List separately in addition to code **99485**)

Code **99485** is used to report the first 16 to 45 minutes of a control physician's documented non–face-to-face supervision of inter-facility critical care transport of a patient 24 months or younger, which includes all 2-way communication between the control physician and the specialized transport team prior to transport, at the referring facility, and during transport to the receiving facility.

Each additional 30-minute period of communication is reported with add-on code **99486**.

- The patient's condition must meet the *CPT* definition of critical care.
- Only report for patients 24 months or younger who are critically ill or injured.
- The control physician does not report any services provided by the specialized transport team.
- The control physician only reports cumulative time spent communicating with the specialty transport team members during an inter-facility transport. Communication between the control physician and the referring facility before or following patient transport *is not* counted.
- Reportable time begins with the initial discussions with the transport team, including discussions of the best mode of transport and strategies for therapy on arrival. Time ends when the patient's care is handed over to the receiving facility team.
- Do not report **99485** or **99486** for services of 15 minutes or less or for any time spent in supervision of a QHP from the same group who is reporting **99466** or **99467**.
- Time spent with the individual patient's transport team and reviewing data submissions should be recorded. Time spent discussing the patient with the referring physician or facility is not counted.
- Total communication time of 15 minutes or less is not reported with code **99485**. Code **99288** (discussed later in this chapter) may be reported when requirements for code **99485** are not met.
- Codes **99485** and **99486** represent preadmission services and may be reported by the same or different individual(s) of the same specialty and same group when neonatal or pediatric critical care services (**99468–99476**) are reported for the same patient on the same day.

Example

➤ **An ED physician requests transfer of an infant with possible sepsis and respiratory distress.** The pediatric intensivist dispatches the transport team, consisting of a hospital-employed transport nurse and a respiratory therapist. On the trip to the referring hospital, the intensivist converses by telephone for 10 minutes with the team, explaining the infant's condition and formulating an initial treatment plan. After arrival, the nurse evaluates the infant and telephones the intensivist to discuss the findings. The decision is made to transport the patient. Because of the critical nature of the infant, the intensivist elects to remain on the telephone until transport is in motion and the patient is critical but stable (15 minutes). On the return trip, another telephone contact lasting 10 minutes is made to receive additional guidance from the intensivist on the infant's worsening respiratory status. The transport is completed and the infant is admitted.

The intensivist spent a total of 35 minutes in direct 2-way telephone communication with the team in 3 discrete episodes. The intensivist carefully documents the time spent in communication with the transport team, the nature of the infant's critical illness, and what decisions were made during each contact in the medical record. Code **99485** is used to report this service.

Direction of Emergency Medical Services

99288   Physician or other qualified health care professional direction of emergency medical systems (EMS) emergency care, advanced life support

See the Non–face-to-face Pediatric Critical Care Patient Transport section earlier in this chapter for discussion of physician non–face-to-face supervision of inter-facility transport of a critically ill or injured pediatric patient 24 months or younger (**99485**, **99486**).

Code **99288**

- May be reported by any physician of any specialty or QHP when advanced life support services are provided via 2-way voice communications (eg, cardiac and/or pulmonary resuscitation; administration of IV fluids, antibiotics, or surfactant).
- This code reflects all the services provided by the directing physician and is not based on any time requirements. Code **99288** may be reported when less than 16 minutes is spent in physician non–face-to-face supervision of inter-facility transport of a critically ill or injured pediatric patient (ie, requirements for reporting **99485** are not met).
- The directing physician should maintain documentation of the times of all contacts, orders, and/or directions for treatment or management of the patient.
- Services or procedures performed by emergency medical services (EMS) personnel are not reported by the physician because he or she was not physically present.

Chapter 18. Critical and Intensive Care

● When an advance practice professional provides and reports face-to-face services during transport, the physician would not report **99288**.
● The appropriate diagnoses are linked to the service.

If, after directing EMS personnel, the physician performs the initial critical care, the appropriate critical care code (eg, **99468**, initial inpatient neonatal critical care) would also be reported with modifier **25** appended to indicate that 2 separate and distinct E/M services were provided by the same physician on the same day of service.

There is no assigned Medicare relative value unit to this service, so it is carrier priced and payments will vary by payer.

Medicare considers code **99288** a bundled service and does not pay separately for the service. Check with your state Medicaid program and other payers to determine their coverage policy.

Total Body Systemic and Selective Head Hypothermia

99184   Initiation of selective head or total body hypothermia in the critically ill neonate, includes appropriate patient selection by review of clinical, imaging and laboratory data, confirmation of esophageal temperature probe location, evaluation of amplitude EEG, supervision of controlled hypothermia, and assessment of patient tolerance of cooling

(Do not report **99184** more than once per hospital stay)

Examples

➤ **A term neonate born with evidence of hypoxic-ischemic encephalopathy is admitted to the NICU and receives critical care services.** Laboratory, EEG, blood gas, and imaging studies confirm the neonate meets objective criteria for *total body cooling*. Continuous total body cooling is undertaken.

Code **99184** is reported for total body systemic hypothermia in addition to **99468**, initial day of neonatal critical care.

➤ **A term neonate born with evidence of hypoxic-ischemic encephalopathy is admitted to the NICU and receives critical care services.** Laboratory, EEG, blood gas, and imaging studies confirm the neonate meets objective criteria for *selective head cooling*. Continuous selective head cooling is undertaken.

Code **99184** is reported for selective head hypothermia in addition to **99468**, initial day of neonatal critical care.

When total body systemic or selective head hypothermia is used in treatment of a critically ill neonate, code **99184** represents the work of initiating the service.

Documentation for use of total body systemic hypothermia and selective head hypothermia should include the neonatal criteria that support initiating this service.

● During either cooling approach, monitoring includes
— Radiographic confirmation of core temperature probe
— Continuous core temperature assessment and adjustment
— Repeated assessment of skin integrity
— Recurrent objective evaluation of evolving neurologic changes (eg, Sarnat stage), which may also include assessment of continuous amplitude EEG monitoring
● In addition, cooling-related laboratory evaluations are required to monitor for cooling-specific complications, including metabolic and coagulation alterations.

Extracorporeal Membrane Oxygenation (ECMO) or Extracorporeal Life Support (ECLS) Services

Prolonged ECMO and extracorporeal life support (ECLS) services commonly involve multiple physicians and supporting health care personnel to manage each patient. ECMO and ECLS codes differentiate components of initiation and daily management of ECMO and ECLS from daily management of a patient's overall medical condition.

These services include cannula insertion (**33951–33956**), ECMO or ECLS initiation (**33946** or **33947**), daily ECMO or ECLS management (**33948** or **33949**), repositioning of the ECMO or ECLS cannula(e) (**33957–33964**), and cannula removal (**33965–33986**). Each physician providing part of the ECMO/ECLS services may report the services they provide except when prohibited by *CPT* instruction (eg, cannula repositioning is not reported by the same or another physician on the same date as initiation of ECMO/ECLS).

Example

➤ **Venoarterial ECMO is initiated for a patient with cardiac and respiratory failure.** Physician A inserts the cannulae. Physician B manages the initial transition to ECMO, including working with physician A, ECMO specialists, and others to initiate an ongoing assessment of anticoagulation, venous return, cannula positioning, and optimal flow. Physician B also provides daily management of the patient's overall care. When ECMO is discontinued, physician A returns and removes the cannulae.

Physician A will report codes for insertion and removal of the ECMO cannulae (eg, **33952** and **33966**) on the date of each service. Physician B will report initiation of venoarterial ECMO (**33947**), the appropriate hospital and/or critical care codes for overall management of the patient for each day provided (eg, **99291**, **99292**, or **99231–99233**), and daily management of ECMO (**33949**) for each day provided.

ECMO/ECLS Cannula Insertion, Repositioning, and Removal

Codes for insertion, repositioning, and removal of ECMO and ECLS are reported based on the patient's age, with separate codes for procedures performed on newborns through 5 years of age and on patients 6 years and older. Codes for these services are shown in **Table 18-5**. While typically only performed by surgeons, other pediatric providers may perform them as well.

> Each physician providing a part of extracorporeal membrane oxygenation/extracorporeal life support services may report the part they provided except as prohibited by *Current Procedural Terminology* instruction.

● Do not separately report repositioning of the ECMO or ECLS cannula(e) (**33957–33964**) at the same session as insertion (**33951–33956**).
● Report replacement of ECMO or ECLS cannula(e) in the same vessel using the insertion code (**33951–33956**) only.

Table 18-5. Extracorporeal Membrane Oxygenation or Extracorporeal Life Support Cannula(e) Procedures			
Approach	**Birth Through 5 Years of Age**	**6 Years and Older**	**Do Not Report With**
Insertion			
Percutaneous peripheral (arterial/venous) cannula(e)[a]	**33951**	**33952**	**33957–33964**
Open peripheral (arterial/venous) cannula(e)	**33953**	**33954**	**33957–33964, 34812, 34820, 34834**
Central cannula(e) by sternotomy or thoracotomy	**33955**	**33956**	**33957–33964, 32100, 39010**
Reposition[b]			
Percutaneous, reposition peripheral (arterial and/or venous) cannula(e)[a]	**33957**	**33958**	**33946, 33947, 34812, 34820, 34834**
Open, reposition peripheral (arterial and/or venous) cannula(e)[a]	**33959**	**33962**	**33946, 33947, 34812, 34820, 34834**
Central cannula(e) reposition by sternotomy or thoracotomy[a]	**33963**	**33964**	**33946, 33947, 32100, 39010**
Removal[c]			
Removal of peripheral (arterial and/or venous) cannula(e), percutaneous	**33965**	**33966**	Not applicable
Removal of peripheral (arterial and/or venous) cannula(e), open	**33969**	**33984**	**34812, 34820, 34834, 35201, 35206, 35211, 35216, 35226**
Removal of central cannula(e) by sternotomy or thoracotomy	**33985**	**33986**	**35201, 35206, 35211, 35216, 35226**

[a] Includes fluoroscopic guidance when performed.
[b] Repositioning of cannula(e) at the same session, as insertion is not separately reported.
[c] Report only the insertion when cannula(e) is replaced in the same vessel.

●=New code   ▲=Revised code   #=Re-sequenced code   +=Add-on code   ★=Telemedicine

- If a cannula(e) is removed from one vessel and a new cannula(e) is placed in a different vessel, report the appropriate cannula(e) removal (33965–33986) and insertion (33951–33956) codes.
- Fluoroscopic guidance used for cannula(e) repositioning (33957–33964) is included in the procedure when performed and should not be separately reported.
- Extensive repair or replacement of an artery may be additionally reported (eg, 35226, 35286, 35371, 35665).
- Direct anastomosis of a prosthetic graft to the artery sidewall to facilitate arterial perfusion for ECMO or ECLS is separately reported with code 33987 in addition to codes 33953–33956.

+33987   Arterial exposure with creation of graft conduit (eg, chimney graft) to facilitate arterial perfusion for ECMO/ECLS (List separately in addition to code for primary procedure)

Do not report 33987 in conjunction with 34833 (open iliac artery exposure with creation of conduit for delivery of aortic or iliac endovascular prosthesis, by abdominal or retroperitoneal incision, unilateral).

ECMO/ECLS Initiation and Daily Management

33946   Extracorporeal membrane oxygenation (ECMO)/extracorporeal life support (ECLS) provided by physician; initiation, venovenous

33947   initiation, venoarterial

33948   daily management, each day, venovenous

33949   daily management, each day, venoarterial

Initiation of the ECMO or ECLS circuit and setting parameters (33946, 33947) involves determining the necessary ECMO or ECLS device components, blood flow, gas exchange, and other necessary parameters to manage the circuit.

Daily care for a patient on ECMO or ECLS includes managing the ECMO or ECLS circuit and related patient issues. These services may be performed by one physician while another physician manages the overall patient medical condition and underlying disorders, but a single physician may provide both services. Regardless of the patient's condition, the basic management of ECMO and ECLS is similar. Documentation for each service should be distinct in the medical record.

- Do not report modifier 63 (procedure performed on infants <4 kg) when reporting codes 33946–33949.
- The physician reporting daily ECMO or ECLS oversees the interaction of the circuit with the patient, management of blood flow, oxygenation, carbon dioxide clearance by the membrane lung, systemic response, anticoagulation and treatment of bleeding, cannula positioning, alarms and safety, and weaning the patient from the ECMO or ECLS circuit when heart and/or lung function has sufficiently recovered.
- Daily management of the patient may be separately reported using the relevant hospital observation services, hospital inpatient services, or critical care E/M codes (99218–99220, 99221–99223, 99231–99233, 99234–99236, 99291, 99292, 99468–99480).
- Daily management (33948 or 33949) or cannula repositioning (33957–33959, 33962–33964) may not be reported on the same date as initiation (33946 or 33947) by the same or different physician.

Sedation

Refer to **Chapter 19**, Common Surgical Procedures and Sedation in Facility Settings, for specific guidelines for reporting sedation services, including moderate (conscious) sedation (99151–99157) and deep sedation.

Car Seat/Bed Testing

94780   Car seat/bed testing for airway integrity, for infants through 12 months of age, with continual clinical staff observation and continuous recording of pulse oximetry, heart rate and respiratory rate, with interpretation and report; 60 minutes

+94781   each additional full 30 minutes (List separately in addition to 94780.)

Neonates who required critical care during their initial hospital stay are most often those patients who require monitoring to determine if they may be safely transported in a car seat or must be transported in a car bed. While these codes are bundled under neonatal and pediatric critical and intensive care codes (99468–99472, 99477–99480), the services most often take place when a neonate is about to go home and, therefore, can be reported if hospital care services (99231–99233) or hospital discharge services (99238, 99239) are being reported instead.

Report codes 94780 and 94781 when the following conditions are met:

- The patient must be an infant (ie, 12 months or younger). Assessment after the patient is 29 days or older may be necessary.

Chapter 18. Critical and Intensive Care

- Continual clinical staff observation with continuous recording of pulse oximetry, heart rate, and respiratory rate is required.
- Inpatient or office-based services are reported.
- Vital signs and observations must be reviewed and interpreted and a written report generated by the physician.
- Codes are reported based on the total observation time spent and documented.
- If less than 60 minutes is spent in the procedure, code **94780** may not be reported.
- Each additional full 30 minutes (ie, not less than 90 minutes) is reported with code **94781**.
- Do not include the time of car seat/bed testing in time attributed to discharge day management services (**99238**, **99239**).
- These codes may be reported with discharge day management (**99238**, **99239**), normal newborn care services (**99460**, **99462**, **99463**), or subsequent hospital care codes (**99231–99233**).

Examples

➤ **A neonate born at 26 weeks' gestation requires a car seat test on the date of discharge from the hospital.**
Code **94780** is reported in addition to hospital discharge management code **99238** or **99239**.

➤ **A neonate born at 26 weeks' gestation requires a car seat test prior to discharge from the hospital.** The newborn has received 60 minutes of testing reported with **94780** and now receives an additional 30 minutes.
Codes **94780** and **94781** are reported.

Values and Payment

The typical times for E/M services most commonly provided to newborns can be used as an excellent and quick internal audit mechanism to judge coding adequacy. The times are based on the American Medical Association/Specialty Society Relative Value Scale Update Committee (RUC) survey results.

Although not exact or applicable for every patient, they are the average times (in minutes) spent by neonatologists for the typical or average patient. RUC Survey Times for Hospital Care and Critical Care Services are available online at www.aap.org/cfp.

Payment Advocacy

The AAP encourages chapter development of pediatric councils as forums to discuss pediatric issues with payers. Pediatric councils have the potential to facilitate better working relationships between pediatricians and health insurance plans and to improve quality of care for children. Learn more about AAP pediatric councils at www.aap.org/en/practice-management/practice-financing/payer-contracting-advocacy-and-other-resources/aap-payer-advocacy/aap-pediatric-councils/.

The AAP Section on Neonatal-Perinatal Medicine, in conjunction with state chapters and councils of the AAP, has developed strategies that have been successful in addressing payment concerns for neonatal care. Contact your state chapter, its pediatric council, your section district AAP Executive Committee representative, a neonatal trainer, or the AAP Committee on Coding and Nomenclature for assistance in addressing any payment inequities for neonatal services in your state.

Resources

Coding Education

AAP Section on Neonatal-Perinatal Medicine coding trainers are available to provide coding education through local educational seminars and continuing education events. Contact section manager Jim Couto (jcouto@aap.org) for additional information about these valuable services.

Critical Care Supervision

Global Per Diem Critical Care Codes: Direct Supervision and Reporting Guideline (www.aap.org/cfp)

ICD-10-CM

"Coding for Abnormalities in Fetal Growth," December 2020 *AAP Pediatric Coding Newsletter* (https://coding.solutions.aap.org/article.aspx?articleid=2765246; subscription required)

Newborn Coding Decision Tool

AAP *Newborn Coding Decision Tool* (available for purchase at https://shop.aap.org)

Payment Advocacy

AAP pediatric councils (www.aap.org/en-us/professional-resources/practice-transformation/getting-paid/Pages/aap-pediatric-councils.aspx)

Test Your Knowledge!

1. **Which of the following is separately reportable in conjunction with critical care services (99291, 99292)?**
   a. Cardiopulmonary resuscitation (**92950**)
   b. X-ray, chest; 2 views (**71046**)
   c. Introduction of needle or intra-catheter, vein (**36000**)
   d. Spinal puncture, lumbar, diagnostic (**62270**)

2. **Which of the following periods is included in code 99291?**
   a. 30–60 minutes
   b. 30–74 minutes
   c. 30–89 minutes
   d. 60–89 minutes

3. **Which of the following is reported by the attending physician when a recovering neonate requires a second episode of critical care (eg, step up from intensive care) during 1 admission?**
   a. Initial inpatient neonatal critical care, per day (**99468**)
   b. Subsequent inpatient neonatal critical care, per day (**99469**)
   c. Critical care, per hour (**99291, 99292**)
   d. Subsequent intensive care, per day (**99478–99480**)

4. **What code is reported when a 29-month-old receives face-to-face critical care services by a physician during interfacility transport?**
   a. **99466, 99467** (critical care face-to-face services, during an interfacility transport)
   b. **99485, 99486** (supervision by a control physician of interfacility transport care of the critically ill or critically injured pediatric patient)
   c. **99468** (initial inpatient neonatal critical care, per day)
   d. **99291, 99292** (hourly critical care services)

5. **For which ages of patients are car seat/bed testing services reported with codes 94780 and 94781?**
   a. 28 days and younger
   b. 24 months and younger
   c. 12 months and younger
   d. Any age when state regulations require use of a car seat/bed

---

Common Surgical Procedures and Sedation in Facility Settings

Contents

Surgical Package Rules 451
    Global Periods and Modifiers for Reporting Postoperative Care 452
    Reporting Postoperative Care 452

Multiple Procedures on the Same Date 452
    Separate Procedure Designation 453

Increased or Decreased Procedural Services 453
    Increased Procedural Service 453
    Reporting Terminated or Partial Procedures 454
    Reporting by Assistant Surgeon 454

Procedures Performed on Infants Less Than 4 kg 455

Physicians at Teaching Hospitals Guidelines for Billing Procedures 456
    Minor Procedures 456
    Interpretation of Diagnostic Radiology and Other Diagnostic Tests 456
    Endoscopy 457
    Complex or High-risk Surgeries and Procedures 457
    Surgery Other Than Minor, Complex, or High-risk Procedures 457
    Postoperative Care 457
    Assistant Surgeon in a Teaching Facility 457

Burn Care 458
    Surgical Preparation and Skin Grafting 458
        Surgical Preparation 458
        Skin Grafts and Skin Graft Substitutes 459

Musculoskeletal Procedures 460
    Fracture and Dislocation Care Codes 460
    Osteotomy Humerus With Intramedullary Lengthening Device 461
    Removal of Musculoskeletal Hardware 461

Respiratory 461
    Intubation and Airway Management 461
    Thoracostomy, Thoracentesis, and Pleural Drainage 462

Cardiovascular Procedures 462
    Echocardiography 462
    Cardiac Catheterization For Congenital Heart Defects 463
        Related Procedures 464
    Pericardiocentesis and Pericardial Drainage 464
    Atrial Septostomy 465
    Valvuloplasty 466
    Transcatheter Pulmonary Valve Implantation 467
    Transcatheter Interventions for Revascularization/Repair for Coarctation of the Aorta ... 467
    Percutaneous Transcatheter Closure of Patent Ductus Arteriosus 468

Vascular Access 469
    Central Venous Access 469
        Insertion or Replacement of Centrally Inserted Central Venous Access Device 470
        Insertion of Peripherally Inserted Central Venous Access Device 471
        Repair of Central Venous Catheters 471
        Removal of Central Venous Catheters 472
    Arterial Access 472

Transfusions 472

Ear, Nose, and Throat Procedures 473
    Laryngoplasty 473
    Adenoidectomy and Tonsillectomy 473

Digestive System Procedures 474
    Gastric Intubation and Aspiration 474
    Appendectomy 474
    Hernia Repair 475

Genitourinary System Procedures 475
    Anogenital Examination 475
    Lysis/Excision of Labial or Penile Adhesions 476
    Repair of Penis 476
        Correction of Chordee and Hypospadias 476

Negative Pressure Wound Therapy 477

Sedation 478
    Moderate Sedation 478
    Deep Sedation/Anesthesia Services 478
    Postoperative Pain Management 479

Resources 480

Test Your Knowledge! 481

Chapter 19. Common Surgical Procedures and Sedation in Facility Settings

● =New code   ▲ =Revised code   # =Re-sequenced code   + =Add-on code   ★ =Telemedicine

Surgical Package Rules

Current Procedural Terminology (*CPT®*) surgical codes (**10004–69990**) are packaged or global codes including all the necessary services normally furnished by a surgeon before, during, and after a procedure. *CPT* defines only a surgical package, whereas the Centers for Medicare & Medicaid Services (CMS) defines the surgical package in terms of global periods based on the pre-, intra-, and postoperative work values assigned to each procedure.

- Most state Medicaid programs follow the CMS definition.
- Each commercial insurance company will have its own policy for billing and payment of global surgical care, and most will designate a specific number of follow-up days for surgical procedures.

  Both *CPT* and the CMS agree that
- Surgical codes include local infiltration, metacarpal/metatarsal/digital block, or topical anesthesia by the physician performing the procedure.
- Preoperative care
  - Includes evaluation and management (E/M) service(s) *subsequent to the decision for surgery* (eg, assessing the site and condition, explanation of procedure, obtaining informed consent) on the day before and/or on the date of the procedure (including history and physical)
  - When the initial decision to perform surgery is made on the day prior to or on the day of surgery, the appropriate-level E/M visit may be reported separately with modifier **57** (decision for surgery) appended. This modifier shows the payer that the E/M service was necessary to make the decision for surgery (ie, not the routine preoperative evaluation).
  - When an E/M service performed on the day of the procedure is unrelated to the decision to perform surgery and is significant and distinct from the usual preoperative care associated with the procedure, it may be reported with modifier **25** (significant, separately identifiable E/M service by the same physician on the same day of the procedure or other service) appended.
  - Medical record documentation must support that the service was significant, separately identifiable, and medically necessary. An E/M service performed prior to the decision to perform the procedure is separately reportable.
  - Different diagnoses are not required when reporting an E/M visit and procedure.

> **Centers for Medicare & Medicaid Services Addresses Preoperative Care Differently for Minor and Major Procedures**
>
> For "minor" procedures (ie, procedures assigned a 0- or 10-day global period or endoscopies), the evaluation and management (E/M) visit on the date of the procedure is considered a routine part of the procedure regardless of whether it is prior or subsequent to the decision for surgery. In these cases, modifier **57** is not recognized.
>
> An E/M code may be reported on the same day as a minor surgical procedure only when a significant, separately identifiable E/M service is performed; modifier **25** is appended to the E/M code.
>
> When the initial decision to perform a major surgical procedure (ie, procedures assigned a 90-day global period) is made on the day prior to or on the day of a procedure, the E/M service may be reported appended with modifier **57**. Medical record documentation should support that the decision for surgery was made during the encounter and that time was spent in performing counseling of the risks, benefits, and outcomes.

- Postoperative care
  - Includes all associated typical postoperative care (eg, dictation of progress notes; counseling with the patient, family, and/or other physicians; writing orders; evaluating the patient in the postanesthesia recovery area).
  - Care for therapeutic surgical procedures includes only the care that is usually part of the surgical service.
  - Care for diagnostic procedures (eg, endoscopies, arthroscopies, injection procedures for radiography) includes only the care that is related to the recovery from the diagnostic procedure.
  - Care resulting from complications of surgery.
  - Any complications, exacerbations, recurrence, treatment of unrelated diseases or injuries, or the presence of other diseases or injuries that require additional services may be reported separately.

> **Centers for Medicare & Medicaid Services Criteria for Reporting Postoperative Medical or Surgical Services**
> - All additional medical or surgical services required of the surgeon during the postoperative period of the surgery because of complications *that do not require additional trips to the operating room* are included in the global package (not separately reported).
> - Does not include treatment for the underlying condition or an added course of treatment that is not part of normal recovery from surgery. (See modifiers **24**, **58**, and **79** discussed in the Global Periods and Modifiers for Reporting Postoperative Care section.)

Global Periods and Modifiers for Reporting Postoperative Care

The CMS-designated global periods for each *CPT* procedure code can be found on the Resource-Based Relative Value Scale of the Medicare Physician Fee Schedule (MPFS) at www.cms.gov/medicare/medicare-fee-for-service-payment/physicianfeesched.

- It designates specific postoperative periods for certain procedure codes (ie, 0, 10, or 90 days). When determining the postoperative period, the day after surgery is day 1 of a 10- or 90-day period.
- In addition to the *CPT* code, physicians use modifier **78** for return to the operating room for a related procedure during a postoperative period. This includes return to the operating room for treatment of complications of the first procedure.
- For return to the operating room for staged or more extensive procedures and therapeutic procedures following a diagnostic procedure, append modifier **58**.
- Report procedures during the postoperative period that are unrelated and not due to complications of the original procedure with modifier **79** and unrelated E/M services with modifier **24** (documentation is typically required prior to payment).
- Other codes are designated YYY, which means the postoperative period is set by the carrier. There are no associated postoperative days included in the payment for codes assigned with status codes XXX (the global concept does not apply) or ZZZ (assigned to an add-on code for a service that is always related to another service to which the global period is assigned).

Reporting Postoperative Care

- Report *CPT* code **99024** (postoperative follow-up visit) for follow-up care provided by the physician who performed a procedure (or the covering physician) during the global surgery period.
  - Reporting of inpatient or observation follow-up visits is typically not required.
  - Reporting code **99024** allows a practice to track the number of visits performed by individuals during the postoperative period of specific procedures, calculate office overhead expenses (eg, supplies, staff, physician time) associated with the procedure, and potentially use the data to negotiate higher payment rates.

Payers track the postoperative care provided. If a physician is not providing or reporting the postoperative care (**99024**) typically performed for a procedure, payers may reduce payment for the surgical service because payment includes postoperative care as part of the procedure.

- Append modifier **24** (unrelated E/M service by the same physician during a postoperative period) to the code for an E/M service provided by the physician who performed a procedure during the postoperative period.
- When physicians from different practices perform part of a surgical package, the procedure should be reported with one of the following modifiers:
  - **54** (surgical care only)
  - **55** (postoperative management only)
  - **56** (preoperative management only)

See Chapter 2 for a more detailed description of modifiers. For critical care following surgery, see the Patients Critically Ill After Surgery section in Chapter 18.

These situations require communication among the surgeon, the physician providing preoperative or postoperative care, and each physician's respective billing personnel to ensure accurate reporting and payment.

- No modifier is required when a physician (different specialty or group practice) other than the surgeon provides unrelated services to a patient during the postoperative period.

Despite the use of different National Provider Identifiers and diagnosis codes, some payers with assigned follow-up surgical periods will deny the service. The claim should be appealed for payment with a letter advising the payer that the service was unrelated to any surgery.

Multiple Procedures on the Same Date

Often, multiple, separately reportable services are provided in one session or on one date of service. However, it is important to recognize which surgical services are considered a component of another procedure and which are separately reported.

- It is not appropriate to report multiple Healthcare Common Procedure Coding System (HCPCS)/*CPT* codes when a single, comprehensive HCPCS/*CPT* code describes the procedures performed.

Example

➤ **Code 42820 describes tonsillectomy and adenoidectomy in a patient younger than 12 years.** It would not be appropriate to separately report **42825** (tonsillectomy) and **42830** (adenoidectomy).

- Surgical access (eg, laparotomy) is integral to more comprehensive procedures (eg, appendectomy) and not separately reported.
- When the surgical approach fails, report only the code for the approach that resulted in the completed procedure. For example, if laparoscopy fails and an open approach is used to complete the procedure, report only the open procedure.
- It is advisable to adopt a process for checking the National Correct Coding Initiative (NCCI) edits prior to submitting multiple procedure codes for services on the same date, as the NCCI edits are used by many payers.

> **See Chapter 2, Coding Edits and Modifiers, for more information on the National Correct Coding Initiative.**

- For Medicaid, the NCCI manual is also informative regarding correct reporting and use of modifiers to override NCCI edits.
- When more than 1 procedure/service is performed on the same date, during the same session, or during a postoperative period, several *CPT* modifiers may apply. Documentation must support the reason for applying a modifier (eg, indicate a separate incision).
  - Modifier **59** is often appended to surgical procedure codes to override payer edits that otherwise would not allow payment for services that may be components of other services.

> **See also modifiers XE (separate encounter), XP (separate provider), XS (separate structure), and XU (unusual nonoverlapping service) in Chapter 2.**

  - It is important to carefully consider whether other modifiers are more appropriate (eg, **50**, bilateral service; an anatomical modifier such as **E4**, lower right eyelid) to indicate a distinct service.

Separate Procedure Designation

One designation in *CPT* helps identify procedures that are commonly performed as an integral component of another procedure. The parenthetical comment "(separate procedure)" follows the code descriptor for these services.
- Services designated as a separate procedure should not be reported in addition to the code for the total procedure or service of which they are considered an integral component.
- A procedure or service that is designated as a separate procedure may be
  - Carried out independently and be the only code reported
  - Considered to be unrelated or distinct from other procedures/services provided at that time and reported in addition to other procedures/services by appending modifier **59** (distinct procedural service)

Increased or Decreased Procedural Services

Increased Procedural Service

Modifier **22** (increased procedural service) may be appended to the code for a surgical procedure when the work required to provide the service was *significantly greater* than typically required for that procedure. To substantiate modifier **22**, documentation must support that the procedure was more difficult due to 1 or more of the following conditions:
- Increased intensity or time
- Technical difficulty
- The severity of the patient's condition
- Significantly increased physical and mental effort

Example

➤ **A child undergoes surgery for acute appendicitis with rupture.** The procedure takes 45 minutes longer than typical due to subhepatic location and rupture of the appendix. The surgeon documents the increased work and time of the procedure and reports

    44970 22   Laparoscopy, surgical, appendectomy

    Teaching Point: Because the work of the procedure was significantly increased by the location and rupture of the appendix, modifier **22** is appropriately appended.

> See Chapter 2 for discussion of other surgical modifiers (eg, **62**, 2 surgeons; **66**, surgical team) and general information on modifiers.

Reporting Terminated or Partial Procedures

- When a procedure is started but cannot be completed due to extenuating circumstances, physicians should consider the individual situation, including the reason for termination of the procedure and the amount of work that was performed, when determining how to report the service rendered.
- When a procedure was performed but not entirely successful (eg, portion of foreign body removed), it may be appropriate to report the procedure code that represents the work performed without modification.
- Only report reduced services (modifier **52**) or discontinued procedure (modifier **53**) when the service was significantly reduced from the typical service and as instructed in *CPT.*

> **Know Payer Policies for Modifiers 52 and 53**
>
> Individual payer policies may specify allowed uses and reporting requirements for discontinued services. Pediatricians should be aware that some payer policies automatically reduce payment to 25% to 50% of the fee schedule amount for the service reported with modifier **52** or **53**.
>
> When indicated, modifier **52** or **53** should always be reported. Documentation should support the reason for termination or reduced service and the extent of the service performed. Payers may audit the patient's medical record or, for facility-based services, use electronic processes to compare a physician's claim to a facility claim for the same service that was reported with modifier **73** or **74** (outpatient hospital/ambulatory surgical center discontinued service). If modifier **52** or **53** was indicated but not reported, a payer may demand return of previous payments.

Examples

➤ *CPT* **instructs to append modifier 52 (reduced service) to code 54150 (circumcision, using clamp or other device with regional dorsal penile or ring block), when performed without dorsal penile or ring block.**

- If the work performed prior to discontinuation was insignificant, it may be appropriate to not report the procedure.
- When not reporting the procedure, consider whether the level of a related E/M service was increased due to the complexity of medical decision-making associated with the attempted procedure, any complicating factors, and the revised management or treatment plan.
- *CPT* includes specific instructions for reporting certain services when they are reduced or discontinued (eg, endoscopy). Be sure to verify *CPT* instructions prior to reporting reduced or terminated services.

> For more information on reporting discontinued or incomplete procedures, see "Discontinued or Reduced Services: Modifier **52** or **53**" in the May 2021 *AAP Pediatric Coding Newsletter*™ (https://coding.solutions.aap.org/article.aspx?articleid=2765344; subscription required).

Reporting by Assistant Surgeon

An assistant surgeon is a physician or other qualified health care professional (QHP) who provides active assistance in the performance of a procedure when clinically indicated (eg, technically complex procedure).

- See the Assistant Surgeon in a Teaching Facility section later in this chapter for guidance on reporting assistant surgeon services by a physician in a teaching facility.

- Global rules do not apply to services performed by an assistant surgeon. Payment is based on a percentage of the fee schedule amount allowed for the procedure performed (eg, Medicare allows 16%).
- Modifiers are appended to the code(s) for the procedure on the assistant's claim. See **Table 19-1** for modifiers for reporting services by an assistant surgeon.
- Reductions for multiple procedures on the same date may apply.
- See individual payer policies for assistant at surgery, as many limit payment to only specific procedures and/or may require documentation substantiating the need for assistance.

Table 19-1. Modifiers for Reporting Assistant Surgeon Services	
80	Assistant surgeon (use for MD or DO)
81	Minimum assistant surgeon
82	Assistant surgeon (when qualified resident surgeon not available)
AS	Physician assistant, nurse practitioner, or clinical nurse specialist services for assistant at surgery

Procedures Performed on Infants Less Than 4 kg

Modifier **63** is used to identify procedures performed on neonates and infants with present body weight of up to 4 kg. This modifier signals significantly increased complexity and physician or other QHP work commonly associated with these patients.
- Append modifier **63** to codes for procedures performed on these infants only when there is no instruction prohibiting reporting.
- Services that cannot be reported with modifier **63** are those that have been valued based on the intensity of the service in patients weighing less than 4 kg. See "Summary of *CPT* Codes Exempt from Modifier **63**" in your *CPT* reference for a list of codes exempt from modifier **63**.
- Unless otherwise designated, this modifier may only be appended to procedures or services listed in the **20100–69999** code series and codes **92920**, **92928**, **92953**, **92960**, **92986**, **92987**, **92990**, **92997**, **92998**, **93312–93318**, **93452**, **93505**, **93593–93598**, **93563**, **93564**, **93568**, **93580**, **93582**, **93590–93592**, **93615**, and **93616**. Modifier **63** is not appended to codes from the E/M, anesthesia, radiology, or pathology/laboratory section of *CPT*.
- Use of modifier **63** may require submission of an operative note with the claim. The operative note should include the patient's weight. It is also beneficial to report the patient's weight on the claim.
- Payer acceptance of modifier **63** may be limited to specific procedures and increased payment allowance (above the payment for the same procedure in a patient weighing more than 4 kg) varies. Verify policies of individual health plans for reporting this modifier.

Examples

➤ **A 13-day-old weighing 2.4 kg requires peripheral cannulae insertion for extracorporeal membrane oxygenation (ECMO).** The physician reports

    33951 63   Extracorporeal membrane oxygenation (ECMO)/extracorporeal life support (ECLS) provided by physician; insertion of peripheral (arterial and/or venous) cannula(e), percutaneous, birth through 5 years of age (includes fluoroscopic guidance, when performed)

    Teaching Point: The patient weighed less than 4 kg, and the procedure is not listed as modifier **63** exempt. Therefore, modifier **63** is appropriately appended to indicate the increased intensity and/or work of performing the procedure on the neonate. Note that modifier **63** cannot be appended to codes for initiation or daily management of ECMO/ECLS (**33646–33949**).

➤ **An infant weighing 3 kg undergoes diagnostic laryngoscopy.** The physician reports

    31520   Laryngoscopy, direct, with or without tracheoscopy; diagnostic newborn

    Teaching Point: The parenthetical instruction below code **31520** ("Do not report modifier **63** in conjunction with **31520**") prohibits reporting modifier **63**, including when this procedure is performed on an infant weighing less than 4 kg.

Physicians at Teaching Hospitals Guidelines for Billing Procedures

The CMS established and maintains guidelines for documentation and billing by teaching physicians. Physicians at Teaching Hospitals guidelines for billing procedures are less complex than those for billing E/M services. Guidelines specify that

- When a procedure is performed by a resident, teaching physician attendance and participation are required and must be documented. See examples of appropriate documentation in **Table 19-2**.
- The level of participation required by the teaching physician depends on the type of procedure being performed.
- A resident, nurse, or teaching physician may document the teaching physician's attendance.

The rules for supervising physicians in teaching settings can be obtained on the CMS website at http://cms.hhs.gov/manuals/downloads/clm104c12.pdf, section 100.

Modifier GC (services have been performed by a resident under the direction of a teaching physician) must be appended to procedure codes for services performed by a resident under the direction of a teaching physician.

Table 19-2. Examples of Appropriate Documentation of Teaching Physician Presence	
Minor procedures	*"Dr Teaching Physician was present during the entire procedure."* —Nurse *"Dr Teaching Physician observed me performing this procedure."* —Dr Resident
Interpretation of diagnostic radiology and other diagnostic tests	*"I personally reviewed the MRI with Dr Resident and agree with his findings."* —Dr Teaching Physician *"I personally reviewed the CAT scan with Dr Resident. Findings are indicative of (insert)."* —Dr Teaching Physician
Endoscopy	*"I was present during the entire viewing of this endoscopy."* —Dr Teaching Physician
Surgery other than minor procedures	*"Dr Teaching Physician was present during entire surgery."* —Dr Resident *"I was present and observed Dr Resident perform the key portion of this procedure."* —Dr Teaching Physician
Complex or high-risk surgeries and procedures	*"I was physically present during this entire procedure with the exception of the [opening and/or closing], as that overlapped with the key portion of another case."* —Dr Teaching Physician *"Dr Y was immediately available during the overlapping portions of this case, which included [cite specifics]."* —Dr Teaching Physician

Abbreviations: CAT, computerized axial tomography; MRI, magnetic resonance imaging.

Minor Procedures

- The CMS defines a minor procedure as one taking *5 minutes or less* to complete with relatively little decision-making once the need for the procedure is determined.
- Minor procedures are usually assigned a 0- to 10-day global period.
- Teaching physicians may bill for a minor procedure when they personally perform the service or when a resident performs the service and they are present for the entire procedure.
- The resident may document the procedure but must attest to the teaching physician's presence.

Interpretation of Diagnostic Radiology and Other Diagnostic Tests

- The teaching physician may bill for interpretation of the diagnostic service if he or she interprets tests or reviews findings with the resident.
- Documentation must support a personal interpretation or a review of the resident's notes with indication of agreement with the resident's interpretation.
- Changes to the resident's interpretation must be documented.

●=New code   ▲=Revised code   #=Re-sequenced code   +=Add-on code   ★=Telemedicine

Endoscopy

- The teaching physician must be present for the entire viewing starting at the time of insertion and ending at the time of removal of the endoscope.
- Viewing the procedure through a monitor located in another room does not meet the requirements for billing.
- The presence of the teaching physician must be documented in the medical record. The teaching physician's presence must be stated.

Complex or High-risk Surgeries and Procedures

- A complex procedure or surgery (eg, cardiac catheterization) requires the direct or personal supervision of a physician as specified in Medicare or local policy or in the *CPT* description.
- A teaching physician must be present with a resident for the entire procedure when billing for a service identified by the CMS or local policy as complex and requiring personal supervision by a physician.
- Documentation must support that the teaching physician was present.

Surgery Other Than Minor, Complex, or High-risk Procedures

- The teaching physician must assume the responsibility of preoperative, operative, and postoperative care of the patient. He or she must be present during all critical and key portions (as determined by the teaching physician) of the procedure. For example, if opening or closing is not considered to be key or critical, the teaching physician does not need to be present.
- The teaching physician must be immediately available to furnish services during the entire procedure.
- If circumstances prevent the physician from being immediately available, arrangements must be made with another qualified surgeon to be immediately available to assist with the procedure.
- The physician's presence for single surgical procedures may be demonstrated in notes made by the teaching physician, resident, or nurse.
- When the teaching physician is present for the entire procedure, only the written attestation of his or her presence is required.
- If the teaching physician is present during only the key or critical portions of the surgery, documentation must indicate his or her presence at those portions of the procedure (the resident may still document the operative report).
- When billing for 2 overlapping (concurrent) surgeries, the teaching physician must be present for the key or critical portions of both procedures and must personally document his or her presence. The surgeon cannot be involved in a second case until all key or critical portions in the first case have been completed.
- Arrangements may be made with another qualified surgeon to be present at one of the surgeries. The name of the other surgeon who was immediately available during overlapping surgeries must be documented.

Postoperative Care

- The teaching physician determines which postoperative visits are considered key or critical and require his or her presence.
- If the teaching physician is not providing postoperative care included in the global surgery package, he or she will report the procedure(s) with modifiers **54** (surgical care only) and **56** (preoperative management only).
- Postoperative care is reported by another physician with the same surgical procedure code with modifier **55** (postoperative management only).
- The surgeon and physician providing postoperative care must keep a copy of a written transfer agreement in the patient's medical record.

Assistant Surgeon in a Teaching Facility

Medicare will not pay for the services of assistants at surgery furnished in a teaching hospital that has a training program related to the medical specialty required for the surgical procedure and has a qualified resident available to perform the service. This policy may be applied by Medicaid and other payers.

- When the MPFS allows payment for an assistant surgeon and a physician assists a teaching physician because no qualified resident was available, modifier **82** (assistant surgeon [when qualified resident surgeon not available]) is appended to the code for the procedure performed on the assistant surgeon's claim.
- The unavailability of a qualified resident surgeon is a prerequisite for use of modifier **82**. Documentation must specify that no qualified resident was available or that there was no residency program related to the medical specialty required for the surgical procedure.

- This modifier is only used in teaching hospitals and only if there is no approved training program related to the medical specialty required for the surgical procedure or no qualified resident was available.

Burn Care

CPT code **16000** (initial treatment, first-degree burn, where no more than local treatment is required) is reported when initial treatment is performed for the symptomatic relief of a first-degree burn that is characterized by erythema and tenderness.

16020	Dressings and/or debridement of partial-thickness burns, initial or subsequent; small or less than 5% total body (eg, finger)
16025	medium or 5%–10% total body surface area (eg, whole face or whole extremity)
16030	large or greater than 10% total body surface area (eg, more than 1 extremity)
16035	Escharotomy; initial incision
+**16036**	each additional incision

Codes **16020–16030**

- Are used to report treatment of burns with dressings and/or debridement of small to large partial-thickness burns (second degree), whether initial or subsequent.
- Are reported based on the percentage of total body surface area (TBSA) affected.
- The percentage of TBSA involved must be calculated and documented when reporting care of second- or third-degree burns.

   Pediatric physicians often use the Lund-Browder classification method for estimating the TBSA based on patient age. (The Lund-Browder diagram and classification method table are in *CPT 2022 Professional Edition*.)

- An E/M visit (critical care, emergency department [ED] services, inpatient or outpatient E/M) may be provided for evaluation of the patient's injuries and management of complications such as dehydration, shock, infection, multiple organ dysfunction syndrome, electrolyte imbalance, cardiac arrhythmias, and respiratory distress.

   Report the E/M code appropriate to the setting and care provided with modifier **25** appended to indicate the significant, separately identifiable E/M service is medically indicated, performed, and documented in addition to the burn care.

- Codes **16000–16036** do not include other services such as pulmonary testing/therapy or procedures such as hyperbaric oxygenation, grafting, or tracheotomy. Separately report other services provided on the same date as burn care.
- Codes **16020–16030** include dressing application (whether initial or subsequent) and any associated debridement or curettement.
- It is advisable to use *International Classification of Diseases, 10th Revision, Clinical Modification* (*ICD-10-CM*) category **T31**, burns classified according to extent of body surface involved, as an additional code for reporting purposes when there is mention of a third-degree burn involving 20% or more of the body surface.
- Codes **16020–16030** include the application of materials (eg, dressings) not described in codes **15100–15278** (skin grafts and substitutes).

Codes **16035** and **16036**

- Are reported per incision of eschar (dead tissue cast off from the surface of the skin in full-thickness burns).
- Are not reported based on anatomical site; report with 1 unit of code **16035** for the first incision only and 1 unit of code **16036** for each additional incision regardless of body area.

Surgical Preparation and Skin Grafting

Surgical Preparation

15002	Surgical preparation or creation of recipient site by excision of open wounds, burn eschar, or scar (including subcutaneous tissues), or incisional release of scar contracture, trunk, arms, legs; first 100 sq cm or 1% of body area of infants and children
+**15003**	each additional 100 sq cm, or part thereof, or each additional 1% of body area of infants and children
15004	Surgical preparation or creation of recipient site by excision of open wounds, burn eschar, or scar (including subcutaneous tissues), or incisional release of scar contracture, face, scalp, eyelids, mouth, neck, ears, orbits, genitalia, hands, feet and/or multiple digits; first 100 sq cm or 1% of body area of infants and children
+**15005**	each additional 100 sq cm, or part thereof, or each additional 1% of body area of infants and children

Chapter 19. Common Surgical Procedures and Sedation in Facility Settings

Surgical preparation codes **15002–15005** for skin replacement surgery describe removal of nonviable tissue to treat a burn, traumatic wound, or necrotizing infection.

Report codes **15002–15005** for preparation of a clean and viable wound surface for placement of an autograft, flap, or skin substitute graft or for negative pressure wound therapy (NPWT).

An incisional release of scar contracture may also be used to create a clean wound bed.

- Code selection for surgical preparation codes is based on the location and size of the defect. Measurements apply to the recipient area.
  — Adults and children 10 years and older: 100 cm^2
  — Infants and children younger than 10 years: each percentage of body surface area
- Codes **15002–15005** are always preparation for healing by primary intention. Do not report codes **15002–15005** for chronic wounds left to heal by secondary intention.
- Report the appropriate codes when closure is achieved by adjacent tissue transfer (codes **14000–14061**) or a complex repair (codes **13100–13153**) rather than skin grafts or substitutes.

Example

➤ **An 8-year-old patient undergoes surgical preparation for skin grafting of face, front of right arm, and right hand.** The body areas are measured as face, 4% of body area; right arm, 4%; and right hand, 1%.

ICD-10-CM	*CPT*
Appropriate codes for burns by depth and body area	**15004** (first 1% of body areas of face and hand) **15005** × 4 (each additional 1%) **15002** 59 (first 1% body area of arm) **15003** × 3 (each additional 1%)

Teaching Point: Because the face and hand are both included in the descriptor for codes **15004** and **15005**, the percentages of body areas are combined. Because the preparation of an area on the arm is described by codes **15002** and **15003**, the body area of the arm is not added to that of the face and hand. Modifier **59** indicates that the procedure reported with code **15002** was performed on distinct body areas not described by code **15004**.

Skin Grafts and Skin Graft Substitutes

See codes for skin grafts online at www.aap.org/cfp.
- When burn wounds are treated and subsequently require skin grafting at the same session, report the burn code along with the appropriate skin graft code.
- A skin graft procedure may be a staged procedure (delayed) with the preparation of the recipient site and the graft procedure being performed on different dates. In these cases, modifier **58** (staged procedure) is appended to the grafting procedure code performed during the global period.
- The appropriate code for harvesting cultured skin autograft is **15040** (harvest of skin for tissue cultured skin autograft, 100 sq cm or less).
- Debridement is considered a separate procedure only when
  — Gross contamination requires prolonged cleansing.
  — Appreciable amounts of devitalized or contaminated tissue are removed.
  — Debridement is carried out separately without immediate primary closure.
- Measurements apply to the recipient area.
  — For patient aged 10 years and older report 1 unit per 100 sq cm.
  — Report 1 unit per 1% of body area of children 9 years and younger.
- Procedures involving the wrist and/or ankle are reported with codes that include "arm" or "leg" in the descriptor.
- The physician should select the skin substitute graft application code based on the actual size of the wound, after wound preparation has been performed, and not the amount of the skin graft substitute used.
- The party supplying skin substitute graft products reports HCPCS codes for the products.

Musculoskeletal Procedures

An object intentionally placed by a physician or other qualified health care professional for any purpose (eg, diagnostic, therapeutic) is considered an implant. If an implant (or part thereof) has moved from its original position, or is structurally broken and no longer serves its intended purpose or presents a hazard to the patient, it qualifies as a foreign body for coding purposes, unless *Current Procedural Terminology* (*CPT*) coding instructions direct otherwise or a specific *CPT* code exists to describe the removal of that broken/moved implant.

Fracture and Dislocation Care Codes

Codes for fracture/dislocation care

- Are listed by anatomical location.
- Are provided (in most cases) for closed or open treatment, with or without manipulation, and with or without internal fixation.
- Typically include a 90-day period of follow-up care under the Medicare global package. Append modifier **57** (decision for surgery) to an E/M code when the decision for the procedure is made during a visit on the day before or day of the procedure.
- Are appended with modifier **54** to the usual procedure code if you provide initial fracture care (with or without manipulation) but transfer to another physician for follow-up care (applies to procedures with a 10- or 90- day global period). The transfer of care should be documented (eg, patient to see Dr X for continuing fracture care Monday morning).

Do not report a fracture care code when stabilization (eg, temporary cast/splint/strap) is performed to protect an injury and provide comfort to the patient until another physician performs initial fracture or dislocation care. Instead, report an evaluation and management service and the application of a cast, splint, or strapping (**29000–29584**), as indicated.

The physician providing follow-up care will report the same date of service and procedure code appended with modifier **55**. The claim will also denote the date of the transfer of care, which should be documented by both physicians.

- Include the initial casting, splinting, or strapping, but do not include radiographs.
- Routine follow-up visits during the global period are reported with no charge with code **99024** (post-op follow-up visit related to the original procedure).
- Are appended with modifier **76** to the usual procedure code to indicate repeat procedure or service by the same physician or other QHP for re-reduction of a fracture and/or dislocation.

Example

➤ **A child is evaluated in the ED for an injury to the left elbow following a fall caused by overturning her bicycle on the sidewalk of her apartment complex.** An orthopedic surgeon is consulted to determine if the injury requires percutaneous fixation. The orthopedic surgeon evaluates the child and diagnoses a displaced supracondylar humerus fracture. A decision is made to proceed with closed reduction and pinning. The procedure takes place on the same date. The child is admitted to the hospital for postoperative monitoring and discharged to home the next day. The orthopedic surgeon provided consultation, procedure, and discharge-day E/M services.

ICD-10-CM	CPT
S42.412A (displaced simple supracondylar fracture without intercondylar fracture of left humerus, initial encounter for closed fracture) **V18.0XXA** (pedal cycle driver injured in noncollision transport accident in nontraffic accident, initial encounter) **Y92.480** (sidewalk as the place of occurrence of the external cause)	**99251–99255 57** (inpatient consultation) or, if the payer does not pay consultation codes, **99221–99223 57** (initial hospital care)
Same as previous	**24538** (percutaneous skeletal fixation of supracondylar or transcondylar humeral fracture, with or without intercondylar extension)

Teaching Point: Because code **24538** is assigned a 90-day global period in the MPFS, many payers may require modifier **57** (decision for surgery) appended to the E/M code reported for the same date of service. Individual payers may have different policies. The postoperative care in the hospital is not separately reported. Follow-up visits in the office should be reported with code **99024** (postoperative follow-up visit).

> See the February 2021 *AAP Pediatric Coding Newsletter* article, "Initial Fracture Care: Musculoskeletal or Evaluation and Management," for additional examples of coding for fracture care (https://coding.solutions.aap.org/article.aspx?articleid=2765276; subscription required).

Osteotomy Humerus With Intramedullary Lengthening Device

A Category III (emerging technology) code is reported for osteotomy with insertion of an externally controlled lengthening device used in treatment of a limb length discrepancy. Note that this code is not reported for insertion of an intramedullary rod in treatment of a fracture.

0594T   Osteotomy, humerus, with insertion of an externally controlled intramedullary lengthening device, including intraoperative imaging, initial and subsequent alignment assessments, computations of adjustment schedules, and management of the intramedullary lengthening device

- Category III codes may not be covered by all health plans or may be covered under limited circumstances. Verify health plan coverage prior to providing these procedures.
- Do not report **0594T** in conjunction with application of multiplane, unilateral, external fixation with stereotactic computer-assisted adjustment (**20696**), osteotomy (**24400**, **24410**), osteoplasty (**24420**), or treatment of humeral shaft fracture with insertion of intramedullary implant (**24516**).
- Revision of externally controlled intramedullary lengthening device is reported with unlisted procedure code **24999**.

Removal of Musculoskeletal Hardware

20665   Removal of tongs or halo applied by another individual
20670   Removal of implant; superficial (eg, buried wire, pin or rod) (separate procedure)
20680   deep (eg, buried wire, pin, screw, metal band, nail, rod or plate)

Removal of a halo or tongs is included in the placement procedure. However, removal of a halo or tongs by another physician is separately reported with code **20665**. (*Note:* Physicians of the same specialty and same group practice are typically considered as the same physician for billing purposes.)

Codes **20670** and **20680** may be reported for removal of orthopedic hardware. If it is necessary to remove an implant within the global period (eg, due to breakage), report the appropriate removal code with modifier **78** (unplanned return to the operating/procedure room by the same physician or other QHP following initial procedure for a related procedure during the postoperative period.)

Respiratory

Intubation and Airway Management

31500   Intubation, endotracheal, emergency

- Moderate sedation (**99151–99157**) may be reported in addition to the intubation if used to sedate the patient prior to and during the intubation procedure (eg, in rapid sequence intubation) and reporting criteria are met.
- See the Sedation section later in this chapter for more on moderate sedation.

31502   Tracheostomy tube change prior to establishment of fistula tract

Report code **31502** only when an indwelling tracheostomy tube is replaced prior to establishment of a fistula tract.

> Routine changing of a tracheostomy tube after a fistula tract has been established is included in a related evaluation and management service. Code **31575** (laryngoscopy, flexible; diagnostic) may be reported when performed to check tracheostomy tube placement.

31505–31520   Indirect laryngoscopy

Report code **31505** for indirect diagnostic laryngoscopy. If, while performing this procedure, a foreign body is removed, report code **31511** (laryngoscopy with removal of foreign body).

31515   Direct laryngoscopy with or without tracheoscopy

Code **31515** is reported when laryngoscopy is performed for aspiration.

When diagnostic direct laryngoscopy, with or without tracheoscopy, is performed on a newborn, report code **31520**. Do not report modifier **63** (procedure performed on infant <4 kg) in conjunction with code **31520**.

31525   Laryngoscopy, direct, with or without tracheoscopy; diagnostic except newborn

Thoracostomy, Thoracentesis, and Pleural Drainage

32551   Tube thoracostomy, includes connection to drainage system (eg, water seal), when performed, open (separate procedure)

32554   Thoracentesis, needle or catheter, aspiration of the pleural space; without imaging guidance

32555   with imaging guidance

32556   Pleural drainage, percutaneous, with insertion of indwelling catheter; without imaging guidance

32557   with imaging guidance

- Thoracostomy (**32551**) represents an open procedure involving incision into a rib interspace with dissection extending through the chest wall muscles and pleura. Thoracentesis and percutaneous pleural drainage may be more commonly performed in pediatrics with the exception of neonatal and pediatric critical care.
- Percutaneous image guidance cannot be reported in conjunction with code **32551**, which represents an open procedure.

  Diagnostic ultrasound performed prior to thoracostomy to localize a collection in the pleural space is separately reportable only when the complete ultrasound study of the chest (**76604**) is performed with permanent recording of images.
- Thoracentesis codes **32554** and **32555** represent a procedure in which the surgical technique is puncture of the pleural space to remove fluid or air. Although a catheter (eg, pigtail catheter) may be used, it is not left in place at the end of the procedure.
- Percutaneous pleural drainage codes **32556** and **32557** represent procedures in which an indwelling catheter is inserted into the pleural space and remains at the end of the procedure. The catheter is secured in place and connected to a suction drainage system.
- Removal of chest tubes and non-tunneled indwelling pleural catheters is included in a related E/M service and not a separately reportable procedure.
- For insertion of a tunneled pleural catheter with cuff, see code **32550**. For removal of a tunneled pleural catheter with cuff, see **32552**.

Cardiovascular Procedures

Echocardiography

> New in 2022, report 3D echocardiographic imaging and postprocessing (**93319**) that is performed during transesophageal echocardiography or during transthoracic echocardiography for congenital cardiac anomalies.

+●93319   3D echocardiographic imaging and postprocessing during transesophageal echocardiography, or during transthoracic echocardiography for congenital cardiac anomalies, for the assessment of cardiac structure(s) (eg, cardiac chambers and valves, left atrial appendage, interatrial septum, interventricular septum) and function, when performed (List separately in addition to code for echocardiographic imaging)

> 3D echocardiographic imaging and postprocessing is reported when performed during transesophageal echocardiography in patients with or without congenital cardiac anomalies. When 3D echocardiographic imaging and postprocessing are performed during transthoracic echocardiography, report code **93319** only if the patient has congenital cardiac anomalies.

When performed, report code **93319** in conjunction with
- Transthoracic echocardiography for congenital cardiac anomalies (complete [**93303**] or follow-up/limited study [**93304**])
- Echocardiography, transesophageal, real time with image documentation (**93312**, **93314**)
- Transesophageal echocardiography for congenital cardiac anomalies (**93315**, **93317**)

Do not report **93319** in conjunction with
- 3D rendering with interpretation and reporting (**76376**, **76377**)
- Doppler echocardiography color flow velocity mapping (**93325**)
- Echocardiography, transesophageal, for guidance of a transcatheter intracardiac or great vessel(s) structural intervention(s) (**93355**)

Cardiac Catheterization for Congenital Heart Defects

New in 2022, codes **93530–93533** for cardiac catheterization for congenital anomalies have been deleted and replaced with codes **93593–93598**.

Modifier **63** may be appended to codes **93593–93598**, **93563**, **93564**, and **93568** (see complete list earlier in this chapter) when procedures are performed on an infant weighing less than 4 kg.

Evaluation of anomalous coronary arteries arising from the pulmonary arterial system is reported with the congenital catheterization codes **93593–93597**.

Codes **93530–93533** are deleted in 2022. New codes **93593–93598** are reported *only when cardiac catheterization is performed for evaluation of congenital cardiac defects.*

Diagnostic heart catheterization in a patient without congenital defect (eg, any acquired heart disease, such as dilated cardiomyopathy secondary to viral myocarditis, coronary artery diagnosis, or intervention in Kawasaki disease) is reported with codes **93451–93456**, **93460**, and **93461**.

There is no age limit for services reported with codes **93593–93598**. As long as there is evaluation of congenital cardiac defects, it is appropriate to report these codes. These codes take into account
- The added technical difficulty presented when structures may be in abnormal positions and locations and access is through abnormal native connections.
- Additional preservice time in discussing the procedure with parents, reviewing noninvasive data, previous cardiac catheterizations, and previous surgeries.
- Procedures may be more time consuming due to small vessels, multiple measurements that must be made, hemodynamic instability of patients, frequency of multiple sites of arterial-venous admixture, and performance of other required interventions.

Imaging guidance by the proceduralist included in heart catheterization includes ultrasound guidance of vascular access, generalized fluoroscopy to guide catheter manipulation, and any limited echocardiographic guidance when performed by the proceduralist. Echocardiography by another cardiologist during the same session is separately reported.

● **93593** Right heart catheterization for congenital heart defect(s) including imaging guidance by the proceduralist to advance the catheter to the target zone; normal native connections

● **93594** abnormal native connections

For reporting purposes, when the morphologic left ventricle or left atrium is in a subpulmonic position due to congenital heart disease (eg, transposition of the great arteries), catheter placement in either of these structures is considered part of right heart catheterization and does not constitute left heart catheterization.

● **93595** Left heart catheterization for congenital heart defect(s) including imaging guidance by the proceduralist to advance the catheter to the target zone, normal or abnormal native connections

● **93596** Right and left heart catheterization for congenital heart defect(s) including imaging guidance by the proceduralist to advance the catheter to the target zone(s); normal native connections

● **93597** abnormal native connections

Report the appropriate code for right and left heart catheterization if catheter placement with hemodynamic assessment of the double outlet ventricle *is performed during the right heart catheterization and separately from the arterial approach.* Catheter placement with hemodynamic assessment of the morphologic left ventricle during right heart catheterization alone (ie, not separately from the arterial approach) is considered part of that procedure.

+●93598   Cardiac output measurement(s), thermodilution or other indicator dilution method, performed during cardiac catheterization for the evaluation of congenital heart defects (List separately in addition to code for primary procedure)

> **Thermodilution cardiac output assessment are not typically included in right heart catheterization for congenital heart defects. Report code 93598 in addition to the code for diagnostic cardiac catheterization, when performed.**

- Codes for right heart or right and left heart catheterization for congenital defects are determined based on access through normal or abnormal native connections.
  - Normal native connections exist when blood flow follows the expected course (ie, superior vena cava/inferior vena cava to right atrium, then right ventricle, then pulmonary arteries for the right heart, and left atrium to left ventricle, then aorta for the left heart). Examples of congenital heart defects with normal connections would include acyanotic defects such as isolated atrial septal defect, ventricular septal defect, or patent ductus arteriosus.
  - Abnormal native connections exist when there are alternative connections for the pathway of blood flow through the heart and great vessels. Abnormal connections are typically present in patients with cyanotic congenital heart defects, any variation of single ventricle anatomy (eg, hypoplastic right or left heart, double outlet right ventricle), unbalanced atrioventricular canal (endocardial cushion) defect, transposition of the great arteries, valvular atresia, tetralogy of Fallot with or without major aortopulmonary collateral arteries, total anomalous pulmonary veins, truncus arteriosus, and any lesions with heterotaxia and/or dextrocardia.
- The work of imaging guidance, including fluoroscopy and ultrasound guidance for vascular access and to guide catheter placement for hemodynamic evaluation, is included in the cardiac catheterization for congenital heart defects codes, when performed by the same operator.
- Procedures such as percutaneous transcatheter closure of patent ductus arteriosus (93582) include right and left heart catheterization for congenital cardiac anomalies. Be sure to read the *CPT* instructions for procedures performed in conjunction with congenital cardiac catheterization to determine if the catheterization is separately reportable.

Related Procedures

Codes 93462–93464 are reported in conjunction with many services, including cardiac catheterization for congenital heart defects, when applicable.

+93462   Left heart catheterization by transseptal puncture through intact septum or by transapical puncture

   Report code 93462 in conjunction with 33477, 93452, 93453, 93458–93461, 93595–93597, 93582, 93653, and 93654.

- Also report code 93462 with 93581 for transseptal or transapical puncture performed for percutaneous transcatheter closure of ventricular septal defect.
- For *transapical puncture* performed for left heart catheterization and percutaneous transcatheter closure of paravalvular leak, report code 93462 in conjunction with 93590 and 93591. However, do not report 93462 in conjunction with 93590 for *transeptal puncture* through intact septum performed for left heart catheterization and percutaneous transcatheter closure of paravalvular leak.

+93463   Pharmacologic agent administration (eg, inhaled nitric oxide, intravenous infusion of nitroprusside, dobutamine, milrinone, or other agent) including assessing hemodynamic measurements before, during, after and repeat pharmacologic agent administration, when performed (List separately in addition to code for primary procedure)

   Report code 93463 in conjunction with 33477, 93451–93453, 93456–93461, 93593–93597, or 93593–93597.

+93464   Physiologic exercise study (eg, bicycle or arm ergometry) including assessing hemodynamic measurements before and after

   Report code 93464 in conjunction with 33477, 93451–93453, 93456–93461, and 93593–93597.

   Table 19-3 provides a quick reference to codes for cardiac catheterization for congenital anomalies with codes included for many services that are separately reported when performed during the catheterization.

Pericardiocentesis and Pericardial Drainage

33016   Pericardiocentesis, including imaging guidance, when performed
33017   Pericardial drainage with insertion of indwelling catheter, percutaneous, including fluoroscopy and/or ultrasound guidance, when performed; 6 years and older without congenital cardiac anomaly
33018   birth through 5 years of age or any age with congenital cardiac anomaly
33019   Pericardial drainage with insertion of indwelling catheter, percutaneous, including CT guidance

Table 19-3. Codes for Cardiac Catheterization for Congenital Heart Defects[a,b]

Type of Catheterization	Right Heart With Normal Native Connections (93593)[c]	Right Heart With Abnormal Native Connections (93594)[c]	Left Heart (Only) (93595)[c]	Right and Left Heart With Normal Native Connections[d] (93596)[c]	Right and Left Heart With Abnormal Native Connections[d] (93597)[c]
Catheterization includes imaging guidance by the proceduralist to advance the catheter to the target zone. See *CPT* reference for complete code descriptors and instructions.					
Separately Reported Services					
With cardiac output measurement(s)	+93598[c]	+93598[c]	+93598[c]	+93598[c]	+93598[c]
With transseptal or transapical access of left atrium	Not applicable	Not applicable	+93462	+93462	+93462
With pharmacologic agent administration	+93463	+93463	+93463	+93463	+93463
With physiologic exercise study	+93464	+93464	+93464	+93464	+93464
With intravascular Doppler velocity and/or pressure derived coronary flow reserve measurement (coronary vessel or graft)	+93571 (first vessel) +93572 (each additional vessel)	+93571 (first vessel) +93572 (each additional vessel)	+93571 (first vessel) +93572 (each additional vessel)	+93571 (first vessel) +93572 (each additional vessel)	+93571 (first vessel) +93572 (each additional vessel)

Abbreviation: *CPT, Current Procedural Terminology.*

[a] Report evaluation of anomalous coronary arteries arising from the pulmonary arterial system with codes for cardiac catheterization for congenital heart defect.

[b] In the absence of other congenital heart defects, report cardiac catheterization services for anomalous coronary arteries arising from the aorta or off of other coronary arteries, patent foramen ovale, mitral valve prolapse, and bicuspid aortic valve with codes **93451–93464** or **93566–93568.**

[c] Report modifier **63** when the procedure is performed on an infant weighing less than 4 kg.

[d] Report the appropriate code for right and left heart catheterization if catheter placement with hemodynamic assessment of double outlet ventricle is performed during the right heart catheterization and separately from the arterial approach. For reporting purposes, when the morphologic left ventricle or left atrium is in a subpulmonic position due to congenital heart disease, catheter placement in either of these structures is considered part of right heart catheterization and does not constitute left heart catheterization.

- Codes **33016–33019** include imaging guidance when performed. Do not separately report imaging guidance (eg, **75989, 76942, 77002, 77012, 77021**) with codes **33016–33019.**

  For thoracoscopic (video assisted) pericardial procedures, see code **32601, 32604, 32658, 32659,** or **32661.**

- Echocardiography, when performed solely for the purpose of pericardiocentesis guidance, is not separately reported in addition to codes **33016–33018.**

- For purposes of reporting percutaneous pericardial drainage with insertion of indwelling catheter (**33017–33019**), congenital cardiac anomaly is defined as
  - Abnormal situs (heterotaxy, dextrocardia, mesocardia)
  - Single ventricle anomaly/physiology
  - Any patient in the first 90-day postoperative period after repair of a congenital cardiac anomaly defect

- Report **33017–33019** only when the catheter remains in place when the procedure is completed and not when a catheter is placed to aspirate fluid and then removed at the conclusion of the procedure.

Atrial Septostomy

33741 Transcatheter atrial septostomy (TAS) for congenital cardiac anomalies to create effective atrial flow, including all imaging guidance by the proceduralist, when performed, any method (eg, Rashkind, Sang-Park, balloon, cutting balloon, blade)

●=New code ▲=Revised code #=Re-sequenced code +=Add-on code ★=Telemedicine

33745 Transcatheter intracardiac shunt (TIS) creation by stent placement for congenital cardiac anomalies to establish effective intracardiac flow, all imaging guidance by the proceduralist when performed, left and right heart diagnostic cardiac catheterization for congenital cardiac anomalies, and target zone angioplasty, when performed (eg, atrial septum, Fontan fenestration, right ventricular outflow tract, Mustard/Senning/Warden baffles); initial intracardiac shunt

+33746 each additional intracardiac shunt location (List separately in addition to code for primary procedure)

Codes 33741–33746 are used to report creation of effective intracardiac blood flow in the setting of congenital heart defects.

> A parenthetical instruction below add-on code 93662 is updated in 2022 to include the codes for transcatheter atrial septostomy (33741, 33745, 33746). Report code 93662 in addition to these codes when intracardiac echocardiography including imaging supervision and interpretation is performed during the services.
>
> Code 93662 is also reported in conjunction with other services such as certain cardiac catheterization codes. See your 2022 *CPT* reference for the current and complete list of codes for services to which 93662 is an add-on code when intracardiac echocardiography is performing during the service.

Code 33741

- Involves the percutaneous creation of improved atrial blood flow (eg, balloon/blade method), typically in infants weighing 4 kg or less with congenital heart disease. Do not append modifier 63 (procedures performed on infants <4 kg) to 33741.
- Ultrasound guidance for vascular access and fluoroscopic guidance for the intervention is included, when performed.
- Use 93462 to report transseptal puncture performed in conjunction with 33741.
- Diagnostic cardiac catheterization is not typically performed at the same session as code 33741; separately report each service when performed. See instructions in *CPT* addressing when it is appropriate to separately report cardiac catheterization.

 Do not separately report cardiac catheterization that is fluoroscopic guidance for the intervention or limited hemodynamic and angiographic data used solely for purposes of accomplishing the intervention.

Codes 33745 and 33746

- Include intracardiac stent placement, target zone angioplasty preceding or after stent implantation, and *complete diagnostic right and left heart catheterization* (not separately reported), when performed.
  - Ultrasound guidance for vascular access and fluoroscopic guidance for the intervention is included, when performed.
  - Includes any and all balloon angioplasties performed in the target lesion, including any pre-dilation or post-dilation following stent placement, or use of larger/smaller balloon to achieve therapeutic result.
  - Angioplasty in a separate and distinct intracardiac lesion may be reported separately with modifier 59 (distinct procedural service) appended to the angioplasty code.
- Although diagnostic angiography (93563, 93565–93568) is typically performed during 33745, target vessels and chambers are highly variable and, *when performed for an evaluation separate and distinct from the stent delivery,* may be reported separately.

 Append modifier 59 to codes for diagnostic angiography performed at the same session for angiographic evaluation separate and distinct from the shunt creation.

- When additional, different intracardiac locations are treated in the same session, code 33746 may be reported for each additional intracardiac shunt creation by stent placement at a separate location.

> Multiple stents placed in a single location may only be reported with a single code and not a first or additional unit of 33746.

Valvuloplasty

33390 Valvuloplasty, aortic valve, open, with cardiopulmonary bypass; simple (ie, valvotomy, debridement, debulking, and/or simple commissural resuspension)

33391 complex (eg, leaflet extension, leaflet resection, leaflet reconstruction, or annuloplasty)

Do not report code 33391 in conjunction with code 33390.

Codes for open valvuloplasty of the aortic valve
- Are descriptive of currently performed valvuloplasty procedures
  - Code **33390** is specifically for reporting valvotomy, debridement, debulking, and/or simple commissural resuspension.
  - Code **33391** represents more complex procedures not limited to the examples in the code descriptor.
- May be reported in conjunction with the code for transmyocardial revascularization (**33141**), operative tissue ablation and reconstruction of atria (**33255–33259**), and reoperation, valve procedure, more than 1 month after original operation (**33530**), when appropriate

Open procedures for aortic valve replacement are reported with codes **33405**, **33406**, and **33410** based on the type of replacement valve (ie, prosthetic, homograft, or stentless).

Transcatheter Pulmonary Valve Implantation

33477   Transcatheter pulmonary valve implantation, percutaneous approach, including pre-stenting of the valve delivery site, when performed

The key instructions for reporting code **33477** are
- Should only be reported once per session
- Includes, when performed
  - Percutaneous access, placing the access sheath, advancing the repair device delivery system into position, repositioning the device as needed and deploying the device(s), angiography, all cardiac catheterization(s) for hemodynamic measurements, intraprocedural contrast injections, radiologic supervision, and interpretation performed to guide transcatheter pulmonary valve implantation.

    Do not separately report diagnostic angiography (**93563**, **93566–93568**) or right heart catheterization (**93451–93461**; **93593**, **93594**; **93596–93598**) that is intrinsic to the procedure.
  - Percutaneous balloon angioplasty of the conduit or treatment zone, valvuloplasty of the pulmonary valve conduit, and stent deployment within the pulmonary conduit or an existing bioprosthetic pulmonary valve.

Diagnostic angiography and right heart catheterization may be separately reported (append modifier **59**) only when one of the following is true:
- No prior study is available and a full diagnostic study is performed.
- A prior study is available, but, as documented in the medical record, one of the following applies:
  - There is inadequate visualization of the anatomy and/or pathology.
  - The patient's condition with respect to the clinical indication has changed since the prior study.
  - There is a clinical change during the procedure that requires new evaluation.

Other cardiac catheterization services may be reported separately when performed for diagnostic purposes not intrinsic to transcatheter pulmonary valve implantation.
- **Does not include** (Report separately, when performed.)
  - Codes **92997** and **92998** when pulmonary artery angioplasty is performed at a site separate from the prosthetic valve delivery site
  - Codes **37236** and **37237** when pulmonary artery stenting is performed at a site separate from the prosthetic valve delivery site
  - Same-session/same-day *diagnostic* cardiac catheterization services (See your *CPT* reference for further instruction and append catheterization code with modifier **59**.)
  - Diagnostic coronary angiography performed at a separate session from an interventional procedure
  - Percutaneous coronary interventional procedures
  - Percutaneous pulmonary artery branch interventions
  - Percutaneous ventricular assist device procedure codes (**33990–33993**), ECMO/ECLS procedure codes (**33946–33989**), or balloon pump insertion codes (**33967**, **33970**, **33973**)
  - Percutaneous peripheral bypass (**33367**), open peripheral bypass (**33368**), or central bypass (**33369**)

Transcatheter Interventions for Revascularization/Repair for Coarctation of the Aorta

- **●33894**   Endovascular stent repair of coarctation of the ascending, transverse, or descending thoracic or abdominal aorta, involving stent placement; across major side branches
- **●33895**   not crossing major side branches
- **●33897**   Percutaneous transluminal angioplasty of native or recurrent coarctation of the aorta

Codes **33894**, **33895**, and **33897** include all fluoroscopic guidance of the intervention, diagnostic congenital left heart catheterization, all catheter and wire introductions and manipulation, and angiography of the target lesion. For additional diagnostic right heart catheterization in the same setting as **33894** and **33895**, see codes **93593** and **93594**.

Code **33897** may be reported in addition to **33894** or **33895** for balloon angioplasty of an additional coarctation of the aorta in a segment *separate from the treatment zone* for the coarctation stent. However, balloon angioplasty *within the target treatment zone*, either before or after stent deployment, is not separately reportable in conjunction with **33894** or **33895**. For angioplasty and other transcatheter revascularization interventions *of additional upper or lower extremity vessels* in same setting as **33897**, use the appropriate code from the Surgery/Cardiovascular System section of *CPT*.

Do not report **33897** in conjunction with open or percutaneous transluminal angioplasty (**37246**) or with transcatheter stent placement for occlusive disease (**37236**).

Codes **33894** and **33895** include stent introduction, manipulation, positioning, and deployment as well as any additional stent delivery in tandem with the initial stent for extension purposes.

- Codes **33894** and **33895** are differentiated by whether or not stent placement crosses major side branches of the aorta. Major side branches include
  — Thoracic aorta: brachiocephalic, carotid, and subclavian arteries
  — Abdominal aorta: celiac, superior mesenteric, inferior mesenteric, and renal arteries
- Do not separately report the following services when reporting codes **33894**, **33895**, and **33897**:
  — Insertion of a temporary pacemaker (**33210**) to facilitate stent positioning, when performed
  — Introduction, positioning, and deployment of an endograft for treatment of abdominal aortic pathology (**34701–34706**)
  — Introduction of catheter, aorta (**36200**)
  — Thoracic or abdominal aortography (**75600, 75605, 75625**)
  — Left heart catheterization for congenital heart defect(s) (**93595**)
  — Right and left heart catheterization for congenital heart defect(s) for normal or abnormal native connections (**93596, 93597**)
- Do not separately report balloon angioplasty of the aorta *within the coarctation treatment zone* (transluminal angioplasty, **37246**; open or percutaneous angioplasty with transcatheter stent placement for occlusive disease, **37236**; or **33897**) when reporting **33894** and **33895**.
- The following services may be separately reported when performed before or after coarctation stent deployment during endovascular repair of coarctation of the aorta (**33894, 33895**):
  — Balloon angioplasty or stenting of the innominate, carotid, subclavian, visceral, iliac, or pulmonary artery
  — Arterial or venous embolization
  — Additional atrial, ventricular, pulmonary, or coronary or bypass graph angiography with injection procedure during cardiac catheterization (**93563–93568**)

For angiography of other vascular structures, use the appropriate code from the Radiology/Diagnostic Radiology section of *CPT*.

Percutaneous Transcatheter Closure of Patent Ductus Arteriosus

93582   Percutaneous transcatheter closure of patent ductus arteriosus

- Includes, when performed (do not separately report)
  — Introduction of catheter, right heart or main pulmonary artery (**36013**)
  — Selective catheter placement, left or right pulmonary artery (**36014**)
  — Introduction of catheter, aorta (**36200**)
  — Aortography, thoracic, without serialography, radiological supervision and interpretation (**75600**)
  — Aortography, thoracic, by serialography, radiological supervision and interpretation (**75605**)
  — Heart catheterization or catheter placement for coronary angiography (**93451–94361**)
  — Heart catheterization for congenital cardiac anomalies (**93593–93598**)
  — Injection procedure during cardiac catheterization including imaging supervision, interpretation, and report; for supravalvular aortography (**93567**)
- Separately report when performed at the time of transcatheter patent ductus arteriosus closure
  — Pharmacologic agent administration (**93463**)
  — Intracardiac echocardiography during therapeutic/diagnostic intervention, including imaging supervision and interpretation (**93662**)

Chapter 19. Common Surgical Procedures and Sedation in Facility Settings

— Add-on codes for injection procedures during cardiac catheterization, including imaging supervision, interpretation, and report, for
- Selective coronary angiography during congenital heart catheterization (**93563**)
- Selective opacification of aortocoronary venous or arterial bypass graft(s) to one or more coronary arteries and in situ arterial conduits, whether native or used for bypass to one or more coronary arteries during congenital heart catheterization, when performed (**93564**)
- Selective left ventricular or left atrial angiography (**93565**)
- Selective right ventricular or right atrial angiography (**93566**)
- Pulmonary angiography (**93568**)

> Modifier **63** may be appended to code **93582** when the procedure is performed on an infant weighing less than 4 kg.

Vascular Access

Many vascular access procedures are included in the services reported with critical or intensive care codes. Please see **Chapter 18** for a list of procedures that are not separately reported by a physician or QHP who is reporting critical care services on the same date.

Central Venous Access

There is no distinction between venous access achieved percutaneously or via cutdown. Report the venous access code (**tables 19-4** and **19-5**) appropriate to the
- Type of insertion (ie, centrally inserted or peripherally inserted)
- Type of catheter (eg, non-tunneled vs tunneled)
- Device (eg, with or without port)
- Age of child

In non-facility settings, code **96522** may be reported for refilling and maintenance of an implantable pump or reservoir for systemic (intravenous, intra-arterial) drug delivery.

Irrigation of an implanted venous access device for drug delivery (**96523**) is only reported in non-facility settings and when no other service is reported by the same individual on the same date.
- Codes for refilling and maintenance and/or irrigation are not reported by physicians in facility settings.

> If an existing central venous access device is removed and a new one *placed via a separate venous access site,* appropriate codes for both procedures (removal of old, if code exists, and insertion of new device) should be reported. See replacement codes for removal with replacement *via the same venous access site.*

Table 19-4. Insertion and Replacement of Central Venous Catheter		
Insertion	**Child <5 y**	**Child ≥5 y**
Insertion non-tunneled centrally inserted central venous catheter	36555	36556
Insertion tunneled centrally inserted central venous catheter, without subcutaneous port or pump	36557	36558
Insertion tunneled centrally inserted central venous access device, with subcutaneous port	36560	36561
Insertion tunneled centrally inserted central venous access device		**Any Age**
with subcutaneous pump		36563
requiring 2 catheters via 2 separate venous access sites; without subcutaneous port or pump (eg, Tesio-type catheter)		36565
requiring 2 catheters via 2 separate venous access sites; with subcutaneous port(s)		36566
Replacement		
Replacement, *catheter only,* of central venous access device, with subcutaneous port or pump, central or peripheral insertion site		36578
Replacement, *complete,* of a non-tunneled centrally inserted central venous catheter, without subcutaneous port or pump, through same venous access		36580

●=New code ▲=Revised code #=Re-sequenced code +=Add-on code ★=Telemedicine

Table 19-4 (*continued*)	
Replacement (*continued*)	
Replacement, *complete*, of a tunneled centrally inserted central venous catheter, without subcutaneous port or pump, through same venous access	**36581**
Replacement, *complete*, of a tunneled centrally inserted central venous access device, with subcutaneous port, through same venous access	**36582**
Replacement, *complete*, of a tunneled centrally inserted central venous access device, with subcutaneous pump, through same venous access	**36583**

Table 19-5. Insertion or Replacement of Peripherally Inserted Central Venous Catheter		
Insertion Procedure	**Child <5 y**	**Child ≥5 y**
Insertion of peripherally inserted central venous catheter, without subcutaneous port or pump, *without imaging guidance*	**36568**	**36569**
Insertion of peripherally inserted central venous access device, with subcutaneous port	**36570**	**36571**
Insertion of peripherally inserted central venous catheter, without subcutaneous port or pump, including all imaging guidance, image documentation, and all associated radiological supervision and interpretation required to perform the insertion	**#36572**	**#36573**
Replacement Procedure	**Any Age**	
Replacement, catheter only, of central venous access device, with subcutaneous port or pump, central or peripheral insertion site	**36578**	
Replacement, complete, of a peripherally inserted central venous catheter, without subcutaneous port or pump, through same venous access, including all imaging guidance, image documentation, and all associated radiological supervision and interpretation required to perform the replacement	**36584**	
Replacement, complete, of a peripherally inserted central venous access device, with subcutaneous port, through same venous access	**36585**	

Insertion or Replacement of Centrally Inserted Central Venous Access Device

- To qualify as a centrally inserted central venous access device, both of the following must be true:
  - The entry site must be the *jugular, subclavian, or femoral vein or the inferior vena cava.*
  - The tip of the catheter must terminate in the *subclavian, brachiocephalic (innominate), or iliac veins; the superior or inferior vena cava; or the right atrium.*
- Moderate sedation services are separately reportable with codes **99151–99157**. For more information on reporting moderate sedation, see the Sedation section later in this chapter.
- Report imaging guidance for gaining access to venous entry site or manipulating the catheter into final central position (in addition to codes **36555–36558**) with either of the following codes:
  - **76937** (ultrasound guidance for vascular access requiring ultrasound evaluation of potential access sites, documentation of selected vessel patency, concurrent real-time ultrasound visualization of vascular needle entry, with permanent recording and reporting)
  - **77001** (fluoroscopic guidance for central venous access device placement, replacement [catheter only or complete], or removal [includes fluoroscopic guidance for vascular access and catheter manipulation, any necessary contrast injections through access site or catheter with related venography radiologic supervision and interpretation, and radiographic documentation of final catheter position])
- Documentation of ultrasound guidance for peripherally inserted central catheter (PICC) placement should include evaluation of the potential puncture sites, patency of the entry vein, and real-time ultrasound visualization of needle entry into the vein.
- *Do not separately report ultrasound for vessel identification only.*

Insertion of Peripherally Inserted Central Venous Access Device

Midline catheters terminate in the peripheral venous system. Midline catheter insertion is not reported as a peripherally inserted central venous catheter insertion. See codes 36400, 36406, and 36410 for midline catheter insertion.

- To qualify as a PICC, both of the following must be true:
  — The entry site must be a peripheral vein (eg, axillary, basilic, or cephalic).
  — The tip of the catheter must terminate in the subclavian, brachiocephalic (innominate), or iliac veins; the superior or inferior vena cava; or the right atrium.
- Codes 36568 and 36569 are reported for PICC insertion without a subcutaneous port *and without imaging guidance* based on the patient's age.
    Do not report imaging guidance (76937, 77001) in conjunction with codes 36568 and 36569.
- If imaging guidance is used in PICC insertion, see codes 36572, 36573, and 36584. Imaging guidance is included in the placement (36572, 36573) or complete replacement (36584) of a PICC without subcutaneous port or pump.
- Using magnetic guidance or any other guidance modality that does not include imaging or image documentation for insertion of a PICC is reported with codes 36568 and 36569.
- Chest radiographs (71045–71048) should not be reported for the purpose of documenting the final catheter position by the same physician on the same day of service as the PICC insertion (36572, 36573, or 36584).
    If PICC insertion is performed without confirmation of the catheter tip location, append modifier 52 (reduced service) to the code for catheter insertion (36572, 36573, or 36584).
- Documentation of services includes
  — Images from all modalities used (eg, ultrasound, fluoroscopy) stored to the patient record
  — Associated supervision and interpretation
  — Venography performed through the same venous puncture
  — The final central position of the catheter with imaging
- Report PICC insertion *with a subcutaneous port* with codes 36570 and 36571.
  — Ultrasound (76937) or fluoroscopic guidance (77001) may be separately reported when performed and documented.
  — Documentation of ultrasound guidance for PICC placement should include evaluation of the potential puncture sites, patency of the entry vein, and real-time ultrasound visualization of needle entry into the vein.

Repair of Central Venous Catheters

36575	Repair of tunneled or non-tunneled central venous access catheter, without subcutaneous port or pump, central or peripheral insertion site
36576	Repair of central venous access device, with subcutaneous port or pump, central or peripheral insertion site
36593	Declotting by thrombolytic agent of implanted vascular access device or catheter
36595	Mechanical removal of pericatheter obstructive material (eg, fibrin sheath) from central venous device via separate venous access

> For radiologic supervision and interpretation of mechanical removal of pericatheter obstructive material from a central venous device via separate venous access, report 75901.

36596	Mechanical removal of intraluminal (intracatheter) obstructive material from central venous device through device lumen
36598	Contrast injection(s) for radiologic evaluation of existing central venous access device, including fluoroscopy, image documentation and report

Repair of a central venous catheter includes fixing the device without replacement of the catheter or port/pump.
- For the repair of a multi-catheter device, with or without subcutaneous ports or pumps, use the appropriate code describing the service with 2 units of service.
- Repair of any central venous access catheter *without a port or pump* is reported with code 36575.
- Repair of any central venous catheter *with a port or pump* is reported with code 36576.
- Code 36593 is reported for declotting of an implanted vascular device or catheter *by thrombolysis.*
- Code 36593 *is not reported* for declotting of a pleural catheter. Use unlisted procedure code 32999 for declotting of a pleural catheter.
- Code 36595 and 36596 are reported for a procedure with *mechanical removal* of pericatheter or intraluminal obstructive material.
  — Radiologic supervision and interpretation are separately reported with code 75901.
  — Do not report code 36595 or 36596 in conjunction with code 36593 or 36598.

- When the patency of a central line is evaluated under fluoroscopy, code **36598** is reported for the contrast injection, image documentation, and report.
  - Fluoroscopy (**76000**) is not separately reported.
  - See codes **75820–75827** for complete venography studies.

Removal of Central Venous Catheters

36589   Removal of tunneled central venous catheter, without subcutaneous port or pump

36590   Removal of tunneled central venous access device, with subcutaneous port or pump, central or peripheral insertion

   Removal codes are reported for removal of the entire device. See replacement codes for partial replacement (catheter only) or complete exchange *in the same venous access site* of central venous access devices.

- For removal of both catheters (placed from separate venous access sites) of a multi-catheter device, with or without subcutaneous ports/pumps, use the appropriate code describing the service with 2 units of service.
- When removal of an existing central venous access device is performed in conjunction with placement of new device *via a separate venous access site,* report both procedures.

Arterial Access

36600   Arterial puncture, withdrawal of blood for diagnosis

36620   Arterial catheterization or cannulation for sampling, monitoring or transfusion (separate procedure); percutaneous

36625   cutdown

- An arterial puncture for diagnosis is reported with code **36600**.
- Code **36620** is reported when a percutaneous peripheral arterial catheterization is performed. Code **36625** is reported when a cutdown is performed.

Transfusions

36430   Transfusion, blood or blood components

36440   Push transfusion; blood, 2 years or younger

> Push transfusion (**36440**) is used only for patients younger than 2 years.

36450   Exchange transfusion, blood, newborn

36455   other than newborn

36456   Partial exchange transfusion, blood, plasma, or crystalloid necessitating the skill of a physician or other qualified health care professional; newborn

> The placement of catheters to support exchange transfusions may be reported separately with the appropriate vascular access codes.

- Transfusion (**36430**) or push transfusion (**36440**) should be used only if the physician personally infuses the substance, and not if the blood is administered by nursing personnel and allowed to enter the vessel via gravity or meter flow.

   Codes **36430** and **36440** are not separately reported when the same physician or physicians of the same specialty and same group practice are reporting neonatal or pediatric critical care (**99468–99472, 99475, 99476**).

- Complete exchange transfusions (double volume) performed during the neonatal period are reported using code **36450**; exchange transfusions for all other age groups are reported using code **36455**.
  - The assumption is that the exchange for the neonate is performed via the umbilical vein, while an exchange for an older child or adult is performed via a peripheral vessel.
  - The actual placement of catheters to support the exchange transfusion may be reported separately with the appropriate vascular access codes.
- Partial exchange transfusions (eg, for hyperviscosity syndrome in the neonate) should be reported using code **36456**.

   Do not report other transfusion codes (**36430, 36440,** or **36450**) with **36456**.

- Do not append modifier **63** (procedure performed on infants <4 kg) when reporting code **36450** or **36456**.

See Chapter 10 for information on coding for hydration and intravenous infusion services.

These services *are not reported by a physician or other QHP when performed in a facility setting* because the physician work associated with these procedures involves only affirmation of the treatment plan and direct supervision of the staff performing the services. These codes may be reported by the facility.

Ear, Nose, and Throat Procedures

69421   Myringotomy including aspiration and/or eustachian tube inflation requiring general anesthesia

69436   Tympanostomy (requiring insertion of ventilating tube), general anesthesia

- For bilateral procedure, report code **69436** with modifier **50**.
- Insertion of ventilation tube(s) is not separately reported when performed in conjunction with another middle ear procedure (eg, tympanoplasty) without significant increase in work.
- Cleaning debris from the lateral drum, including a pars flaccida retraction pocket, is inclusive to the tube placement code.
- Use of an operating microscope is included in the procedure described by **69436**.

92511   Nasopharyngoscopy with endoscope (separate procedure)

Code **92511** is designated as a "separate procedure" and should not be reported in addition to the code for the total procedure or service of which it is considered an integral component.

- When carried out independently, report code **92511**.
- When considered to be unrelated or distinct from other procedures or services provided at that time, report code **92511 59** in addition to other procedures or services.

Laryngoplasty

#31551   Laryngoplasty; for laryngeal stenosis, with graft, without indwelling stent placement, younger than 12 years of age

#31552   age 12 years or older

#31553   Laryngoplasty; for laryngeal stenosis, with graft, with indwelling stent placement, younger than 12 years of age

#31554   age 12 years or older

31580   Laryngoplasty; for laryngeal web, with indwelling keel or stent insertion

31584   Laryngoplasty; with open reduction and fixation of (eg, plating) fracture, includes tracheostomy, if performed

- Do not report graft separately if harvested through the laryngoplasty incision (eg, thyroid cartilage graft).
- Report only one of the following codes for a single operative session: **31551–31554** or **31580**.
- Codes for treatment of laryngeal stenosis by laryngoplasty with graft are selected based on whether or not the procedure includes indwelling stent placement and by the age of the patient (<12 years or ≥12 years).
- Open treatment of a hyoid fracture is reported with code **31584** (repair procedure on the larynx).
- To report tracheostomy, see code **31600**, **31601**, **31603**, **31605**, or **31610**.
- Report laryngoplasty, not otherwise specified or for removal of a keel or stent, with code **31599**.

Adenoidectomy and Tonsillectomy

42820   Tonsillectomy and adenoidectomy; younger than age 12

42821   age 12 or over

42825   Tonsillectomy, primary or secondary; younger than age 12

42826   age 12 or over

42830   Adenoidectomy, primary; younger than age 12

42831   age 12 or over

42835   Adenoidectomy, secondary; younger than age 12

42836   age 12 or over

For partial ablation of tonsils with laser, report the appropriate code from **42820** or **42821**, or **42825** or **42826**, with modifier **52** (reduced service).

For control of hemorrhage following tonsillectomy or adenoidectomy, see codes **42960–42972**.

Digestive System Procedures

Gastric Intubation and Aspiration

43752	Naso- or orogastric tube placement, requiring physician's skill and fluoroscopic guidance (includes fluoroscopy, image documentation and report)
43753	Gastric intubation and aspiration(s), therapeutic (eg, for ingested poisons), including lavage if performed

Do not report code **43752** or **43753** in conjunction with critical or intensive care services (**99291**, **99292**; **99466–99469**; **99471–99476**; or **99477–99480**). Append modifier **25** to codes for other significant, separately identifiable E/M services (eg, hospital care, consultation).

Note that code **43752** is reported when a physician's skill is required for placement of a nasogastric or orogastric tube using fluoroscopic guidance.

- This service is not separately reported when a physician's skill is not required or placement is performed without fluoroscopic guidance.
- Replacement of a nasogastric tube requiring physician's skill and fluoroscopic guidance may also be reported with code **43752**.
- Do not separately report **43752** for tube placement to insufflate the stomach prior to percutaneous gastrointestinal tube placement.

Examples

➤ **A 10-year-old is brought to the ED after having ingested drugs.** Gastric intubation and lavage are performed.

Code **43753** would be reported in addition to the appropriate E/M service (eg, ED services **99281–99285**).

➤ **A patient requires placement of a nasogastric tube.** Attempts by nursing staff are unsuccessful, so placement by the physician is required. The physician places the tube using fluoroscopic guidance.

Code **43752** would be reported in addition to the appropriate E/M service but is not reported when the service is performed by the physician out of convenience rather than necessity for a physician's skill. Use of fluoroscopic guidance is required and must be documented (ie, image documentation and report).

Appendectomy

44950	Appendectomy
+44955	when done for indicated purpose at time of other major procedure
44960	for ruptured appendix with abscess or generalized peritonitis
44970	Laparoscopy, surgical, appendectomy
44979	Unlisted laparoscopy procedure, appendix

As a sole procedure, appendectomy coding is fairly straightforward, with 3 code choices: **44950**, **44960**, and **44970**.

CPT instructs that incidental appendectomy (ie, not due to disease or symptom) during intra-abdominal surgery does not usually warrant reporting a code for the appendectomy procedure.

- If it is necessary to report an incidental appendectomy performed during another intra-abdominal procedure, append modifier **52** (reduced service).
- The Medicaid NCCI manual also instructs that incidental removal of a normal appendix during another abdominal surgery is not separately reportable. This instruction is likely followed by other payers.

Appendectomy performed for an indicated purpose (ie, problem with the appendix) in conjunction with another procedure is separately reported.

- Report add-on code **44955** in addition the code for the primary procedure when open appendectomy is performed (due to clinical indication) in conjunction with another procedure.
- For a laparoscopic appendectomy when done for an indicated purpose at the time of another major procedure, report code **44979**.
- A separate diagnosis code (distinct from the diagnoses for which other intra-abdominal procedures were performed) should be linked to the appendectomy procedure code to indicate the medical necessity of the procedure.

Hernia Repair

49491	Repair, initial inguinal hernia, preterm infant (younger than 37 weeks gestation at birth), performed from birth up to 50 weeks postconception age, with or without hydrocelectomy; reducible
49492	incarcerated or strangulated
49495	Repair, initial inguinal hernia, full term infant younger than age 6 months, or preterm infant older than 50 weeks postconception age and younger than age 6 months at the time of surgery, with or without hydrocelectomy; reducible
49496	incarcerated or strangulated
49500	Repair initial inguinal hernia, age 6 months to younger than 5 years, with or without hydrocelectomy; reducible
49501	incarcerated or strangulated
49505	Repair initial inguinal hernia, age 5 years or older; reducible
49507	incarcerated or strangulated
49520	Repair recurrent inguinal hernia, any age; reducible
49521	incarcerated or strangulated

- For purposes of reporting inguinal hernia repair, postconception age equals gestational age at birth plus age of newborn/infant in weeks at the time of the hernia repair. **Table 19-6** includes criteria for determining initial hernia repair codes by patient birth status, age, and hernia status.
- Initial inguinal hernia repair performed on preterm newborns and infants who are older than 50 weeks' postconception age and younger than 6 months at the time of surgery should be reported using codes 49495 and 49496.
- Modifier 63 (procedure performed on infants <4 kg) is not appended to code 49491, 49492, 49495, or 49496.
- Separately report inguinal hernia repair (49495–49525) performed in conjunction with inguinal orchiopexy (54640).

Table 19-6. Code Selection for Initial Hernia Repair in Infants

Patient Status	Hernia Reducible	Hernia Incarcerated or Strangulated
Preterm, <37 weeks gestation at birth, performed from birth up to 50 weeks postconception age	49491	49492
Term infant age <6 months, or preterm infant >50 weeks postconception age and <6 months at the time of surgery	49495	49496

Genitourinary System Procedures

Anogenital Examination

99170	Anogenital examination, magnified, in childhood for suspected trauma including image recording when performed

Moderate sedation of 10 minutes or more may be separately reported when performed by the same physician performing the anogenital examination.

Example

➤ **A child is brought to the ED for concern of sexual molestation after blood was found in the child's underpants.**
The physician performs a comprehensive history and physical examination. Because of the findings on general examination, the physician elects to further examine the child's genitalia with magnification to document findings that may be consistent with abuse or trauma.

CPT copyright 2021 American Medical Association. All rights reserved. ● =New code ▲ =Revised code # =Re-sequenced code + =Add-on code ★ =Telemedicine

Chapter 19. Common Surgical Procedures and Sedation in Facility Settings

ICD-10-CM	CPT
Report confirmed abuse with all of the following: **T74.22XA** (child sexual abuse, confirmed, initial encounter) An appropriate injury code (eg, **S39.848A**, other specified injuries of external genitals, initial encounter) A code from categories **X92–Y06** or **Y08** for assault A code from category **Y07** to identify the perpetrator of assault If abuse is suspected but not confirmed, report **T76.22XA** (child sexual abuse, suspected, initial encounter) and a code for injury. If there are no findings, report **Z04.42** (encounter for examination and observation following alleged child rape or sexual abuse).	**99285** (comprehensive ED examination) **99170** (anogenital examination) If the same physician performs moderate (conscious) sedation, also report code **99152**. See more on moderate sedation in the Sedation section later in this chapter.

Lysis/Excision of Labial or Penile Adhesions

54162 Lysis or excision of penile post-circumcision adhesions
56441 Lysis of labial adhesions

Lysis of labial or penile adhesions performed by the application of manual pressure without the use of an instrument to cut the adhesions is considered part of the E/M visit and not reported separately.

Code **54162** is only reported when lysis is performed under general anesthesia or regional block, with an instrument, and under sterile conditions.

- This code has a 2021 total relative value of 5.83 when performed in a facility setting and a Medicare 10-day global surgery period, which payers may or may not use.
- If post-circumcision adhesions are manually broken during the postoperative period by the physician or physician of the same group and specialty who performed the procedure, it would be considered part of the global surgical package.

> An integumentary repair performed in conjunction with lysis or excision of penile post-circumcision adhesion is not reported in addition to code **54162**.

- Report the service with *ICD-10-CM* code **N47.0**, adherent prepuce in a newborn, or **N47.5**, adhesions of prepuce and glans penis (patients older than 28 days).

> For repair of incomplete circumcision with removal of excessive residual foreskin, see code **54163**.

Code **56441** is performed by using a blunt instrument or scissors under general or local anesthesia.
- The 2021 total relative value units for this procedure in a facility setting are 4.48, and the procedure is assigned a Medicare 10-day global surgery period, which may or may not be used by payers.
- *ICD-10-CM* code **Q52.5** (fusion of labia) would be reported with *CPT* code **56441**.
- When provided without anesthesia, modifier **52** may be appended to indicate reduced services. Payer guidance may vary with regard to use of modifier **52**.

Repair of Penis

> New in 2022, codes **54340–54348** are revised to improve terminology describing revision of prior hypospadias repair (removing the term "hypospadias cripple"). Additionally, code **54340** is changed to reflect complication(s) rather than complications to allow reporting for correction of 1 complication.

Correction of Chordee and Hypospadias

54300 Plastic operation of penis for straightening of chordee (eg, hypospadias), with or without mobilization of urethra

54304   Plastic operation on penis for correction of chordee or for first stage hypospadias repair with or without transplantation of prepuce and/or skin flaps

▲**54340**   Repair of hypospadias complication(s) (ie, fistula, stricture, diverticula); by closure, incision, or excision, simple

▲**54344**   requiring mobilization of skin flaps and urethroplasty with flap or patch graft

▲**54348**   requiring extensive dissection, and urethroplasty with flap, patch or tubed graft (including urinary diversion, when performed)

▲**54352**   Revision of prior hypospadias repair requiring extensive dissection and excision of previously constructed structures including re-release of chordee and reconstruction of urethra and penis by use of local skin as grafts and island flaps and skin brought in as flaps or grafts

Code **54300** is appropriately reported for *straightening* of the chordee to correct congenital concealed penis (**Q55.64**). This procedure may also be performed to correct an entrapped penis after newborn circumcision (eg, release of concealed penis with coverage of deficient penile ventral skin using penile skin-raised Byars flaps and re-circumcision).

Codes **54304–54336** describe procedures performed to *correct* hypospadias in either single-stage or multiple-stage procedures.

- Do not separately report codes **54300**, **54304**, or **54360** (plastic operation on penis to correct angulation) when reporting single-stage repair of hypospadias.

  Correction of penile chordee or penile curvature is included in all single-stage repairs of hypospadias.

- For more detailed information on reporting procedures to repair hypospadias, see the American Urological Association policy and advocacy brief, "Pediatric Hypospadias Repair: A New Consensus Document on Coding," at www.auanet. org/Documents/practices-resources/coding-tips/Pediatric-Hypospadias-Repair.pdf.

  Repair or revision of hypospadias complication is reported with codes **54340–54352**.

  The following procedures are not separately reported when reporting code **54352**.

- Application of skin substitute graft (**15275**)
- Formation of direct or tubed pedicle (**15574**)
- Island pedicle flap (**15740**)
- Excision of urethral diverticulum (**53235**)
- One-stage urethroplasty of anterior urethra (**53410**)
- Repair of hypospadias or hypospadias correction described by codes **54300**, **54336**, **54340**, **54344**, and **54348**
- Plastic operation to correct penile angulation (**54360**)

Negative Pressure Wound Therapy

97605   Negative pressure wound therapy (eg, vacuum assisted drainage collection), utilizing durable medical equipment (DME), including topical application(s), wound assessment, and instruction(s) for ongoing care, per session; total wound(s) surface area less than or equal to 50 square centimeters

97606   total wound(s) surface area greater than 50 square centimeters

97607   Negative pressure wound therapy (eg, vacuum assisted drainage collection), utilizing disposable, non-durable medical equipment including provision of exudate management collection system, topical application(s), wound assessment, and instructions for ongoing care, per session; total wound(s) surface area less than or equal to 50 square centimeters

97608   total wound(s) surface area greater than 50 square centimeters

Negative pressure wound therapy

- Requires direct (one-on-one) physician or QHP contact with the patient.
- May be initiated in a hospital or surgical center setting and continued in the home setting after discharge.
- Includes application of dressings.
- Is separately reported when performed in conjunction with surgical debridement (**11042–11047**).
- Documentation should include current wound assessment, including
  — Quantitative measurements of wound characteristics (eg, site, surface area and depth)
  — Any previous treatment regimens
  — Debridement (when performed)
  — Prescribed length of treatment
  — Dressing types and frequency of changes
  — Other concerns that affect healing
- Encounters for ongoing NPWT may include documentation of progress of healing and changes in the wound, including measurement, amount of exudate, and presence of granulation or necrotic tissue.

- Codes **97605** and **97606** represent NPWT provided via a system that includes a *non-disposable* suction pump and drainage collection device.

  Supplies, including dressings, are reportable with HCPCS codes (eg, **A6550**, wound care set, for NPWT electrical pump, includes all supplies and accessories).

- Codes **97607** and **97608**
  - Report NPWT that utilizes a *disposable* suction pump and collection system.
  - Are not reported in conjunction with codes **97605** and **97606**.
  - Payer policies may limit coverage to care of specific types of wounds that require NPWT to improve granulation tissue formation and to certain types of NPWT equipment.
  - Be sure to verify the coverage policy of the patient's health plan prior to provision of services.
  - Supplies for a disposable system are reported with code **A9272**, which also includes all dressings and accessories.

Sedation

Moderate Sedation

Moderate sedation is reported with codes **99151–99153** (provided by the same physician or QHP performing the diagnostic or therapeutic service) and **99155–99157** (provided by different physician or QHP who is not performing the diagnostic or therapeutic service). See **Table 10-5** for full code descriptors and time requirements.

Moderate sedation codes are not used to report administration of medications for pain control, minimal sedation (anxiolysis), deep sedation, or monitored anesthesia care (**00100–01999**).

Moderate sedation is discussed in more detail in **Chapter 10**.

Deep Sedation/Anesthesia Services

Deep sedation/analgesia is a drug-induced depression of consciousness during which patients cannot be easily aroused but respond purposefully after repeated verbal or painful stimulation (eg, purposefully pushing away the noxious stimuli). A state of deep sedation may be accompanied by partial or complete loss of protective airway reflexes. Cardiovascular function is usually maintained.

CPT codes for reporting anesthesia services, including deep sedation, monitored anesthesia care, or general anesthesia, are **00100–01999**. These codes are not as specific as codes for other services and generally identify a body area or type of procedure.

00102   Anesthesia for procedures involving plastic repair of cleft lip

01820   Anesthesia for all closed procedures on radius, ulna, wrist, or hand bones

  Anesthesia services include
- Preoperative evaluation of the patient
- Administration of anesthetic, other medications, blood, and fluids
- Monitoring of physiologic parameters
- Other supportive services
- Postoperative E/M related to the surgery (Ongoing critical care services by an anesthesiologist may be separately reportable.)

  Pediatricians who provide deep sedation services for procedures performed outside the operating suite should follow the same anesthesia policies and coding instructions as other providers of anesthesia services.

> If surgery is canceled, subsequent to the preoperative evaluation, payment may be allowed to the anesthesiologist for an evaluation and management (E/M) service and the appropriate E/M code (eg, consultation) may be reported. See Chapter 16 for information on reporting these services.

  Add-on codes may be reported to identify special circumstances that increase the complexity of providing anesthesia care, including

+99100   Patient under 1 year or older than 70 years (not reported in conjunction with codes **00326**, **00561**, **00834**, or **00836**)

+99116   Anesthesia complicated by total body hypothermia

+99135   Anesthesia complicated by controlled hypotension

+99140   Emergency conditions

Emergency is defined by *CPT* as a situation in which delay in treatment of the patient would lead to a significant increase in the threat to life or body part.

Modifiers are reported in addition to anesthesia codes to indicate the physical status of the patient. The American Society of Anesthesiologists (ASA) classification of the patient's physical status is represented by the following HCPCS modifiers:

P1	Normal healthy patient
P2	Patient with mild systemic disease
P3	Patient with severe systemic disease
P4	Patient with severe systemic disease that is a constant threat to life
P5	Moribund patient who is not expected to survive without the operation
P6	Declared brain-dead patient whose organs are being removed for donor purposes

Base units for anesthesia services are published in the ASA *Relative Value Guide* and by the CMS for each anesthesia procedure code. Payers typically do not require reporting of base units on the claim for services.

- Many private payers will allow additional base units for physical status modifiers **P3** (1 unit), **P4** (2 units), and **P5** (3 units).
- Anesthesia time is reported in minutes unless a payer directs to report units (1 unit per 15 minutes). Start and stop times must be documented, including multiple start and stop times when anesthesia services are discontinuous.

Other modifiers that may be required by payers for anesthesia services by pediatric physicians are those identifying the type of anesthesia or anesthesia provider.

AA	Anesthesia services performed personally by anesthesiologist

> **Payers may require this modifier for services personally rendered by physicians other than anesthesiologists. This signifies that services were not rendered by a nonphysician provider, such as a certified registered nurse anesthetist.**

GC	This service has been performed in part by a resident under the direction of a teaching physician
G8	Monitored anesthesia care for deep complex, complicated, or markedly invasive surgical procedure
G9	Monitored anesthesia care for patient who has history of severe cardiopulmonary condition
QS	Monitored anesthesia care service

> **Medicare considers deep sedation equivalent to monitored anesthesia care. Private payers may vary.**

Postoperative Pain Management

Generally, the surgeon is responsible for postoperative pain management. However, a surgeon may request assistance with postoperative pain management (eg, epidural or peripheral nerve block).

- Payers may require a written request by the surgeon for postoperative pain management by the anesthesia provider.
- When a catheter is placed as the mode of anesthesia (eg, epidural catheter) and retained for use in postoperative pain management, this is not separately reported.
- When separately reporting postoperative pain management, append modifier **59** (distinct procedural service) to indicate the separate service and document this service distinctly (and preferably separately) from the anesthesia record.
- When an epidural catheter is used for postoperative pain management, code **01996** (daily management of epidural) may be reported on days subsequent to the day of surgery. Daily management of other postoperative pain management devices may be reported with subsequent hospital care codes (**99231–99233**).

Example

➤ **An orthopedic surgeon requests preanesthetic insertion of a catheter to provide a continuous infusion of the femoral nerve for postoperative pain relief for a patient undergoing an arthroscopy of the knee with lateral meniscectomy.** The anesthesiologist uses ultrasound guidance to insert a catheter for continuous infusion prior to inducing general anesthesia for the surgical procedure.

ICD-10-CM	CPT
Appropriate diagnosis code	**01400** (anesthesia for open or surgical arthroscopic procedures on knee joint; not otherwise specified) **64448 59** (injection, anesthetic agent[s] and/or steroid; femoral nerve, continuous infusion by catheter [including catheter placement])

Teaching Point: Because the anesthetist provided a distinct service separate from the anesthesia for the procedure, the catheter insertion is separately reported with modifier **59.** Had the procedure been performed under an epidural block and the epidural catheter left in place for postoperative pain management, no additional code would be reported.

Resources

Fracture Care

"Initial Fracture Care: Musculoskeletal or Evaluation and Management," February 2021 *AAP Pediatric Coding Newsletter* (https://coding.solutions.aap.org/article.aspx?articleid=2765276; subscription required)

Sedation

"Beyond Moderate Sedation: Coding for Anesthesia Services," April 2014 *AAP Pediatric Coding Newsletter* (https://coding.solutions.aap.org/article.aspx?articleid=1906504; subscription required)

"Documentation of Deep Sedation Services (Online Exclusive)," May 2014 *AAP Pediatric Coding Newsletter* (https://coding.solutions.aap.org/article.aspx?articleid=1906514; subscription required)

Surgery

CMS-designated global periods, Medicare Resource-Based Relative Value Scale Physician Fee Schedule (www.cms.gov/Medicare/Medicare-Fee-for-Service-Payment/PhysicianFeeSched/PFS-Relative-Value-Files.html; see column O)

"The Surgical Package and Related Services," May 2018 *AAP Pediatric Coding Newsletter* (https://coding.solutions.aap.org/article.aspx?articleid=2679119; subscription required)

"Coding Challenge: Modifiers and Procedural Services (Online Exclusive)," May 2018 *AAP Pediatric Coding Newsletter* (https://coding.solutions.aap.org/article.aspx?articleid=2679120; subscription required)

"Discontinued or Reduced Services: Modifier **52** or **53**," May 2021 *AAP Pediatric Coding Newsletter* (https://coding.solutions.aap.org/article.aspx?articleid=2765344; subscription required)

"Subspecialty Corner: Coding for Complications of Neonatal Circumcision," June 2017 *AAP Pediatric Coding Newsletter* (https://coding.solutions.aap.org/article.aspx?articleid=2629478; subscription required)

American Urological Association, "Pediatric Hypospadias Repair: A New Consensus Document on Coding" (www.auanet.org/Documents/practices-resources/coding-tips/Pediatric-Hypospadias-Repair.pdf)

Teaching Physician

Medicare Teaching Physician Services rules (http://cms.hhs.gov/manuals/downloads/clm104c12.pdf; see section 100)

Test Your Knowledge!

1. **Which is not an indication for appending modifier 22?**
   a. Increased intensity or time
   b. Technical difficulty
   c. The patient weighs less than 4 kg.
   d. The severity of the patient's condition

2. **What is the *Current Procedural Terminology* instruction for reporting a related evaluation and management (E/M) service during the postoperative global period?**
   a. No modifier is required. Report the E/M code supported by the documentation.
   b. Append modifier 24.
   c. Do not report the service.
   d. Report code 99024.

3. **Which of the following is true of cardiac catheterization codes 93593–93598?**
   a. Codes 93593–93598 are reported only when the patient is a neonate.
   b. Echocardiography by another cardiologist during the same session is separately reported.
   c. Modifier 63 (performed on an infant weighing less than 4 kg) is not appended to codes 93593–93598.
   d. Codes 93593–93598 are reported only when there are abnormal native connections.

4. **Which is correct when a central venous access device is removed and a new one is placed at the same access site?**
   a. Report codes for removal and introduction.
   b. Report a code for removal only.
   c. Report a code for introduction only.
   d. Report a code for replacement.

5. **Which of the following would prohibit reporting of code 49491 for initial inguinal hernia repair?**
   a. The patient was younger than 37 weeks' gestation at birth.
   b. The patient is younger than 50 weeks' postconception age.
   c. The hernia is reducible.
   d. The patient was 37 weeks, 1 day gestation at birth.

Part 4
Digital Medicine Services

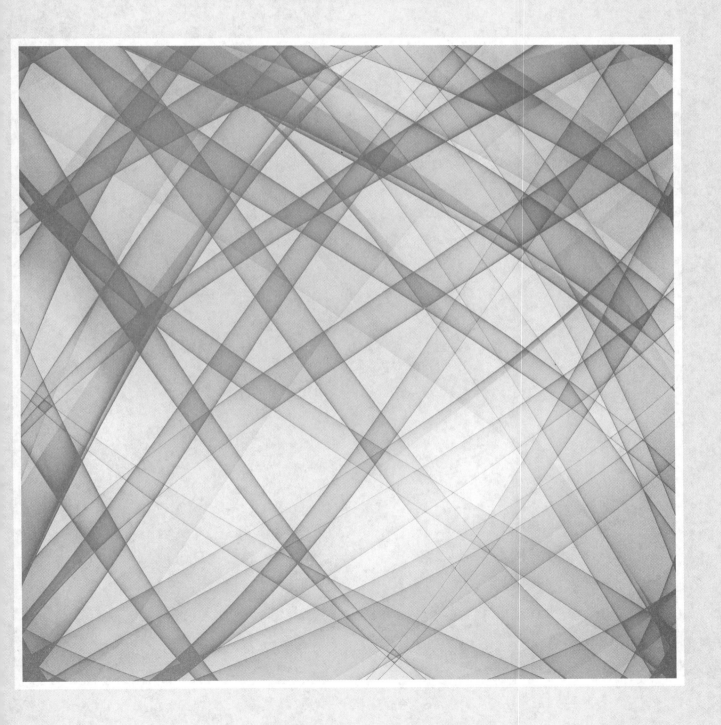

Part 4: Digital Medicine Services

Chapter 20
Telemedicine Services 485

Chapter 21
Remote Data Collection and Monitoring Services 497

Telemedicine Services

Contents

Telemedicine Services 487

    Payer Coverage 487

        Medicaid Payment 490

Reporting Telemedicine Services 490

    Documentation of Services 490

    Place of Service Codes 491

    Telemedicine Modifiers 491

    Healthcare Common Procedure Coding System (HCPCS) Telehealth Codes 492

    Examples of Coding for Telemedicine Services (*Current Procedural Terminology*, HCPCS) 492

    Critical Care Via Telemedicine 494

    Continuing Changes in Digital Medicine Services 495

Resources 495

Test Your Knowledge! 496

● =New code ▲ =Revised code # =Re-sequenced code + =Add-on code ★ =Telemedicine

Telemedicine Services

This chapter provides information on coding for telemedicine—virtual face-to-face care facilitated by digital technology providing simultaneous audiovisual communication between a patient and a physician or other qualified health care professional (QHP) at remote locations. Telemedicine brings a physician in a distant location to a patient without the need for either party to physically travel.

Telemedicine Terminology

Key terms in differentiating telemedicine services from other digital services are *synchronous* and *asynchronous*. Telemedicine services (other than a special Medicare demonstration project) always include synchronous communication.

- Synchronous telemedicine services include simultaneous interaction between a physician or other qualified health care professional and a patient who is located at a distant site.
- Asynchronous communication does not require simultaneous interaction from both parties. Examples of asynchronous communication are email and data and/or images transferred for review and subsequent response.

Telemedicine may also be referred to as *telehealth;* definitions for each vary by state and payer, but telehealth is more commonly used to reference any health service provided via telecommunications. Telemedicine may be more appropriate to describe services of physicians and other QHPs and is the terminology used by *Current Procedural Terminology (CPT®)*.

Current Procedural Terminology (CPT) describes synchronous virtual face-to-face care as telemedicine. *CPT* requires *real-time* interaction between a physician or other qualified health care professional (QHP) and a patient who is located at a distant site from the physician or QHP for telemedicine. Payer policy may also include coverage of asynchronous or store-and-forward telehealth services (eg, remote interpretation and report of images).

During the COVID-19 public health emergency (PHE), allowances were made to use and report certain codes outside of *CPT* instruction and/or typical payment policy. However, these allowances were limited to the duration of the emergency or a specified period beyond the end of the PHE. Check with your payers before reporting telemedicine services outside of current *CPT* guidelines.

Before providing telemedicine or any digital medicine service, understand local and state laws, ensure that communications will be Health Insurance Portability and Accountability Act (HIPAA) of 1996 compliant, establish written guidelines and procedures, educate payers and negotiate for payment, and educate patients. Note that many popular communication platforms, such as FaceTime, Google Talk, and Skype, are not HIPAA compliant and should not be used for health care communications (except when specifically allowed by an emergency use authorization declared by state and federal authorities).

See Chapter 9 for information on coding for telephone or online digital assessment and management services that are not telemedicine services for purposes of code assignment.

Payer Coverage

The PHE declared in 2020 not only prompted immediate growth in the provision of telemedicine services but also brought about changes in how health plans designed or redesigned payment policies for telehealth. Some plans now offer payment parity for telemedicine services (ie, payment is equal to that of in-person services). Review the payment policies of health plans and payers such as Medicaid prior to initiating telemedicine services, as coverage and payment policies may vary.

Medicare has published a list of codes (**Table 20-1** and online at www.aap.org/cfp) that are covered when provided via telemedicine, but this list may be more restrictive than the lists used by Medicaid plans and other payers. Private payers may limit telemedicine services to those described by specific codes with benefit policy based on state telemedicine or telehealth regulations. It is important to verify the services and sites of service that are covered by each patient's health plan.

Table 20-1 includes the Medicare list of codes eligible for payment when provided via telemedicine and those codes included in *Current Procedural Terminology* Appendix P in 2021 (updates for 2022 were not yet available at time of publication).

Table 20-1. 2021 Telemedicine Services

CY 2021 Telehealth Services (Please see coding reference for code descriptors.)	HCPCS/CPT Code	CPT Allows[a]	Medicare Allows
Advanced care planning	**99497** and **99498**	√	√
Annual alcohol misuse screening, 15 min	**G0442**		√
Annual behavioral therapy for cardiovascular disease, 15 min	**G0446**		√
Annual depression screening, 15 min	**G0444**		√
Annual wellness visit, first visit	**G0438**		√
Annual wellness visit, subsequent visit	**G0439**		√
Behavioral counseling for alcohol misuse, 15 min	**G0443**		√
Behavioral counseling for obesity, 15 min	**G0447**		√
Comprehensive assessment and care planning for chronic care management	**G0506**		√
Diabetes self-management training services	**G0108** and **G0109**		√
Electrocardiographic rhythm derived event recording	**93268, 93270–93272**	√	
ESRD-related services[b]	**90951, 90952, 90954, 90955, 90957, 90958, 90960,** and **90961**	√	√
ESRD-related services for home dialysis[b]	**90963–90970**	√	√
External mobile cardiovascular telemetry with electrocardiographic recording, concurrent computerized real-time data analysis	**93228** and **93229**	√	
Genetic counseling	**96040**	√	
Health and behavior assessment/re-assessment and intervention	**96158, 96159,** and **96164–96171**		√
Health risk assessment	**96160** and **96161**	√	√
High-intensity behavioral counseling to prevent sexually transmitted infection; 30 min	**G0445**		√
Hospital subsequent care services (payer may limit to 1 telehealth visit every 3 days)	**99231–99233**	√	√
Inpatient consultation	**99251–99255**	√	
Kidney disease education services	**G0420** and **G0421**		√
Medical nutrition therapy	**G0270**		√
	97802–97804	√	√
Neurobehavioral status exam	**96116**	√	√
Nursing facility subsequent care services (payer may limit to 1 telehealth visit every 30 days)	**99307–99310**	√	√
Office consultation	**99241–99245**	√	
Office or other outpatient visits	**99202–99215**	√	√
Pharmacologic management, telehealth, inpatient	**G0459**		√
Pharmacologic management performed with psychotherapy services	**90863**	√	
Prolonged office or other outpatient E/M on the date of the primary service (report with **99202–99215**)	**99417**	√	

Table 20-1 (*continued*)

CY 2021 Telehealth Services (Please see coding reference for code descriptors.)	HCPCS/*CPT* Code	*CPT* Allows[a]	Medicare Allows
Prolonged preventive services	G0513 and G0514		√
Prolonged service in an outpatient setting other than an office or other outpatient visit (99202–99215)	99354 and 99355	√	√
Prolonged service in the inpatient or observation setting	99356 and 99357	√	√
Psychiatric diagnostic interview examination	90791 and 90792	√	√
Psychiatric services with interactive complexity	+90785	√	√
Psychoanalysis	90845	√	√
Psychotherapy, family	90846 and 90847	√	√
Psychotherapy, individual	90832–90834 and 90836–90838	√	√
Psychotherapy for crisis	90839 and 90840	√	√
Remote imaging for detection of retinal disease	92227	√	
Remote imaging for monitoring and management of active retinal disease	92228	√	
Self-management education and training	98960–98962	√	
Smoking cessation services	G0436 and G0437		√
	99406 and 99407	√	√
Structured assessment and intervention services for alcohol and/or substance (other than tobacco) abuse	G0396 and G0397		√
	99408 and 99409	√	
Telehealth consultation, critical care, initial, physicians typically spend 60 minutes	G0508		√
Telehealth consultation, critical care, subsequent, physicians typically spend 50 minutes	G0509		√
Telehealth consultations, emergency department or initial inpatient	G0425–G0427		√
Telehealth consultations, follow-up inpatient hospital or SNF	G0406–G0408		√
Transitional care management services	99495 and 99496	√	√

Abbreviations: *CPT, Current Procedural Terminology*; CY, calendar year; E/M, evaluation and management; ESRD, end-stage renal disease; HCPCS, Healthcare Common Procedure Coding System; SNF, skilled nursing facility.

[a] Append modifier 95 (telemedicine service rendered via a real-time interactive audio and video telecommunications system).

[b] For ESRD-related services, a physician, nurse practitioner, physician assistant, or clinical nurse specialist must furnish at least 1 hands-on visit (not telehealth) each month to examine the vascular access site.

Many health plans develop policies that designate covered and non-covered telemedicine services. Services that are most often not reportable as a telemedicine service include

- A service provided on the same day as an in-person visit, when performed by the same provider and for the same condition

> Typically, the work of 2 evaluation and management (E/M) services provided by the same physician (or physicians of the same group practice and same specialty) addressing the same problem at different times on the same date may be combined and reported as a single E/M service. If reporting 2 E/M services by the same physician addressing different problems, the services may be separately reported with modifier 25 (significant and separately identifiable E/M service) appended to the code for the second E/M service.

- A service that is incidental to an E/M service and limited to clinical staff communication of test results, scheduling additional services, or providing educational resources

- Any service that is not a covered benefit, such as travel vaccines or travel counseling
- Any service that is not separately paid because the service is included in the postoperative work of a procedure (eg, E/M services within 90 days of a major surgery)

Medicaid Payment

For purposes of Medicaid, telemedicine is a service that includes 2-way, real-time interactive communication between the patient and the physician or practitioner including, at a minimum, audio and video technology. Although exceptions were made during the PHE, Medicaid plans may limit telemedicine services to those provided to patients who are located in an originating site that is a physician office or other health care facility at the time of service (ie, exclude services to patients in their home).

State telehealth laws often include mandates for coverage of telemedicine services, and some include parity of payment (ie, equal to in-person services). Medicaid payment policies often align with state regulations. Policies vary widely by state and may vary between Medicaid managed care plans (eg, a specific plan may allow more than is required by standard Medicaid policy or regulation).

> ### Medicare and Medicaid Telemedicine Terminology
>
> *Originating site:* location of the patient at the time of service
> *Distant site:* location of the physician or other qualified health care professional at the time of service

Medicaid plans may pay the physician or other QHP at the distant site for each service rendered via telemedicine and pay a facility fee to the originating site (eg, hospital), when applicable. States can also pay any additional costs, such as technical support, transmission charges, and equipment. These add-on costs can be incorporated into the fee-for-service rates or separately paid as an administrative cost by the state. If they are separately billed and paid, the costs must be linked to a covered Medicaid service.

States may also choose to pay for services delivered using technology that does not meet the definition of telemedicine services (eg, telephones, facsimile machines, email systems, remote patient monitoring).

> **See Chapter 21 for information on remote patient monitoring services.**

States may cover telemedicine services reported with a variety of *CPT* and Healthcare Common Procedure Coding System (HCPCS) codes. Plans may also pay **T1014** (telehealth transmission, per minute) to originating sites (other than patient's home) or **Q3014** (telehealth originating site facility fee). Modifiers are often required to designate a telemedicine service, as discussed later in this chapter.

Reporting Telemedicine Services

From a *CPT* coding perspective, telemedicine services are face-to-face services reported using the same E/M codes that would be appropriate for in-person encounters. *CPT* codes for services that are typically performed face-to-face but may be rendered via a real-time (synchronous) interactive audio and video telecommunications system are preceded by a star (★) and listed in Appendix P of the *CPT* manual.

Synchronous telemedicine service is defined by *CPT* as a real-time interaction between a physician or QHP and a patient who is located at a separate site. The total communication between the physician or QHP and the patient during the course of the synchronous telemedicine service must be of an amount and nature that would be sufficient to meet the requirements of the same service when rendered via a face-to-face interaction.

Documentation of Services

Documentation of telemedicine services should be similar to that of services provided in traditional patient care settings. For E/M services, *other than* **99202–99205** and **99211–99215**, this means that documentation supports reporting of services based on the required key components (ie, history, examination, and/or medical decision-making [MDM]) or typical time of service (when >50% of the face-to-face time of the encounter is spent in counseling and/or coordination of care). The MDM or total time of service on the date of service should support telemedicine E/M services reported with **99202–99205** and **99211–99215**.

See Chapter 7 for more information on documentation of office and other outpatient evaluation and management services and instructions for reporting based on time.

Place of Service Codes

Use of the correct place of service (POS) code on claims for telemedicine services is important to appropriate payment. Place of service code 02 (telehealth) is described by Medicare as the location where health services and health-related services are provided or received through a telecommunication system. However, some payers accept the POS code for distant site where the physician or QHP would provide the service if performed in person (eg, 11, office) in addition to appending modifier 95 to the procedure code to indicate the service was delivered via telemedicine.

Payment for claims reported with place of service (POS) code 02 may be set at a facility rate that does not include a physician's practice expense. For instance, a level 3 office evaluation and management service (99213) reported with POS code 02 might be paid based on 1.95 total facility relative value units (RVUs) versus 2.65 total non-facility RVUs if reported with POS code 11 (office).

See Chapter 4 for more information on POS codes.

See an individual payer's telemedicine policy to determine if there are reporting requirements for the specific site of service (eg, physical location from which services were rendered or received).

Field 32 of the 1500 paper claim form and its electronic equivalent is used to report the site of service (eg, hospital name, address, National Provider Identifier). This is typically the physical location of the physician or other provider of service at the time of service when payment is influenced by geographic location.

Telemedicine Modifiers

Modifiers are used to indicate that a service was somehow modified from what is typical (ie, reduced or increased service). *CPT* and HCPCS include modifiers for indicating that a service was provided by telemedicine. It is important to append an indicated modifier as directed by *CPT* or, when applicable, in compliance with an individual health plan's payment policy.

95   Telemedicine service rendered via a real-time interactive audio and video telecommunications system

Modifier 95 may only be appended to the codes listed in *CPT* Appendix P (see **Table 20-1**). Appending modifier 95 to the appropriate procedure code identifies to the payer that telemedicine services were rendered via real-time interactive audio and video telecommunications. This modifier is not applied if the communication is not real-time interactive audio and video. Telephone care is not telemedicine.

Appendix P codes that may be of particular interest to pediatricians include

- New and established patient office or other outpatient E/M services (99202–99205, 99212–99215, 99417)
- Subsequent hospital care (99231–99233)
- Inpatient (99251–99255) and outpatient (99241–99245) consultations
- Administration of patient-focused health risk assessment instrument (eg, health hazard appraisal) with scoring and documentation, per standardized instrument (96160)
- Administration of caregiver-focused health risk assessment instrument (eg, depression inventory) for the benefit of the patient, with scoring and documentation, per standardized instrument (96161)
- Prolonged services in the outpatient setting (99354, 99355)
- Individual behavior change interventions (99406–99409)
- Transitional care management services (99495, 99496)

Appendix P also includes codes for services such as psychotherapy, health and behavior assessment and intervention, medical nutrition therapy, and education and training for patient self-management, allowing for telemedicine services provided by certain qualified nonphysician health care professionals in addition to subspecialty physicians.

GT   Via interactive audio and video telecommunication systems

Some payers accept modifier GT in lieu of modifier 95. Critical access hospitals billing under Method II report modifier GT (via interactive audio and video telecommunication systems) because no POS code is reported on Method II claims to identify telemedicine services. Some health plans may also require modifier GT.

State Medicaid plans may also use modifiers U1–UD (as defined by the state) to identify, track, and pay for telemedicine services.

Healthcare Common Procedure Coding System (HCPCS) Telehealth Codes

While *CPT* codes are accepted by most plans covering telemedicine services, payers may require HCPCS codes that are used in the Medicare program for consultations and other services with specific coverage policies (eg, telehealth critical care consultation).

● HCPCS codes are used for telemedicine consultations with Medicare beneficiaries because *CPT* consultation codes are not payable under the Medicare Physician Fee Schedule.

● Only specific services are eligible for Medicare payment when provided via telemedicine. The following codes do not apply in all potential settings where telemedicine might be provided (eg, Medicare does not cover telemedicine services to patients in observation settings).

● Exceptions apply for telemedicine services rendered as part of certain demonstration projects (eg, under telehealth waiver for patients associated with a Next Generation accountable care organization).

G0406	Follow-up inpatient consultation, limited, physicians typically spend 15 minutes communicating with the patient via telehealth
G0407	intermediate, physicians typically spend 25 minutes communicating with the patient via telehealth
G0408	complex, physicians typically spend 35 minutes communicating with the patient via telehealth
G0425	Telehealth consultation, emergency department or initial inpatient, typically 30 minutes communicating with the patient via telehealth
G0426	typically 50 minutes communicating with the patient via telehealth
G0427	typically 70 minutes or more communicating with the patient via telehealth
G0459	Inpatient telehealth pharmacologic management, including prescription, use, and review of medication with no more than minimal medical psychotherapy
G0508	Telehealth consultation, critical care, physicians typically spend 60 minutes communicating with the patient via telehealth (initial)
G0509	Telehealth consultation, critical care, physicians typically spend 50 minutes communicating with the patient via telehealth (subsequent)

> **Please see further discussion of critical care provided via telemedicine later in this chapter.**

When a payer uses Medicare program policies for telemedicine services, it is important to learn which services are and are not covered when delivered via telemedicine. A current listing of services covered under the Medicare program is available at https://www.cms.gov/Medicare/Medicare-General-Information/Telehealth.

Examples of Coding for Telemedicine Services (*Current Procedural Terminology,* HCPCS)

Examples

➤ **A consultation is requested of a physician at a children's hospital for an inpatient in a rural hospital, 75 miles away.** Through real-time interactive technology, the physician performs a consultation, including a comprehensive history, comprehensive examination (assisted by clinical staff of the facility), and MDM of moderate complexity. The total time of the interactive communication is 30 minutes. A written report to the requesting physician is transmitted via secure electronic health information exchange.

MDM: Moderate *History:* Comprehensive *Physical examination:* Comprehensive	**CPT** **99254 95** (initial inpatient consultation, which requires these 3 key components: a comprehensive history; a comprehensive examination; MDM of moderate complexity) or, if payer requires HCPCS codes, **G0425** (telehealth consultation, emergency department [ED] or initial inpatient, typically 30 minutes communicating with the patient via telehealth)

Teaching Point: If payer policy allows payment for overhead expenses related to telemedicine services, also report **T1014**, telehealth transmission, per minute, professional services bill separately. Because this is billed per minute, 30 units are reported. The rural hospital, as the originating facility, may also report **Q3014**, telehealth originating site facility fee.

A payer that does not accept consultation codes may require that the physician report a code for initial hospital care (**99221–99223 95**) in lieu of the previous codes.

➤ **A parent requests an established patient telemedicine appointment with her 8-year-old's physician for evaluation of side effects of medication prescribed for predominantly hyperactive attention-deficit/hyperactivity disorder (ADHD).** The physician's staff verify that the child's health plan covers telemedicine services provided to patients in their home, advise the parent of any out-of-pocket costs, and schedule an appointment for later that morning. At the appointment, the physician establishes a secure audiovisual connection with the parent. The physician obtains a history from the parent, who reports that the child has had no appetite and has been "acting like a zombie" since the child's methylphenidate dose was increased last week. The physician counsels that the symptoms are a side-effect of the medication, and the physician decreases the child's dose. The child is present during the visit and appears well on examination. The physician's total time directed to this patient was 15 minutes including time spent documenting the service.

ICD-10-CM	CPT
R63.0 (anorexia) **R41.89** (other symptoms and signs involving cognitive functions and awareness) **T43.635A** (adverse effect of methylphenidate, initial encounter) **F90.1** (ADHD, predominantly hyperactive)	**99214 95** (office or other outpatient visit for an established patient, moderate complexity MDM)

Teaching Point: The physician's total time on the date of the encounter (15 minutes) would support code **99212**. However, the MDM supports code **99214** based on a moderate-complexity problem of 1 chronic illness with side effects of treatment and moderate risk of prescription drug management. The service was provided in real-time audiovisual communication with the caregiver and patient, so modifier **95** is appended.

➤ **A parent requests an established patient telemedicine appointment with her 6-year-old's physician for evaluation of a day's worth of coughing and wheezing.** Health plan coverage of telemedicine services provided to patients in their home is verified, and an appointment is scheduled for later that morning. At the appointment, the physician establishes a secure audiovisual connection with the parent. The parent reports the child, who has a history of intermittent asthma, does not have albuterol at home. On examination, the child has minimal subcostal retractions. The physician decides to bring the child into the office for further evaluation and treatment. Time of the telemedicine evaluation is 10 minutes.

Once in the office, the physician examines the patient and determines the child requires albuterol treatment and oral steroids. A medical assistant provides albuterol treatment and education using a metered-dose inhaler (MDI) with spacer. Overall, the physician spends an additional 25 minutes directing this patient's care, including ordering medications and documenting the service.

ICD-10-CM	CPT
J45.21 (mild intermittent asthma with [acute] exacerbation)	**99214** (office or other outpatient visit for an established patient with moderate complexity MDM or 30–39 minutes total physician time on the date of the encounter) **94640** (pressurized or nonpressurized inhalation treatment for acute airway obstruction for therapeutic purposes and/or for diagnostic purposes such as sputum induction with an aerosol generator, nebulizer, MDI or intermittent positive pressure breathing [IPPB] device) **J3535** (drug administered via MDI)

●=New code   ▲=Revised code   #=Re-sequenced code   +=Add-on code   ★=Telemedicine

Teaching Point: Although this encounter began as a telemedicine visit, the conversion to an in-person visit negates the need for modifier **95**. The total time for the visit is 35 minutes, 10 minutes during the telemedicine portion and 25 minutes during the in-person portion. Moderate MDM is also supported by 1 chronic condition with exacerbation and prescription drug management.

When a medication is administered via MDI, do not report other HCPCS codes (eg, **J7613**, albuterol, inhalation solution, US Food and Drug Administration–approved final product, non-compounded, administered through durable medical equipment [DME], unit dose, 1 mg) that represent inhalation solutions administered via DME. Code **J3535** may be used to report the medication administered via MDI. This is a nonspecific code, so the inclusion of the National Drug Code and grams of the medication provided should be included on the claim. (Some practices do not charge for the medication when provided with an MDI that will be cleaned and reused.) The patient education is not separately reported when provided for use of the same equipment used in treatment.

➤ **A parent requests an established patient telemedicine appointment with her 6-year-old's physician for evaluation of chronic idiopathic urticaria.** The physician's staff verify that the child's health plan covers telemedicine services provided to a patient at home and schedules an appointment for later that morning. At the appointment, the physician attempts to establish a secure audiovisual connection with the parent. However, the connection could not be established. Instead, the physician and parent spoke by telephone, and the parent sent digital photographs of the rash through the electronic health record (EHR). Based on the history and severity of the rash, the physician prescribes steroids and long-acting antihistamines. The physician spends a total of 20 minutes, of which 12 minutes were spent on the telephone visit and 8 minutes in review of the photographs and documentation of the encounter.

ICD-10-CM	CPT
L50.1 (idiopathic urticaria)	99442 (telephone E/M service provided by a physician to an established patient, parent, or guardian not originating from a related E/M service provided within the previous 7 days nor leading to an E/M service or procedure within the next 24 hours or soonest available appointment [2.66 total non-facility RVUs])

Teaching Point: A telephone encounter is not considered a telemedicine encounter because a telemedicine encounter must include real-time (synchronous) audiovisual communication. The combination of a telephone encounter and a photo does not meet the requirements of a synchronous audiovisual telemedicine encounter. Telephone encounter codes (**99441–99443**) are based solely on time spent on the telephone in medical discussion. Although the MDM is moderately complex (**99214**) due to chronic illness with exacerbation and prescription drug management, MDM plays no role in selecting telephone visit codes. Ensure that telephone encounter codes are accepted by the patient's plan before billing these codes.

Had this service been conducted entirely via EHR, online digital E/M code **99422** would be reported for the physician's cumulative service time of 11 to 20 minutes. Codes **99421–99423** are assigned lower RVUs than services provided via telephone or telemedicine.

> **Learn more about** evaluation and management services provided by telephone or online digital communication in Chapter 9.

Critical Care Via Telemedicine

CPT codes for critical and intensive care services are not included in Appendix P. *CPT* instructs to report unlisted E/M service code **99499** for critical care provided via telemedicine. (Payers may instruct to append modifier **95** when reporting **99499**.) Alternatively, payers may include HCPCS codes **G0508** and **G0509** as covered critical care consultation services when provided via telemedicine.

Example

➤ **A pediatric intensivist is contacted via live audiovisual telecommunications to provide remote critical care to an infant who presented with fever, lethargy, and suspected sepsis.** The intensivist views radiographs and other data from monitoring devices in addition to performing visual and audio examination of the infant. The attending physician at the hospital where the infant is an inpatient performs necessary procedures as advised by the intensivist (eg, lumbar puncture). The infant remains at the same hospital under the care of the pediatrician. A total of 65 minutes of remote critical care service is provided.

| The consulting physician reports | **G0508** (telehealth consultation, critical care, physicians typically spend 60 minutes communicating with the patient via telehealth [initial]) Or, if a payer does not accept this code, **99499 95** (unlisted E/M service) (Enter description of service on claim or attachment.) |
| The attending physician reports | *CPT* codes for services personally performed (eg, initial hospital care, intubation, lumbar puncture) |

Teaching Point: Code **G0508** is reported only once per date of service per patient. Alternatively, the neonatologist may report an inpatient consultation (**99251–99255**) as allowed under the specific payer's policy for telemedicine.

Continuing Changes in Digital Medicine Services

Physicians providing digital medicine services may find that coding and payment policies for these services change from year to year. As adoption of technology increases and evidence of the value of digital medicine services is further demonstrated, codes and payment policies will likely be adapted. It is important that physician practices monitor local and regional payer policies for opportunities to use data in patient management and get paid for the physician work and practice expense of providing these services.

Resources

CPT Telemedicine Code List

CPT list of codes that may be reported with modifier **95** (See Appendix P of your *CPT* coding reference.)

Medicare Telehealth Policies and Service List

Medicare telehealth service list (www.cms.gov/Medicare/Medicare-General-Information/Telehealth)

Telemedicine Originating Site Eligibility Analyzer

Health Resources and Services Administration Medicare Telehealth Payment Eligibility Analyzer for originating site payment (https://data.hrsa.gov/tools/medicare/telehealth)

Test Your Knowledge!

1. **Which of the following is a telemedicine service?**
   a. An email exchange with a patient to provide clinical advice
   b. A consultation provided to patient via secure audiovisual technology
   c. A consultation with another physician (patient not present) via secure audiovisual technology
   d. All of the above

2. **Which term describes the location of the patient receiving a telemedicine service?**
   a. Distant site
   b. Place of service code
   c. Originating site
   d. Modifier

3. **Which of the following is true of Medicaid coverage of telemedicine services?**
   a. Medicaid plans typically align with state regulations for telemedicine services.
   b. Medicaid coverage of telemedicine services is the same across all states.
   c. Medicaid always covers telemedicine services regardless of patient location.
   d. Only asynchronous store-and-forward technology is covered under Medicaid.

4. **Which is a *Current Procedural Terminology* (*CPT*) instruction for reporting telemedicine services?**
   a. Any service represented by a *CPT* code may be reported as a telemedicine service.
   b. Only consultations are provided via telemedicine.
   c. Modifier **95** should be appended to codes found in Appendix P when provided via telemedicine.
   d. Telemedicine is limited based on patient location.

5. **What determines code selection for any service provided via telemedicine?**
   a. Only a physician's time communicating with the patient
   b. The same requirements required by the code descriptor and guidelines that apply when provided in person
   c. Only history and medical decision-making
   d. The physician's total time on the date of service is always used in code selection.

CHAPTER 21

Remote Data Collection and Monitoring Services

Contents

Types of Remote Data Collection and Monitoring Services 499

Collection and Interpretation of Digitally Stored Physiologic Data 499

    Self-measured Blood Pressure Monitoring 499

    Nonspecific Physiologic Data Collection and Interpretation 500

    Circadian Respiratory Pattern Recording 501

    Pediatric Home Apnea Monitoring Event Recording 501

    Ambulatory Continuous Glucose Monitoring 502

Remote Physiologic Monitoring Services 503

    Remote Monitoring Setup and Device Supply 503

    Remote Physiologic Monitoring Treatment Management Services 504

Remote Therapeutic Monitoring Services 505

    Remote Therapeutic Monitoring Setup and Device Supply 505

        Initial Setup and Patient Education 505

        Therapeutic Monitoring Device Supply and Transmission 506

    Remote Therapeutic Monitoring Treatment Management Services 506

Resource 507

Test Your Knowledge! 507

This chapter reviews codes for reporting services that include collection of data over a period of time with submission/transmission of data for review and report at the conclusion of the service period, and for remote monitoring of patient data with concurrent treatment management services.

Codes are included to describe the following related services:
- Device supply and data capture/transfer services
- Patient education/training and device calibration

Appendix R of *Current Procedural Terminology* (*CPT*) is a digital medicine taxonomy table providing an at-a-glance resource for identifying and differentiating digital medicine services including clinical data monitoring services. (Note that the taxonomy table is not all-inclusive of services that may be considered digital medicine services and does not supersede the specific coding guidance found elsewhere in *CPT*.)

Types of Remote Data Collection and Monitoring Services

CPT describes multiple services that may include utilization of data acquired remotely by
- Patient self-collection and data transmission/submission to a physician for review and interpretation outside of a face-to-face visit
- Remote physiologic monitoring with treatment management services
- Remote therapeutic monitoring of non-physiologic data (eg, level of function, compliance with treatment plan) with treatment management services

Devices used for digitally storing data and/or remote physiologic or therapeutic monitoring must be medical devices as defined by the US Food and Drug Administration (FDA). Medical devices may be listed as *FDA approved* or *FDA cleared*.

Collection and Interpretation of Digitally Stored Physiologic Data

Certain codes describe specific physiologic data collection/monitoring (eg, apnea monitoring), while other codes describe more generalized services (eg, remote monitoring of physiologic parameter[s] [eg, weight, blood pressure, pulse oximetry, respiratory flow rate]). The code that most specifically describes a service should be selected.

Self-measured Blood Pressure Monitoring

#99473   Self-measured blood pressure using a device validated for clinical accuracy; patient education/training and device calibration

#99474   separate self-measurements of two readings one minute apart, twice daily over a 30-day period (minimum of 12 readings), collection of data reported by the patient and/or caregiver to the physician or other qualified health care professional, with report of average systolic and diastolic pressures and subsequent communication of a treatment plan to the patient

Self-measured blood pressure monitoring is a non–face-to-face service in which the patient or caregiver uses a home blood pressure measurement device to measure and record readings that are then provided to the ordering physician on paper or digitally (eg, email). As technology changes, these data are increasingly available for electronic transmission from the device to an application that allows the patient to directly share data with the ordering physician.

Self-measured blood pressure monitoring is used for
- Ruling out white coat hypertension, which can avoid unnecessary treatment, adverse medication effects, and laboratory or diagnostic costs
- Identifying masked hypertension, which, if left untreated, carries a higher risk of cardiovascular disease and stroke
- Assessing control of hypertension and ensuring appropriate treatment is being ordered

Table 21-1 provides an overview of work included in each code.

Codes **99473** and **99474** are not reported for automated ambulatory blood pressure monitoring using report-generating software worn continuously for 24 hours or longer; see codes **93784–93790**.

Do not report **99473** or **99474** when reporting ambulatory blood pressure monitoring (**93784**, **93786**, **93788**, **93790**), collection and interpretation of physiologic data (**99091**), remote physiologic monitoring and treatment management (**99453**, **99454**, **99457**), remote therapeutic monitoring treatment management services (**98980**, **98981**), chronic care management (**99487**, **99489**, **99490**, **99439**, **99491**, **99437**), or principal care management (**99424–99427**) in the same calendar month.

Table 21-1. Self-measured Blood Pressure Monitoring by Patient	
#99473	Clinical staff or physician work ● Patient education/training on self-measurement and reading collection ● Home blood pressure monitoring device calibration Report once per device.
#99474	Physician work ● Review report of individual and average systolic/diastolic blood pressure readings (must include ≥12 readings; patient performs/documents 2 readings 1 minute apart at each measurement). ● Communicate treatment plan to clinical staff or patient/caregiver. Report for a 30-day period.

Example

➤ **A 16-year-old patient with moderate obesity presents with primary hypertension that is not responsive to life-style management.** The patient is struggling with dietary guidelines and exercises only during physical education. A low-dose medication is prescribed with instruction to continue the previously agreed-on diet and exercise regimen. The patient has previously been intolerant of ambulatory blood pressure monitoring but agrees to monitoring by self-measurement. The physician orders a blood pressure device validated for clinical accuracy and instructs the patient to obtain 2 readings twice daily for a 30-day period and send the results to the physician's clinical staff. The physician's documented evaluation and management (E/M) service supports moderate medical decision-making (MDM).

After the instrument is received by the patient, clinical staff calibrate the device and provide training for measurement and download and transmission of readings via the practice patient portal.

At the end of the 30-day period, the clinical staff review the patient's transmitted readings and average the systolic and diastolic pressures. The readings and calculated averages are reviewed by the physician, who communicates an ongoing treatment plan to the patient and/or caregivers.

International Classification of Diseases, 10th Revision, Clinical Modification (ICD-10-CM)	I10 (hypertension)
CPT	*Initial date of service* **99214** (office or other outpatient E/M service with moderate MDM) *Return visit for device setup after receipt of blood pressure device* **99473** (patient education/training and device calibration) *Data analysis and patient communication after 30-day period* **99474** (collection and averaging of blood pressure readings with communication of plan of care)

Teaching Point: At least 12 blood pressure readings must be obtained and averaged to create a treatment plan for the patient. Code **99474** includes collection, analysis, and communication of treatment plan(s) within a 30-day period.

If the patient returned for an office or other outpatient E/M service to review the readings and obtain the physician's recommended care plan, an E/M service (eg, **99214**) would be reported in lieu of **99474**.

Nonspecific Physiologic Data Collection and Interpretation

#99091 Collection and interpretation of physiologic data (eg, ECG, blood pressure, glucose monitoring) digitally stored and/or transmitted by the patient and/or caregiver to the physician or other qualified health care professional, qualified by education, training, licensure/regulation (when applicable) requiring a minimum of 30 minutes of time, each 30 days

Code **99091** *does not require active monitoring of physiologic data* or live interactive communication with the patient during the service period as is required for remote physiologic monitoring treatment management service codes **99457** and **99458** (discussed later in this chapter).

Code **99091** represents a 30-day episode of care. Time spent by a physician or other qualified health care professional (QHP) in activities listed in **Table 21-2** is included in the time supporting code **99091**.

Table 21-2. Collection and Interpretation of Physiologic Data	
#**99091**	Physician work ● Data access, review, and interpretation. ● Modify care plan as necessary and communicate to patient/caregiver. ● Associated documentation. ● Report for minimum of 30 minutes, each 30 days.

● Do not report **99091** if other, more specific *CPT* codes exist (eg, **93227**, **93272** for electrocardiographic services; **95250** for continuous glucose monitoring).
● If the services described by code **99091** are provided on the same day the patient presents for an E/M service, these services should be considered part of the E/M service and not separately reported.
● Do not report **99091** for transfer and interpretation of data from hospital or clinical laboratory computers.
● Do not report **99091** for time used to meet the criteria for care plan oversight services (**99374–99380**, **99339**, **99340**), personally performed chronic (**99491**, **99437**) or principal care management (**99424–99427**), or remote physiologic monitoring treatment management services (**99457**, **99458**).
● Code **99091** was assigned 1.63 relative value units (RVUs) in 2021 (facility or non-facility, not geographically adjusted).

Current Procedural Terminology **does not require use of a medical device as defined by the US Food and Drug Administration for services reported with code 99091. Live interactive contact during the reporting period is also not a required element of service for code 99091.**

Example

➤ **A child with epilepsy is prescribed a wearable device that detects seizures and notifies caregivers.** The data collected by the device is transmitted to a server from which the child's physician downloads a report at the end of each 30-day period that provides the frequency of seizure detection; detailed physiologic data collected before, during, and after each seizure; and information on the patient's sleep and wake times. An additional report provides information the patient or caregiver has entered into the device diary during the reporting period. The physician spends 30 minutes or more reviewing and interpreting the data and communicating by phone with the patient or caregiver about the treatment plan. The physician reports **99091** linked to a diagnosis code for the epilepsy.

Circadian Respiratory Pattern Recording

94772   Circadian respiratory pattern recording (pediatric pneumogram), 12–24-hour continuous recording, infant

● Report code **94772** when circadian respiratory pattern recording (pediatric pneumogram), 12- to 24-hour continuous recording, is performed on an infant.
● Physicians may be required to append modifier **26** to indicate only the professional component of this service was provided.
● Report 1 unit per recording period unless otherwise instructed by a payer.
● This code is not assigned RVUs in the Medicare Physician Fee Schedule (used by many payers). Allowable fees are determined by the payer.

Pediatric Home Apnea Monitoring Event Recording

94774   Pediatric home apnea monitoring event recording including respiratory rate, pattern and heart rate per 30-day period of time; includes monitor attachment, download of data, review, interpretation, and preparation of a report by a physician or other qualified health care professional

94775   monitor attachment only (includes hook-up, initiation of recording and disconnection)
94776   monitoring, download of information, receipt of transmission(s) and analyses by computer only
94777   review, interpretation and preparation of report only by a physician or other qualified health care professional

- Codes **94774–94777** are reported once per 30-day period.
- Codes **94775** and **94776** are reported by the home health agency because there is no physician work involved.
- Codes **94774** and **94777** are reported by the physician.
  - Code **94774** is reported by the physician when he or she orders home monitoring, chooses the monitor limits, and arranges for a home health care provider to teach the parents. It includes reviewing and interpreting data and preparation of the report.
  - Code **94777** is reported when the physician receives the downloaded information on disc or hard copy or electronically, reviews the patterns and periods of abnormal respiratory or heart rate, and summarizes, in a written report, the findings and recommendations for continuation or discontinuation of monitoring. This information is provided to the primary care physician and/or the family.
  - Codes **94774–94777** are not reported in conjunction with codes **93224–93272** (electrocardiographic monitoring). The apnea recording device cannot be reported separately. When oxygen saturation monitoring is used in addition to heart rate and respiratory monitoring, it is not reported separately.

Example

➤ **An infant born at 23 weeks' gestation, now 38 weeks old, has chronic lung disease and requires prolonged low-flow oxygen.** She continues to have occasional episodes of self-stimulated apnea lasting less than 15 seconds. She goes home with heart rate and respiratory monitoring during unattended periods and sleep. The physician orders the monitor, contacts the home health agency for its provision, and instructs the home health agency to teach the parents about cardiopulmonary resuscitation, proper attachment of the monitor leads, and resetting of the monitor. The home health agency provides the physician with the downloaded recordings. The first month's data are interpreted by the physician and a written report generated. The physician counsels the parents about the need to continue monitoring.

Teaching Point: Report code **94774** and the appropriate *ICD-10-CM* code (eg, **G47.35** for congenital central alveolar hypoventilation/hypoxemia).

In subsequent months, the physician receives the downloaded recordings, interprets them, and generates reports with recommendations for continued or discontinuation of monitoring. These services are reported with code **94777**.

Ambulatory Continuous Glucose Monitoring

95250	Ambulatory continuous glucose monitoring of interstitial tissue fluid via a subcutaneous sensor for a minimum of 72 hours; physician or other qualified health care professional (office) provided equipment, sensor placement, hook-up, calibration of monitor, patient training, removal of sensor, and printout of record
#95249	patient-provided equipment, sensor placement, hook-up, calibration of monitor, patient training, and printout of recording
95251	Ambulatory continuous glucose monitoring of interstitial tissue fluid via a subcutaneous sensor for a minimum of 72 hours; analysis, interpretation and report

- When use of an ambulatory glucose monitor is initiated and data are captured for a minimum of 72 hours, report code **95249** or **95250** based on the supplier of the equipment (patient or physician office).
- Codes **95249** and **95250** do not include physician work (ie, valued for practice expense and liability only). **Table 21-3** lists the physician and clinical staff work components of codes **95249–95251**.

Table 21-3. Ambulatory Continuous Glucose Monitoring of Interstitial Tissue Fluid Via a Subcutaneous Sensor *(A minimum of 72 hours of monitoring is required for each code.)*	
95251	Physician work includes correlation of individual data points with the patient daily log and interpretation and report. Do not report more than once per month.
#95249 (patient provided equipment only)	Clinical staff work includes sensor placement, hookup, calibration of the monitor, patient training, and printout of record. Report only once during the time a patient owns a given data receiver.
95250 (physician office provided equipment only)	Clinical staff work includes sensor placement, hookup, calibration of the monitor, patient training, removal of the sensor, and printout of the record. Do not report more than once per month.

- Physicians report code 95249 only if the patient brings the data receiver into the physician's or other QHP's office with the entire initial data collection procedure conducted in the office.
- Report code 95249 only once for the entire duration that a patient has a receiver, even if the patient receives a new sensor and/or transmitter. If a patient receives a new or different model of receiver, code 95249 may be reported again when the entire initial data collection procedure is conducted in the office.
  — Report 95249 on the date the continuous glucose monitoring recording is printed in the office.
  — Removal of a sensor is not a required component of 95249.
- Analysis, interpretation, and report (95251) may be performed without a face-to-face encounter on the same date of service. This service is reported only once per month.
- Code 95251 was assigned 1.02 RVUs in either a facility or non-facility setting in 2021 (not geographically adjusted).

Remote Physiologic Monitoring Services

Remote physiologic monitoring services include use of a medical device approved by the US Food and Drug Administration (FDA) to record and transmit daily recordings or programmed alerts. The transmitted data is used to manage the patient's care under a specific care plan. Codes distinguish equipment setup and patient education, device supply with transmission of data, and use of results to manage a patient under a specific treatment plan.

Do not report codes 99453, 99454, 99457, and 99458 for remote physiologic monitoring services when the parameters monitored are more specifically identified by other codes.

- A physician practice may provide all components (eg, equipment supply, initial setup, calibration, training, monitoring, treatment management services) or, perhaps more frequently, only the remote physiologic monitoring treatment management component (ie, 99457 and 99458).

Remote Monitoring Setup and Device Supply

#99453   Remote monitoring of physiologic parameter(s) (eg, weight, blood pressure, pulse oximetry, respiratory flow rate), initial; set-up and patient education on use of equipment

#99454   device(s) supply with daily recording(s) or programmed alert(s) transmission, each 30 days

To report codes 99453 and 99454, the device used must be a medical device as defined by the FDA (eg, blood glucose monitor) and the service must be ordered by a physician or QHP. Do not report when monitoring is fewer than 16 days.

- Codes 99453 and 99454 represent practice expense only; no physician work is valued in these codes. The time spent by a physician or QHP in activities listed in **Table 21-4** is included in the time supporting codes 99453 and 99454.

Table 21-4. Remote Monitoring of Physiologic Parameters: Setup and Device Supply	
Report only when the monitoring period is 16 days or longer.	
#99453	Clinical staff work includes setup and patient education on use of equipment. Report once per episode of care.[a]
#99454	Supply expense Supplies for daily recordings or programmed-alert transmissions Report once per episode of care.[a]

[a] An episode of care begins when the remote monitoring physiologic service is initiated and ends with attainment of targeted treatment goals.

- Do not report codes 99453 and 99454 in conjunction with codes for more specific physiologic parameters (eg, home apnea monitoring [94762]).
- Do not report 99453 and 99454 when these services are included in other *CPT* codes for the duration of time of the physiologic monitoring service (eg, 95250, ambulatory continuous glucose monitoring of interstitial tissue fluid via a subcutaneous sensor).
- Initial setup and patient education on use of equipment (99453) is reported for each episode of care (begins when the remote monitoring physiologic service is initiated and ends with attainment of targeted treatment goals).

Examples

➤ **A child with epilepsy is prescribed an FDA-approved wearable device that detects seizures and notifies caregivers in addition to transmitting data to the prescribing physician.** The patient is provided with setup and education for use of the device and the program's monitoring application. The practice directly receives and monitors daily recordings and/or programmed alerts for at least a 16-day period. Education on equipment use is provided as needed. Codes **99453** and **99454** are reported.

   Teaching Point: The device must be used for monitoring for at least 16 days to report **99453** and/or **99454**. The patient and caregivers are provided separately reported treatment management services (**99457**, **99458**) of at least 20 minutes in the month, as indicated.

➤ **A child with poorly controlled asthma is enrolled in a remote monitoring program.** A Bluetooth-enabled device that promotes and monitors effective inhaler use and measures forced expiratory volume in 1 second (FEV_1) and peak expiratory flow is provided to the patient by a remote monitoring technology provider. The patient's physician and/or clinical staff provide education to the patient and caregivers on device use. The physician reports code **99453**.

   Teaching Point: Because the physician practice furnishes only the initial setup and patient education, only code **99453** is reported for setup and education encounter. This service is reported only at the time of the initial 16 to 30 days of monitoring. Code **99454** would be reported by the provider of the equipment and monitoring service. See codes **99457** and **99458** for reporting 20 or more minutes of remote physiologic monitoring treatment management services during a calendar month.

Remote Physiologic Monitoring Treatment Management Services

#99457 Remote physiologic monitoring treatment management services, clinical staff/physician/other qualified health care professional time in a calendar month requiring interactive communication with the patient/caregiver during the month; first 20 minutes

#+99458   each additional 20 minutes

Remote physiologic monitoring treatment management services include time spent in a calendar month using the results of transmitted physiologic data to manage a patient under a specific treatment plan. These services may be rendered by physicians, QHPs, and/or clinical staff working under supervision of a physician or QHP.

> The reporting period for codes 99457 and 99458 is a calendar month. At least 20 minutes must be spent in treatment management services to report 99457.

The time spent in activities listed in **Table 21-5** is included in the time supporting codes **99457** and **99458**.

Table 21-5. Remote Physiologic Monitoring Treatment Management Services	
#99457	Physician work (personally performed or by clinical staff under physician or QHP supervision) • Data access, review, and interpretation. • Modify care plan as necessary and communication to patient/caregiver. • Associated documentation. • Report for minimum of 20 min, each calendar month.
#+99458	Physician work Each additional period of no less than 20 min (as previous)
Abbreviation: QHP, qualified health care professional.	

Documentation of remote physiologic monitoring treatment management must include
• An order by a physician or QHP
• *Live interactive communication* (eg, 2-way conversation via telephone or secure messaging) with the patient and/or caregiver
• Time of service of 20 or more minutes in a calendar month, including time in live interactive communication, data access, review and interpretation, and documentation

Reporting instructions

- Report code **99457** once with 1 unit of service for the initial 20 minutes of service regardless of the number of physiologic monitoring modalities performed in a given calendar month. When the time of service extends a full 20 minutes beyond the first 20 minutes, report code **99458** in addition to **99457**.
- Do not count any time on a day when the physician or QHP reports an E/M service (office or other outpatient services [**99202–99205, 99211–99215**]; domiciliary, rest home services [**99324–99328, 99334–99337**]; home services [**99341–99345, 99347–99350**]).
- Do not count any time related to other reported services (eg, **93290**, interrogation of implantable cardiovascular physiologic monitor system).
- Do not report **99457** or **99458** in conjunction with collection and interpretation of physiologic data (**99091**).
- Codes **99457** and **99458** may be reported during the same service period as chronic care management (**99439, 99487–99491, 99437**), principal care management (**99424–99427**), transitional care management (**99495, 99496**), and behavioral health integration services (**99492–99494, 99484**). However, the time for each service must be distinct and not overlapping and must be separately documented.
- Code **99457** was assigned 0.91 RVUs in a facility setting and 1.46 in a non-facility setting in 2021. Code **99458** was assigned 0.91 RVUs in a facility setting and 1.18 in a non-facility setting. Relative value units are not geographically adjusted. 2022 RVUs were not available at the time of publication.

Example

➤ **Data are received for a child with poorly controlled asthma who is enrolled in a remote physiologic monitoring program.** Clinical staff of the ordering physician review the data and note that the patient's plan of care calls for patient contact because FEV_1 and/or peak expiratory flow measurements are outside a specific range. A care coordinator contacts the patient's parent to inquire about medication use and signs and symptoms. The child's physician is consulted by the care coordinator and advice or orders for a change in management are relayed to the parent. At the end of the calendar month, documentation supports 25 minutes spent in remote physiologic monitoring treatment management services with at least 1 episode of live interactive communication with the patient's caregiver. Code **99457** is reported.

Remote Therapeutic Monitoring Services

Remote therapeutic monitoring services (eg, musculoskeletal function, therapy adherence, therapy response) represent the review and monitoring of transmitted data related to signs, symptoms, and functions of a therapeutic response as opposed to physiologic data such as heart rate and rhythm. These data may represent objective device-generated integrated data or subjective inputs reported by a patient. These data are reflective of therapeutic responses that provide a functionally integrative representation of patient status.

Remote Therapeutic Monitoring Setup and Device Supply

Initial Setup and Patient Education

●**98975**   Remote therapeutic monitoring (eg, respiratory system status, musculoskeletal system status, therapy adherence, therapy response); initial set-up and patient education on use of equipment

Code **98975** is reported once per episode of care for the initial setup and patient education on use of the equipment. An *episode of care* is defined as beginning when the remote therapeutic monitoring service is initiated and ending with attainment of targeted treatment goals.

- **98975** is not reported for a period of monitoring of less than 16 days.

> Codes **98975–98977** are specific to remote therapeutic monitoring services and are not used in conjunction with other physiologic monitoring services (eg, **95250**, ambulatory continuous glucose monitoring).

Therapeutic Monitoring Device Supply and Transmission

●**98976**   Remote therapeutic monitoring (eg, respiratory system status, musculoskeletal system status, therapy adherence, therapy response); device(s) supply with scheduled (eg, daily) recording(s) and/or programmed alert(s) transmission to monitor respiratory system, each 30 days

●**98977**   device(s) supply with scheduled (eg, daily) recording(s) and/or programmed alert(s) transmission to monitor musculoskeletal system, each 30 days

Codes **98976** and **98977** are reported for 16 to 30 days of device supply (ie, do not report <16 days of monitoring). Report **98976** and **98977** only in conjunction with remote therapeutic monitoring treatment management services **98980** and **98981**.

Remote Therapeutic Monitoring Treatment Management Services

●**98980**   Remote therapeutic monitoring treatment management services, physician/other qualified health care professional time in a calendar month requiring at least one interactive communication with the patient/caregiver during the calendar month; first 20 minutes

+●**98981**   each additional 20 minutes

Remote therapeutic monitoring treatment management service codes **98980** and **98981** are reported for a physician's or other QHP's cumulative time in a calendar month spent in remote therapeutic monitoring to manage a patient under a specific treatment plan. *At least 1 interactive communication with the patient/caregiver is required* in the calendar month. Time of interactive communication with the patient/caregiver contributes to the cumulative time of remote therapeutic monitoring treatment management services.

- Code **98980** is reported once per calendar month regardless of the number of therapeutic parameters monitored.
- If the time spent in remote therapeutic monitoring treatment management services during a calendar month is less than 20 minutes, do not report **98980**.
- Report add-on code **98981** in addition to **98980** when the service time of **98980** is exceeded by at least 20 minutes. Report 1 unit of **98981** for each additional 20-minute period. Do not report **98981** for a period of less than 20 minutes.
- Do not include any time spent on the date of an E/M service (including home, office or other outpatient, domiciliary, rest home, or inpatient services) in the time of remote therapeutic monitoring treatment management services.

  Do not report **98980** and **98981**

- In conjunction with remote monitoring of a wireless pulmonary artery pressure sensor (**93264**), collection and interpretation of physiologic data (**99091**), or remote physiologic data monitoring treatment management (**99457, 99458**)
- In the same calendar month as self-measured blood pressure (**99473, 99474**)
- For time counted toward separately reported chronic care management services (**99439, 99487–99491, 99437**), principal care management services (**99424–99427**), transitional care management services (**99495, 99496**), or behavioral health integration services (**99484, 99492–99494**) (When provided in the same time period, each service must be separately documented and no time should be counted toward the required time for both services.)
- Any time related to other reported services during the calendar month of reporting remote therapeutic monitoring treatment management (See a listing of other services that may be reported in your *CPT* reference.)

  Documentation of remote physiologic monitoring treatment management must include

- An order by a physician or QHP
- *Live interactive communication* (eg, 2-way conversation via telephone or secure messaging) with the patient and/or caregiver
- Time of service of 20 or more minutes in a calendar month

Example

➤ **An adolescent patient with moderate persistent asthma is learning to take responsibility for following a QHP's orders for use of control medication, identification and avoidance of triggers, and response to symptoms.** The QHP has prescribed remote therapeutic monitoring using an FDA-cleared medical device that automatically transmits the patient's use of an inhaler. The QHP reviews the transmissions and, at least once during the calendar month, telephones the patient to discuss medication compliance. The QHP's total time spent in remote therapeutic monitoring treatment management during the calendar month is 35 minutes. Code **98980** is reported. Had time during the calendar month exceeded 39 minutes, code **98981** would also be reported (ie, for 20 minutes beyond the first 20-minute service period).

Resource

Digital Medicine Taxonomy: Appendix R of *CPT 2022*

Test Your Knowledge!

1. **Which of the following is not a required component of self-measured blood pressure (99474)?**
   a. Minimum of 12 readings over a 30-day period
   b. A report of average systolic and diastolic pressures personally developed by a physician or qualified health care professional
   c. Communication of a treatment plan to the patient
   d. Use of a device validated for clinical accuracy

2. **Which describes the work reported with code 99091?**
   a. Transfer and interpretation of data from hospital or clinical laboratory computers
   b. Collection and interpretation of physiologic data collected over a 30-day period occurring on the date of an E/M service
   c. Collection and interpretation of physiologic data collected over a 30-day period not occurring on the date of an E/M visit
   d. Monitoring of physiologic data over a 30-day period

3. **Which of the following components of ambulatory continuous glucose monitoring of interstitial tissue fluid may be reported once per month?**
   a. Patient-provided equipment sensor placement, hookup, calibration of monitor, patient training, removal of sensor, and printout of recording
   b. Physician-provided equipment sensor placement, hookup, calibration of monitor, patient training, removal of sensor, and printout of recording
   c. Analysis, interpretation, and report of ambulatory continuous glucose monitoring
   d. b and c

4. **Which of the following is included in pediatric home apnea monitoring services described by code 94777?**
   a. Monitoring, download of information, receipt of transmission(s), and analyses by computer only
   b. Monitor attachment with parent education
   c. Monitor attachment, download of data, physician review, interpretation, and preparation of a report
   d. Physician review, interpretation, and preparation of a report

5. **Which statement represents a key difference between codes 99457 and 99458 and codes 98980 and 98981?**
   a. The services are differentiated by the type of data monitored and whether or not provision by clinical staff is included in the service.
   b. A requirement for live interactive communication
   c. A minimum time of service is required for reporting.
   d. Results of remote monitoring are used to manage a patient under a specific treatment plan.

Appendixes

More coding resources can be accessed at www.aap.org/cfp.

I. Quick Reference to 2022 *ICD-10-CM* Pediatric Code Changes 511

II. Quick Reference to 2022 *CPT®* Pediatric Code Changes 514

III. Vaccine Products: Commonly Administered Pediatric Vaccines 518

IV. Test Your Knowledge! Answer Key 522

I. Quick Reference to 2022 *ICD-10-CM* Pediatric Code Changes

This quick reference list does not include all changes made to *International Classification of Diseases, 10th Revision, Clinical Modification (ICD-10-CM)*. We have made every effort to include the diagnosis code changes that are most applicable to pediatric practices. However, revisions and/or additional codes may have been published subsequent to the date of this printing. Refer to your 2022 *ICD-10-CM* coding reference (eg, manual, data files) for a complete listing of new and revised codes, complete descriptions, and instructions for reporting. Always begin in the *ICD-10-CM* alphabetic index to locate the code most specific to the condition or other reason for encounter. Codes are valid as of October 1, 2021, unless otherwise noted.

Quick Reference to 2022 *ICD-10-CM* Pediatric Code Changes	
Codes followed by a dash (-) require an additional character. See an *ICD-10-CM* coding reference to complete these codes.	
R79.83	Abnormal findings of blood amino-acid level
P09.2	Abnormal findings on neonatal screening for congenital endocrine disease
P09.3	Abnormal findings on neonatal screening for congenital hematologic disorders
P09.5	Abnormal findings on neonatal screening for critical congenital heart disease
P09.4	Abnormal findings on neonatal screening for cystic fibrosis
P09.1	Abnormal findings on neonatal screening for inborn errors of metabolism
P09.6	Abnormal findings on neonatal screening for neonatal hearing loss
P09.8	Abnormal findings on neonatal screening, Other
P09.9	Abnormal findings on neonatal screening, unspecified
G04.82	Acute flaccid myelitis
T40.715-	Adverse effect of cannabis
T40.725-	Adverse effect of synthetic cannabinoids
Z91.014	Allergy to mammalian meats
A79.82	Anaplasmosis [A. phagocytophilum]
D55.29	Anemia due to other disorders of glycolytic enzymes
D55.21	Anemia due to pyruvate kinase deficiency
M54.59	Back (lower) pain, other
G44.86	Cervicogenic headache
T80.82X-	Complication of immune effector cellular therapy
Z20.822*	Contact with and (suspected) exposure to COVID- 19
R05.4	Cough syncope
R05.1	Cough, acute
R05.3	Cough, chronic
R05.8	Cough, other specified
R05.9	Cough, unspecified
F32.A	Depression, unspecified
K22.89	Disease of esophagus, other specified
Z71.85	Encounter for immunization safety counseling
Z11.52*	Encounter for screening for COVID-19

* Became effective Jan 1, 2021

Appendixes

Quick Reference to 2022 *ICD-10-CM* Pediatric Code Changes (*continued*)

Codes followed by a dash (-) require an additional character. See an *ICD-10-CM* coding reference to complete these codes.

K22.8-	Esophageal polyp
R63.39	Feeding difficulties, other specified
R63.30	Feeding difficulties, unspecified
Z59.41	Food insecurity
K31.A-	Gastric intestinal metaplasia
F78.A9	Genetic related intellectual disability, other
M31.11	Hematopoietic stem cell transplantation-associated thrombotic microangiopathy [HSCT-TMA]
D89.44	Hereditary alpha tryptasemia
Z59.02	Homelessness, sheltered
Z59.01	Homelessness, unsheltered
Z59.00	Homelessness, unspecified
Z59.81-	Housing instability
G92.0-	Immune effector cell-associated neurotoxicity syndrome
Z58.6	Inadequate drinking-water supply
L24.A-	Irritant contact dermatitis due friction or contact with body fluids
L24.B-	Irritant contact dermatitis related to (specified) stoma or fistula
Z59.48	Lack of adequate food (other specified)
M54.50	Low back pain, unspecified
M35.81	Multisystem inflammatory syndrome
P00.82	Newborn affected by (positive) maternal group B streptococcus (GBS) colonization
E75.244	Niemann-Pick disease type A/B
R35.81	Nocturnal polyuria
I5A	Non-ischemic myocardial injury (non-traumatic)
R45.88	Nonsuicidal self-harm
M35.89	Other specified systemic involvement of connective tissue
R63.31	Pediatric feeding disorder, acute
R63.32	Pediatric feeding disorder, chronic
Z92.859	Personal history of cellular therapy, unspecified
Z92.850	Personal history of Chimeric Antigen Receptor T-cell therapy
Z86.16*	Personal history of COVID-19
Z92.86	Personal history of gene therapy
Z91.52	Personal history of nonsuicidal self-harm
Z92.858	Personal history of other cellular therapy
Z91.51	Personal history of suicidal behavior
J12.82*	Pneumonia due to coronavirus disease 2019

*Became effective Jan 1, 2021

Quick Reference to 2022 *ICD-10-CM* Pediatric Code Changes (*continued*)

Codes followed by a dash (-) require an additional character. See an *ICD-10-CM* coding reference to complete these codes.

T40.71-	Poisoning by cannabis (derivatives)
T40.72-	Poisoning by synthetic cannabinoids
R35.89	Polyuria, other
U09.9	Post COVID-19 condition, unspecified
M35.0-	Sjogren syndrome with central nervous system involvement
R05.2	Subacute cough
F78.A1	SYNGAP1-related intellectual disability
D75.83-	Thrombocytosis
M31.19	Thrombotic microangiopathy, other
M31.10	Thrombotic microangiopathy, unspecified
G92.8	Toxic encephalopathy, other
G92.9	Toxic encephalopathy, unspecified
S06.A1X-	Traumatic brain compression with herniation
S06.A0X-	Traumatic brain compression without herniation
M54.51	Vertebrogenic low back pain

Abbreviation: NEC, not elsewhere classified

ᵃ Seventh character required (A, D, or S). See *ICD-10-CM* tabular list for full codes.

Appendixes

II. Quick Reference to 2022 *CPT*® Pediatric Code Changes

We have made every effort to include changes to procedures and services that are applicable to pediatric practices in this appendix. However, revisions and/or additional codes may have been published subsequent to the date of this printing. This list does not include all changes made to *Current Procedural Terminology* (*CPT*) *2022.* Also, not all codes included in the quick reference table are further discussed in this publication (typically due to limited use by most pediatricians). Codes not discussed elsewhere are shaded in gray. Always refer to *CPT 2022* for a complete listing of new codes, complete descriptions, and revisions. For questions or additional information on codes not discussed in this publication, please contact the American Academy of Pediatrics Coding Hotline (https://form.jotform.com/Subspecialty/aapcodinghotline). Any errata to *CPT 2022* will be posted to the American Medical Association website, https://www.ama-assn.org/practice-management/cpt/errata-technical-corrections. These changes take effect January 1, 2022. Do not report the changes or codes prior to that date.

Quick Reference to 2022 *CPT* Pediatric Code Changes

The following codes are listed as "revised" (▲). However, the only changes made were to punctuation (no changes were made to code definition or application): **99439**, **99483**, **99487**, **99489**, **99490**, **99492**, **99493**, and **99484**.

2021	2022
Evaluation and Management	
99211 Office or other outpatient visit for the evaluation and management of an established patient, that may not require the presence of a physician or other qualified health care professional. Usually, the presenting problem(s) are minimal.	▲**99211** Office or other outpatient visit for the evaluation and management of an established patient, that may not require the presence of a physician or other qualified health care professional.
#**99491** Chronic care management services, provided personally by a physician or other qualified health care professional, at least 30 minutes of physician or other qualified health care professional time, per calendar month, with the following required elements: • multiple (two or more) chronic conditions expected to last at least 12 months, or until the death of the patient; • chronic conditions place the patient at significant risk of death, acute exacerbation/decompensation, or functional decline; • comprehensive care plan established, implemented, revised, or monitored.	#▲**99491** Chronic care management services, with the following required elements: • multiple (two or more) chronic conditions expected to last at least 12 months, or until the death of the patient, • chronic conditions place the patient at significant risk of death, acute exacerbation/decompensation, or functional decline, • comprehensive care plan established, implemented, revised, or monitored; first 30 minutes, provided personally by a physician or other qualified health care professional, per calendar month +●**99437** each additional 30 minutes by a physician or other qualified health care professional, per calendar month
No specific code	●**99424** Principal care management services, for a single high-risk disease, with the following required elements: • one complex chronic condition expected to last at least 3 months, and which places the patient at significant risk of hospitalization, acute exacerbation/decompensation, functional decline, or death, • the condition requires development, monitoring, or revision of disease-specific care plan, • the condition requires frequent adjustments in the medication regimen, and/or the management of the condition is unusually complex due to comorbidities, • ongoing communication and care coordination between relevant practitioners furnishing care; first 30 minutes provided personally by a physician or other qualified health care professional, per calendar month +●**99425** additional 30 minutes provided personally by a physician or other qualified health care professional, per calendar month

Quick Reference to 2022 *CPT* Pediatric Code Changes (*continued*)

2021	2022
Evaluation and Management (*continued*)	
No specific code	●**99426** Principal care management services, for a single high-risk disease, with the following required elements;
	● one complex chronic condition expected to last at least 3 months, and which places the patient at significant risk of hospitalization, acute exacerbation/decompensation, functional decline, or death,
	● the condition requires development, monitoring, or revision of disease-specific care plan,
	● the condition requires frequent adjustments in the medication regimen, and/or the management of the condition is unusually complex due to comorbidities,
	● ongoing communication and care coordination between relevant practitioners furnishing care;
	first 30 minutes of clinical staff time directed by physician or other qualified health care professional, per calendar month
	+●**99427** each additional 30 minutes of clinical staff time directed by a physician or other qualified health care professional, per calendar month
Musculoskeletal System	
21310 Closed treatment of nasal bone fracture without manipulation	Evaluation and management appropriate to site of service
21315 Closed treatment of nasal bone fracture; without stabilization **21320** with stabilization	▲**21315** Closed treatment of nasal bone fracture with manipulation; without stabilization ▲**21320** with stabilization
Cardiovascular	
None	●**33894** Endovascular stent repair of coarctation of the ascending, transverse, or descending thoracic or abdominal aorta, involving stent placement; across major side branches +●**33895** not crossing major side branches ●**33897** Percutaneous transluminal angioplasty of native or recurrent coarctation of the aorta
33470 Valvotomy, pulmonary valve, closed heart; transventricular	None (procedure no longer performed)
33471 Valvotomy, pulmonary valve, closed heart; via pulmonary artery	▲**33471** Valvotomy, pulmonary valve, closed heart, via pulmonary artery
Digestive	
No specific code	●**43497** Lower esophageal myotomy, transoral (ie, peroral endoscopic myotomy [POEM])

Appendixes

Quick Reference to 2022 *CPT* Pediatric Code Changes (*continued*)

2021	2022
Male Genital System	
54340 Repair of hypospadias complications (ie, fistula, stricture, diverticula); by closure, incision, or excision, simple	▲**54340** Repair of hypospadias complication(s) (ie, fistula, stricture, diverticula); by closure, incision, or excision, simple
54344 requiring mobilization of skin flaps and urethroplasty with flap or patch graft	▲**54344** requiring mobilization of skin flaps and urethroplasty with flap or patch graft
54348 requiring extensive dissection and urethroplasty with flap, patch or tubed graft (includes urinary diversion)	▲**54348** requiring extensive dissection and urethroplasty with flap, patch or tubed graft (including urinary diversion, when performed)
54352 Repair of hypospadias cripple requiring extensive dissection and excision of previously constructed structures including re-release of chordee and reconstruction of urethra and penis by use of local skin as grafts and island flaps and skin brought in as flaps or grafts	▲**54352** Revision of prior hypospadias repair requiring extensive dissection and excision of previously constructed structures including re-release of chordee and reconstruction of urethra and penis by use of local skin as grafts and island flaps and skin brought in as flaps or grafts
Radiology	
75573 Computed tomography, heart, with contrast material, for evaluation of cardiac structure and morphology in the setting of congenital heart disease (including 3D image postprocessing, assessment of LV cardiac function, RV structure and function and evaluation of venous structures, if performed)	▲**75573** Computed tomography, heart, with contrast material, for evaluation of cardiac structure and morphology in the setting of congenital heart disease (including 3D image postprocessing, assessment of left ventricular [LV] cardiac function, right ventricular [RV] structure and function and evaluation of vascular structures, if performed)
Medicine: Cardiovascular	
No specific code	+●**93319** 3D echocardiographic imaging and postprocessing during transesophageal echocardiography, or during transthoracic echocardiography for congenital cardiac anomalies, for the assessment of cardiac structure(s) (eg, cardiac chambers and valves, left atrial appendage, interatrial septum, interventricular septum) and function, when performed (List separately in addition to code for echocardiographic imaging)
93530 Right heart catheterization, for congenital cardiac anomalies	●**93593** Right heart catheterization for congenital heart defect(s) including imaging guidance by the proceduralist to advance the catheter to the target zone; normal native connections
93531 Combined right heart catheterization and retrograde left heart catheterization, for congenital cardiac anomalies	●**93594** abnormal native connections
93532 Combined right heart catheterization and transseptal left heart catheterization through intact septum with or without retrograde left heart catheterization, for congenital cardiac anomalies	●**93595** Left heart catheterization for congenital heart defect(s) including imaging guidance by the proceduralist to advance the catheter to the target zone; normal or abnormal native connections
93533 Combined right heart catheterization and transseptal left heart catheterization through existing septal opening, with or without retrograde left heart catheterization, for congenital cardiac anomalies	●**93596** Right and left heart catheterization for congenital heart defect(s) including imaging guidance by the proceduralist to advance the catheter to the target zone(s); normal native connections
93561 Indicator dilution studies such as dye or thermodilution, including arterial and/or venous catheterization; with cardiac output measurement (separate procedure)	●**93597** abnormal native connections
93562 subsequent measurement of cardiac output	+●**93598** Cardiac output measurement(s), thermodilution or other indicator dilution method, performed during cardiac catheterization for the evaluation of congenital heart defects (List separately in addition to code for primary procedure)

Quick Reference to 2022 *CPT* Pediatric Code Changes (*continued*)	
2021	**2022**
Medicine: Non–face-to-face	
No specific code	● **98975** Remote therapeutic monitoring (eg, respiratory system status, musculoskeletal system status, therapy adherence, therapy response); initial set-up and patient education on use of equipment ● **98976** device(s) supply with scheduled (eg, daily) recording(s) and/or programmed alert(s) transmission to monitor respiratory system, each 30 days ● **98977** device(s) supply with scheduled (eg, daily) recording(s) and/or programmed alert(s) transmission to monitor musculoskeletal system, each 30 days ● **98980** Remote therapeutic monitoring treatment management services, physician/other qualified health care professional time in a calendar month requiring at least one interactive communication with the patient/caregiver during the calendar month; first 20 minutes +● **98981** each additional 20 minutes
Medicine: Miscellaneous Services	
No specific code	**99072** Additional supplies, materials, and preparation time required and provided by the physician or other qualified health care professional and/or clinical staff over and above those usually included in an office visit or other service(s), when performed during a nationally declared public health emergency due to respiratory transmitted infectious disease
Category III	
No specific codes	● **0652T** Esophagogastroduodenoscopy, flexible, transnasal; diagnostic, including collection of specimen(s) by brushing or washing, when performed (separate procedure) ● **0653T** with biopsy, single or multiple ● **0654T** with insertion of intraluminal tube or catheter
No specific code	● **0647T** Insertion of gastrostomy tube, percutaneous, with magnetic gastropexy, under ultrasound guidance, image documentation and report
No specific code	● **0656T** Vertebral body tethering, anterior; up to 7 vertebral segments ● **0657T** 8 or more vertebral segments
No specific code	● **0704T** Remote treatment of amblyopia using an eye tracking device; device supply with initial set-up and patient education on use of equipment ● **0705T** surveillance center technical support including data transmission with analysis, with a minimum of 18 training hours, each 30 days ● **0706T** interpretation and report by physician or other qualified health care professional, per calendar month

Appendixes

●=New code   ▲=Revised code   #=Re-sequenced code   +=Add-on code   ★=Telemedicine

III. Vaccine Products: Commonly Administered Pediatric Vaccines

This list was current as of September 1, 2021. For updates, visit www.aap.org/cfp. For COVID-19 vaccines, see page 520.

CPT® Product Code	Separately report the administration with CPT® codes 90460–90461 or 90471–90474.	Manufacturer	Brand	# of Vaccine Components
90702	Diphtheria and tetanus toxoids (**DT**), adsorbed when administered to <7 years, for IM use	SP	**Diphtheria and tetanus toxoids adsorbed (no trade name)**	2
90700	Diphtheria, tetanus toxoids, and acellular pertussis vaccine (**DTaP**), when administered to <7 years, for IM use	SP GSK	**DAPTACEL Infanrix**	3
90696	Diphtheria, tetanus toxoids, and acellular pertussis vaccine and inactivated poliovirus vaccine (**DTaP-IPV**), when administered to children 4–6 years of age, for IM use	GSK SP	**KINRIX Quadracel**	4
90697	Diphtheria, tetanus toxoids, acellular pertussis vaccine, inactivated poliovirus vaccine, Haemophilus influenza type b PRP-OMP conjugate vaccine, and hepatitis B vaccine (**DTaP-IPV-Hib-HepB**), for IM use	Merck/SP	**VAXELIS**	6
90723	Diphtheria, tetanus toxoids, acellular pertussis vaccine, Hepatitis B, and inactivated poliovirus vaccine (**DTaP-HepB-IPV**), for IM use	GSK	**Pediarix**	5
90698	Diphtheria, tetanus toxoids, acellular pertussis vaccine, haemophilus influenza Type B, and inactivated poliovirus vaccine (**DTaP-IPV/Hib**), for IM use	SP	**Pentacel**	5
90633	Hepatitis A vaccine (**HepA**), pediatric/adolescent dosage, 2 dose, for IM use	GSK Merck	**Havrix VAQTA**	1
90740	Hepatitis B vaccine (**HepB**), dialysis or immunosuppressed patient dosage, 3 dose, for IM use	Merck	**Recombivax HB**	1
90743	Hepatitis B vaccine (**HepB**), adolescent, 2 dose, for IM use	Merck	**Recombivax HB**	1
90744	Hepatitis B vaccine (**HepB**), pediatric/adolescent dosage, 3 dose, for IM use	Merck GSK	**Recombivax HB Engerix-B**	1
90746	Hepatitis B vaccine (**HepB**), adult dosage, for IM use	Merck GSK	**Recombivax HB Engerix-B**	1
90747	Hepatitis B vaccine (**HepB**), dialysis or immunosuppressed patient dosage, 4 dose, for IM use	GSK	**Engerix-B**	1
90647	Hemophilus influenza B vaccine (**Hib**), PRP-OMP conjugate, 3 dose, for IM use	Merck	**PedvaxHIB**	1
90648	Hemophilus influenza B vaccine (**Hib**), PRP-T conjugate, 4 dose, for IM use	SP GSK	**ActHIB Hiberix**	1
90651	Human Papillomavirus vaccine types 6, 11, 16, 18, 31, 33, 45, 52, 58, nonavalent (9v **HPV**), 2 or 3 dose schedule, for IM use	Merck	**Gardasil**	1
#90672	**Influenza** virus vaccine, quad (LAIV), live, intranasal use	AstraZeneca	**FluMist Quadrivalent**	1

Appendixes

CPT® Product Code	Separately report the administration with CPT® codes 90460–90461 or 90471–90474.	Manufacturer	Brand	# of Vaccine Components
#90674	**Influenza** virus vaccine, quad (ccIIV4), derived from cell cultures, subunit, preservative and antibiotic free, 0.5 mL dosage, IM	Seqirus	**Flucelvax Quadrivalent**	1
90682	**Influenza** virus vaccine, quad (RIV4), derived from recombinant DNA, HA protein only, preservative and antibiotic free, IM use	Seqirus	**Flublok Quadrivalent**	1
90685	**Influenza** virus vaccine, quad (IIV4), split virus, preservative free, 0.25mL dose, for IM use	Seqirus GSK SP	**AFLURIA Quadrivalent** **Fluzone Quadrivalent**	1
90686	**Influenza** virus vaccine, quad (IIV4), split virus, preservative free, 0.5mL dose, for IM use	Seqirus SP GSK GSK	**AFLURIA Quadrivalent** **Fluzone Quadrivalent** **FluLaval Quadrivalent**	1
90687	**Influenza** virus vaccine, quad (IIV4), split virus, 0.25mL dose, for IM use	Seqirus SP	**AFLURIA Quadrivalent** **Fluzone Quadrivalent**	1
90688	**Influenza** virus vaccine, quad (IIV4), split virus, 0.5mL dose, for IM use	Seqirus SP	**AFLURIA Quadrivalent** **Fluzone Quadrivalent**	1
#90756	**Influenza** virus vaccine, quad (ccIIV4), derived from cell cultures, subunit, antibiotic free, 0.5mL dose, for IM use	Seqirus	**Flucelvax Quadrivalent**	1
90707	Measles, mumps, and rubella virus vaccine (**MMR**), live, for subcutaneous use	Merck	**M-M-R II**	3
90710	Measles, mumps, rubella, and varicella vaccine (**MMRV**), live, for subcutaneous use	Merck	**ProQuad**	4
#90620	**Meningococcal** recombinant protein and outer membrane vesicle vaccine, serogroup B (MenB-4C), 2 dose schedule, for IM use	GSK	**Bexsero**	1
#90621	**Meningococcal** recombinant lipoprotein vaccine, serogroup B, 2 or 3 dose schedule, for IM use	Pfizer	**TRUMENBA**	1
90734	**Meningococcal** conjugate vaccine, serogroups A, C, W, and Y, quad, diphtheria toxoid carrier (MenACWY-D) or CRM197 carrier (MenACWY-CRM), for IM use	SP GSK	**Menactra** **Menveo**	1
#90619	**Meningococcal** conjugate vaccine, serogroups A, C, W, Y, quad, tetanus toxoid carrier (MenACWY-TT), for IM use	SP	**MenQuadfi**	1
90670	**Pneumococcal** conjugate vaccine, 13 valent (PCV13), for IM use	Pfizer	**Prevnar 13**	1
90732	**Pneumococcal** polysaccharide vaccine, 23 valent (PPSV23), adult or immunosuppressed patient dosage, when administered to ≥2 years, for subcutaneous or IM use	Merck	**Pneumovax 23**	1
90713	**Poliovirus** vaccine (IPV), inactivated, for subcutaneous or IM use	SP	**IPOL**	1
90680	**Rotavirus** vaccine, pentavalent (RV5), 3 dose schedule, live, for oral use	Merck	**RotaTeq**	1

Appendixes

Appendixes

CPT® Product Code	Separately report the administration with CPT® codes 90460–90461 or 90471–90474.	Manufacturer	Brand	# of Vaccine Components
90681	**Rotavirus** vaccine, human, attenuated (RV1), 2 dose schedule, live, for oral use	GSK	**ROTARIX**	1
90714	Tetanus and diphtheria toxoids (**Td**) adsorbed, preservative free, when administered to ≥7 years, for IM use	MBL SP	**TDVAX** **TENIVAC**	2
90715	Tetanus, diphtheria toxoids and acellular pertussis vaccine (**Tdap**), when administered to ≥7 years, for IM use	SP GSK	**Adacel** **Boostrix**	3
90716	**Varicella** virus vaccine (VAR), live, for subcutaneous use	Merck	**Varivax**	1
90749	**Unlisted vaccine or toxoid**	Please see *CPT* manual.		

Immunization Administration (IA) Codes

IA Through Age 18 With Counseling

90460	IA through 18 years of age via any route of administration, with counseling by physician or other QHP; first or only component of each vaccine or toxoid component administered (Do not report with **90471** or **90473**)
+90461	IA through 18 years of age via any route of administration, with counseling by physician or other qualified health care professional; each additional vaccine or toxoid component administered

Immunization Administration

90471	IA, one injected vaccine (*Do not report with* **90460** *or* **90473**)
+90472	IA, each additional injected vaccine
90473	IA by intranasal/oral route; one vaccine (Do not report with **90460** or **90471**)
+90474	IA by intranasal/oral route; each additional vaccine

Product Codes for COVID-19 Vaccines

91300	SARS-CoV-2 COVID-19 vaccine, mRNA-LNP, spike protein, PF, 30 mcg/ 0.3mL dosage, diluent reconstituted, IM
91301	SARS-CoV-2 COVID-19 vaccine, mRNA-LNP, spike protein, PF, 100 mcg/0.5mL dosage, for IM use
91303	SARS-CoV-2 COVID-19 vaccine, DNA, spike protein, adenovirus type 26 (Ad26) vector, PF, 5×10^{10} viral particles/0.5mL dosage, for IM use
⁄⁄ 91304	SARS-CoV-2 COVID-19 vaccine, recombinant spike protein nanoparticle, saponin-based adjuvant, PF, 5 mcg/0.5mL dosage, for IM use
⁄⁄ 91305	SARS-CoV-2 COVID-19 vaccine, mRNA-LNP, spike protein, PF, 30 mcg/0.3 mL dosage, tris-sucrose formulation, for IM use
⁄⁄ 91306	SARS-CoV-2 COVID-19 vaccine, mRNA-LNP, spike protein, PF, 50 mcg/0.25 mL dosage, for IM use

COVID-19 Vaccine Administration

CPT Product Code	Manufacturer	Initial IA	Second IA	Third IA	Booster	Dosing Interval
91300	Pfizer-BioNTech	0001A	0002A	0003A	0004A	1st Dose to 2nd Dose: **21 Days** 2nd Dose to 3rd Dose*: **28 or More Days** Booster: **Refer to FDA/CDC Guidance**
91301	Moderna	0011A	0012A	0013A	N/A	1st Dose to 2nd Dose: 28 Days 2nd Dose to 3rd Dose*: 28 or More Days
91303	Janssen	0031A	N/A	N/A	N/A	—
⁄⁄ 91304	Novavax	0041A	0042A	N/A	N/A	21 Days

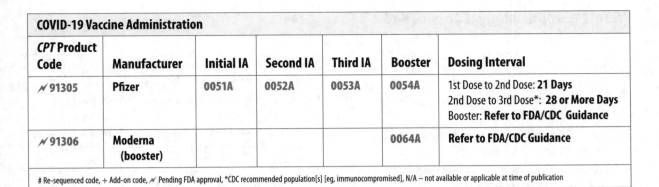

COVID-19 Vaccine Administration

CPT Product Code	Manufacturer	Initial IA	Second IA	Third IA	Booster	Dosing Interval
⟋ 91305	Pfizer	0051A	0052A	0053A	0054A	1st Dose to 2nd Dose: **21 Days** 2nd Dose to 3rd Dose*: **28 or More Days** Booster: **Refer to FDA/CDC Guidance**
⟋ 91306	Moderna (booster)				0064A	**Refer to FDA/CDC Guidance**

Re-sequenced code, + Add-on code, ⟋ Pending FDA approval, *CDC recommended population[s] [eg, immunocompromised], N/A – not available or applicable at time of publication

Appendixes

IV. Test Your Knowledge! Answer Key

Chapter 1

1. **c.** An Excludes2 note means "not included here" in *International Classification of Diseases, 10th Revision, Clinical Modification.*

2. **b.** The seventh character **D** indicates subsequent care during the healing phase.

3. **d.** When provided, category- or code-specific instructions are followed in lieu of the midpoint rule.

4. **b.** National Drug Codes must be submitted on a claim with 11 digits in 5-4-2 format.

5. **a.** The diagnosis code may be the same for each service performed.

Chapter 2

1. **c.** A National Correct Coding Initiative modifier indicator of 0 indicates that the edit for this code pair cannot be overridden with a modifier.

2. **c.** Modifier **26** indicates that the reporting physician provided only the professional component.

3. **c.** Often, modifier **51** is not required by payers.

4. **c.** Modifier **80** indicates a second physician provided assistance throughout a procedure.

5. **c.** Modifier **95** indicates that real-time audiovisual technology was used to provide a service.

Chapter 3

1. **c.** Hierarchical condition categories are used to calculate a patient's risk of increased health care use or risk adjustment.

2. **d.** Many health plans provide specific information on documentation and codes that do or do not support Healthcare Effectiveness Data and Information Set measurement.

3. **b.** False. Medicaid and Children's Health Insurance Program plans do participate in performance measurement programs.

4. **d.** Allergy to a vaccine or its components excludes a patient from performance measurement for immunization.

Chapter 4

1. **b.** Fully read and ask questions, as necessary, about the terms of the contract.

2. **d.** All of the above; accurate listing of diagnoses, selection of complete codes, and procedure code selection based on work performed and documented are basic parts of charge capture in an electronic health record.

3. **a.** A clean claim contains sufficient and correct information for processing without further investigation or development by the payer.

4. **c.** Requesting payer guidance on codes that are more likely to be paid is seldom beneficial and would be more appropriate for preparing to submit a corrected claim (although payers seldom directly offer coding guidance).

5. **c.** Assignment refers to the patients that a payer lists on your panel roster.

Chapter 5

1. **c.** Physician Self-Referral Law (Stark law) affects how a practice distributes income from designated health services.

2. **d.** All of the above; an auditor may be alerted to possible fraud or abuse by analysis of claim data across payers and care settings, inconsistency in billing by the physician and facility, and number of services reported exceeding the hours in a day.

3. **b.** An overpayment must be refunded to Medicaid within 60 days of the date when the overpayment was identified.

4. **a.** Request identification of each claim included in the extrapolation in response to a payer's request for refunds based on extrapolation.

5. **b.** False; physicians in all practices should be concerned about auditors.

Chapter 6

1. **d.** All of the above; past, family, and social history is not required for a problem-focused, an expanded problem-focused, or an interval history.

2. **c.** Eight systems must be examined to support a general multisystem examination.

3. **c.** Differential diagnoses may be in the assessment or clinical impression of a presenting problem without an established diagnosis.

4. **b.** Documentation of "old records reviewed" without further description of relevant findings or lack thereof is not sufficient per the evaluation and management (E/M) guidelines.

5. **a.** Presence via real-time audiovisual technology is sufficient to support presence for the key portion of an E/M service provided by a resident in a rural location.

Chapter 7

1. *a.* Code **99211** is appropriately reported when clinical staff provide dietary education to an established patient on a date when no physician service is provided.

2. *b.* Discussion between a treating qualified health care professional (QHP) and a physician working in the same group and same specialty is not an example of discussion with an external physician as defined for office E/M.

3. *d.* Two acute, uncomplicated illnesses or injuries do not support a moderate number and complexity of problems addressed.

4. *c.* Ordering 3 unique tests and discussing management with an external physician or external source supports an extensive amount and/or complexity of data to be reviewed and analyzed.

5. *b.* Prolonged office E/M service (**99417**) is reported when a physician's total time on the date of the encounter exceeds the minimum time of the range of total time assigned to **99205** or **99215** by at least 15 minutes.

Chapter 8

1. *c.* A newborn who was cared for by a physician of a different group practice or different specialty during the birth admission is a new patient when a preventive medicine service is provided.

2. *b.* Immunization administration on a date different from the date physician counseling was provided is reported with code **90471**.

3. *c.* A preventive medicine E/M code and **99188** are reported when a preventive medicine service and counseling for oral health with application of fluoride varnish are provided at the same encounter.

4. *d.* Code **96161** is appropriate for reporting maternal depression screening.

5. *c.* The midpoint rule applies to codes **99401–99404**.

Chapter 9

1. *b.* Codes **99241–99245** may be selected based on typical time when more than 50% of the physician's face-to-face time is spent in counseling and/or coordination of care.

2. *b.* False; **99324–99337** are reported for E/M services in a group home setting.

3. *c.* A physician spends at least 5 minutes speaking to an established patient who requested a telephone service for a new problem unrelated to and not resulting in any face-to-face visit.

4. *d.* Time of online digital E/M services begins with a physician's personal review of the patient's initial inquiry.

5. *b.* Code **99291** includes the first 30 to 74 minutes, and code **99292** is reported for each additional period of up to 30 minutes.

Chapter 10

1. *a.* Modifier **24** (unrelated E/M service by the same physician during a postoperative period) would be appended to the E/M code to signify an unrelated E/M service provided during the global surgical period.

2. *a.* A zero (0)-day global period applies to simple skin wound repair.

3. *c.* Layered closure of 1 or more of the deeper layers of subcutaneous tissue and superficial (non-muscle) fascia is an intermediate repair.

4. *c.* Codes **96360** and **96361** describe the initial infusion of hydration (prepackaged fluid and electrolytes) for the initial 31 minutes to 1 hour and each additional hour.

5. *b.* One unit of service is reported per injection (**96372**). Multiple units of service would be reported in conjunction with a Healthcare Common Procedure Coding System code describing the medication.

Chapter 11

1. *d.* No modifier is required to indicate a physician provided both professional and technical components of a service.

2. *c.* Direct optical observation describes a laboratory testing platform that provides a result (ie, positive or negative) by producing a signal on the reaction chamber.

3. *b.* Modifier **QW** is appended to most Clinical Laboratory Improvement Amendments–waived tests.

4. *c.* Modifier **52** is appended to the code for the audiometry service to indicate it was performed unilaterally.

5. *b.* Code **95117** is reported for 3 injections of previously prepared allergy extracts.

Chapter 12

1 *c.* A care plan must be established, implemented, revised, or monitored for principal care management.

2. *a.* Clinical staff time is not included in the time of service of code **99491**.

3. *a.* A face-to-face visit must occur prior to provision of the care plan oversight (CPO) service.

4. *c.* Principal care management and CPO are never reported by the same individual in the same calendar month.

5. *d.* Transitional care management includes a face-to-face service that is not separately reported.

Appendixes

●=New code   ▲=Revised code   #=Re-sequenced code   +=Add-on code   ★=Telemedicine

Chapter 13

1. **b.** National Provider Identifier describes a unique identification number for covered health care professionals.

2. **c.** Only 99211 may be reported for a nurse's assessment of a patient when Medicare incident-to billing requirements are met.

3. **a.** Use of a standardized curriculum is a required component of education and training for patient self-management.

4. **c.** Code Z39.1 is appropriately reported in the absence of feeding problems of an infant or health problems of the mother.

5. **d.** Medication therapy management services (99605–99607) are reported by a pharmacist.

Chapter 14

1. **b.** Code 96110 and the preventive medicine service (eg, 99391) are used to report developmental screening using a standardized instrument during a well-child visit.

2. **c.** Codes 96132, 96133 × 2 are reported for 2 hours and 40 minutes spent in neuropsychological testing data interpretation, interactive feedback, and report creation.

3. **b.** False; family members may act as informants during individual psychotherapy, but family psychotherapy (90846–90847) is reported only when family psychotherapy techniques are used.

4. **c.** A code for dependence is reported for abusive alcohol use with dependence.

5. **d.** Brief emotional/behavioral assessment using a standardized instrument is not separately reported when reporting general behavioral health integration care management (99484).

Chapter 15

1. **c.** A neonate born on January 1 is 28 days old on January 29th.

2. **a.** 99460; the attending physician reports initial newborn care on the date that the face-to-face service is provided.

3. **b.** A category Z38 code (liveborn infant) is the attending physician's first-listed code during the birth admission.

4. **d.** The attending physician reports 99462 25 and the appropriate code for the circumcision (eg, 54150) when providing both services on the same date.

5. **a.** The pediatrician reports 99231–99233 (subsequent hospital care) for continuing care of a newborn who no longer requires critical or intensive care.

Chapter 16

1. **c.** Hospital services may be selected based on time when more than 50% of the total unit/floor time was spent in counseling and/or coordinating care.

2. **b.** Split/shared describes an E/M service in which a physician and a QHP from the same group practice/same specialty each personally perform and document a substantive portion of 1 or more face-to-face E/M encounters on the same date.

3. **d.** All of the above; observation care is not reported on the same date as inpatient care by the same physician and requires at least detailed history and examination.

4. **a.** Code 99217 represents all E/M services provided by an attending physician to a patient on discharge from observation status if the discharge is on other than the initial date of observation status.

5. **d.** A second consultation during one admission is reported with codes 99231–99233.

Chapter 17

1. **a.** Codes for reporting abuse or neglect describe suspected, ruled out, or confirmed abuse.

2. **d.** Codes 99281–99285 are only reported for care in an emergency department as defined by *Current Procedural Terminology* or state regulation.

3. **d.** Both codes 99283 and 99284 include moderate-complexity medical decision-making.

4. **b.** Initial fracture care is reported with modifier 54 if another physician will provide follow-up care.

5. **c.** Thirty to 74 minutes is included in the service reported with code 99291.

Chapter 18

1. **a.** Cardiopulmonary resuscitation (92950) is separately reported when provided in conjunction with critical care services.

2. **b.** Thirty to 74 minutes of service time are included in 99291.

3. **b.** Subsequent inpatient neonatal critical care, per day (99469) is reported.

4. **d.** Codes 99291 and 99292 are reported because the child is outside the age range for codes 99466 and 99467 and codes 99485 and 99486. Code 99468 is reported only for services after the patient is admitted.

5. **c.** Car seat/bed testing services are reported with codes 94780 and 94781 when provided to patients 12 months and younger.

Chapter 19

1. *c.* Modifier **22** is not indicated solely on a patient weighing less than 4 kg (reportable with modifier **63**, when appropriate).

2. *d.* Report code **99024** for a related E/M service during the postoperative global period.

3. *b.* Echocardiography by another cardiologist during the same session as cardiac catheterization is separately reported.

4. *d.* Report a code for replacement when a central venous access device is removed and a new one is placed at the same access site.

5. *d.* Code **49491** is reported for initial hernia repair on a patient who was younger than 37 weeks' gestation at birth when the procedure is performed from birth up to 50 weeks' postconception age.

Chapter 20

1. *b.* A consultation provided to patient via secure audiovisual technology is an example of a telemedicine service.

2. *c.* Originating site describes the location of the patient receiving a telemedicine service.

3. *a.* Medicaid plans typically align with state regulations for telemedicine services.

4. *c.* Modifier **95** should be appended to codes found in Appendix P when provided via telemedicine.

5. *b.* The same requirements required by the code descriptor and guidelines that apply when provided in person are required when provided via telemedicine.

Chapter 21

1. *b.* The physician or other qualified health care professional is not required to personally develop the report of average blood pressures. Clinical staff may develop the report.

2. *c.* Code **99091** includes collection and interpretation of physiologic data collected over a 30-day period not occurring on the date of an E/M visit

3. *d.* Physician-provided equipment sensor placement, hookup, calibration of monitor, patient training, removal of sensor, and printout of recording and analysis, interpretation, and report of ambulatory continuous glucose monitoring are reported once per month.

4. *d.* Physician review, interpretation, and preparation of a report is included in pediatric home apnea monitoring services described by code **94777**.

5. *a.* The services described by codes **99457** and **99458** and codes **98980** and **98981** are differentiated by the type of data monitored and whether or not provision by clinical staff is included in the service.

Appendixes

Subject Index
Code Index

A

AAP. See American Academy of Pediatrics (AAP)
AAP Pediatric Coding Newsletter, 12, 83, 96
Abdominal radiographs, 281
Abuse, reporting suspected or confirmed, 404
Accountable care organizations (ACOs), 71, 86
ACIP. See Advisory Committee on Immunization Practices (ACIP)
ACO. See Accountable care organizations (ACOs)
Adaptive behavior assessment and treatment services, 336–340
Adenoidectomy, 473
Administrative services and supplies, 282
Advance care planning
    chronic and complex conditions and, 303–304
    in inpatient settings, 399
Advisory Committee on Immunization Practices (ACIP), 173
After-hours services, 165–166, 306
Agency for Healthcare Research and Quality (AHRQ), 59
AHRQ. See Agency for Healthcare Research and Quality (AHRQ)
Airway management, 461–462
Alcohol use disorders, 349–351
Allergy and clinical immunology, 275–278
    allergen immunotherapy, 276–277
    allergy testing, 275–276
    epinephrine auto-injector administration, 278
    immunoglobulins, 278
Alternative laboratory platform testing modifier, 45
Ambulatory continuous glucose monitoring, 502–503
American Academy of Pediatrics (AAP)
    on accountable care organizations (ACOs), 86
    appeal letters, 82
    Bright Futures: Guidelines for Health Supervision of Infants, Children, and Adolescents, 173
    coding and payment tools, 82–83
    Council on Children With Disabilities and the Medical Home Implementation Project Advisory Committee, 288
    Council on Early Childhood, Committee on Psychosocial Aspects of Child and Family Health, and Section on Developmental and Behavioral Pediatrics, 329
    Initial History Questionnaire, 174
    payment advocacy, 445
    Section on Neonatal-Perinatal Medicine, 361, 445
Amount and/or complexity of data to be reviewed, 132, 150–153
Anatomical modifiers, 46–47
Anesthesia by surgeon modifier, 36
Anesthesia services, 478–479
Annual child and adolescent well-care visits, 62
Annual nursing facility assessment, 222
Anogenital examination, 475–476
Anti-Kickback Statute, 91
Apnea, 501–502
Appeals, claim, 81–82
Appendectomy, 474
Arterial access, 472
Arterial puncture, 265
Assessment
    adaptive behavior, 336–340
    annual nursing facility, 222
    central nervous system, 331

child/adolescent weight assessment and counseling for nutrition and physical activity, 62
    emotional/behavioral, 188, 280
    health and behavior interventions and, 340–342
    health assessment screening, 187–190
    health risk, 189–190
    medical nutrition assessment and intervention, 321–322
    nonphysician assessment and management services, 315–318
    online medical, 315–316
Assistant surgeon
    modifier, 45
    modifier, minimum, 45
    modifier, when qualified resident surgeon not available, 45
    reporting by, 454–455
    in teaching facility, 457–458
Asthma, 166–167
Atrial septostomy, 465–466
Attendance at delivery, 364–366, 431
Attention-deficit/hyperactivity disorder, 167–168
Audiometry, 185–186, 278–280
Audits
    activities following, 102
    advice for, 103–104
    documentation and coding, 82, 100
    performance of, 100
    preparing for, 100–101
    and review process in compliance programs, 99–100
Automated neuropsychological testing and result, 335–336

B

Behavioral health integration, 351–355
    general behavioral health integration care management, 287, 354–355
    psychiatric collaborative care management services, 287, 351–354
Behavior change intervention, 194–196
Benign lesions, destruction of, 234
Bilateral procedure modifier, 36–37
Bilirubin testing, 271
Biofeedback, 347
Blood pressure monitoring, self-measured, 499–500
Blood sampling for diagnostic study, 262–265
Blood transfusion, 472–473
Bones. See Fracture and/or dislocation care
Boston Children's Hospital Care Coordination Curriculum, 288
Brackets, 7
Breastfeeding support/lactation services, 320
Bright Futures: Guidelines for Health Supervision of Infants, Children, and Adolescents, 173
Bundled payments, 83
Burn care, 238, 458–459
    skin grafts and skin graft substitutes, 459
    surgical preparation, 458–459

C

Cannula insertion, repositioning, and removal, 443–444
Cardiac catheterization, 463–464
Cardiovascular examination, 121, 123
Cardiovascular procedures, 462–469
    atrial septostomy, 465–466
    cardiac catheterization for congenital heart defects, 463–464

echocardiography, 462–463
    percutaneous transcatheter closure of patent ductus arteriosus, 468–469
    pericardiocentesis and pericardial drainage, 464–465
    transcatheter interventions for revascularization/repair for coarctation of the aorta, 467–468
    transcatheter pulmonary valve implantation, 467
    valvuloplasty, 466–467
Care plan, 295, 296
    oversight services, 298–301
Care plan oversight (CPO), 287, 288
Car seat/bed testing, 274–275, 374, 444–445
Casts/strapping/splints, 241–242
Catastrophe/disaster-related modifiers, 47
Catheterization
    arterial access, 472
    cardiac, 463–464
    central venous access, 469–472
    urinary, 246
Cauterization, chemical, 234–235
CC. See Chief complaint (CC)
CDT. See Code on Dental Procedures and Nomenclature (CDT)
Centers for Disease Control and Prevention (CDC)
    Advisory Committee on Immunization Practices (ACIP), 173
Centers for Medicare & Medicaid Services (CMS), 27
    documentation guidelines for E/M services, 110
    Healthcare Effectiveness Data and Information Set (HEDIS) and, 58
    on safe harbors and exceptions, 92
    surgical package rules, 451
Central nervous system assessments/tests, 331
Central venous access, 469–472
Cerumen removal, 243–245
Chemical cauterization of granulation tissue, 234–235
Chemotherapy and other highly complex drug/biologic agent administration, 252
Chest (breasts) examination, 121
Chest radiographs, 281
Chief complaint (CC), 114–116
Child abuse, 404
Child/adolescent weight assessment and counseling for nutrition and physical activity, 62
Children's Health Insurance Program (CHIP), 60
Chronic and complex conditions
    advance care planning for, 303–304
    care plan oversight services, 298–301
    chronic care management (CCM), 295–297
    coding for management of, 289–292
    complex chronic care management (CCCM), 295–297
    monthly care management services, 292–301
    outpatient management of, 287–289
    principal care management (PCM), 298
    prolonged services without direct patient contact, 304–305
    related services discussed in other chapters, 305–307
    reporting a combination of complex medical management services, 306–307
    tracking time of periodic services in, 288–289
    transitional care management (TCM), 287–292
Chronic care management (CCM), 287–289, 295–297
    monthly care management services, 292–301
    reporting, 297, 306–307

Circadian respiratory pattern recording, 501
Circumcision, newborn, 247, 373
Civil Monetary Penalties Law, 91
Clean claims, 73–83
    capturing charges in the electronic health
        record (EHR), 74–75
    encounter forms and other coding tools for,
        75–77
    Medicare, 79
    monitoring status of, 79
    place of service codes in, 77–78
    submitting, 78–79
CLIA. *See* Clinical Laboratory Improvement
        Amendments (CLIA)
Clinical Laboratory Improvement Amendments
        (CLIA), 265
    CLIA-waived tests modifier, 49
Clinical staff members, 311. *See also* Qualified
        nonphysician health care professionals
        (QNHCPs)
    scope of practice laws, 312–313
Clinical staff service, prolonged, 162–164
CMS. *See* Centers for Medicare & Medicaid Services
        (CMS)
Coarctation of the aorta, 467–468
Code on Dental Procedures and Nomenclature
        (*CDT*), 5, 191
Code sets
    Current Procedural Terminology (*CPT*), 13–18
    Healthcare Common Procedure Coding System
        (HCPCS), 12–13
    International Classification of Diseases,
        10th Revision, Clinical Modification
        (*ICD-10-CM*), 6–12
    National Drug Code (NDC), 18–19
    official, 5
    reporting codes for payment, 19–21
    who assigns codes for, 19
Coding. *See also Current Procedural Terminology*
        (*CPT*); Healthcare Common Procedure
        Coding System (HCPCS); *International*
        Classification of Diseases, 10th Revision,
        Clinical Modification (*ICD-10-CM*);
        National Correct Coding Initiative (NCCI);
        National Drug Code (NDC)
    edits to. *See* Coding edits
    E/M services. *See* Evaluation and management
        (E/M) services
    encounter story told through, 5–6
    official code sets, 5
Coding Clinic for ICD-10-CM and ICD-10-PCS, 6
Coding edits
    appropriate NCCI modifiers, 27–29
    Medically Unlikely Edits (MUEs), 27, 28–29
    National Correct Coding Initiative (NCCI), 27
    procedure-to-procedure, 27
    reviewing and using, 30
Comanagement of emergency department patients,
        409–410
Common office procedures and global days, 232–233
Complex chronic care management (CCCM),
        287–289, 295–297
    monthly care management services, 292–301
    reporting, 297
Compliance officers, 98–99
Compliance programs, 94–95
    audit/review process in, 99–104
    coding and billing and, 95–96
    compliance officers and, 98–99
    document advice from payers and, 98

documentation and coding audits and, 100
medical record documentation and, 96–97
necessity of, 103
responding to repayment demands and, 103
retention of records and, 98
steps to developing, 95–104
written policies and procedures in, 95
Comprehensive examination, 120
Concurrent care, 392–393
Concurrent infusion, 251
Congenital accessory digits, removal of, 234
Congenital heart defects, 463–464
Constitutional examination, 121
Consultations
    hospital services by other than admitting
        physicians, 392–393
    interprofessional telephone/internet/electronic
        health record, 211–213, 306, 396–397
    Medicare guidelines, 208–210, 393–396
    newborn hospital care, 371–372
    office and outpatient, 207–213
        expectant parent, 210
        Medicare guidelines, 208–210
        remote interprofessional, 211–213, 306
Consumer Assessment of Healthcare Providers and
        Systems (CAHPS), 59–60
Continuing care after hospitalization, 399
Continuum models
    asthma, 166–167
    attention-deficit/hyperactivity disorder, 167–168
    fever, 419–420
    otitis media, 168
    problem-oriented and preventive E/M on same
        date, 199
Contracting with payers, 71–72
Contributory factors, 112
Conventions, *ICD-10-CM*, 7–8
Coordination of care, 134
Coronavirus (SARS-CoV-2)
    COVID-19 vaccine, 179–180
    laboratory testing, 267–268
Counseling, 134
    genetic, 323
    group, 193–194
    immunization, 183–185
    and/or risk-factor reduction, 192–194
CPT. See Current Procedural Terminology (*CPT*)
Crisis, psychotherapy for, 347
Critical and intensive care services, 223–224
    attendance at delivery and newborn
        resuscitation, 431–432
    car seat/bed testing, 444–445
    critical illness or injury, 425
    definition of neonatal/perinatal periods and,
        430–431
    ECLS and ECMO services, 442–444
    in the emergency department, 416–418
    emergency medical services supervision and
        patient transport, 439–442
    hourly, 425–428
    initial and continuing intensive care, 437–439
    neonatal and pediatric daily critical care codes,
        432–437
    procedures not bundled with, 428–429
    remote, 436–437, 494–495
    sedation, 444
    total body systemic and selective head
        hypothermia, 442
    values and payment, 445
Cultures, 266

Current Procedural Terminology (*CPT*), 5
    add-on codes, 15
    Category II codes, 55–56
    on clinical staff members, 311
    conventions and guidelines, 13–15
    E/M services guidelines, 109–110
    Healthcare Common Procedure Coding System
        (HCPCS) Level I and Level II codes, 12–13
    mental/behavioral health services add-on
        codes, 331
    modifiers, 30–46
        alternative laboratory platform testing, 45
        anesthesia by surgeon, 36
        assistant surgeon, 45
        assistant surgeon, minimum, 45
        assistant surgeon, when qualified resident
            surgeon not available, 45
        bilateral procedure, 36–37
        decision for surgery, 40
        discontinued procedure, 38–39
        distinct procedural service, 41–42
        increased procedural services, 31–32
        mandated services, 35
        multiple, 46
        multiple procedures, 37–38
        postoperative management only, 39
        preoperative management only, 39–40
        preventive services, 35–36
        procedure performed on infants less than
            4 kg, 42–43
        professional component, 34–35
        reduced services, 38
        reference (outside) laboratory, 45
        repeat procedure or service by another
            physician or other qualified health
            care professional, 44
        repeat procedure or service by same
            physician or other qualified health
            care professional, 43
        significant, separately identifiable E/M
            service by the same physician or other
            qualified health care professional on
            the same day of the procedure or other
            service, 32–34
        staged or related procedure or service by
            the same physician or other qualified
            health care professional during the
            postoperative period, 40–41
        surgical care only, 39
        surgical team, 43
        synchronous telemedicine service
            rendered via a real-time interactive
            audio and video telecommunications
            system, 46
        two surgeons, 42
        unplanned return to the operating/
            procedure room by the same
            physician or other qualified health
            care professional following initial
            procedure for a related procedure
            during a postoperative period, 44
        unrelated E/M service by the same
            physician or other qualified health care
            professional during a postoperative
            period, 32
        unrelated procedure or service by the
            same physician or other qualified
            health care professional during the
            postoperative period, 44
        on normal newborn care, 361

Current Procedural Terminology (CPT) (continued)
    outpatient management of chronic and
        complex conditions, 287–289
    parenthetical instructions, 13
    on plan of care, 295
    provider terminology, 15
    quick reference to 2022 pediatric code changes,
        514–517
    surgical package rules, 229, 451–452
    symbols, 14
    telemedicine definition, 487
    updates, 13
    use of time in procedure coding, 15–18
Custodial care services, 215–216

D

Dash, 7
Decision for surgery modifier, 40
Deep sedation, 416, 478–479
Definitive drug testing, 351
Dental caries, prevention of, 190–191
Dental codes, 5
Destruction of benign lesions, 234
Detailed examination, 120
Developmental screening, 187–190, 331–332
    in first 3 years of life, 62
Diagnosis coding tips, 10–11
Diagnostic evaluation, psychiatric, 343–344
Diagnostic radiology, 456
Digestive system procedures, 245–246, 474–475
    appendectomy, 474
    gastric intubation and aspiration, 474
    gastrostomy tube replacement, 246
    hernia repair, 475
    incision in lingual frenulum, 245–246
Digital medicine services. See Telemedicine services
Direct optical observation, 266
Direct patient contact
    prolonged service with, 222
    prolonged service without, 223, 304–305
Discharge services
    hospital discharge day management, 391–392
    newborn hospital care, 369–370
    nursing facility care, 222
    observation care, 386
        same date admission and, 386–388
    versus subsequent hospital services, 392
Discontinued procedure modifier, 38–39
Disease management program, 319
Dislocations. See Fracture and/or dislocation care
Distinct procedure service modifier, 41–42
Documentation
    and coding audits, 82, 100
    compliance programs and medical record,
        96–97
    E/M services. See Evaluation and management
        (E/M) services
    incident-to services by qualified nonphysician
        health care professionals (QNHCPs), 314
    medical student, 136
    performance measures, 61–64
    retention of records, 98
    teaching physician E/M services, 135–137
    of telemedicine services, 490
Domiciliary, rest home, or custodial care services,
    215–216
Drug amount discarded/not administered to any
    patient modifier, 48–49

E

Ear, nose, and throat
    control of nasal hemorrhage, 243
    examination of, 121, 124
    hearing screening, 185–186, 278–280
    procedures of, 243–245, 473
    removal of impacted cerumen, 243–245
Early and Periodic Screening, Diagnostic, and
    Treatment (EPSDT) program, 47–48
Echocardiography, 462–463
ECLS. See Extracorporeal life support (ECLS)
ECMO. See Extracorporeal membrane oxygenation
    (ECMO)
Education and training, patient self-management,
    318–319
Effectiveness of care, 63–64
Electronic health records (EHRs), 73
    capturing charges in, 74–75
    compliance programs and, 96–97
    encounter forms and other coding tools for,
        75–77
    pitfalls of, 97
Emergency department (ED) services
    code modifiers, 410–411
    comanagement of patients, 409–410
    common procedures, 411–415
        fracture care, 412–413
        point-of-care ultrasound, 413–415
    continuum model for fever, 419–420
    critical care, 416–418
    directing emergency medical technicians, 416
    evaluation and management codes, 404–410
    reporting diagnosis code for, 403–404
    reporting external cause of injury, 403–404
    reporting suspected or confirmed abuse, 404
    sedation, 415–416
    special service codes, 418–419
Emergency medical services (EMS), 416
    direction of, 441–442
    supervision and patient transport, 439–442
Emergency medical technicians, 416
Emergency services in office, 166
Emotional/behavioral assessment, 188, 280
E/M services. See Evaluation and management
    (E/M) services
Encounter forms, 75–77
Encounter story told through code sets, 5–6
Endoscopy, 457
Epinephrine auto-injector administration, 278
Established versus new patients, 109–110, 144–145
    consultation codes, 208
    home care services, 213–215
Evaluation and management (E/M) services
    after-hours services, 165–166, 306
    clinical perspective on coding, 111
    CMS documentation guidelines for, 110
    code categories, 111, 205
    code components, 111–112
    comparison of 1995 and 1997 documentation
        guidelines for, 118–120
    complexity of medical decision-making,
        131–133
    consultations, 207–213
    contributory factors, 112
    CPT guidelines, 109–110, 205
    critical care, 223–224
    documentation guidelines, 112–134
    documentation of encounter dominated by
        counseling or coordination of care, 134
    domiciliary, rest home, or custodial care
        services, 215–216

emergency department (ED) services, 404–410
    examination documentation, 118–131
    general multisystem examinations, 120–122
    general principles of medical record
        documentation, 113
    history, 113–118
    home care services, 213–215
    with immunization administration, 198
    introduction, 112
    medical student documentation, 136
    more coding tips and, 134
    newborn hospital, 367
    new versus established patients, 109–110
    noncritical hospital. See Noncritical hospital
        E/M services
    nursing facility care, 219–222
    office and other outpatient. See Office and other
        outpatient E/M services
    online digital, 218–219, 305
    out-of-office service add-on codes, 216
    preventive medicine, 173–178
    primary care exception rule, 137
    significant surgical service and procedure,
        230–231
    single organ system examinations, 122–131
    split/shared, 134
    teaching physician guidelines for reporting,
        135–137
    telephone services, 217–218
    time component, 112, 205–207
Exclusion authorities, 91
Expanded problem-focused examination, 120
Expectant parents
    consultations, 210
    visits, 361
Explanation of benefits (EOB), 80
External cause of injury reporting, 403–404
Extracorporeal life support (ECLS), 442–444
    cannula insertion, repositioning, and removal,
        443–444
    initiation and daily management, 444
Extracorporeal membrane oxygenation (ECMO),
    442–444
    cannula insertion, repositioning, and removal,
        443–444
    initiation and daily management, 444
Eye examination, 121, 125
    vision screening, 186–187

F

Face-to-face critical care patient transport, 439–440
Face-to-face visit in transitional care management,
    291–292
False Claims Act, 91
Family adaptive behavior treatment guidance,
    339–340
Family and group psychotherapy, 348
Fever, 419–420
First drug of a multiple drug unit dose formulation
    modifier, 49
Fluoride varnish application, 190
Foreign bodies, removal of, 238–239
Foster care, 216
Fracture and/or dislocation care, 240–243, 460–461
    casts/strapping/splints, 241–242
    emergency department (ED) services, 412–413
    nasal, 413
    supplies, 242–243

Subject Index

Fraud and abuse
    additional liability insurance and, 105
    anti-fraud and anti-abuse activities, 93–94
    areas of specific concern, 94
    audits for, 99–104
    compliance programs for preventing. See
        Compliance programs
    defining, 91–94
    safe harbors and exceptions and, 92–93
Frenotomy, 374

G

Gastric intubation and aspiration, 474
Gastrointestinal (abdomen) examination, 121
Gastrostomy tube replacement, 246
General behavioral health integration care
    management, 287, 354–355
General multisystem examinations, 120–122
Genetic counseling services, 323
Genitourinary system
    anogenital examination, 475–476
    examination, 121–122, 125–126
    lysis/excision of labial or penile adhesions,
        246–247, 476
    newborn circumcision, 247
    procedures, 246–247, 475–477
    repair of penis, 476–477
    urinary catheterization, 246
Glucose monitoring, 502–503
Glucose tests, 269
Granulation tissue, chemical cauterization of,
    234–235
Group counseling, 193–194

H

Habilitative and rehabilitative modifiers, 340
HCPCS. See Healthcare Common Procedure Coding
    System (HCPCS)
Health assessment screening, 187–190
Healthcare Common Procedure Coding System
    (HCPCS), 5, 12–13
    coding for nutrition assessment and
        intervention, 322–323
    coding for services under disease management
        program, 319
    on mental/behavioral health services, 330
    modifiers, 46–50
        anatomical, 46–47
        catastrophe/disaster related, 47
        Clinical Laboratory Improvement
            Amendments–waived tests, 49
        drug amount discarded/not administered
            to any patient, 48–49
        first drug of a multiple drug unit dose
            formulation, 49
        patient relationship, 50
        second or subsequent drug of a multiple
            drug unit dose formulation, 49
        service has been performed in part by
            a resident under the direction of a
            teaching physician, 48
        service provided as part of Medicaid Early
            and Periodic Screening, Diagnostic,
            and Treatment (EPSDT) program,
            47–48
        this service has been performed by a
            resident without the presence of a
            teaching physician under the primary
            care exception, 48

    via interactive audio and video
        telecommunication systems, 48
    waiver of liability statement issued as
        required by payer policy
        individual case, 48
        routine notice, 48
    X {E, P, S, U}, 47
    telehealth codes, 492–494
Healthcare Effectiveness Data and Information Set
    (HEDIS), 57–59
    preventive care and, 176
Health Insurance Portability and Accountability Act
    (HIPAA), 5
Health Resources and Services Administration
    (HRSA), 173
Health risk assessment, 189–190
Hearing screening, 185–186, 278–280
HEDIS. See Healthcare Effectiveness Data and
    Information Set (HEDIS)
Hematologic/lymphatic/immunologic examination,
    122, 126–127
Hematology tests, 269
Hernia repair, 475
Heterophile antibodies screening, 270
Hierarchical condition categories, 56–57
HIPAA. See Health Insurance Portability and
    Accountability Act (HIPAA)
Hip radiographs, 281
History, documentation of, 113–118
History of present illness (HPI), 114–116
Home care services, 213–215
Home health procedures/services, 323–324
Home ventilator management, 301
Hospital care of newborns, 373–374
    car safety seat testing, 274–275, 374
    circumcision, 247, 373
    frenotomy, 374
Hospital care of the ill newborn, 364–373
    attendance at delivery, 364–366
    coding for transitions to different levels of
        neonatal care, 372–373
    consultations, 371–372
    diagnosis codes for perinatal conditions,
        366–367
    discharge day management, 369–370
    hospital E/M services, 367
    initial, 367–368
    versus normal newborn care, 367–372
    prolonged services, 370–371
    stillborn deliveries and unsuccessful
        resuscitation, 366
    subsequent, 369
Hospital-mandated on-call services, 399
Hospital services, noncritical. See Noncritical
    hospital E/M services
Hourly critical care, 425–428
HPI. See History of present illness (HPI)
HRSA. See Health Resources and Services
    Administration (HRSA)
Hydration, 249
Hypothermia, 442

I

ICD-10-CM. See International Classification
    of Diseases, 10th Revision, Clinical
    Modification (ICD-10-CM)
Imaging guidance, 281
Immunizations
    administration of, 179–185, 198
    coding for counseling when immunizations not
        carried out, 183–185

    commonly administered pediatric vaccines,
        518–520
    COVID-19, 179–180
    National Drug Code (NDC), 179
    vaccine refusal, 61
    vaccines and toxoids, 178–179
    Vaccines for Children (VFC) program, 185
Immunization status, 62–63
Immunoglobulins, 278
Immunotherapy, allergy, 276–277
Impacted cerumen removal, 243–245
Incision, lingual frenulum, 245–246
Incision and drainage, integumentary system, 234
Increased or decreased surgical procedure services,
    453–455
Increased procedural services modifier, 31–32
Indexes, 9
Inducements, 92–93
Influenza testing, 269–270
Infusions
    concurrent, 251
    hydration, 249
    initial, 250–251
    intra-arterial and intravenous push injections,
        249
    irrigation of implanted venous access device for
        drug delivery systems, 251
    sequential, 251
    therapeutic, prophylactic, and diagnostic, 250
Inhalation solutions, 263
Inhalation treatment, 273
Initial and continuing intensive care, 437–439
Initial hospital care of newborn, 367–368
Initial infusion, 250–251
Initial inpatient hospital care, 388–390
Initial nursing facility care, 220–221
Initial observation care, 382–384
Injections
    intravenous push, 249
    medication, 263–264
    subcutaneous or intramuscular, 247–248
Injury
    critical care services for, 425
    reporting external cause of, 403–404
Inpatient hospital care, 388–392
    advance care planning and, 399
    discharge versus subsequent hospital services,
        392
    hospital discharge day management, 391–392
    hospital services by other physicians, 392–397
    initial, 388–390
    prolonged E/M services in, 397–398
    subsequent, 390–391
Integumentary procedures, 234–238
    burn care, 238
    chemical cauterization of granulation tissue,
        234–235
    destruction of benign lesions, 234
    incision and drainage, 234
    laceration repairs, 235–236
    other repairs, 237–238
    removal of foreign bodies, 238–239
    removal of skin tags and congenital accessory
        digits, 234
    suture removal, 237
Interactive audio and video telecommunication
    systems modifier, 48
Interactive complexity in psychiatric services,
    342–343

Subject Index

International Classification of Diseases, 10th Revision, Clinical Modification (ICD-10-CM), 5, 6
  chapter-specific guidelines, 8
  code selection, 8–9
  coding for use, abuse, and dependence, 349
  conventions, 7–8
  diagnosis coding tips, 10–11
  on external cause of injury, 403
  general coding guidelines, 8
  hierarchical condition codes, 56–57
  indexes, 9
  mental/behavioral health services codes, 330–331
  neonatal critical care, 430–431
  newborn services codes, 363–364
  pathway to code selection, 9–12
  preventive care visits codes, 175–176
  quick reference to 2022 pediatric code changes, 511–513
  tabular list, 9–10
  unspecified codes, 11–12
Interprofessional telephone/internet consultations, 211–213, 306
  hospital services by other than admitting physicians, 396–397
Interventions
  behavior change preventive care, 194–196
  coding for nutrition assessment and, 322–323
  health behavior, 340–342
  medical nutrition, 321–322
  substance use, 348–351
  transcatheter, for revascularization/repair for coarctation of the aorta, 467–468
Intra-arterial injections, 249
Intramuscular injections, 247–248
Intravenous push injections, 249
Intubation and airway management, 461–462
Irrigation of implanted venous access device for drug delivery systems, 251

K

Kickbacks, 92–93

L

Labial adhesions, 246–247, 476
Laboratory procedures. *See also* Testing
  general guidance for reporting, 265–266
  laboratory panel coding, 266
  pathology and, 265–266
  performed in the office, 267–272
  screening, 191
Laceration repairs, 235–236
Laryngoplasty, 473
Lead screening, 63, 270
Lingual frenulum incision, 245–246
Lip repair, 237
Lymphatic examination, 122, 126–127
Lysis/excision of labial or penile adhesions, 246–247, 476

M

MAAA. *See* Multianalyte assays with algorithmic analyses (MAAA)
Mandated services modifier, 35
Mandatory reporting, 404
MDM. *See* Medical decision-making (MDM)
Medicaid
  Children's Health Insurance Program (CHIP) quality measures and, 60

Early and Periodic Screening, Diagnostic, and Treatment (EPSDT) program, 47–48
  fraud cases, 104
  NCCI edits, 27, 29–30
  telemedicine payment, 490
Medical decision-making (MDM), 131–133
  office or other outpatient E/M services, 148–155
    amount and/or complexity of data to be reviewed and analyzed, 150–153
    number and complexity of problems addressed in, 148–150
    risk of complications and/or morbidity or mortality of patient management, 153–155
    selection of level 2 through 5 codes, 155–160
  in transitional care management, 291–292
Medical liability insurance, 105
Medically Unlikely Edits (MUEs), 27, 28–29
Medical nutrition assessment and intervention, 321–322
Medical student documentation, 136
Medical team conferences, 301–303
  inpatient hospital setting, 398
  qualified nonphysician health care professionals (QNHCPs) and, 317–318
Medicare
  clean claims, 79
  consultation guidelines, 208–210, 393–396
  NCCI edits, 27, 29–30
  observation policy, 386–388
  Physician Fee Schedule (MPFS), 70
  Resource-Based Relative Value Scale (RBRVS), 69
  surgical package, 229–230
Medications
  chemotherapy and other highly complex drug/biologic agent administration, 252
  epinephrine auto-injector administration, 278
  immunoglobulins, 278
  testing, 262, 263–264
Medication therapy management services by pharmacist, 323
Mental/behavioral health services
  adaptive behavior assessment and treatment services, 336–340
  behavioral health integration, 351–355
  central nervous system assessments/tests, 331
  CPT add-on-codes, 331
  developmental testing, 62, 187–190, 331–332
  health and behavior assessments/interventions, 340–342
  neuropsychological and psychological testing, 332–336
  physicians and other providers of, 329–330
  psychiatric services, 342–348
  reporting codes F01–F99, 330–331
  substance use evaluation and treatment, 348–351
Mini-mental status examination, 333
Minimum assistant surgeon modifier, 45
Minor procedures, 456
  with no codes, 232
Mistreatment, child, 404
Moderate sedation, 252–255, 415–416, 478
Modifiers
  Current Procedural Terminology (CPT), 30–46
  emergency department codes, 410–411
  National Correct Coding Initiative (NCCI), 27–30
  preventive medicine, 196–197
  telemedicine, 491

Monitoring of payments, 80–82
Mononucleosis testing, 270
Monthly care management services, 292–301
  activities of, 294
  plan of care, 295, 296
  required practice capabilities, 294–295
Multianalyte assays with algorithmic analyses (MAAA), 266
Multiple modifiers, 46
Multiple procedures modifier, 37–38
Multiple surgical procedures on the same date, 452–453
Musculoskeletal examination, 122, 127
  osteotomy humerus with intramedullary lengthening device, 461
Musculoskeletal foreign bodies, 239
Musculoskeletal procedures, 460–461. *See also* Fracture and/or dislocation care
  removal of musculoskeletal hardware, 461

N

Nail bed repair, 237
Nasal fractures, 413
Nasal hemorrhage, 243
National Correct Coding Initiative (NCCI), 27
  appropriate modifiers, 27–29
  keeping up to date with, 29–30
  Medically Unlikely Edits (MUEs), 27, 28–29
  procedure-to-procedure edits, 27
National Drug Code (NDC), 5, 18–19
  vaccines, 179
National Provider Identifier (NPI), 146, 313
National Uniform Claim Committee 1500 claim form, 19–20
NCCI. *See* National Correct Coding Initiative (NCCI)
NDC. *See* National Drug Code (NDC)
Nebulizer demonstration or evaluation, 273–274
Neck examination, 121
Negative pressure wound therapy, 477–478
Neglect, child, 404
Negotiating with payers, 71–72
Neonatal and pediatric critical care, 432–437
  neonatal critical care, 433–435
  patients critically ill after surgery, 436
  pediatric critical care, 435–436
  remote critical care services, 436–437
  supervision requirements, 432–433
Neonatal period, 361, 430–431
Neonatal resuscitation, 431–432
Neurobehavioral status examination, 332–333
Neurological examination, 122, 128
Neuropsychological and psychological testing, 332–336
  neurobehavioral status examination, 332–333
  testing administration services, 334–336
  testing evaluation services by physician or other qualified health care professional with interpretation and report, 333–334
Newborns
  attendance at delivery and resuscitation of, 364–366, 431–432
  car seat/bed testing, 274–275, 374
  circumcision, 247, 373
  excision, 247
  frenotomy, 374
  hospital care of ill, 364–373
  ICD-10-CM codes for, 363–364
  neonatal and pediatric daily critical care codes, 432–437

normal care, 361–364
other hospital care, 373–374
perinatal care, 361
surgical procedures performed on infants less
than 4 kg, 455
New versus established patients, 109–110, 144–145
consultation codes, 208
home care services, 213–215
Noncritical hospital E/M services
coding for, 379–381
key components, 380
progression of care, 379
split/shared billing, 381
time-based code selection, 380–381
continuing care after hospitalization, 399
hospital-mandated on-call services, 399
hospital services by other physicians, 392–397
concurrent care, 392–393
consultations, 393
interprofessional telephone/internet/
electronic health record consultation,
396–397
Medicare consultation guidelines, 393–396
inpatient hospital care, 388–392
advance care planning, 399
discharge versus subsequent hospital
services, 392
hospital discharge day management,
391–392
initial, 389–390
medical team conferences, 398
subsequent, 390–391
medical team conferences, 398
observation care, 382–386
discharge day management, 386
initial, 382–384
subsequent, 385
prolonged E/M services, 397–398
same date admission and discharge services,
386–388
Nonphysician assessment and management
services, 315–318
online medical assessment, 315–316
Nonphysician providers (NPPs), 15
mental/behavioral services by, 329–330
supervision of, 314
Nonspecific physiologic data collection and
interpretation, 500–501
Normal newborn care, 361–364
versus hospital care, 367–372
Nose. See Ear, nose, and throat
Number and complexity of problems addressed in
office or other outpatient settings, 148–150
Number of diagnoses or management options,
131–132
Nursing evaluation and management visit, 314–315
Nursing facility care, 219–222
annual assessment, 222
critical care, 223–224
discharge services, 222
initial, 220–221
subsequent, 221
Nutritional support services, 320–323
breastfeeding support/lactation services, 320
medical nutrition assessment and intervention,
321–322
payer-specific coding for, 322–323

O

Observation care, 382–386
discharge day management, 386
initial, 382–384
Medicare policy, 386–388
subsequent, 385
Occult blood testing, 271
Office and other outpatient E/M services
after-hours, 165–166
chronic and complex conditions management,
287–289
consultations, 207–213
continuum models
asthma, 166–167
attention-deficit/hyperactivity disorder,
167–168
otitis media, 168
critical care, 223–224
domiciliary, rest home, or custodial care
services, 215–216
guidelines, 144–147
medical decision-making, 148–155
for selecting level of service, 145
time, 147–148
home care services, 213–215
laboratory tests, 267–272
new versus established patients, 144–145
nursing facility care, 219–222
online digital, 218–219
overview of, 143
prolonged, 160–164
selection of level 2 through 5 codes, 155–160
split/shared, 164–165
telephone services, 217–218
visits not requiring a physician's or qualified
health care professional's presence,
146–147
Office hours, 165–166
Office of Inspector General (OIG), 92
on compliance programs, 94–95
On-call services, hospital-mandated, 399
Online digital E/M services, 218–219, 305
Online medical assessment, 315–316
Osteotomy humerus with intramedullary
lengthening device, 461
Otitis media, 168
Out-of-office service add-on codes, 216

P

Pain management, postoperative, 479–480
Papanicolaou (Pap) tests, 270
Parentheses, 7
Past, family, and/or social history (PFSH), 114–117
Patent ductus arteriosus, 468–469
Pathology and laboratory procedures, 265–266
Patient Protection and Affordable Care Act
(PPACA), 35, 56, 86, 94, 102, 173, 320, 340
Patient relationship modifiers, 50
Patient self-management training services, 318–319
Pay for performance, 84
Payment
accountable care organizations (ACOs) and, 86
clean claims to correct, 73–83
contracting and negotiating with payers for,
71–72
documentation and coding audits, 82
emerging methodologies for, 83–86
filing appeals for, 81–82
monitoring of, 80–82

preparing for new models of, 84–86
repayment demands and, 103
tools for pediatric practice, 82–83
value-based models of, 83, 84–85
values assigned to physician services for, 69–71
PCER. See Primary care exception rule (PCER)
Pediatric Coding Basics, 10
Pediatric daily critical care codes, 432–437
Pediatric home apnea monitoring event recording,
501–502
Pediatric ICD-10-CM: A Manual for Provider-Based
Coding, 12
Penile adhesions, 246–247, 476
Penis, repair of, 476–477
Percutaneous transcatheter closure of patent ductus
arteriosus, 468–469
Pericardial drainage, 464–465
Pericardiocentesis, 464–465
Perinatal care, 361
diagnosis codes for, 366–367
Perinatal period, 361, 430–431
Periodic services time tracking, 288–289
PFSH. See Past, family, and/or social history (PFSH)
Pharmacist, medication therapy management
services by, 323
Physician group education services, 282
Physician Self-Referral Law, 91
Physician services
hospital services by other than admitting
physician, 392–397
mental/behavioral health, 329–330
physician arrival after delivery, 365
prolonged, 160–162
scope of practice laws, 312–313
values assigned to, 69–71
visits not requiring, 146
Physician work, 69
Physiologic data, digitally stored, 499–503
ambulatory continuous glucose monitoring,
502–503
circadian respiratory pattern recording, 501
nonspecific, 500–501
pediatric home apnea monitoring event
recording, 501–502
self-measured blood pressure monitoring,
499–500
PLA. See Proprietary laboratory analysis (PLA)
Place of service codes, 77–78, 491
Plan of care. See Care plan
Pleural drainage, 462
Point-of-care ultrasound, 413–415
Postoperative care, 231, 457. See also Surgery
global periods and modifiers for reporting, 452
pain management, 479–480
reporting, 452
Postoperative management only modifier, 39
Post-service work, 69
PPACA. See Patient Protection and Affordable Care
Act (PPACA)
Practice expense, 70
Pregnancy consultations, 210
Preoperative management only modifier, 39–40
Presumptive drug tests, 271, 350–351
Preventive care
behavior change intervention, 194–196
dental caries, 190–191
developmental screening and health
assessment, 187–190
E/M services, 173–178
health plan coverage for, 173

Preventive care (continued)
    ICD-10-CM codes, 175–176
    immunizations, 178–185
    preventive medicine services modifier, 196–197
    in problem-oriented visit, 197–199
    provided outside preventive visit, 192–197
    quality initiatives and, 176–177
    screening laboratory tests, 191
    screening tests and procedures, 185–187
    sports/camp physicals, 177–178
Preventive screening and utilization measures, 61–62
Preventive services modifier, 35–36
Primary care exception rule (PCER), 137
Principal care management (PCM), 287–289, 298
    monthly care management services, 292–301
Problem-focused examination, 120
    preventive medicine and, 197–199
Procedure performed on infants less than 4 kg modifier, 42–43
Professional components
    modifier, 34–35
    testing, 261–262
Professional liability, 70
Prolonged services
    with direct patient contact, 222
    in inpatient setting, 397–398
    newborn hospital care, 370–371
    office E/M services, 160–164
    without direct patient contact, 223, 304–305
Proprietary laboratory analysis (PLA), 266
Psychiatric collaborative care management, 287, 351–354
Psychiatric examination, 122, 128–129
Psychiatric services, 342–348
    diagnostic evaluation, 343–344
    interactive complexity, 342–343
    psychotherapy, 345–348
Psychological testing. See Neuropsychological and psychological testing
Psychotherapy, 345–348
Pulmonary function tests, 272–273

Q

QHPs. See Qualified health care professionals (QHPs)
QNHCPs. See Qualified nonphysician health care professionals (QNHCPs)
Qualified health care professionals (QHPs), 13, 15. See also Qualified nonphysician health care professionals (QNHCPs)
    documentation requirements, 314
    nonphysician assessment and management services, 315–318
    nursing evaluation and management visit, 314–315
    prolonged service by, 160–162
    scope of practice laws, 312–313
    supervision of, 313–314
    terminology, 311
    visits not requiring presence of physician or, 146
Qualified nonphysician health care professionals (QNHCPs)
    documentation requirements, 314
    genetic counseling services, 323
    home health procedures/services, 323–324
    included in physician's practice, 311–313
    medical team conferences and, 317–318

    medication therapy management services by pharmacist, 323
    mental/behavioral health services by, 329–330
    nonphysician assessment and management services, 315–318
    nursing evaluation and management visit, 314–315
    nutritional support services by, 320–323
    patient self-management training services by, 318–319
    payer-specific coding for services under a disease management program, 319
    scope of practice laws, 312–313
    supervision of, 313–314
    telephone calls by, 316–317
    terminology, 311
Quality and performance measurement, 55
    coding and documentation for, 61–64
    Consumer Assessment of Healthcare Providers and Systems (CAHPS), 59–60
    CPT Category II codes, 55–56
    Healthcare Effectiveness Data and Information Set (HEDIS), 57–59
    hierarchical condition categories, 56–57
    Medicaid and Children's Health Insurance Program Quality Measures, 60
    preventive care and, 176–177

R

Radiology services, 280–281
    abdominal radiographs, 281
    chest radiographs, 281
    diagnostic, 456
    hip radiographs, 281
    imaging guidance, 281
    total spine radiographs, 281
Reduced services modifier, 38
Reference (outside) laboratory modifier, 45
Relative Value Scale Update Committee (RUC), 71
Relative value units (RVUs), 69–71
    surgical package, 229–230
Remote data collection and monitoring services
    collection and interpretation of digitally stored physiologic data, 499–503
    remote monitoring setup and device supply, 503–504
    therapeutic monitoring services, 505–506
    treatment management services, 504–505, 506
    types of, 499
Remote services
    critical care, 436–437, 494–495
    interprofessional consultations, 211–213, 306
    physiologic monitoring, 306
Removal of
    foreign bodies, 238–239
    skin tags and congenital accessory digits, 234
Repayment demands, 103
Repeat procedure or service by another physician or other qualified health care professional modifier, 44
Repeat procedure or service by same physician or other qualified health care professional modifier, 43
Resource-Based Relative Value Scale (RBRVS), 69, 70
Respiratory examination, 121, 129–130
    car seat/bed testing, 274–275

Respiratory function tests and treatments, 272–275
    inhalation treatment, 273
    nebulizer demonstration or evaluation, 273–274
    pulmonary function tests, 272–273
Respiratory procedures, 461–462
    intubation and airway management, 461–462
    thoracostomy, thoracentesis, and pleural drainage, 462
Respiratory syncytial virus test, 271
Rest home services, 215–216
Retention of records, 98
Revascularization/repair for coarctation of the aorta, 467–468
Review of systems (ROS), 114–117
Risk-factor reduction, 192
Risk of significant complications, morbidity, and/or mortality, 132–133, 153–155
ROS. See Review of systems (ROS)

S

Safe harbors and exceptions, 92–93
Same date admission and discharge services, 386–388
Scope of practice laws, 312–313
Screening tests and procedures. See also Laboratory procedures; Testing
    alcohol and/or substance use, 350–351
    health assessment and developmental, 62, 187–190, 331–332
    hearing, 185–186, 278–280
    vision, 186–187
Second or subsequent drug of a multiple drug unit dose formulation modifier, 49
Sedation, 415–416, 478–480
    critical and intensive care services, 444
    deep, 416, 478–479
    moderate, 252–255, 415–416, 478
Selective head hypothermia, 442
Self-measured blood pressure monitoring, 499–500
Self-referrals, 92–93
Separate procedure designation, surgical, 453
Sequential infusion, 251
Serum and transcutaneous bilirubin testing, 271
Service has been performed by a resident without the presence of a teaching physician under the primary care exception modifier, 48
Service has been performed in part by a resident under the direction of a teaching physician modifier, 48
Seventh character, 10
Sexual abuse, 404
Shared savings, 83–84
Significant, separately identifiable E/M service by the same physician or other qualified health care professional on the same day of the procedure or other service modifier, 32–34
Single organ system examinations, 122
    cardiovascular, 123
    ear, nose, and throat, 124
    eye, 125
    genitourinary, 125–126
    hematologic/lymphatic/immunologic, 126–127
    musculoskeletal, 127
    neurological, 128
    psychiatric examination, 128–129
    respiratory, 129–130
    skin, 130–131

Skin examination, 122, 130–131. *See also* Integumentary procedures
Skin grafts and skin graft substitutes, 459
Skin tag removal, 234
Special service codes, emergency department, 418–419
Spine radiographs, 281
Splints, 241–242
Split/shared E/M services, 134
noncritical hospital E/M services, 381
office or other outpatient settings, 164–165
Sports/camp physicals, 177–178
Staged or related procedure or service by the same physician or other qualified health care professional during the postoperative period modifier, 40–41
Stark Law, 91
Stillborn deliveries, 366
Stool occult blood testing, 271
Strapping, 241–242
Subcutaneous injections, 247–248
Subsequent hospital care of newborn, 369
Subsequent inpatient hospital care, 390–391
Subsequent nursing facility care, 221
Subsequent observation care, 385
Substance use evaluation and treatment, 348–351
Supervision of qualified nonphysician health care professionals (QNHCPs), 313–314
Supplies and materials
administrative services and, 282
fracture care, 242–243
surgical, 232
testing, 262
Surgery. *See also* Postoperative care
assistant surgeon
modifier, 45
modifier, minimum, 45
modifier, when qualified resident surgeon not available, 45
reporting by, 454–455
in teaching facility, 457–458
burn care, 238, 458–459
cardiovascular procedures, 462–469
atrial septostomy, 465–466
cardiac catheterization for congenital heart defects, 463–464
echocardiography, 462–463
percutaneous transcatheter closure of patent ductus arteriosus, 468–469
pericardiocentesis and pericardial drainage, 464–465
transcatheter interventions for revascularization/repair for coarctation of the aorta, 467–468
transcatheter pulmonary valve implantation, 467
valvuloplasty, 466–467
common pediatric procedures, 232–233
complex or high-risk surgeries and procedures, 457
digestive system procedures, 245–246, 474–475
appendectomy, 474
gastric intubation and aspiration, 474
gastrostomy tube replacement, 246
hernia repair, 475
incision in lingual frenulum, 245–246
ear, nose, and throat procedures, 243–245, 473
endoscopy, 457

genitourinary system procedures, 246–247, 475–477
anogenital examination, 475–476
lysis/excision of labial or penile adhesions, 246–247, 476
global periods and modifiers for reporting postoperative care, 452
increased procedural service, 453–454
integumentary procedures, 234–238
burn care, 238
chemical cauterization of granulation tissue, 234–235
destruction of benign lesions, 234
incision and drainage, 234
laceration repairs, 235–236
other repairs, 237–238
removal of foreign bodies, 238–239
removal of skin tags and congenital accessory digits, 234
suture removal, 237
interpretation of diagnostic radiology or other diagnostic tests, 456
Medicare surgical package, 229–230
minor procedures, 456
multiple procedures on the same date, 452–453
musculoskeletal procedures, 460–461
osteotomy humerus with intramedullary lengthening device, 461
removal of musculoskeletal hardware, 461
negative pressure wound therapy, 477–478
other than minor, complex, or high-risk procedures, 457
patients critically ill after, 436
Physicians at Teaching Hospitals guidelines for billing procedures, 456–458
postoperative pain management, 479–480
procedures performed on infants less than 4 kg, 455
reporting by assistant surgeon, 454–455
reporting postoperative care after, 231
reporting terminated procedures, 232, 454
respiratory procedures, 461–462
intubation and airway management, 461–462
thoracostomy, thoracentesis, and pleural drainage, 462
sedation for, 478–480
significant E/M service and procedure, 230–231
supplies and materials, 232
surgical package rules, 229–232, 451–452
transfusions, 472–473
vascular access procedures, 469–472
arterial access, 472
central venous access, 469–472
Surgical care only modifier, 39
Surgical team modifier, 43
Suspected or confirmed abuse, reporting, 404
Suture removal, 237
Synchronous telemedicine service rendered via a real-time interactive audio and video telecommunications system modifier, 46

T

Tabular list, 9–10
Teaching physician guidelines for reporting E/M services, 135–137, 456–458
Technical components, testing, 261–262
Technician-administered neuropsychological testing, 335

Telemedicine services. *See also* Remote data collection and monitoring services; Remote services
critical care via, 436–437, 494–495
Medicaid payment, 490
online digital E/M services, 218–219
online medical assessment, 315–316
payer coverage, 487–490
by qualified nonphysician health care professionals (QNHCPs), 315–317
remote critical care services, 436–437
remote interprofessional consultations, 211–213, 306
reporting, 490–495
documentation of services, 490
Healthcare Common Procedure Coding System (HCPCS) telehealth codes, 492–494
modifiers, 491
place of service codes, 491
telephone services, 217–218, 306, 316–317
terminology, 487
Telephone services, 217–218, 306
by qualified nonphysician health care professional (QNHCP), 316–317
Terminated procedures, reporting, 232, 454
Testing. *See also* Laboratory procedures; Screening tests and procedures
alcohol and/or substance use, 350–351
allergy, 275–276
arterial puncture, 265
blood sampling for diagnostic study, 262–265
central nervous system, 331
coronavirus (SARS-CoV-2), 267–268
developmental, 62, 187–190, 331–332
emotional/behavioral assessment, 188, 280
glucose, 269
hearing, 185–186, 278–280
hematology, 269
influenza, 269–270
interpretation and report, 261
lead, 63, 270
mononucleosis, 270
neuropsychological and psychological, 332–336
Papanicolaou, 270
pathology and laboratory procedures, 265–266
performed in the office, 267–272
presumptive drug, 271
professional and technical components, 261–262
respiratory function treatments and, 272–275
respiratory syncytial virus, 271
screening, 191
serum and transcutaneous bilirubin, 271
stool occult blood, 271
supplies and medications, 262, 263–264
tuberculosis skin (Mantoux), 272
urinalysis, 269
urine pregnancy test, 269
venipuncture, 191, 262–264
Zika virus, 272
Therapeutic, prophylactic
or diagnostic infusions, 250
or diagnostic injections, 247–248
Thoracentesis, 462
Thoracostomy, 462
Throat. *See* Ear, nose, and throat

Time
    in *CPT* procedure coding, 15–18
    in critical care services, 427–428
    documentation of, 17–18
    as explicit component in E/M services, 112,
        205–207
    general guidelines for reporting, 16–17
    guidelines for office or other outpatient E/M
        services, 147–148
    in noncritical hospital E/M services, 380–381
    periodic services tracking, 288–289
    value of documenting, 16
Tongue repair, 238
Tonsillectomy, 473
Total body systemic and selective head
        hypothermia, 442
Total spine radiographs, 281
Transcatheter atrial septostomy (TAS), 465
Transcatheter interventions for revascularization/
        repair for coarctation of the aorta, 467–468
Transcatheter intracardiac shunt (TIS), 466
Transcatheter pulmonary valve implantation, 467
Transfusions, 472–473
Transitional care management (TCM), 287–292,
        306–307
Transitions
    critical and intensive care, 438–439
    different levels of neonatal care, 372–373

Transport, critical care pediatric patient
        face-to-face, 439–440
        non–face-to-face, 440–441
Tuberculosis skin test (Mantoux), 272
Two surgeons modifier, 42

U

Ultrasound, point-of-care, 413–415
Unplanned return to the operating/procedure room
        by the same physician or other qualified
        health care professional following initial
        procedure for a related procedure during a
        postoperative period modifier, 44
Unrelated E/M service by the same physician or
        other qualified health care professional
        during a postoperative period modifier, 32
Unrelated procedure or service by the same
        physician or other qualified health care
        professional during the postoperative
        period modifier, 44
Unspecified codes, 11–12
Urinalysis, 269
Urinary catheterization, 246
Urine pregnancy test, 269

V

Vaccine refusal, 61
Vaccines and toxoids, 178–179
        commonly administered pediatric, 518–520
Vaccines for Children (VFC) program, 185
Value-based payment models, 83, 84–85
Values and payment, critical care services, 445
Values assigned to physician services, 69–71
Valvuloplasty, 466–467
Vascular access procedures, 469–472
        arterial access, 472
        central venous access, 469–472
Venipuncture, 191, 262–264
VFC. *See* Vaccines for Children (VFC) program
Vision screening, 186–187

W

Waiver of liability statement issued as required by
        payer policy
        individual case modifier, 48
        routine notice modifier, 48
Warts, 234
Well-child visits, 61

Z

Zika virus testing, 272

CODE INDEX

References are to pages. **Boldfaced** page numbers indicate the pages on which the primary code descriptions reside. *Current Procedural Terminology (CPT*) codes begin on this page; International Classification of Diseases 10th Revision, Clinical Modification (ICD-10-CM) codes begin on page 542; and Healthcare Common Procedure Coding System (HCPCS) codes begin on page 545.*

CPT Codes

0001A , 179, 520
0002A , 179, 520
0003A , 179, 520
00100–01999 , 36, 252, 478
00102 , 478
0011A , 520
0012A , 520
0013A , 520
0031A , 520
00326 , 478
0041A , 520
0042A , 520
0051A , 521
0052A , 521
0053A , 521
0054A , 521
00561 , 478
0064A , 521
00834 , 478
00836 , 478
01400 , 480
01820 , 478
01996 , 479
0202U , 267
0208T–0212T , 186, 279
0223U , 268
0224U , 268
0225U , 266, **268**
0226U , 268
0240U , 268
0241U , 268
0333T , 186–187
0362T , 331, **336–337**, 343, 345, 348
0373T , 331, **338–339**, 343, 345, 348
0469T , 186–187
0485T , 279
0486T , 279
0594T , 461
0647T , 517
0652T , 517
0653T , 517
0654T , 517
0656T , 517
0657T , 517
0704T , 517
0705T , 517
0706T , 517
10004–69990 , 229
10060 , **233–234**, 412
10061 , 233–234
10120 , 28, 231, 233, **238–239**, 407, 412
10121 , 28, 233, **238–239**, 254–255, 407
10160 , 412
11042–11047 , 236, 477
11200 , 233–234
11601 , 41
11602 , 41
11730 , 47
11740 , 47, 412
11760 , 233, 237, 412

12001 , 233, 236, 411–412
12001–12018 , **235**, 237
12001–13160 , 235
12002 , 412
12011 , 31, 233, 237, 412
12013 , 412
12031 , 233, 412
12031–12057 , **235**, 237
12032 , 236, 411–412
12041 , 233, 412
12042 , 412
12051 , 233, 412
12052 , 412
13100–13153 , 237, 459
13100–13160 , 235
14000–14061 , 459
15002 , 458–459
15002–15005 , 459
15003 , 458–459
15004 , 458–459
15005 , 458–459
15040 , 459
15100–15278 , 458
15275 , 477
15574 , 477
15740 , 477
16000 , 233, 238, 458
16000–16036 , 458
16020 , 233, **238**, 412, 458
16020–16030 , 458
16025 , 412, **458**
16030 , 412, **458**
16035 , 458
16036 , 458
17110 , 233–234
17111 , 233–234
17250 , 233–235
20100–69990 , 42
20100–69999 , 455
20665 , 461
20670 , 461
20680 , 461
20696 , 461
21310 , 240, 413, 515
21315 , 240, **413**, 515
21320 , 240, **413**, 515
23500 , 233, 240–241, 412
23650 , 412–413
24200 , 239
24201 , 239
24400 , 461
24410 , 461
24420 , 461
24516 , 461
24538 , 460–461
24640 , 233, 240–241, 412
24999 , 461
25111 , 36
25500 , 240
25565 , 43–44
25600 , 39, 240
25622 , 242
26011 , 412
26720 , 240, 412
26750 , 240, 412
26990 , 44
27603 , 40
28190 , 233, 239
28192 , 239
28470 , 40, 240
28490 , 233, 240

28510 , 240
29000–29590 , 241
29000–29799 , 41, 240
29085 , 242
29125 , 241, 412
29126 , 241
29130 , 241, 412
29131 , 241
29240 , 241, 412
29260 , 241
29515 , 241, 412
29530 , 412
29540 , 412
3008F , 56, 62, 177
3016F , 56
30300 , 233, 239, 412
30310 , 239
30901 , 233, **243**
30903 , 243
31231 , 37
31500 , 17, 412, 417–418, 426, 428, 431–432, 440, **461**
31502 , 461
31505 , 461
31505–31520 , 461
31511 , 461
31515 , 431, **462**
31520 , 455
31525 , 462
31551 , 473
31551–31554 , 473
31552 , 473
31553 , 473
31554 , 473
31580 , 473
31584 , 473
31599 , 473
31600 , 473
31601 , 473
31603 , 473
31605 , 473
31610 , 473
32100 , 443
32550 , 462
32551 , 412, **462**
32554 , 412, 428, **462**
32555 , 412, 428, **462**
32556 , 412, 428, **462**
32557 , 412, 428, **462**
32601 , 465
32604 , 465
32658 , 465
32659 , 465
32661 , 465
32999 , 471
33016 , 464
33016–33018 , 465
33016–33019 , 465
33017 , 464
33017–33019 , 465
33018 , 464
33019 , 464
33141 , 467
33210 , 468
33255–33259 , 467
33367 , 467
33368 , 467
33369 , 467
33390 , 466–467
33391 , 466–467
33405 , 467
33406 , 467

Code Index

33410, 467
33470, 515
33471, 515
33477, 464, **467**
33530, 467
33646–33949, 455
33741, 465–466
33741–33746, 466
33745, 466
33746, 466
33820, 43
33894, **467–468**, 515
33895, **467–468**, 515
33897, **467–468**, 515
33946, 442, **444**
33946–33949, 429, 444
33946–33989, 467
33947, 442–444
33948, 442, 444
33949, 442–444
33951, 443, 455
33951–33956, 442–444
33952, 443
33953, 443
33953–33956, 444
33954, 443
33955, 443
33956, 443
33957, 443
33957–33959, 444
33957–33964, 442–444
33958, 443
33959, 443
33962, 443
33962–33964, 444
33963, 443
33964, 443
33965, 443
33965–33986, 442, 444
33966, 443
33967, 467
33969, 443
33970, 467
33973, 467
33984, 443
33985, 443
33986, 443
33987, 444
33990–33993, 467
34701–34706, 468
34812, 443
34820, 443
34833, 444
34834, 443
35201, 443
35206, 443
35211, 443
35216, 443
35226, 443–444
35371, 444
35665, 444
35840, 44
36000, 426
36013, 468
36014, 468
36140, 426
36200, 468
36400, 191, **262**, 412, 426, 471
36400–36406, 191, 264
36400–36416, 191, 265
36405, 191, **264**, 426

36406, 191, **264**, 426, 471
36410, 191, **264**, 426, 471
36415, 146, 191, **264–266**, 271–272, 350, 426
36416, 63, 146, 191, **264–265**
36420, 426
36430, 426, **472**
36440, 426, **472**
36450, 429, 432, **472**
36455, 429, **472**
36456, 429, **472**
36510, 426, 428, 431–432
36511–36514, 429
36555, 39, 414, 426, 469
36555–36558, 470
36556, 429, 469
36557, 469
36558, 469
36560, 469
36561, 469
36563, 469
36565, 469
36566, 469
36568, 470–471
36568–36573, 429
36569, 470–471
36570, 470
36571, 470
36572, 38, 471
36573, 471
36575, 471
36576, 471
36578, 469–470
36580, 429, 469
36581, 470
36582, 470
36583, 470
36584, 470–471
36585, 470
36589, 472
36590, 472
36591, **264**, 426
36593, 471
36595, 471
36596, 471
36598, 471
36600, **265**, 412, 426, 472
36620, 426, **472**
36625, 472
36660, 426
36680, 412, 417, 429
36800, 429
37236, 467–468
37237, 467
37246, 468
38220, 429
39010, 443
39503, 436
40650, 237
40652, 237
40654, 237
40806, 374
41010, 233, **245**, 374
41115, 374
41250–41252, 238
42820, 453, **473**
42821, 473
42825, 453, **473**
42826, 473
42830, 38, 453, **473**
42831, 473
42835, 473

42836, 473
42960–42972, 473
43246, 246
43314, 436
43497, 515
43752, 426, **474**
43753, 412, 426, **474**
43762, 246
43763, 246
44950, 32, **474**
44955, 474
44960, 474
44970, 44, 454, **474**
44979, 474
45999, 239
46050, 412
49082, 429
49083, 429
49450, 246
49491, **475**, 524
49492, 475
49495, 475
49495–49525, 475
49496, 475
49500, 475
49501, 475
49505, 475
49507, 475
49520, 475
49521, 475
49605, 436
51100, 412, 426, 429
51701, 233, **246**, 426
51702, 233, **246**, 426
53235, 477
53410, 477
54150, 38–40, 233, **247**, 373, 429, 454, 523
54160, 247, 373
54161, 247, 373
54162, **246**, 476
54300, 477
54304, 477
54304–54336, 477
54336, 477
54340, **476–477**, 516
54340–54348, 476
54340–54352, 477
54344, **477**, 516
54348, **477**, 516
54352, **477**, 516
54360, 477
54450, 246
54640, 475
56441, **246–247**, 476
57415, 239
58999, 239
62223, 42
62270, 412, 426, 429
62328, 412, 429
64415, 36
64448, 480
64936, 37
65205, 239, 412
65220, 239
69200, 37, 239, 412
69209, **243–245**, 279
69210, 34, 76, 231, **243–245**, 279
69421, 473
69436, 38, **473**
71045, **281**, 426
71045–71048, 471

71046, 261, **281**, 426
71047, 281
71048, 281
72081, 281
72081–72084, 281
72082, 281
72083, 281
72084, 281
72170, 281
73000, 37
73080, 49
73110, 49, 242
73501, 281
73501–73523, 281
73502, 281
73503, 281
73521, 281
73522, 281
73523, 281
73525, 281
73592, 281
73620, 34
74018, 281
74019, 281
74021, 281
74022, 281
75573, 516
75600, 468
75605, 468
75625, 468
75820–75827, 472
75901, 471
75989, 465
76000, 472
76376, 463
76377, 463
76536, 414
76604, 414, 462
76700, 414
76705, 414–415
76770, 414
76775, 414
76857, 414
76870, 414
76881, 414
76882, 414
76885, 414
76886, 414
76937, 414, 470–471
76942, 414, 465
77001, 470–471
77002, 465
77012, 465
77021, 465
80000, 49
80047–80076, 266
80061, 266
80305, **271**, 350–351
80306, **271**, 351
80307, 271, 351
81000, 269
81001, 269
81002, 21, 49, 265, **269**
81003, 269
81007, 266
81025, 265, **269**
82135, 270
82247, 271
82248, 271
82272, 49, 265, **271**
82465, 266

82947, 45, **269**
82948, 269
82951, 269
82952, 269
82962, 269
83036, 269
83037, 269
83655, 63, **270**
83718, 266
84202, 270
84203, 270
84478, 266
85013, 269
85018, 269
85025–85027, 269
86308, 270
86328, 268
86408, 268
86409, 268
86413, 268
86480, 272
86580, 272
86701–86703, 45
86703, 36
86769, 268
86794, 272
87046, 266
87070, 266
87081, 266, **271**
87086, 266
87088, 266
87389, 45
87426, 267
87428, 267
87430, 271
87502, 269
87631–87633, 267, 271
87634, 271
87635, 267
87636, 267
87637, 267
87651, 271
87662, 272
87804, 266, **270**
87807, 266, **271**
87811, 267
87880, 49, 64, 266, **271**
88141–88155, 270
88164–88167, 270
88174, 270
88175, 270
88720, 271
88738, 269
89190, 276
90281–90399, 278
90378, 49, 278
90460, 32–33, 82, 102, **179–182**, 185, 190, 313–314, 520
90460–90474, 189
90461, 33, 82, **179–182**, 185, 313, 520
90471, 102, 182–183, 185, 520, 522
90471–90474, 82, 146, **179–182**
90472, **181**, 183, 520
90473, **182**, 520
90474, **182**, 520
90476–90758, 178
90619, 177, 520
90620, 183, 519
90621, 519
90633, 518
90640, 177

90647, 519
90648, 519
90649–90651, 177
90651, 177, 519
90670, 181, 520
90672, 181, 314, 519
90674, 519
90680, 520
90682, 519
90685, 181, 190, 519
90686, 5, 182, 519
90687, 519
90688, 519
90694, 33
90696, 518
90697, 518
90698, 518
90700, 181, 518
90702, 518
90707, 178, 183, 519
90710, 519
90713, 520
90714, 520
90715, 33, 177, 520
90716, 178, 183, 520
90723, 518
90732, 520
90734, 33, 177, 519
90740, 518
90743, 518
90744, 518
90746, 518
90747, 519
90749, 520
90756, 519
90785, **342–343**, 489
90785–90899, 341, 347
90791, **343–344**, 353, 489
90792, **343–344**, 353, 489
90832, **346–347**, 354
90832–90834, 489
90832–90838, 348
90832–90839, 344
90832–90853, 303
90833, 345–347
90834, **346–347**, 354
90836, 345–346
90836–90838, 343, 489
90837, 222, **346**, 354, 397
90838, 345–346
90839, 343, 345, **347**, 489
90840, 343, 345, **347**, 489
90845, 489
90846, 345–346, **348**, 489
90846–90847, 523
90847, 345–346, **348**, 397, 489
90849, 348
90853, 343, 348
90863, **346–347**, 488
90875, 345, **347**
90876, 345, **347**
90882, 348
90885, 348
90887, 348
90889, 348
90901, 347
90951–90970, 294, 488
90952, 488
90954, 488
90955, 488
90957, 488

Code Index

90958, 488
90960, 488
90961, 488
90963–90970, 488
91300, 179, 518
91301, 518
91303, 518
91304, 518
91305, 521
91306, 521
92002–92700, 187
92227, 489
92228, 489
92511, 473
92550, 279
92551, **185–186**, 279
92552, **185–186**, 279
92553, 279
92558, **185–186**, 279
92567, **185–186**, 244, 279
92568, 185–186
92583, **185–186**, 279
92587, 279
92588, 279
92620, 278
92621, 278
92920, 455
92928, 455
92950, 412, 417, 429, 523
92953, 426, 455
92960, 412, 429, 455
92986, 455
92987, 455
92990, 455
92997, 455, 467
92998, 455, 467
93000–93010, 34
93005, 261
93010, 261
93040–93042, 429
93228, 488
93229, 488
93268, 488
93270–93272, 488
93303, 462
93304, 462
93306, 35
93308, 414–415
93312, 462
93312–93318, 455
93314, 462
93315, 462
93317, 462
93318, 429
93319, **462–463**, 516
93325, 463
93355, 463
93451–93453, 464
93451–93456, 463
93451–93461, 467
93452, 455, 464
93453, 464
93456–93461, 464
93458–93461, 464
93460, 463
93461, 463
93462, 464–466
93462–93464, 464
93463, **464–465**, 468
93464, 464–465
93505, 455

93530, 516
93530–93533, 463
93531, 516
93533, 516
93561, 516
93562, 516
93563, 455, 463, 466–467, 469
93563–93564, 42
93563–93568, 468
93564, 455, 463, 469
93565–93568, 466, 469
93566–93568, 467, 469
93567, 468
93568, 42, 455, 463, 469
93571, 465
93572, 465
93580, 42, 455
93581, 464
93582, 42, 455, 464, **468–469**
93590, 464
93590–93592, 42, 455
93591, 464
93593, **463**, 465, 467, 516
93593–93597, 464
93593–93598, 42, 455, 463, 468
93594, **463**, 465, 467–468, 516
93595, **463**, 465, 516
93595–93597, 464
93596, 42, **463**, 465, 516
93596–93598, 467
93597, **463**, 465, 516
93598, 426, **464**, 516
93615, 42, 455
93616, 42, 455
93653, 464
93654, 464
93662, 466, 468
93784, 499
93784–93790, 499
93786, 499
93788, 499
93790, 499
93792, 305
93793, 305
93976, 414
94002, 427
94003, 427
94004, 427
94005, 300–301
94010, 273
94010–94799, 272
94011, 15, 272
94012, 272
94013, 272
94060, 272
94150, 272
94375, 427
94610, 427, 431
94618, 273
94640, 43, 164, 263, **272–274**, 493
94644, 263, **273**
94645, 273
94660, 427
94662, 427
94664, 146, **273–274**
94760, 426
94760–94762, 254
94761, 274, 426
94762, 426
94772, 501
94774, 501–502

94775, 501–502
94776, 501–502
94777, 501–502, 524
94780, **274–275**, 374, 427, 444–445, 523
94781, **274–275**, 374, 427, 444–445, 523
94799, 276
95004, 275–276
95012, 276
95017, 275
95018, 275
95024, 275
95027, 275
95028, 275
95044–95056, 276
95060–95079, 276
95115, 277
95117, **277**, 522
95120, 277
95120–95134, 277
95131, 277
95131–95134, 277
95144, 276
95144–95170, 276–277
95145, 276
95145–95170, 276–277
95146, 276
95146–95149, 276
95147, 276
95148, 276
95149, 276
95165, 276–277
95170, 276
95180, 277
95201, 443
95249, 502–503
95249–95251, 269
95250, 502
95251, 502–503
95930, 187
96040, **323**, 488
96105, 280
96110, 29, 47–48, 62–63, **187–188**, 190, 332, 523
96112, 331–332
96113, 331–332
96116, **332–333**, 488
96121, 332–333
96125, 280
96127, 29, 41, 64, 187–189, 212, **280**, 334, 336, 352, 355
96130, 333
96130–96133, 334–335
96130–96134, 343
96130–96139, 188, 333
96131, 333
96132, **333–334**, 523
96133, **333–334**, 523
96136, 334–335
96136–96137, 334
96136–96139, 333–334, 343
96137, 334–335
96138, 334–335
96139, 334–335
96146, 188, **335–336**, 343
96156, 318, 320, **340–341**
96158, 318, 320, 340–342, 488
96159, 318, 320, 340–342, 488
96160, 158, 187, **189**, 195, 274, 488, 491
96161, 187, **189–190**, 488, 491, 522
96164–96171, 318, 320, 340–342, 488
96360, 249, 522
96360–96379, 247, 411

96361, 249, 251, 522
96365, 249–251
96365–96368, 178, **250**
96366, 250
96367, 250
96368, 250
96369, 250
96369–96371, 250
96370, 250
96372, 12, 33, 146, 178, **247–248**, 252, 263–264, 278, 522
96373, 249
96374, 178, **249–251**, 263–264, 278
96375, 178, **249**, 251
96376, 249, 251
96401–96549, 252
96409, 249–250
96413, 249–250
96415, 250
96416, 250
96522, 469
96523, 251
97151, 336–337
97151–97158, 331, 343, 348
97152, 336–337
97153, 338
97153–97158, 345
97154, 338
97155, 338
97156, 339–340
97157, 339–340
97158, 338–339
97597, 236
97598, 236
97605, 238, **477–478**
97606, 238, **477–478**
97607, 238, **477–478**
97608, 238, **477–478**
97802, 321
97802–97804, 321, 324, 488
97803, 321
97804, 321–322
98960, 318–320
98960–98962, 318–319, 489
98961, **318**, 323
98962, **318**, 323
98966, 217, 316
98966–98968, 205, 211, **217–218**, 300, 306, 316
98967, **217**, 317
98968, 217, 316
98970, 218, 315
98970–98972, 211, 218, 300, 305, 315–316
98971, 218, 315
98972, 218, 315
98975, **505**, 517
98976, **506**, 517
98977, **506**, 517
98980, 499, **506**, 517, 524
98981, 499, **506**, 517, 524
99000, 63, 265–266, 270
99024, 76, 231, 234, 236, 242, 245, 461, 524
99026, 364–365, **399**
99027, 364–365, **399**
99050, 165–166
99050–99058, 165
99050–99060, 306
99051, 165–166
99053, 418–419
99056, 418–419
99056–99060, 205, **216**
99058, **165–166**, 168

99060, 418–419
99070, 164, 232, 235, 242–243, 247, **262**
99071, 282
99071–99082, 282
99072, 517
99075, 282
99078, 193, **282**
99082, 215, **282**
99091, 294, 300, 316, **500–501**, 524
99100, 478
99116, 478
99135, 478
99140, 478
99151, 253–254, **415**
99151–99153, 252–253, 478
99151–99157, 252, 415, 444, 461, 470
99152, 253, **415**, 476
99153, 253–254, **415**
99155, 253, 255, **415**
99155–99157, 252, 478
99156, 253, **415–416**
99157, 253, 255, **415–416**
99170, 475–476
99172, 187
99173, 14, **186–187**
99174, 186–187
99177, 186–187
99184, 429, **442**
99188, **190**, 522
99201–99215, 379
99202, 102, 137, 143, **156–157**, 162, 183
99202–99204, 161
99202–99205, 16, 46, 69, 109, 134, 143–145, 160, 195, 197, 205, 208, 241, 273, 313, 315, 348, 393–394, 398, 490–491
99202–99215, 40, 82, 143, 162, 166, 191, 194, 198, 245, 382, 393, 404, 410, 428, 488
99202–99499, 32, 218, 303
99203, 137, 143, **156–158**, 162
99204, 143, 156, **158–159**, 162–163, 209, 395
99205, 143, **160–163**, 209, 211, 304, 393, 522
99211, 143, 146, 148–149, 166–168, 198, 264–265, 272, 311–315, 320, 323, 514, 522–523
99211–99213, 137
99211–99214, 161
99211–99215, 75, 109, 143–144, 160, 205, 490
99212, 28, 32, 102, 143, **156–157**, 162, 166–168, 186, 193, 198–199, 237, 493
99212–99215, 16, 33, 46, 69, 134, 145, 178, 197, 208, 273, 291, 304, 313, 315, 348, 384, 387, 394, 398, 427, 491
99213, 16, 21, 32, 76, 102, 143, **156–158**, 162, 166–168, 175, 198–199, 212, 218–219, 231, 233, 237, 240–241, 243–244, 246, 248, 274, 279, 336, 345–346, 355, 491
99214, 16, 33, 64, 70, 102, 143, 156, **158–159**, 162–163, 167–168, 176, 188, 197, 199, 212, 248, 251, 274, 395, 493–494, 500
99215, 143, 147–148, **160–162**, 164, 167–168, 194, 199, 211, 274, 304, 393, 522
99217, 28, 220, 290, 382, **386**, 523
99217–99499, 313
99218, 383–384
99218–99220, 379, 382–384, 386, 397, 405, 409, 436, 444
99219, 383–384
99220, 383
99221, 28, 368, 372, 384
99221–99223, 28, 75, 364–366, 370, 372–373, 379, 382, 384, 386, 388–389, 393–394, 397, 405, 428, 433, 437–438, 444, 460, 493

99222, 368, 371, 387, 390
99223, 368, 390, 396, 398, 437
99224, 383
99224–99226, 379, 382, 385, 394, 397
99225, 383, 385
99226, 383
99231, 369, 391, 428
99231–99233, 46, 368–369, 373, 390–398, 433, 436, 438–439, 443–445, 479, 488, 491, 523
99232, 369–370, 373, 390
99233, 369, 373, 391
99234, 383
99234–99236, 220, 379, 382–383, 386–387, 397, 405, 444
99235, 383, 387
99236, 383, 388
99238, 17, 40, 220, 290, **361–364**, 369–370, 373, 391–392, 396, 438–439, 444–445
99239, 17, 220, 290, **361–362**, 369–370, 391–392, 396, 438–439, 444–445
99241–99245, 46, 178, 205, **207–208**, 210, 303–304, 370, 379, 382, 394, 396, 410, 488, 491, 522
99242, 210
99243, 209
99244, 209, 395, 409
99245, 409
99251–99255, 46, 370, 394–395, 397, 434, 460, 488, 491, 495
99253, 372
99254, 492
99281, 406–407, 419
99281–99285, 39, 143, 379, 403–404, 406, 416, 419, 427, 474, 523
99282, 406–407, 419
99283, 240, 403, 406, 408, 411, 413, 419, 523
99284, 403, 406, 408–409, 413, 418–420, 523
99285, 403, 405–406, 409, 417–420, 476
99288, **416**, 441–442
99291, 5, 15, 17, 205, **223**, 304, 364, 369, 372, 399, 410, **416–418**, 420, 425–429, 431–432, 434–436, 440, 443–444, 474, 522–523
99292, 15, 17, 205, **223**, 304, 364, 369, 372, 399, 410, **416–417**, 420, 425–429, 431–432, 434, 436, 440, 443–444, 474, 522–523
99304–99306, 208, **220–221**
99304–99310, 205, 397
99306, 220
99307–99310, 46, 208, **221**, 488
99309, 220
99315, 205, 220, **222**
99316, 205, 220, **222**
99318, 205, 220, **222**
99324, 214
99324–99328, 109, 208, 213
99324–99337, 205, **215–216**, 522
99325, 214
99326, 214
99327, 214
99328, 214
99334–99336, 208
99334–99337, 109, 213, 215
99335, 210
99336, 215–216
99339, 217, 219, 287, 294, 299–301, 305, 316
99340, 217, 219, 287, 294, 299–301, 305, 316
99341–99345, 109, 208
99341–99350, 205, **213–214**, 324
99345, 214
99347, 214
99347–99350, 109, 208
99348, 214–215

Code Index

99349, 214
99350, 214
99354, 160–161, 211, 215, **222**, 303, 394, 489, 491
99354–99357, 211, **222**, 370
99354–99359, 205, 303
99355, 160–161, 211, 215, **222**, 303, 394, 489, 491
99356, 211, 220, **222**, **370**, 373, 397–398, 489
99357, 211, 220, **222**, **370**, 397, 489
99358, 76, 161, 211–212, **223**, 300, 305, **370–371**, 398
99359, 161, 211–212, **223**, 300, 304–305, **370–371**, 398
99366, 302–303, **317**, 398
99366–99368, 302, 305
99367, 301–303, 317, **398**
99368, 302–303, **317–318**, 398
99374, 287, 299–301
99374–99378, 301
99374–99380, 217, 294, 303, 305
99375, 219, 287, 299–301, 316
99377, 287, 299–301
99377–99380, 219, 316
99378, 299–301
99379, 287, 300–301
99380, 287, 300–301
99381, 174
99381–99385, 70, 82, 109, 137, 192
99381–99395, 173, 175, 177, 191–192, 198
99381–99397, 192
99382, 174, 199
99383, 62, 174, 184–185
99384, 174
99385, 174
99388, 287
99391, 47–48, 174, 181, 235, 523
99391–99395, 70, 109, 137, 192
99392, 35, 47, 63, 174, 188, 190, 199
99393, 32, 174–176, 190, 198
99394, 33, 174, 177, 186, 188, 196
99395, 174, 183
99401, 17, 36, 173, 184, 192–193, 198
99401–99404, 17, 183, 185, 188, 192–193, 198, 210, 312, 320, 522
99402, 17, 192–193
99403, 17, 192
99404, 17, 192
99406, 353, 489
99406–99409, 46, 194–195, 491
99407, 195, 353, 489
99408, 189, 195–196, 353, 489
99409, 189, 195, 353, 489
99411, **192–194**, 282
99411–99412, 192
99412, **192–194**, 282
99415, **161–163**, 370
99416, **161–163**, 370
99417, 46, **160–162**, 164, 168, 211, 303–304, 393, 488, 491, 522
99421, 218–219
99421–99423, 205, 211, 300–301, 305, 494
99422, **218**, 494
99423, 218–219
99424, 293, 298–299, 305, 514
99424–99427, 217, 219, 287, 300, 302, 353, 355, 499
99425, 293, 298–299, 305, 514
99426, 289, 293, 298, 515
99427, 293, 298
99429, 14, **197**
99437, 217, 219, 287, 293, 295, 297, 299, 302, 305, 353, 355, 499, 514
99439, 217, 219, 287, 293, 295, 297, 302, 353, 355

99441, 217
99441–99443, 205, 211, **217–218**, 300–301, 306, 316, 494
99442, **217**, 494
99443, 217
99446, 211
99446–99449, 211, 306, 396
99446–99451, 212, 396
99446–99452, 305
99447, 211
99448, 211
99449, 211–213
99451, **211**, 306, 397
99452, **211–212**, 396
99453, 499, **503–504**
99454, 499, **503–504**
99457, **306**, 499, **504–505**, 524
99458, **306**, **504–505**, 524
99460, 361–365, 367–368, 372–373, 431, 434, 445, 523
99460–99462, 437
99461, 361–362
99462, 28, **361–362**, 364, 367–369, 372–373, 434, 445, 523
99463, 17, **361–362**, 373, 445
99464, **364–365**, 431, 437
99465, 365–366, **431–432**, 437, 439
99466, 425–427, 433, **439–440**, 523
99466–99469, 474
99467, 425–427, 433, **439–441**, 523
99468, 17, 304, 364, 372, 399, 425, **430–434**, 438–440, 442
99468–99472, 429, 444, 472
99468–99476, 426–427, 437, 441
99468–99480, 444
99469, 304, 399, 425, 430, **432–433**, 435, 438–439, 523
99471, 425, 432–433, **435–436**, 440
99471–99476, 304, 399, 432, 435, 474
99472, 425, 432–433, **435–436**
99473, 499–500
99474, 499–500
99475, 425, 429, 432–433, **435–436**, 472
99476, 425, 429, 432–433, **435–436**, 472
99477, 364, 372–373, 430–431, 433, **437–439**
99477–99480, 304, 367, 372, 399, 426–427, 429, 437, 444, 474
99478, 437–438
99478–99480, 373, 433, 437–439
99479, 437–438
99480, 437–438
99483, 280
99484, 287, 294, 350, **354–355**
99485, 416, 433, **440–441**, 523
99486, 416, 433, **440–441**, 523
99487, 219, 287, 293, 295, 297, 300, 302, 316, 353, 355, 499
99487–99490, 217
99487–99491, 303
99489, 219, 287, 293, 295, 297, 302, 499
99489–99491, 316, 353, 355
99490, 219, 287, 293, 295, 297, 300, 302, 499
99491, 217, 219, 293, 295, 297, 299–300, 305, 499, 514, 522
99492, 351–354
99492–99494, 287, 294, 351–352
99493, 352–353
99494, 352–353
99495, 46, 217, 287, 289–292, 294, 316, 489, 491
99496, 46, 217, 287, 289–292, 294, 316, 489, 491
99497, **303–304**, **399**, 488

99498, **303–304**, **399**, 488
99499, 436, 440, 494–495
99500–99600, 324
99501, 323
99502, 323
99503, 323
99504, 323
99505, 323
99506, 323
99507, 323
99509, 323–324
99510, 324
99511, 324
99512, 324
99600, 324
99605, **323**
99605–99607, 294, 323, 523
99606, **323**
99607, **323**

ICD-10-CM Codes

A08.4, 12, 163
A09, 12
A38, 7
A41.9, 417
A79.82, 511
B07.0, 234
B07.8, 234
B08.1, 234
B20, 62
B96.5, 292, 297–298
D55.21, 511
D55.29, 511
D75.83, 513
D80–D84, 278
D81.31, 63
D81.9, 62
D84.9, 63
D89.44, 512
E10, 322, 342
E10.10, 160
E66.9, 146, 197, 209
E75.244, 512
E78.00, 321
E84.0, 297–298, 303
E84.8, 297–298, 303, 305
E86.0, 163–164, 251, 384, 390
F01–F99, 330–331
F10, 349
F10–F19, 349–350
F10.9, 349
F10.99, 196
F11–F16, 349
F11.9, 349
F12.188, 351
F12.21, 351
F13.9, 349
F14.9, 349
F15.9, 349
F16.9, 349
F17.29, 195
F18, 349
F19, 349
F19.9, 349
F32.0, 188
F32.1, 64, 210, 280, 344, 354
F32.A, 511
F33.2, 344
F41.9, 212, 341
F41.96, 198
F43.22, 212

F78.A1 , 513
F78.A9 , 512
F80–F88 , 318
F81.2 , 333
F84.0 , 330, 403
F84.2 , 330
F84.5 , 330
F90.0 , 212, 333
F90.1 , 493
G04.82 , 511
G44.309 , 385
G44.86 , 511
G92.0 , 512
G92.8 , 513
G92.9 , 513
H60.331 , 158
H61.2 , 34
H61.21 , 76, 245
H61.22 , 231
H61.23 , 245
H62.40 , 7
H62.41 , 7
H62.42 , 7
H62.43 , 7
H65.23 , 209
H66.001 , 76, 248
H66.003 , 251
H66.009 , 12
H66.90 , 12
I5A , 512
I10 , 146, 500
I34.1 , 209
I46.8 , 417
I46.9 , 417
J00 , 64
J02.0 , 7
J02.0–J02.9 , 7
J02.9 , 12, 231
J05.0 , 248, 418
J06.0 , 64
J06.9 , 7, 64, 166
J09.X2 , 7
J11.1 , 7, 215
J12.82 , 512
J18.9 , 12
J21.9 , 7
J22 , 7
J30.1 , 277
J30.2 , 231
J30.5 , 277
J31.2 , 7
J35.2 , 209
J45.2 , 75
J45.20 , 158
J45.21 , 493
J45.3 , 75
J45.30 , 32, 102, 175
J45.31 , 102, 159, 176, 274
J45.4 , 75
J45.41 , 164, 166, 215–216, 387–388
J45.42 , 418
J45.5 , 75
J45.50 , 252
J45.909 , 11
J96.00 , 160, 418
J96.01 , 223, 418
K02 , 190
K22.8 , 512
K22.89 , 511
K31.A , 512
K35.80 , 396

K52.9 , 163
K55.30–K55.33 , 366
K56.41 , 387
K86 , 297–298, 303, 305
L01.00 , 7
L02.415 , 40
L02.419 , 12
L21.0 , 193
L23.7 , 159
L24.A , 512
L24.B , 512
L50.1 , 494
L55.0 , 238
L90.5 , 10
M25.50 , 11
M25.561 , 11
M30.3 , 278
M31.10 , 513
M31.11 , 512
M31.19 , 513
M35.0 , 513
M35.81 , 512
M35.89 , 512
M54.50 , 512
M54.51 , 513
M54.59 , 511
N10 , 384
N39.0 , 21
N47.0 , 246, 476
N47.5 , 246, 476
O92.5 , 320
P00–P04 , 366
P00–P96 , 366, 430
P00.82 , 512
P00.89 , 367
P05 , 430–431
P05.0 , 430
P05.1 , 430
P05.2 , 430
P07 , 366, 430–431
P07.0 , 431
P07.00 , 12
P07.1 , 431
P07.2 , 431
P07.3 , 431
P07.37 , 275
P07.38 , 372
P08 , 10
P08.0 , 10
P08.1 , 10
P08.2 , 10
P08.21 , 10
P08.22 , 10
P09.1 , 511
P09.2 , 511
P09.3 , 511
P09.4 , 511
P09.5 , 511
P09.6 , 60, 511
P09.8 , 511
P22.9 , 39
P27 , 366
P55.0 , 368
P55.1 , 369
P59.9 , 364
P70.4 , 372
P77 , 366
P83.81 , 235
P92.5 , 245, 374
Q00–Q99 , 366
Q16.1 , 8

Q38.1 , 245, 374
Q52.5 , 247, 476
Q55.64 , 477
Q69.0 , 234
Q69.1 , 234
Q69.2 , 234
Q69.9 , 234
Q90.9 , 209
R04.0 , 243
R05.1 , 511
R05.2 , 513
R05.3 , 511
R05.4 , 511
R05.8 , 511
R05.9 , 511
R06.03 , 384
R09.02 , 274, 384
R10 , 7
R10.84 , 11, 395
R11 , 344
R11.10 , 251, 385
R11.2 , 351
R35.81 , 512
R35.89 , 513
R40.2412 , 409
R41.89 , 493
R45.88 , 512
R50.81 , 248, 251
R50.9 , 160, 390
R51.9 , 408
R53.83 , 390
R62.51 , 297–298, 303
R63.0 , 493
R63.30 , 512
R63.31 , 512
R63.32 , 512
R63.39 , 512
R65.20 , 418
R65.21 , 417–418
R76.11 , 10
R78 , 350
R78.0 , 350
R78.1 , 350
R78.2 , 350
R78.3 , 350
R78.4 , 350
R78.5 , 350
R78.6 , 350
R78.89 , 350
R78.9 , 350
R79.83 , 511
R94.120 , 279–280, 364
S00.31XA , 243
S01.81XA , 10, 237
S01.81XD , 10, 237
S01.81XS , 10
S02.0XXA , 409
S04.811 , 7
S06.0X1A , 385–386
S06.A0X , 513
S06.A1X , 513
S39.848A , 476
S42.021A , 409
S42.022A , 241
S42.412A , 460
S43.014A , 413
S50.12XA , 408
S51.812A , 236
S51.812D , 237
S53.032A , 241
S61.411A , 404

Code Index

S62.001A, 242
S62.025D, 242
S70.12XA, 408
S81.012A, 236
S81.811A, 411
S83.91X, 12
S90.851A, 407
S90.851D, 231
S91.011A, 411
S91.341A, 254–255
S93.412A, 408
S93.492A, 407–408
T23.221A, 238
T31, 458
T40.71, 513
T40.715, 511
T40.72, 513
T40.725, 511
T43.635A, 493
T52.92XA, 331
T58.11XA, 404
T74, 404
T74.02X, 405
T74.12X, 405
T74.22X, 405
T74.22XA, 476
T74.32X, 405
T74.4XX, 405
T74.52X, 405
T74.62X, 405
T75.0, 403
T76, 404
T76.02X, 405
T76.12X, 405
T76.22XA, 476
T76.32X, 405
T76.52X, 405
T76.62X, 405
T80.82X, 511
U09.9, 513
V18.0XXA, 460
V48.5XXA, 409
V86.55XA, 408
W01.0XXA, 243, 407–408
W01.0XXD, 242
W09.8XXA, 236
W10.9XXA, 241
W13.0XXA, 403
W18.0, 403
W18.30XA, 413
W21.03, 403
W21.07XA, 385–386
W25.XXXA, 411
X15.3XXA, 238
X92–Y04, 404
X92–Y06, 476
Y07, 404, 476
Y08, 404, 476
Y08.02, 403
Y09, 404
Y90, 350
Y90.0, 350
Y90.1, 350
Y90.2, 350
Y90.3, 350
Y90.4, 350
Y90.5, 350
Y90.6, 350
Y90.7, 350
Y90.8, 350
Y90.9, 350

Y92.007, 411
Y92.310, 407–408
Y92.322, 413
Y92.413, 409
Y92.480, 243, 460
Y92.73XA, 408
Y92.838, 236
Y93.01, 243
Y93.64, 385–386
Y93.66, 413
Y93.67, 407–408
Y99.8, 407–408
Z00, 63
Z00–Z99, 9
Z00.00, 175, 183
Z00.01, 175
Z00.110, 5, 175, 247
Z00.111, 5, 175
Z00.121, 19, 33, 175–176, 178, 188, 190, 197–198, **235**, 270
Z00.129, 19, 63, 175–178, 181, 184, 186, 188–190, **196**, 199, 270
Z01.11, 186
Z01.110, 186, 279–280, 364
Z01.118, 186, 279–280
Z01.411, 270
Z01.419, 270
Z01.81, 9
Z01.89, 9
Z02, 63, 183
Z02.0, 35, 63, 183
Z02.5, 178
Z02.83, 350–351
Z03.89, 11
Z04.1, 404
Z04.42, 405, 476
Z04.72, 404–405
Z04.81, 404–405
Z04.82, 404–405
Z05, 367
Z05.0–Z05.9, 11
Z05.1, 367
Z09, 11, 157
Z11–Z13, 191, 270
Z11.1, 11, 272
Z11.3, 36
Z11.4, 36
Z11.52, 511
Z12.4, 270
Z13.31, 188
Z13.40–Z13.49, 187
Z13.41, 63, 188
Z13.42, 62–63, 187–188
Z13.84, 191
Z13.88, 63, 270
Z20, 11
Z20.822, 511
Z21, 62
Z23, 19, 33, 175, 177, 179, 181–183, 193
Z28, 183–184
Z28.0, 184
Z28.01, 184
Z28.02, 184
Z28.03, 184
Z28.04, 61, 184
Z28.09, 184
Z28.1, 184
Z28.20, 184
Z28.21, 184, 193
Z28.29, 184
Z28.3, 159, 183, 184, 193

Z28.81, 184
Z28.82, 159, 184
Z28.83, 184
Z29.3, 190
Z30.09, 36, 194
Z32.00–Z32.02, 269
Z38, 363, 366, 374, 523
Z38.00, 40, 363–364, 367–369, 373
Z38.01, 363, 364
Z38.1, 363
Z38.2, 363
Z38.30, 363
Z38.31, 363
Z38.4, 363
Z38.5, 363
Z39.1, 320
Z41.2, 39–40, 247
Z42–Z49, 11
Z48.02, 237
Z51, 11
Z58.6, 512
Z59.0, 403
Z59.00, 512
Z59.01, 512
Z59.02, 512
Z59.41, 512
Z59.48, 512
Z59.81, 512
Z63.79, 198
Z63.8, 344
Z68.51–Z68.54, 62, 176–177
Z68.53, 321
Z68.54, 197
Z71.3, 62, 173, 176–177, 321–322
Z71.41, 349
Z71.51, 349–351
Z71.6, 195
Z71.82, 62, 176–177
Z71.84, 193
Z71.85, 511
Z71.89, 184, 195–196
Z72.0, 195
Z72.40, 344
Z76.2, 363
Z76.81, 210
Z77.011, 270
Z77.99, 270
Z80–Z84, 9
Z82.79, 210
Z83.3, 197
Z85–Z87, 9
Z86, 11
Z86.16, 512
Z86.69, 11
Z86.898, 157
Z87, 11
Z87.74, 199
Z87.892, 61–62
Z88.7, 61–62
Z91.010, 341
Z91.014, 511
Z91.51, 512
Z91.52, 512
Z92.850, 512
Z92.858, 512
Z92.859, 512
Z92.86, 512
Z92.89, 270
Z93.1, 305

HCPCS Codes

A4450, 235
A4565, 243
A4570, 243
A4580, 242
A4590, 242
A6550, 478
A7003, 164
A9272, 478
E1800–E1841, 242
G0108, 322, 488
G0109, 322, 488
G0168, 235
G0181, 299, 301
G0182, 299, 301
G0270, 322, 488
G0271, 322
G0396, 489
G0397, 489
G0406, 492
G0406–G0408, 489
G0407, 492
G0408, 492
G0420, 488
G0421, 488
G0425, 492
G0425–G0427, 489
G0426, 492
G0427, 492
G0436, 489
G0437, 489
G0438, 488
G0439, 488
G0442, 488
G0443, 488
G0444, 488
G0445, 488
G0446, 488
G0447, 62, 488
G0459, 488, 492

G0506, 488
G0508, 436, 489, 492, 494–495
G0509, 436, 489, 492, 494
G0513, 489
G0514, 489
G2212, 161–162, 393
G8431, 64
G8510, 64
G9717, 64
H0003, 351
H0016, 349
H0048, 351
J0171, 5, 263, 278
J0290, 263
J0461, 263
J0558, 263
J0561, 264
J0696, 12, 248, 251, 263
J0698, 263
J0702, 263
J1094, 263
J1100, 248, 263
J1165, 264
J1200, 263
J1460, 263
J1560, 263
J1566, 263
J1580, 263
J1610, 263
J1642, 263
J1720, 263
J2357, 252
J2550, 264
J3490, 262
J3535, 493–494
J7030, 251
J7510, 264
J7512, 264
J7611, 263
J7612, 263

J7613, 262–263, 272, 494
J7614, 263
J7615, 263
J7620, 263
J7626, 263
J7627, 263
J8498, 264
J8540, 264
L3650–L3678, 243
Q0091, 270
Q3014, 490, 493
Q4001–Q4051, 232, 242–243
Q4011, 12
Q4013, 242
Q4014, 242
S0315, 319
S0316, 319
S0317, 319
S0320, 319
S0630, 5, 12, 237
S8450–S8452, 243
S9083, 143
S9088, 143
S9441, 319
S9443, 320
S9445, 319–320
S9446, 319–320
S9449, 322
S9452, 322
S9455, 322
S9460, 322
S9465, 322
S9470, 322
S9981, 282
S9982, 282
T1007, 349
T1014, 490, 493
U0001–U0004, 267

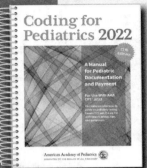
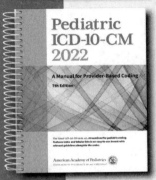
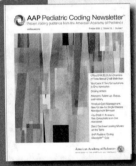
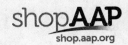